80p

Geriatric Anesthesia

Geriatric Anesthesia

Frederick E. Sieber, MD
Director of Anesthesia Department
Johns Hopkins Bayview Medical Center
Associate Professor
Anesthesia and Critical Care Medicine
Johns Hopkins University School of Medicine
Baltimore, Maryland

McGraw-Hill
Medical Publishing Division

New York   Chicago   San Francisco   Lisbon   London   Madrid
Mexico City   Milan   New Delhi   San Juan   Seoul   Singapore   Sydney   Toronto

Geriatric Anesthesia

Copyright © 2007 by The McGraw-Hill Companies, Inc. All rights reserved. Printed in the United States of America. Except as permitted under the United States Copyright Act of 1976, no part of this publication may be reproduced or distributed in any form or by any means, or stored in a database or retrieval system, without the prior written permission of the publisher.

1 2 3 4 5 6 7 8 9 0   QPD/QPD   0 9 8 7 6

ISBN-13: 978-0-07-146308-9
ISBN-10: 0-07-146308-9

This book was set in Minion by International Typesetting and Composition, Inc.
The editors were Joseph Rusko, Lawrence Greenberg, and Peter J. Boyle.
The production supervisor was Catherine H. Saggese.
Project management was provided by International Typesetting and Composition, Inc.
The index was prepared by Susan Hunter.
Cover design by Elizabeth Pisacreta.
Cover photo: Jonas Strandberg-Ringh/Gettyimages
Quebecor World Dubuque was printer and binder.

This book is printed on acid-free paper.

Library of Congress Cataloging-in-Publication Data

Geriatric anesthesia /[edited by] Frederick E. Sieber.
         p. ; cm.
    Includes bibliographical references and index.
    ISBN 0-07-068291-7 (alk. paper)
    1. Geriatric anesthesia.   I. Sieber, Frederick E.
    [DNLM: 1. Aged.   2. Anesthesia—methods. WO 445 G3685 2006]
  RD145.G47   2006
  617.9′600849—dc22

                                    2006043804

I dedicate this book to my loving wife, Elizabeth,
and to my parents, Bill and Ann Sieber.

CONTENTS

CONTRIBUTORS

Dan E. Berkowitz, MD
Associate Professor
Department of Anesthesiology and Critical Care Medicine
Johns Hopkins Medical Institutions
Baltimore, Maryland

Renee Blanding, MD, MPH
Assistant Professor
Department of Anesthesiology and Critical Care Medicine
Johns Hopkins University School of Medicine
Johns Hopkins Bayview Medical Center
Baltimore, Maryland

Manfred Blobner, MD
Professor
Clinic for Anesthesiology of the Technical University of Munich
Clinical Center on the Right of the Isar
Munich, Germany

Ali Chandani, MD
Assistant Professor
Department of Anesthesiology and Critical Care Medicine
Johns Hopkins University School of Medicine
Johns Hopkins Bayview Medical Center
Baltimore, Maryland

Barbara Eckel, MD
Clinic for Psychiatry, Technical University of Munich
Clinical Center on the Right of the Isar
Munich, Germany

Neal S. Fedarko, PhD
Associate Professor of Medicine
Division of Geriatric Medicine and Gerontology
Department of Medicine
Johns Hopkins University School of Medicine
Baltimore, Maryland

Lee A. Fleisher, MD, FACC
Robert D. Dripps Professor and Chair of Anesthesiology and Critical Care
Professor of Medicine
University of Pennsylvania
Philadelphia, Pennsylvania

Steven M. Frank, MD
Staff Anesthesiologist
Department of Anesthesiology
Greater Baltimore Medical Center (GBMC)
Baltimore, Maryland

Kevin Gerold, DO, JD
Assistant Professor
Department of Anesthesiology and Critical Care Medicine
Johns Hopkins University School of Medicine
Johns Hopkins Bayview Medical Center
Baltimore, Maryland

Peter S.A. Glass, MB, ChB
Professor and Chair
Department of Anesthesiology
State University of New York at Stony Brook
Stony Brook, New York

Jian Hang, MD, PhD
Assistant Professor
Department of Anesthesiology and Critical Care Medicine
Johns Hopkins University School of Medicine
Johns Hopkins Bayview Medical Center
Baltimore, Maryland

James E. Heavner, DVM, PhD
Professor of Anesthesiology and Physiology
Director of Anesthesia and Pain Research
Texas Tech University Health Sciences Center (TTUHSC)
Lubbock, Texas

Mahmood Jaberi, MD
Assistant Professor of Anesthesiology
Department of Anesthesiology and Critical Care Medicine
Johns Hopkins University School of Medicine
Johns Hopkins Bayview Medical Center
Baltimore, Maryland

Christopher J. Jankowski, MD
Assistant Professor of Anesthesiology
Mayo Clinic College of Medicine
Consultant in Anesthesiology
Mayo Clinic and Foundation
Rochester, Minnesota

Ambullar D. John, MD
Assistant Professor
Department of Anesthesiology and Critical Care Medicine
Johns Hopkins University School of Medicine
Johns Hopkins Bayview Medical Center
Baltimore, Maryland

Sean X. Leng, MD, PhD
Assistant Professor of Medicine
Division of Geriatric Medicine and Gerontology
Department of Medicine
Johns Hopkins University School of Medicine
Baltimore, Maryland

Richard J. Lofrumento, MD
Clinical Associate
Department of Anesthesiology and Critical Care Medicine
Johns Hopkins University School of Medicine
Johns Hopkins Bayview Medical Center
Baltimore, Maryland

Brice Lortat-Jacob
Resident
Departement d'Anesthésie Réanimation Chirurgicale
Hopital Bichat
Paris, France

Elizabeth Martinez, MD
Assistant Professor
Department of Anesthesiology and Critical
Care Medicine
Johns Hopkins Medical Institutions
Baltimore, Maryland

Daniel Nyhan, MD
Professor
Department of Anesthesiology and Critical Care Medicine
Johns Hopkins Medical Institutions
Baltimore, Maryland

Asha Padmanabhan, MD
Instructor
Department of Anesthesiology and Critical Care Medicine
Johns Hopkins University School of Medicine
Johns Hopkins Bayview Medical Center
Baltimore, Maryland

L. Reuven Pasternak, MD, MPH, MBA
Executive Vice President and Chief Medical Officer
Health Alliance of Greater Cincinnati
Cincinnati, OH
Clinical Professor of Anesthesiology
University of Cincinnati College of Medicine
Cincinnati, OH
Associate Professor of Anesthesiology and Critical
Care Medicine, Health Policy and Management
(Adjunct)
Johns Hopkins University School of Medicine
Bloomberg School of Public Health of the Johns Hopkins
University
Baltimore, Maryland

Ronald Pauldine, MD
Assistant Professor
Department of Anesthesiology and Critical Care Medicine
Johns Hopkins University School of Medicine
Vice Chairman
Johns Hopkins Bayview Medical Center
Baltimore, Maryland

Srinivasa N. Raja, MD
Professor, Director
Division of Pain Medicine
Department of Anesthesiology and Critical
Care Medicine
Johns Hopkins University
Baltimore, Maryland

Frédérique Servin, MD
Staff Anesthesiologist
Departement d'Anesthésie Réanimation Chirurgicale
Hopital Bichat
Paris, France

Amit Sharma, MD
Assistant Professor
Department of Anesthesiology
College of Physicians and Surgeons of Columbia University
New York

Punita T. Sharma, MD
Assistant Professor
Department of Anesthesiology and Critical Care Medicine
Johns Hopkins University School of Medicine
Johns Hopkins Bayview Medical Center
Baltimore, Maryland

Frederick E. Sieber, MD
Associate Professor
Department of Anesthesiology and Critical Care Medicine
Johns Hopkins University School of Medicine
Director of Anesthesiology
Johns Hopkins Bayview Medical Center
Baltimore, Maryland

Roy G. Soto, MD
Associate Professor
Department of Anesthesiology
State University of New York at Stony Brook
Stony Brook, New York

Jochen Steppan
Research Associate
Department of Anesthesiology and Critical Care Medicine
Johns Hopkins Medical Institutions
Baltimore, Maryland

Robert William Thomsen, MD
Assistant Professor
Johns Hopkins University School of Medicine
Baltimore, Maryland

William Vernick, MD
Assistant Professor of Anesthesiology and Critical Care
University of Pennsylvania
Philadelphia, Pennsylvania

Weili Weng, MD
Assistant Professor
Department of Anesthesiology and Critical Care Medicine
Johns Hopkins University School of Medicine
Johns Hopkins Bayview Medical Center
Baltimore, Maryland

Orion Whitaker, MD
Clinical Associate
Department of Anesthesiology and Critical Care Medicine
Johns Hopkins University School of Medicine
Johns Hopkins Bayview Medical Center
Baltimore, Maryland

Khwaja Javaid Zakriya, MBBS, MD
Assistant Professor
Department of Anesthesiology and Critical Care Medicine
Johns Hopkins University School of Medicine
Johns Hopkins Bayview Medical Center
Baltimore, Maryland

The purpose of this book is to provide an up-to-date review of pertinent information focused on the geriatric population. The stages of life—childhood, adult, and old age—have been well-recognized since ancient times. The medical profession has acknowledged the unique attributes of each stage of life, and specialties (pediatrics, internal medicine, geriatrics) that are primarily devoted to serving the special needs of each patient population have developed. Subspecialty areas in other medical disciplines have also begun to emerge, as information concerning the fundamental differences between these patient populations has continued to increase. This evolution in medicine is occurring at an ever-increasing pace in the field of geriatrics, particularly as the population continues to age. The book provides a basic fund of knowledge in the developing field of geriatric anesthesiology.

The intended audience for *Geriatric Anesthesia* is residents, students, and persons in clinical practice. The material is not focused on a basic science level. Rather, the text is clinically oriented and pays attention to information that is critical to managing the elderly patient undergoing surgery and anesthesia.

The book is divided into seven sections that provide an overview of the unique issues in anesthetizing the geriatric patient: general information; aging and its effects on organ reserve; pharmacology; preoperative assessment; controversies in intraoperative management; postoperative issues specific to the elderly; and special topics. It is important to emphasize that this book is not meant to provide an exhaustive resource of all possible scenarios that may be encountered when anesthetizing the elderly. I have made a conscious decision in editing this book to include material that is unique to the blossoming subspecialty of geriatric anesthesia.

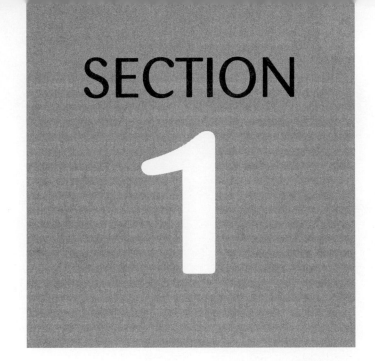

SECTION 1

GENERAL INFORMATION

Overview of Aging and its Demographics

Richard J. Lofrumento

INTRODUCTION: GERIATRIC PATIENTS AND GERIATRIC ANESTHESIA

The riddle of the sphinx asked the question: "Which creature walks on four legs in the morning, two legs in the afternoon, and three legs in the evening?" The answer to this question is man. Even in ancient times, the aging of humanity was recognized. Many societies like the ancient Chinese revered their elders holding them in high esteem. Today, humanity is facing a graying of our species, which will lead to many challenges. One of the greatest challenges will be how we care for our future selves. As physicians, we must address these needs by learning about the changes caused by aging, and how these changes influence care. A selected generalized picture from human studies of the geriatric patient, our modern geriatric everyman, shall be developed to illustrate the variability in physiologic aging between organ systems. From this picture of the geriatric everyman we will discuss the definition of the geriatric patient. World demographics of the geriatric patient and the aging population will be reviewed. These viewpoints will serve as a framework for succeeding chapters.

THE GERIATRIC EVERYMAN: OVERVIEW OF ANATOMIC AND PHYSIOLOGICAL AGING AND CHANGES

▶ The nervous system: brain

"Cogito ergo sum (I think therefore I am)," Rene Descartes' existential statement that has inspired much philosophical debate, could also be for us the demarcation for the examination of our everyman.[1] As anesthesiologists, we manipulate both the conscious state and nervous functions of our patients. Important to our practice are the changes that occur in the brain with aging.

Quantitative magnetic resonance imaging (MRI) studies reveal age-related changes in brain microstructure and metabolism of both gray and white matter. Whole brain volume is greatest in adolescence (12–15 years), having grown by 25% from childhood. Prior to age 50, age-related changes in brain volumes are small. Thereafter, whole brain volume decreases, reaching a volume of 25% less in the 70–80-year-old group.[2] From childhood to adolescence (12–15 years) intracranial space increases by 27%. Thereafter, intracranial space remains relatively constant between 16 and 80 years.[2] Cerebral spinal fluid volume increases from 7.1% to 13.4% of intracranial space when comparing 18–39-year-olds with those ≥ 69 years.[3]

Examination of autopsy material from different age groups has demonstrated changes in the gross anatomy of the cerebellum and cellular layers of the cerebellar cortex. The aging effects on anatomical specimens above 65 years consist of a 26% reduction of white matter, which is most prominent in the flocculonodullar lobes. On a cellular level, there is a 26% reduction in the perikaryon mean volume of Purkinje cells without significant differences in nuclear volume. The age effect is most striking in the anterior cortex, which shows a 28.7% overall reduction in volume with a 40% reduction in Purkinje and granular cell volumes.

Researchers have attempted to relate these observed morphological changes with functional changes. Studies of the supratentorial region relate white matter changes to decline in executive function (function involving working memory, problem solving, and dual memory) and demonstrate a greater age-associated decline in function of the anterior cingulum and middle frontal gyrus.[4] Function of the posterior cerebral regions is largely unchanged with age. In the corpus callosum, interhemispheric function shows decreased function occurring between the ages of 40 and 55 years. After age 60, this effect is characterized by decreased speed of interhemispheric transfer, which undergoes no further diminution with advancing age.[5]

▶ The nervous system: peripheral nerve

As the population grays and interventions in the geriatric population become more numerous, there will be an increasing use of regional anesthesia in an attempt to help rapidly mobilize this age group for early discharge. The changes seen in the peripheral nerves should be of interest to our practice. Various studies have shown that with aging there is a linear decrease in nerve conduction velocity. Nerve responsiveness becomes increasingly absent, but this effect varies by the individual nerve stimulated. The compound muscle potential also shows decreasing response amplitudes that have a strong negative correlation with age.[5]

▶ The respiratory system

Equally important as the nervous system to our practice is the respiratory system. The respiratory system is another element that ages and can affect our patient care. Respiratory reserve decreases with aging as a result of many physiologic changes. Of importance, the elderly have decreased respiratory muscle strength. Between the ages of 20 and 80 years, the strength of muscular contraction is gradually reduced by 15–35%. In general, diaphragm strength is reduced by about 25% in healthy elderly individuals compared with young adults.[6] With aging, a widening of the alveolar-to-arterial gradient occurs in conjunction with increased ventilation/perfusion (V/Q) mismatch as closing capacity begins to exceed functional residual capacity. At about 44 years of age, closing capacity reaches functional residual capacity in the supine position. By age 66, closing capacity equals functional residual capacity in the erect position. In addition, aging brings about a shift of intrapulmonary gas volume from the alveoli to the alveolar duct and respiratory bronchioles. As a result, the alveolar surface area decreases 15% by age 70.[7] These observations can have significance in the conduction of our general anesthetics as well as how the geriatric patient tolerates general anesthesia.

The cardiovascular system

Numerous research articles on caring for the cardiac patient undergoing noncardiac surgery illustrate the importance of the cardiovascular system to the anesthesiologist. These studies emphasize the diseased cardiovascular system. Many elderly patients have cardiovascular systems that are not diseased but show the physiological changes of aging. These changes are important both in the care of our modern everyman and the geriatric patient with physiological changes of aging superimposed upon disease changes.

The aging heart shows changes in the myocyte composition of the myocardium. The number of myocytes decreases and the size of myocytes increases. From middle to old age, the myocardium has two other changes associated with aging: the deposit of lipofusin in the myocardium and the increase in interstitial collagen in the myocardium and subendocardium.[8]

Examination of the ventricular septal wall thickness, when indexed to body surface, reveals a wall thickness increase that is age related. In patients over 60 years, this thickness between septal wall and free left ventricular wall can reach a 3:1 ratio.[8] The aging heart geometry undergoes changes which result in a mild decrease in both systolic and diastolic left ventricular dimensions plus a dilation and rightward shift of the aortic root. Each decade the heart ages results in thickening of the aortic and mitral valve leaflets. After age 70, the mitral annular ring calcifies and 40% of the women > 90 years old have mitral annular ring calcification. In both the semilunar valves and to a lesser extent in the atrioventricular valves, this calcification has a 4:1 ratio of women to men.[8] The aging heart also demonstrates dilation of the coronary arteries, and the number and size of coronary collateral arteries increase. The resting myocardial blood flow of the aging heart is higher in people > 50 years.. This is associated with an increase in cardiac work and a markedly lower myocardial blood flow reserve, which declines as a function of age.[9] There exists in the very old a universal finding of medial calcification of the coronary arteries, Monckeberg's medial calcification.[8] The conducting system shows a loss of pacemaker cells between 20 and 75 years. Studies have demonstrated an increase in atrioventricular (AV) block where 6.1% of patients > 69 years have AV block regardless of the presence of cardiovascular disease.[10]

The immune system and aging

As the human organism ages, there is a concurrent deterioration of the immune system. There are reduced humeral and cellular immune responses that can be seen throughout the immune system. The thymus as early as 1 year of age begins an involutionary process that proceeds at the rate of 3% per year until middle age. From this period, involution continues at 1% per year for the remainder of life. The thymus secretes thymulin, a hormone that is responsible for progenitor phenotypic cell maturation and mature T-cell modulation. Physiological aging has been correlated with decreased thymulin production. After age 30, an inhibitory factor affects the peripheral action of activated thymulin; this effect reaches maximal levels after 70 years of age. The thymus atrophies with aging and even with this atrophy studies have shown that older individuals contribute reduced numbers of T lymphocytes to the circulation.[11]

The kidneys and aging

There is a 20% decrease in renal mass between the age of 30 and 80 years.[12] Renal blood flow is maintained up to the fourth decade. Thereafter it is reduced by approximately 10% per decade. This decline is associated with a 50% reduction in glomerular filtration rate by the age of 90.[13] Maximum ability to concentrate urine decreases by approximately 30%, between age 30 and age 80.[14] The elderly may also display impairment of renal diluting capacity. Both plasma renin activity and aldosterone levels decrease after age 50.

When the geriatric everyman should be considered such?

From our development of the geriatric everyman, it is evident that the time at which the changes of aging occur varies among organ systems from the earliest period in life to periods above 70 years of age. For instance, the thymus starts the aging process in the very first year of life. In contrast, prior to the age of 50, age-related changes in brain volumes are small. Aging of the lung, kidney, and cardiovascular system all occur in an organ system–specific manner. Because of the variability in the timing of the aging process among organ systems, it becomes evident that there is no defined age at which we can say that a patient becomes a geriatric patient. Because it is difficult to define a geriatric patient on the basis of physiologic changes, the geriatric patient will be defined by age. Based on the ages used in the literature and by Medicare, this age structure transcends the range: 65 years old ≤ geriatric patient ≤ 75 years old. It is obvious that our definition ignores the population aged > 75 years . However, it is not obvious that this age group > 75 is homogeneous with the defined geriatric group and that each decade above does not present with unique changes that are important to us. All the time, patients present for treatment whose chronological age is either younger or older than the stated physiological age. In the past, anesthesia literature has not been specific in the use of the term geriatric patient because, in general when speaking about the geriatric patient this included the cohort group age 65 and above. Perhaps we should classify the whole population above 65 as the geriatric cohort group. This cohort group would be subdivided into age groups starting at 65 using a progressive nomenclature as young-old for 65–75 (our definition of the geriatric patient), aged for 75–85, oldest-old or very old for 85–100, and centenarian for 100 years and greater. For now, we have this limited chronological demographic definition.

THE DEMOGRAPHICS OF THE GERIATRIC COHORT POPULATION

Our world is a beacon as seen from space (Map 1-1) and the lights represent part of the density of the world population (Map 1-2).

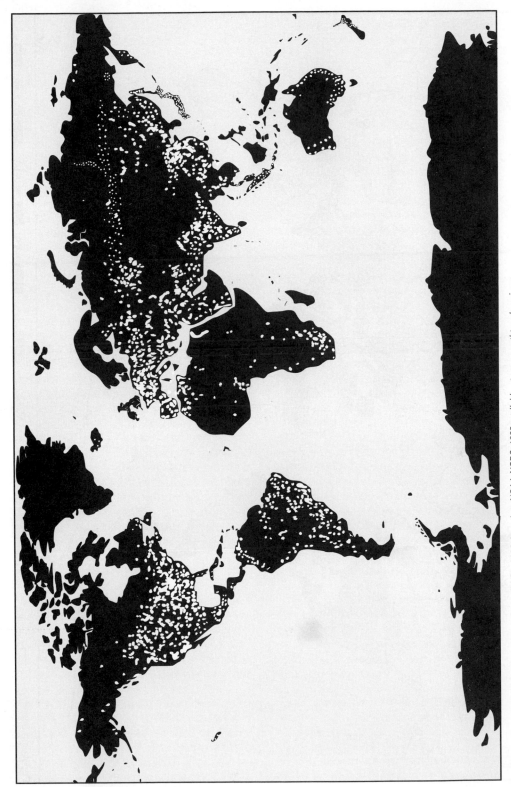

MAP 1-1 The world as seen from space. *Source: WRI, 2000, based on NOAA-NGDC, 1998 available at www.earthtrends.wri.org.*

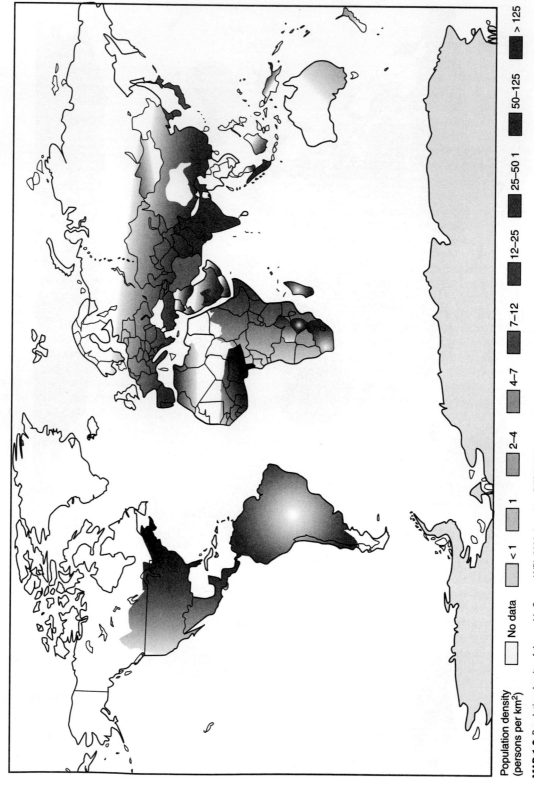

Population density
(persons per km²)

| No data | <1 | 1 | 2–4 | 4–7 | 7–12 | 12–25 | 25–50 1 | 50–125 | > 125 |

MAP 1-2 Population density of the world. *Source:* WRI, 2000, based on CIESIN 2000 available at www.earthtrends.wri.org.

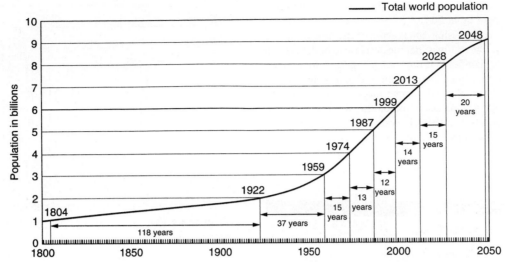

FIGURE 1-1 Time to successive billions in world population: 1800–2050. *Source:* United Nations (1995 b); U.S. Census Bureau, International Programs Center, International Database and Unpublished Tables.

The geriatric everyman forms part of the demographics of the world population. The world population is increasing in size. From 1804, the world population took 118 years to double. Fifty-two years were required for the population to double again. In 1999, the population reached 6 billion. This represented the shortest period for the population to increase by 1 billion. The estimated population will reach 9 billion by 2048. However, the time interval to add 1 billion people will increase for each billion people in the ensuing years (Fig. 1-1).[15] This may represent the high watermark for the human population since the population growth will drop below replacement level as a result of decreased fertility. In 2002, the population replacement level was only slightly greater than a half child or in terms of fertility levels, this represents 2.6 children per woman. The fertility level will continue to decline over the next four decades (Fig. 1-2).[16] Yet, population momentum will continue to cause an increase in population growth albeit at a slower rate. This population momentum phenomenon is a result of both relative and absolute increase in the number of women in the childbearing age. This phenomenon in 2002 was the principal cause of three-quarters of the population growth. This growth will lead to realignment in the 10 countries with the largest population.[16] By 2050, Japan and Russia will no longer be among the 10 most populated countries. China will yield

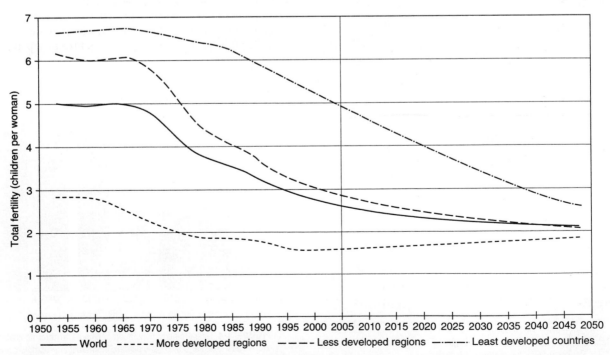

FIGURE 1-2 Total fertility for the world and development groups: 1950–2050.

the number one spot to India while the United States will maintain the number three spot (Table 1-1).

If the population is increasing, the graying of the human species seems contradictory. The reality is that the decrease in both the birth rate and fertility rate signifies that the younger age groups make up a smaller portion of the population meaning a relative increase in the older age groups. The resulting decreased mortality in age-specific middle and older age groups accounts for the absolute increased numbers in these cohorts. Increasing life expectancy has added three decades to human life from that of 150 years ago (Fig. 1-3).[15]

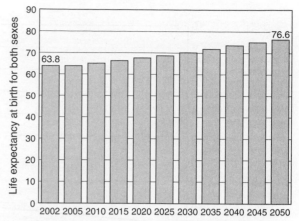

FIGURE 1-3 World life expectancy at birth: 2002–2050. *Source:* U.S. census bureau, international programs center, international database.

Table 1-1

Countries Ranked by Population

Rank Country	2000 Population
1 China	1,268,853,362
2 India	1,002,708,291
3 United States	282,338,631
4 Indonesia	224,138,438
5 Brazil	175,552,771
6 Russia	146,731,774
7 Pakistan	146,342,958
8 Bangladesh	130,406,594
9 Japan	126,699,784
10 Nigeria	114,306,700

Rank Country	2025 Population
1 China	1,453,123,817
2 India	1,361,625,090
3 United States	349,666,199
4 Indonesia	300,277,490
5 Pakistan	228,822,199
6 Brazil	217,825,222
7 Nigeria	206,165,946
8 Bangladesh	204,538,715
9 Russia	130,534,651
10 Mexico	130,198,692

Rank Country	2050 Population
1 India	1,601,004,572
2 China	1,424,161,948
3 United States	420,080,587
4 Nigeria	356,523,597
5 Indonesia	336,247,428
6.Pakistan	294,995,104
7 Bangladesh	279,955,405
8 Brazil	228,426,737
9 Congo (Kinshasa)	183,177,415
10 Mexico	147,907,650

Note: Data updated 4-26-2005 (Release notes).
Source: U.S. Census Bureau, International Database.

Decreasing infant and child mortality have accomplished some of this change. This change relates to increased sanitation and better water supplies. Moreover, advances in medicine, vaccination, and antibiotics have also contributed to this increased life expectancy. Another factor contributing to increased life expectancy is decreasing death rates. In the nineteenth century, this declining death rate did not relate to a country's economic level. In the twentieth century, there occurred a divergence between developed and less developed countries secondary to lower infant death rates.

This graying of the world's population will cause a doubling of the number of people in the geriatric cohort group (65 years of age or older)—from 420 million in 2000 to an estimated 973 million in 2030 (Fig. 1-4).[15] The graying of the human species implies that the geriatric cohort group will also undergo demographic aging. The population of people aged 80 or more is increasing at an annual rate of 3.8%. This rate is twice the rate of people above 60, which is 1.9%. The projected growth rate of these age cohorts will decrease to 3% and 1.6% in people ≥ 80 years and > 60 years, respectively, over the next 50 years. The cohort from 80 years old or above will increase from 1% of the total population to 4.1% of the total population in

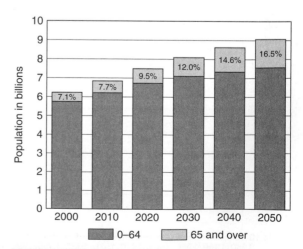

FIGURE 1-4 Global elderly population compared to total population: 2002–2050. *Source:* U.S. census bureau, international programs center, international database.

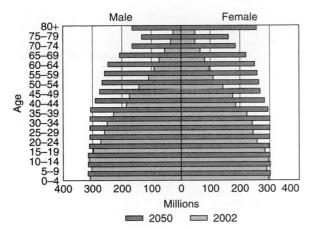

FIGURE 1-5 Pyramids of global population: 2002–2050. *Source:* U.S. census bureau, international programs center, international database.

50 years. A similar age distribution exists in Sweden where this cohort group currently represents 5% of the population. From the approximately 80 million people in the 80 and above cohort presently in the world, this group will increase to greater than 400 million by 2050, and continue to increase steadily (Fig. 1-5). Coincidental with the increase in the 80 and above cohort group, the centenarian group will increase from an estimated 180,000 people to 3.2 million people worldwide.

The future distribution of the graying population is important to the world's health services. The population of North America consists of a distribution where the 80 or older cohort comprises more than 3% of the population. The European cohort population of 80 or older is 3%. Examinations of other parts of the world show an 80 or older cohort population of less than 0.9% in areas like the Caribbean, Latin America, and Asia. Population estimates for the year 2050 reveal that 19 countries will have 80 or older cohort groups of 10%. By 2050, it is estimated that 1 in every 10 people living in developed regions will be 80 years or older. The less developed regions estimations are that 1 in 30 people of the population will be 80 years or older. This favorable ratio of population cohort will still mean that from the population cohort of 80 and older there will be a shift from the 2000 figure of 53% in the developed countries to an estimated 57% in the less developed countries.[15] However, this population shift in the 80-year-old cohort group does not hold true for the centenarian cohort. In 2000, 78% of this cohort group was living in developed countries while 69% of the centenarian cohort group will be living in developed countries by 2050.

CONCLUSIONS

The population will increase barring natural or man-made disasters as well as if the assumptions on growth and death rates hold to 9 billion people in the year 2048. At this time, the geriatric cohort (people above 65 years old) has been projected to be greater than 1 billion people worldwide. This increase will see proportionate increase in the 65–75 geriatric group (young-old), the 75–85 group (aged), and even the groups above 85 (oldest-old). These groups should be defined in similar manners and included in study methodology so that differences can be compared on an equal basis among studies and different age groups.

The aging process renders changes in the anatomy and physiology of many organ systems. The changes that occur have importance to

the practice of anesthesia. For the present, some of these changes are of intellectual curiosity. However, as the fund of knowledge increases these changes may have impact on the practice of anesthesia. Certainly, there will be as occurred in pediatric anesthesia a better appreciation that our patients are not just older adults but an entity with distinct requirements that are different from the normal adult demands. As geriatric medicine continues to mature, the knowledge needed to care for this patient group will increase, and with this increased knowledge, the education of future anesthesiologists will include training specifically aimed at the geriatric population. As the geriatric population continues to represent an ever-increasing percentage of our population and patient base, there will be those that specialize in newly developed geriatric fellowships. The sequential chapters contribute to this educational process and aid the anesthesiologist in caring for this aging population.

KEY POINTS

▶ Because of the variability in the timing of the aging process among organ systems, it becomes evident that there is no defined age at which we can say that a patient becomes a geriatric patient on a physiologic basis.

▶ The world fertility level will continue to decline over the next four decades. Yet, population momentum will continue to cause an increase in population growth albeit at a slower rate.

▶ The decrease in both the birth rate and fertility rate signifies that the younger age groups make up a smaller portion of the population meaning a relative increase in the older age groups. Increasing life expectancy in age-specific middle and older age groups accounts for the absolute increased numbers in these cohorts.

▶ Over the next half-century, the aging of the world population will have its greatest effect in less developed countries.

KEY WEBSITES

▶ http:/www.census.gov/ipc/www/wp02.html

▶ http:/www.un.org/esa/population/publications/WPP2004/wpp2004.htm

REFERENCES

1. Albuquerque J, Deshauer D, Grof P. Descartes' passions of the soul—seeds of psychiatry? *J Affect Disord*. 2003;76:285–291.
2. Courchesne E, Chisum HJ, Townsend J, et al. Normal brain development and aging: quantitative analysis at in vivo MR imaging in healthy volunteers. *Radiology*. 2000;216:672–682.
3. Guttmann CR, Jolesz FA, Kikinis R, et al. White matter changes with normal aging. *Neurology*. 1998;50:972–978.
4. Pfefferbaum A, Adalsteinsson E, Sullivan EV. Frontal circuitry degradation marks healthy adult aging: evidence from diffusion tensor imaging. *Neuroimage*. 2005;26:891–899.
5. Bellis TJ, Wilber LA. Effects of aging and gender on interhemispheric function. *J Speech Lang Hear Res*. 2001;44:246–263.
6. Tolep K, Higgins N, Muza S, et al. Comparison of diaphragm strength between healthy adult elderly and young men. *Am J Respir Crit Care Med*. 1995;152:677–682.
7. Thurlbeck WM, Angus GE. Growth and aging of the normal human lung. *Chest*. 1975;67:3S–6S.
8. Kitzman DW, Edwards WD. Age-related changes in the anatomy of the normal human heart. *J Gerontol*. 1990;45:M33-M39.
9. Czernin J, Muller P, Chan S, et al. Influence of age and hemodynamics on myocardial blood flow and flow reserve. *Circulation*. 1993;88:62–69.
10. Fleg JL, Das DN, Wright J, et al. Age-associated changes in the components of atrioventricular conduction in apparently healthy volunteers. *J Gerontol*. 1990;45:M95-M100.

11. Pido-Lopez J, Imami N, Aspinall R. Both age and gender affect thymic output: more recent thymic migrants in females than males as they age. *Clin Exp Immunol.* 2001;125:409–413.

12. Beck LH. Changes in renal function with aging. *Clin Geriatr Med.* 1998; 14:199–209.

13. Lubran MM. Renal function in the elderly. *Ann Clin Lab Sci.* 1995; 25:122–133.

14. Rowe JW, Shock NW, DeFronzo RA. The influence of age on the renal response to water deprivation in man. *Nephron.* 1976;17:270–278.

15. U.S. Census Bureau. Global population profile: 2002.

16. U.N. Population Division. The world population prospects: the 2004 revision.

Mechanisms of Aging

Sean X. Leng
Neal S. Fedarko

The fact that many surgically treatable diseases become more common with age and that age is associated with increased risk for anesthesia-related morbidity and mortality highlights the critical importance of careful evaluation and management of older patients during pre-, peri-, and postoperative periods. This daunting task will be impossible to accomplish unless the health-care providers understand age-related physiological changes and their impact on older patients' risk for adverse outcomes and reserves for recovery. To better understand physiological alterations in specific organ systems during aging, which will be reviewed in the subsequent chapters of this text, an overview of current knowledge on mechanisms of aging is in order. This chapter focuses its brief discussion on definition of aging, theories of aging, and aging and physiologic reserve.

DEFINITION OF AGING

A discussion about the mechanisms of aging demands that one first address how aging is defined. Broadly defined, aging refers to all time-associated events that occur during the postmaturation period in the life span of an organism. For humans, aging is defined as a universal biological process that manifests itself as a decline in functional capacity and an increased risk for morbidity and mortality over time. However, measuring an age-related increase in health risk in older patients is not as easy as it seems. This is because, at least in part, not all age-related changes are necessarily present in an older person, and no two individuals age at the same rate. Diseases accumulated during aging, other extrinsic environmental, psychological, and social-economical factors, and their impacts (negative or positive) on one's health and functional capacity have further complicated the situation. In discussing aging, terms commonly encountered include chronological age, physiological age, and clinical age.

▶ Chronological age

This is probably the most convenient measure and is widely used in clinical settings and in aging research. Medicare, arguably the most important mechanism of payment of health care for older adults in the United States, sets its current eligibility threshold at 65 years of age. Because the average life expectancy dramatically increased during the last century, some propose to group older adults into the young-old (aged 65–74 years), the mid-old (aged 75–84 years), and the oldest-old (aged 85 years and above), suggesting different levels of clinical risk among these age groups. However, this measure is seriously flawed due to significant heterogeneity of the older adult population. It is conceivable and commonly encountered by clinicians that a healthy 85-year-old has physiologic reserve and recovers from surgery just as well as or better than a 65-year-old with many diseases and poor health. Therefore, it is quite evident that chronological age is not a reliable estimate of age-related surgical risk in older patients. Furthermore, denial of surgical intervention based on a patient's old age alone is ageism.

▶ Physiological age

Physiological aging, or biological aging, is intended to describe the progressive changes of the physiological systems with age during the postmaturation period of life. It usually refers to changes resulting from the intrinsic biological aging process and thus, although it is much less accepted now, is also termed as *normal* aging. Some of the crude markers of physiological aging are quite evident to clinicians, such as loss of height, graying of hair, wrinkling of skin, changes in eyesight, and to some extent reduced coordination of movement. More importantly, biological aging attempts to address the age-related decrease in physiologic reserve in older adults. Older persons may do just as well as young individuals under normal or unstressful circumstances. With decreased physiologic reserve, however, older adults cannot mount an adequate compensatory response to an insult (injury, new onset of disease process, or catastrophic psychosocial event) and they have a much lower threshold to become decompensated and ill. Furthermore, older patients likely have a decreased ability to tolerate surgical procedures and/or to recover from surgery, especially when their physiologic reserve is further depleted by a disease process regardless of whether this disease process is the primary indication for the surgical intervention.

However, physiological aging, per se, only addresses the intrinsic biological aging process with the following two limitations: (a) Evaluation of intrinsic physiological aging independent of extrinsic factors and disease processes requires the identification of older individuals free of diseases and health habits issues (such as smoking), which is methodologically challenging. This is because the screening process is cumbersome and costly and, in addition, only a small fraction of older persons would meet the above criteria. For example, almost all individuals in their eighth decade of life suffer from one or more chronic conditions, such as osteoarthritis, osteoporosis, type 2 diabetes, coronary heart disease, dementia, cancer, benign prostate hypertrophy, or cataracts, to name just a few. (b) Although it is important to understand intrinsic biological aging, the applicability of this information to the general older patient population is questionable.

Therefore, merely knowing physiological aging is not enough. Clinicians are often confronted with how to apply or incorporate this basic knowledge into their daily practice when caring for ordinary older patients who suffer from multiple comorbid conditions and are affected by many other extrinsic, environmental, and psychosocial factors. In addition, not all the physiological changes during aging are deleterious. For example, graying of hair is considered neutral, at least physiologically speaking.

▶ Clinical age

Clinical aging is a relatively newer term and perhaps, at least conceptually, a more useful one to clinicians. Although geriatricians, scientists, and bureaucrats have long debated the distinction between aging and disease, it is abundantly clear that the physiologic reserve and vulnerability of older patients are affected by biological aging as well as age-related diseases and other extrinsic factors. In addition, there is general agreement that much of the physiological deterioration of older patients is secondary to age-associated diseases and that the occurrence and progression of many chronic diseases are strongly influenced by physiological aging. Clinical age emphasizes that intrinsic physiological aging, extrinsic factors, as well as disease processes, all contribute significantly to decreased physiologic reserve, reduced functional capacity, and altered homeostasis in older adults. Therefore, these adverse consequences during aging can be modified by altering lifestyle and environmental factors. They can also be modulated by presently available medical and public health measures and undoubtedly much more by those that will be developed in the future.

THEORIES OF AGING

Theories on mechanisms of aging are general statements proposed to address the following two fundamental questions: why we age and how we age. Making such general statements is no easy task for numerous reasons. These include, but are not limited to, the lack of agreement on the definition of aging; the limited information about aging processes; the multitude of possible causes of aging; the complexity of aging within one species or one organism; the diverse ways aging reveals itself in different species; and the interactions among aging processes, environmental influences, and diseases. Although current theories of aging cannot explain all aspects of aging, they are valuable in giving broad logical perspectives on mechanisms of aging based on diverse bits of information; giving direction to further research; and helping to envision applications of current knowledge in clinical practice and develop interventional strategies for older patients. Based on the two fundamental questions they are intended to address, the theories on mechanisms of aging can be grouped into two categories: evolutionary theories and physiological theories.

▶ Evolutionary theories

As defined above, aging is a gradual process characterized by decline in functional capacity and increased risk for morbidity and mortality over time. This suggests that aging does not provide survival advantage to individual persons. How, then, can aging exist through the action of natural selection? In other words, why do we age? Over the past century, many theories have been proposed to address this fundamental question. Several major theories and their arguments and drawbacks are discussed below.

Theory of programmed death

This theory was proposed over 100 years ago by August Weismann.[1-3] Selective pressure occurs in areas affecting *fitness* of the organism. Fitness is the capability to reproduce successfully. Aging can be viewed as either an adaptive trait or a nonadaptive trait. In Weismann's argument, aging was an adaptive response. Aging was a specific mechanism designed by natural selection to eliminate the old and free up resources. Arguments against this theory include that (a) it is rare in natural populations for individuals to survive long enough (from predation) to die from a postulated death mechanism; and (b) how could natural selection act against an aging phenomenon in nature where old age is typically not found. While the theory has been out of favor for many years, there has recently been renewed interest in looking at aging as an evolved characteristic.[4] A facet of the theory (programmed obsolescence) has survived in a number of the mechanistic theories presented below.

Mutation accumulation theory

This theory was first proposed by Peter Medawar more than 70 years after Weissmann.[5,6] It states that alleles (genes) with purely detrimental effects can accumulate if those effects are confined to late life when selection against them is weak. With this theory, genetic or evolutionary changes in senescence need not be accompanied by changes in early-life fitness. Aging is a nonadaptive trait, a by-product. Aging is an inevitable result of declining force of natural selection. No selective pressure is brought to bear on organisms expressing a mutation at older postreproductive ages. In an evolutionary context, aging is neutral, not selected for or against. Recent evidence in support of mutation accumulation theory has arisen from studies of age-specific reproductive success of *Drosophila melanogaster*[7] and in transgenic mice where mutation rates in different kinds of tissues have been quantified.[8,9]

Disposable soma theory

The disposable soma theory arose from a molecular theory concerning the stability of protein synthesis.[10,11] The theory is mainly based on two concepts: (a) Homeostasis maintenance is required for an organism to survive day-to-day wear and tear, disease, and environmental hazards; and (b) natural selection favors investment in this maintenance when it promotes the fitness of the species (ability to successfully reproduce). In a natural environment, homeostasis maintenance at a certain level keeps the body in good condition and functional until an age after which most individuals will have died from accidental causes. A greater investment in this maintenance would be disadvantageous because resources are finite and are better used for reproduction. Thus, the disposable soma theory concludes that the optimum course is to invest fewer resources in the maintenance of somatic tissues than are necessary for indefinite survival. The result is that aging occurs through the gradual accumulation of unrepaired somatic defects when the ability of the body to maintain homeostasis becomes less robust after the reproductive age. This theory can be viewed as a special, more narrowly defined variant of the antagonistic pleiotropy theory.

Antagonistic pleiotropic gene theory

The antagonistic pleiotropic gene theory was first proposed by Williams in 1957.[12] This theory is based on the genetics principle that genes direct the body's activities during all stages of life including fetal development, maturation, and aging. It further states that effects from certain genes may be beneficial early in life but detrimental later in life. Because of the declining force of natural selection with age (selective pressure decreases as the reproductive age is passed), any gene that conferred an advantage early in life would be favored by selection even if the same gene could cause deleterious effects at an older age. The deleterious effects of such pleiotropic genes result in aging. For example, certain genes may promote rapid metabolism leading to rapid successful reproduction early in life. However, rapid metabolism may also cause damage to a variety of molecules of the body. The damaged molecules may accumulate, resulting in aging. According to this theory, the decline in the force of natural selection with age would ensure that even quite modest early benefits would outweigh severe harmful side effects, provided the latter occurred late enough.

The success of artificial selection for increased longevity in *Drosophila* has provided supportive evidence for trade-offs between early and late fitness components predicted by both the disposable soma and antagonistic pleiotropic gene theories. These studies have shown reduced fecundity as a general correlate of delayed senescence in the long-lived flies.[13] A similar trade-off has also been reported for a human population, based on analysis of birth and death records of British aristocrats.[14] In addition, active genetic research in the nematode *Caenorhabditis elegans* has recently yielded a growing number of long-lived mutants in which increased longevity has been consistently associated with increased resistance to biochemical and other stresses.[15] Many of the affected genes are linked to pathways that control a switch between the normal developmental process of the worm and an alternative long-lived form called the *dauer* larva, which is invoked during stressful times, such as food shortage. This and other emerging evidence suggest a fundamental link between metabolic control, growth and reproduction, and homeostasis maintenance, as predicted by both of the above theories. The physiological theories of aging discussed in the section below attempt to address the above areas at the genetic, cellular, and molecular levels.

▶ Physiological theories of aging

The next fundamental question on mechanisms of aging is how we age. With rapid advances in biomedical research, a great deal of information on changes during aging at the organ system, cellular, molecular, and genetic levels has been gathered. Based on this wealth of information, dozens of physiological theories have been proposed. While it is impossible and unnecessary to include all of them in this section, some of the major physiological theories on mechanisms of aging are selected, with special emphasis on genetic and free radical theories.

Genetic theories

Genetic principles suggest that genes direct the body's activities during all stages of life including fetal development, maturation, and aging. However, it is unlikely that humans are genetically *programmed* to die. In other words, aging is nonadaptive; being programmed to die by genes offers no evolutionary advantage to the individual organism or to the species as a whole. Therefore, the effect of genes on aging is clearly distinct from the effect of genes on the other two stages of life. While genes driving development and maturation have evolved roles that define highly ordered sequential events, the major effect of *aging genes* is likely to be on processes other than aging. Such processes include an effect on homeostasis maintenance as suggested by the disposable soma theory, or detrimental effect from pleiotropic

genes as suggested by the antagonistic pleiotropic gene theory. Another key point is the interactions among genes, diseases, and environmental factors in their influence on aging (nature vs. nurture). For example, it is estimated that only about 35% of variance among human life spans can be accounted for by variations among genes. For identical twins, the estimate is 40–70%. The same seems true for many animal models. The remaining variation in life span and age-related diseases is due to lifestyle, environmental factors, and occasional incidents (e.g., accidents). Keeping such perspectives in mind, the genetic theories are, nevertheless, among the principle theories on mechanisms of aging.

Currently, there are many genetic theories. Based on their individual emphasis, the genetic theories can be grouped into the following categories.

Genetic Biography Category   The genetic theories in this category emphasize that genes act as the genetic timers that provide instructions, directly or indirectly, on how to progress in all stages of life including aging. Aging begins at birth or even at conception and all that follows is programmed within the genetic material.

Antagonistic pleiotropic gene theory   The antagonistic pleiotropic gene theory is a classic example in this category and is discussed in detail in the previous section.

Genetic clock theory   This theory suggests that some genes keep track of the body's progress and perhaps the passage of time or number of cell divisions. In this way, genes can control the age at which certain events occur. The observations that life expectancy is consistent across members of a species and that females tend to live longer than males support a genetic clock theory. The genetic contribution to human aging is evident from studies showing that long-lived parents tend to have long-lived children, centenarians and nonagenarians occur with high frequency in some families, and the life expectancies of identical twins are more closely related than those of other siblings.

Telomere theory   The replication of linear chromosome DNA by DNA polymerase leads to the loss of terminal sequences, in the absence of a special mechanism to maintain ends or telomeres. This mechanism involves short terminal repeats and the enzyme telomerase. In normal cells, telomeric DNA continually decreases in size in the absence of telomerase, and this is followed by cellular senescence. The telomere theory of cellular senescence appears to provide a molecular basis for the *Hayflick limit* to human fibroblast growth.[16] The telomere theory predicts that different rates of aging could occur in different cells or parts of the body because the telomeres in some cells shorten faster than those of other cells.

Limited Gene Usage Category   The genetic theories in this category emphasize that there is a limited number of times that the instructions in genes can be read with high fidelity. After many years of being read and reread some genes may become unreadable and instructions are lost. Other genes may be read poorly, causing mistakes to the body. In either case, detrimental changes result in aging.

Somatic mutation theory   Mutations that occur not in egg or sperm cells, but in somatic cells of an individual will affect that individual but not be passed on to future generations. While most somatic mutations may be corrected or eliminated, some will not and will accumulate over time. This accumulation eventually causes cells to malfunction and die. This theory proposes that harmful environmental factors injure the genes. Possible harmful factors include radiation, toxic chemicals, free radicals, and certain microorganisms. Somatic mutations can be in the form of deletions, insertions, or point mutations. The theory posits that these somatic mutations have a deleterious effect later in life.[9,17] Such mutations can also occur within the cell when transposable elements move between the mitochondrial DNA (mtDNA) and the nuclear DNA, resulting in genetic disruption. Somatic mutations in the DNA of mitochondria are also included in this theory (see below).

Faulty DNA repair theory This theory states that although genes are being damaged throughout life, cells also have mechanisms to repair the damage as quickly as it occurs. The intact repair mechanisms ensure that the genes are read accurately. After many years, however, the mechanisms begin to fail. The faulty repair mechanisms cannot keep up and DNA damage accumulates over time, resulting in detrimental genetic disruption.

Mitochondrial DNA Category

Mitochondrial DNA theory The mtDNA theory in this category emphasizes genetic material in the mitochondria rather than that in the nucleus.[18,19] According to this theory, mtDNA damage occurs much faster than does damage to nuclear DNA. mtDNA sustains damage 10–20 times faster than does nuclear DNA because (a) mtDNA is attached to the inner mitochondrial membrane, where most free radicals are produced; (b) mtDNA is not protected by proteins (e.g., histones); and (c) mtDNA cannot repair itself. In addition, damaged mtDNA accumulates in cells because (a) damaged mitochondria replicate faster than undamaged mitochondria; (b) mitochondria that replicate retain damaged mtDNA; (c) mitochondria with damaged mtDNA are eliminated slower than normal mitochondria; and (d) nondividing or slowly dividing cells accumulate a high percentage of damaged mitochondria. The damaged mtDNA has more deleterious effects than does damaged nuclear DNA because each cell uses almost all its mtDNA genes while using only approximately 7% of its nuclear DNA. Thus, nearly any adverse change in mtDNA will have adverse effects on mitochondrial function. These effects include less energy production, more free radical formation, reduced control of other cell processes, and accumulation of damaged harmful molecules, leading to aging and certain age-related diseases.

Molecular theories

Molecular theories focus on molecules other than DNA and modification of molecules. Such molecules include free radical species and calcium. Types of modification of molecules included are cross-linking and glycation.

Error Catastrophe Theory This theory proposes that the damage is not to the genes themselves but to the protein molecules that are the products of the genes. Specifically, protein synthesis fidelity in somatic cells becomes progressively inaccurate propagating errors.[20] These damaged molecules spread increasing numbers of mistakes (altered physical, chemical, or biological properties) throughout the cell and the body and result in aging.

Free Radical Theory The free radical theory was proposed by Harman in 1956 and is probably the most widely accepted among the molecular theories.[21] Free radicals are chemical species that have unpaired electrons in an outer orbital. They are extremely reactive and unstable. In the context of biological damage, oxygen or oxidative free radicals are the most important, including superoxide ($O_2 \bullet -$), hydrogen peroxide (H_2O_2), and hydroxyl ions ($\bullet OH$). Oxidative reactions in mitochondria are a major source of oxygen free radicals. In the normal respiratory pathway to energy (in the form of adenosine triphosphate [ATP]) production, oxygen is reduced to water. The

above partially reduced oxygen free radicals are also produced in this process. Figure 2-1 illustrates the formation, removal, and detrimental effects of oxygen free radicals.

Oxygen free radicals can react with a variety of inorganic and organic molecules including nucleic acids, lipids, proteins, and carbohydrates. Damage to DNA by oxygen free radicals includes the formation of several base adducts, which has been convincingly demonstrated by Ames and his colleagues. Using sensitive chromatographic techniques, they measured the quantities excreted by animals with different metabolic rates, and found that the amount adduct per kilogram of body weight was proportional to metabolic rate. This is expected if oxygen free radicals are generated primarily by respiration. More importantly, the results also show that DNA is a real target for damage. Damage to DNA slows DNA replication for cell reproduction, adversely affects numerous cell processes by interrupting the structure and regulation of genes, and promotes cancer. Oxygen free radicals react with lipids and produce lipid peroxidation that results in structural and functional damage to the membranes of cells and organelles. This is likely to be particularly important in long-lived, nondividing cells such as neurons. Lipid peroxidation is believed to be the major source of the so-called age pigment lipofuscin, which accumulates in the brain and other tissues. Oxidation of proteins by oxygen free radicals is one of the major abnormal postsynthetic changes that lead to protein damage. Such damage disturbs and distorts much bodily structure, inactivates or reduces enzyme activity, and accelerates protein degradation. Therefore, the free radical theory suggests that free radical damage, primarily by targeting to DNA, protein, and lipids, is the main reason for true aging and age-related diseases.

Rate of Living Theory This theory has at its basis the belief that organisms possess a finite amount of some vital substance. When this substance has been consumed, aging and death occurs. The number of breaths and heartbeats has been proposed as limiting substances. More recently, the theory has been adapted to include oxygen metabolism. This theory states that aging is determined by the rate of metabolism because aerobic metabolism causes damage, primarily through the production of oxygen free radicals.[22,23] The rate of living theory predicts that the higher the rate of metabolism, the faster the

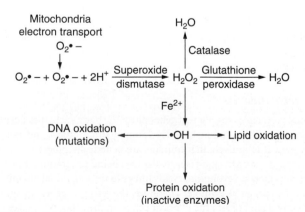

FIGURE 2-1 Superoxide anions ($O_2 \bullet -$) produced by the respiratory electron transport in the mitochondria form hydrogen peroxide (H_2O_2) under superoxide dismutase. H_2O_2 can be metabolized by glutathione peroxidase or catalase into water. In the presence of iron (Fe^{2+}), H_2O_2 is converted to hydroxyl radical ($\bullet OH$), which causes oxidation of DNA, lipids, proteins, and other vital molecules of the body.

rate of aging and the shorter the life span. Most animals follow this prediction. Two major exceptions are mammals and birds, which have life spans longer than their rates of metabolism would predict. Proposed explanations for these discrepancies include that mammals and birds have more efficient metabolism resulting in less damage and/or they have better repair mechanisms.

Data supportive of this theory come from experiments of caloric restriction in a variety of animals including primates. Animals placed on caloric restriction consume less food with slower rate of metabolism. These animals live 25–30% longer compared to their littermates ad libitum. Data against the rate of living theory come from observations that humans that live to be centenarians have metabolized more oxygen than the longest-lived animals. Centenarians are also equally likely to have lived physically active lives as sedentary ones.

Calcium Theory Many of the mechanisms regulating activities and processes in the body rely on calcium as a signaling molecule. The calcium theory proposes that abnormal levels and movements of calcium, resulting from free radical damage to membranes in cells and a variety of other causes, lead to cell malfunctions and inadequate regulation of adaptive mechanisms.[24,25] These include dysregulation in the functions of numerous enzymes, muscle cells, nerve cells, and blood vessels, which result in aging.

Cross-Linkage Theory The fact that DNA, proteins (such as collagen), and other structural macromolecules develop inappropriate covalent attachments (cross-links) with increasing age has led to the cross-linkage theory. Cross-links reduce the mobility, elasticity, and resiliency of these molecules. Normally, damaged molecules are broken down and removed by proteases. Cross-links inhibit the ability of proteases to break down altered macromolecules. Proteins and other components that have cross-links are not readily degraded and accumulate over time. Free radicals, glucose, and even light seem to promote the formation of bonds between molecules. The cross-linkage theory maintains that such bonding leads to reduced resiliency of body parts, increased wear and tear, and malfunction that result in aging.[26] Evidence in support of this theory includes the observation that cross-linking of collagen in skin contributes to wrinkling and other age-related skin changes. Age-related cataract formation is associated with cross-linking of proteins in the lens of the eye.

Glycation Theory This theory is related to the cross-linkage theory but is more focused on glycation. Glycation is a process of nonenzymatic addition of sugars to amino acid residues in proteins. The initial reaction involves amino groups, particularly that in the lysine side chain of proteins, and the aldehyde group of sugars to form a ketoamine or Amadori product. This is subject to a series of higher-order reactions (collectively known as the *Maillard reaction*) to give a complex mixture of products, which are referred to as advanced glycation end products (AGE). Collagen and other long-lived proteins can become glycated, and thickening of the basement membranes seen in diabetic patients is in part due to glycation. Glycated proteins are likely to form cross-links with other proteins, producing large aggregates of materials that are not soluble and cannot be degraded. Accumulation of these materials and toxic AGE in cells and tissues over time leads to structural and functional damage to the body. In addition, glycation process produces free radicals. Therefore, the glycation theory suggests that most aging is caused by glycation and its resulting AGE and free radicals.[27–29]

Cellular theories

Cellular theories are based on either a specific organelle or a cellular phenotype expressed over time, as represented by the mitochondrial theory and cellular senescence theory, respectively.

Mitochondrial Theory The mitochondrial theory was proposed by Ozawa and colleagues in 1989.[30] It states that mitochondrial activities and damage to mitochondria result in aging. This theory is developed from the free radical theory. Further discussions can be found in sections on the mitochondrial DNA and free radical theories above.

Cellular Senescence Theory The cellular senescence theory is based on the phenomenon described by Hayflick and Moorhead in 1961 that after finite numbers of division in tissue culture, human fibroblasts stop dividing, become senescent, and gradually die.[31,32] This phenomenon has been observed in cultures of many other cell types from both humans and other animals, and is now commonly referred as Hayflick limit or replicative senescence. In addition, the number of times the cells can divide decreases as the age of the person who donated the cells increases. While they do not die quickly, cells with senescent phenotype demonstrate significant functional impairment. The cellular senescence theory suggests that aging is caused by decreased ability of cells to divide and renew as well as accumulation of senescent cells in the body.

Organ system theories

Organ system theories are based on an underlying pacemaker or biological clock foundation, but the concept is applied to a complex system as opposed to a specific gene, protein, or tissue. Systems are set at birth to run for a finite period of time and then wind down leading to aging and death. The two pivotal communication systems of the body—the neuroendocrine and the immune systems—are most often discussed as the clocks or pacemakers. In the neuroendocrine theory, the system includes the hypothalamus that stimulates or inhibits the pituitary gland that, in turn, regulates other components of the endocrine system (thyroid, adrenal glands, testes, or ovaries) and modulates the release of their hormones into circulation, which in turn affect target organs. During aging, this system becomes dysfunctional, resulting in high blood pressure, impaired sugar metabolism, and sleep abnormalities, all of which have further cascading downstream adverse effects.

Hormone Theories Hormones are chemical messengers that are carried in the circulation and give instructions to almost all cells and tissues in the body. The *insulin theory* and *growth hormone theory* focus on these two individual hormones.[33,34] These theories propose that aging results from excess stimulation of growth by insulin and growth hormone. The results are faster cell reproduction, larger cell size, larger body size, and the decline in physiologic reserve that marks aging. The *glucocorticoid theory* focuses on glucocorticoid steroid hormones. It suggests that aging results from improper levels of glucocorticoid steroid hormones. When levels are low, adaptive mechanisms become inadequate. When levels are high, damage results from excess suppression of defense mechanisms, such as inflammatory and immune responses, and stimulation of high blood glucose levels. The *reproductive hormone theory* emphasizes the importance of sex hormones. It states that aging results when sex hormone levels decline after reproductive years. With lower sex hormones, genes receive inadequate or detrimental signals. The result is declining production of desirable proteins and excess production of deleterious proteins, leading to aging.

Immune System Theories In addition to the communicating capability by circulating immune cells and cytokines, the immune system is one of the major defense systems in the body. The immune system is able to distinguish normal self from foreign materials. Those identified as normal parts of the body self are left undisturbed and those as foreign objects are attacked and destroyed by immune mechanisms. The *autoimmune theory* proposes that aging results from weakened ability of the immune system to distinguish normal self from foreign objects so that important self-components of the body are attacked and destroyed by inappropriately mounted and/or dysregulated immune mechanisms.[35] The *immune deficiency theory* suggests that aging results from the deficient immune system, because either the body is born with less than optimal indefinite capability as suggested by evolutionary theory or weakened by persistent use over time.[36] A deficient immune system is not able to defend the body against foreign toxins and pathogens. These noxious agents are allowed to injure the cells of the body and to disrupt their function, leading to aging.

This section has briefly introduced major physiological theories on mechanisms of aging categorized by different levels (genetic, molecular, cellular, and organ system). However, this categorization is arbitrary because many of them overlap. For example, mitochondrial theory (cellular level) may incorporate aspects of mitochondrial DNA theory (genetic level) and free radical theory (molecular level). Furthermore, since aging likely results from combinations of physiological processes like those stated in the above theories, it is not surprising for complex interactions to occur among these physiological processes in the body. For example, free radicals from mitochondria damage the mitochondria, cause somatic mutations, cause membrane damage that leads to calcium leakage, and promote glycation. These changes also reduce the production and effectiveness of enzymes that remove free radicals and that repair molecules damaged by free radicals. Still, glycation increases free radical production. With more free radicals and less defenses (removal and repair) against them, the rate of damage to mitochondria increases and faster free radical production results, leading to an exponentially expanding spiral of damage to multiple components throughout the body. *Network theory* has been proposed to capture these complex interactions.[37] The network theory for human aging may include all the genetic, molecular, and cellular theories described above plus their effects on the endocrine and immune systems. Damage to these systems leads to disruption in regulatory and defense mechanisms needed to maintain homeostasis. Figure 2-2 further illustrates the normal biological processes at the genetic, molecular, and cellular levels and time-related alterations of the critical components of these processes resulting in aging.

AGING AND PHYSIOLOGIC RESERVE

The sheer number and diversity of the theories of aging described in the previous section clearly demonstrate the complexity and multidimensionality of the mechanisms of aging. Each theory is supported by some evidence and each can explain certain aspects of aging. However, none tells the complete story. This is because aging likely results from multiple mechanisms or causes. Some may be more important than others, some may act at different times, and some may affect different parts of the body. For gerontologists, however, it is important to formulate, test, and revise these theories if mechanisms of aging are to be elucidated. Once they are delineated, influencing the processes in human aging might be possible. It might also be possible to identify and minimize undesirable but not inevitable changes that frequently occur along with aging. For clinicians, understanding current theories on mechanisms of aging helps to learn age-related physiological changes in each organ system detailed in the subsequent chapters of this text. Since many diseases are not part of aging but intimately associated with aging, it is equally important for clinicians to incorporate current knowledge on aging into their comprehensive assessment and treatment of age-related medical and surgical conditions in older patients.

The changes in physiological processes from primary aging result in little clinically significant change in function and overall condition of an older individual in the unstressed state, but these age changes become readily evident when the older person is stressed or moved away from homeostasis. Most physiological systems of the body build a significant amount of redundancy and reserve. This physiologic reserve enables us to tolerate and defend against numerous external insults (e.g., accidental injuries, bad choice of lifestyles, environmental hazards, and social and behavioral stressors) and disease conditions. As shown in Fig. 2-3, however, with primary aging changes and numerous acute and/or chronic diseases experienced over the years, the physiologic reserve of an older patient is severely depleted and extremely limited, especially if the patient seeks care for an acute medical or surgical condition at the time of evaluation. If the concept of primary physiological changes of aging seems too remote, clinicians should be well aware of the age-related depletion

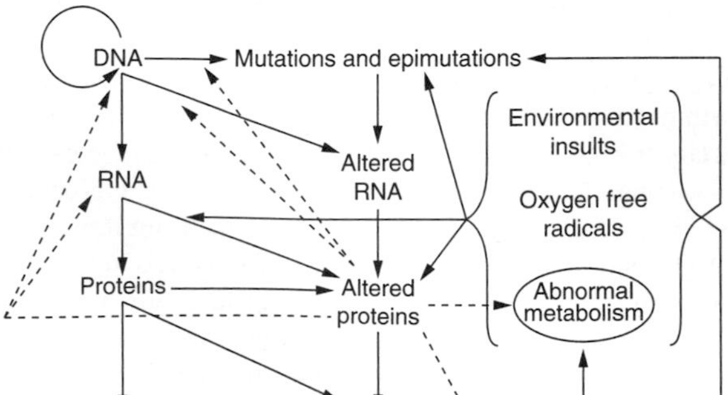

FIGURE 2-2 Normal biological processes at the genetic, molecular, and cellular levels (left side) and time-related alterations of the critical components of these processes (mid and right side), result in aging.

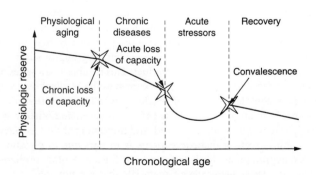

FIGURE 2-3 Primary aging changes (physiological aging), multiple comorbid chronic conditions (chronic diseases), and numerous acute insults (acute stressors) over the years lead to age-related depletion in physiologic reserve of older patients. Older patients also have resounding resiliency. They can recover most of the physiologic reserve lost from acute insults (recovery) but unlikely to the previous level.

in physiologic reserve of their older patients and integrate that into their clinical assessment. How to provide the best care to our ever-growing older patient population in the context of numerous subtle and not-so-subtle primary physiological changes of aging, along with the increasing comorbid medical and surgical conditions as well as social and behavioral issues, will be a daunting challenge for our health-care system in the twenty-first century.

SUMMARY AND KEY POINTS

Human aging is defined as a universal and progressive physiological process that manifests itself as decreased functional capacity, reduced physiologic reserve, and disturbed homeostasis over time. Several terms, including chronological age, physiological age, and clinical age, are commonly used to describe human aging. Intrinsic biological aging as well as age-associated diseases and other extrinsic factors all contribute to this process. This complex etiology is likely the reason for significant heterogeneity of the older patient population. This complexity also impacts interventional strategies and care for older patients. Therefore, clinicians are obligated to carefully assess health risk and reserve for recovery and not to deny otherwise indicated surgical intervention, or other types of treatment, merely based on chronological age of their older patients.

Many theories on mechanisms of aging have been proposed to address two fundamental questions: why we age and how we age. Accordingly, they are categorized into evolutionary theories and physiological theories. The disposable soma theory and the antagonistic pleiotropic gene theory are two widely accepted evolutionary theories at present. Physiological theories attempt to explain physiological changes during aging at different levels, namely, at the genetic, molecular, cellular, and organ system levels. Although the genetic and free radical theories are probably the most widely accepted theories in aging research, the key for clinicians is to understand age-related physiological changes at different levels across these theories so that appropriate assessment and treatment strategies can be developed for older patients.

Understanding the complex mechanisms of aging should improve clinicians' knowledge about physiological changes during aging. Physiologic reserve is a useful concept that further integrates the potential impact of these age-related physiological changes, multiple comorbid disease conditions, and environmental, social, and behavioral factors on the overall health status and surgical risk of older patients. Accurate assessment of the physiologic reserve and, ultimately, prevention of its depletion will benefit our older patients who need surgical intervention.

REFERENCES

1. Weismann A. *Über die Dauer des Lebens*. Jena, Germany: Verlag von Gustav Fisher; 1882.
2. Weismann A. *Essays Upon Heredity and Kindred Biological Problems*. Oxford: Clarendon Press; 1889.
3. Weismann A. *Über Leben und Tod*. Jena, Germany: Verlag von Gustav Fisher; 1892.
4. Goldsmith TC. Aging as an evolved characteristic—Weismann's theory reconsidered. *Med Hypotheses*. 2004;62(2):304–308.
5. Medawar P. *An Unsolved Problem in Biology*. London: HK Lewis; 1952.
6. Medawar PB. Old age and natural death. *Modern Q*. 1946;1:30–56.
7. Hughes KA, Alipaz JA, Drnevich JM, et al. A test of evolutionary theories of aging. *Proc Natl Acad Sci USA*. 2002;99(22):14286–14291.
8. Ono T, Uehara Y, Saito Y, et al. Mutation theory of aging, assessed in transgenic mice and knockout mice. *Mech Ageing Dev*. 2002;123(12):1543–1552.
9. Vijg J. Somatic mutations and aging: a reevaluation. *Mutat Res*. 2000;447(1):117–135.
10. Kirkwood TBL. Evolution of ageing. *Nature*. 1977;270:301–304.
11. Kirkwood TBL, Holliday R. The evolution of ageing and longevity. *Proc R Soc London Ser B Biol Sci*. 1979;205:531–546.
12. Williams GC. Pleiotropy, natural selection, and the evolution of senescence. *Evolution*. 1957;11:398–411.
13. Rose MR, Drapeau MD, Yazdi PG, et al. Evolution of late-life mortality in Drosophila melanogaster. *Evol Int J Org Evol*. 2002;56(10):1982–1991.
14. Westendorp RGJ, Kirkwood TBL. Human longevity at the cost of reproductive success. *Nature*. 1998;396:743–746.
15. Hughes KA, Reynolds RM. Evolutionary and mechanistic theories of aging. *Ann Rev Entomol*. 2005;50:421–445.
16. Olovnikov AM. Telomeres, telomerase, and aging: origin of the theory. *Exp Gerontol*. 1996;31(4):443–448.
17. Morley A. Somatic mutation and aging. *Ann NY Acad Sci*. 1998;854:20–22.
18. Jacobs HT. The mitochondrial theory of aging: dead or alive? *Aging Cell*. 2003;2(1):11–17.
19. Lenaz G. Role of mitochondria in oxidative stress and ageing. *Biochim Biophys Acta*. 1998;1366(1-2):53–67.
20. Orgel LE. The maintenance of the accuracy of protein synthesis and its relevance to ageing. *Proc Natl Acad Sci USA*. 1963;49:517–521.
21. Harman D. Aging: a theory based on free radical and radiation chemistry. *J Gerontol*. 1956;11(3):298–300.
22. Economos AC. Beyond rate of living. *Gerontology*. 1981;27(5):258–265.
23. Lints FA. The rate of living theory revisited. *Gerontology*. 1989;35(1):36–57.
24. Kanowski S. Aging, dementia, and calcium metabolism. *J Neural Transm Suppl*. 1998;54:195–200.
25. Khachaturian ZS. The role of calcium regulation in brain aging: reexamination of a hypothesis. *Aging (Milano)*. 1989;1(1):17–34.
26. Bjorksten J. The cross-linkage theory of aging. *J Am Geriatr Soc*. 1968;16(4):408–427.
27. Kristal BS, Yu BP. An emerging hypothesis: synergistic induction of aging by free radicals and Maillard reactions. *J Gerontol*. 1992;47(4):B107–B114.
28. Miksik I, Struzinsky R, Deyl Z. Change with age of UV absorbance and fluorescence of collagen and accumulation of epsilon-hexosyllysine in collagen from Wistar rats living on different food restriction regimes. *Mech Ageing Dev*. 1991;57(2):163–174.
29. Ulrich P, Cerami A. Protein glycation, diabetes, and aging. *Recent Prog Horm Res*. 2001;56:1–21.
30. Linnane AW, Marzuki S, Ozawa T, et al. Mitochondrial DNA mutations as an important contributor to ageing and degenerative diseases. *Lancet*. 1989;1(8639):642–645.
31. Hayflick L, Moorhead PS. The serial cultivation of human diploid cell strains. *Exp Cell Res*. 1961;25:585–621.
32. Hayflick L. The cell biology of aging. *J Invest Dermatol*. 1979;73(1):8–14.
33. Parr T. Insulin exposure and aging theory. *Gerontology*. 1997;43(3):182–200.
34. Parr T. Insulin exposure and unifying aging. *Gerontology*. 1999;45(3):121–135.
35. Walford RL. Immunologic theory of aging: current status. *Fed Proc*. 1974;33(9):2020–2027.
36. Kent S. Can normal aging be explained by the immunologic theory? *Geriatrics*. 1977;32(5):111–116.
37. Ying W. Deleterious network hypothesis of aging. *Med Hypotheses*. 1997;48(2):143–148.

SECTION

2

AGING AND ITS EFFECTS ON ORGAN RESERVE

Central/Peripheral nervous System

Khwaja Javaid Zakriya

The nervous system of the elderly individual differs both quantitatively and qualitatively from that of a younger individual. These changes in the elderly brain have to be considered during the preoperative evaluation. Changes in the central and peripheral nervous system (CNS and PNS) may affect functional outcome both in the immediate postoperative period and later during the recovery phase. This chapter reviews the changes which occur in the CNS and PNS with aging. The effect of aging on functional reserve of the CNS/PNS and its anesthetic ramifications are discussed. In addition, preoperative evaluation of some common neurologic diseases of the elderly are presented.

CHANGES WHICH OCCUR IN THE CENTRAL NERVOUS SYSTEM WITH AGING

▶ Brain

Anatomical changes occur in the brain during normal aging. The volume of the cortical gray matter and thalamus decreases with age. In comparison, the white matter volume of the cerebrum, cerebellum, corpus callosum, and pons remains fairly intact across ages 20 to 90. (Fig. 3-1).[1] Although in the past it was generally believed that loss of gray matter volume was caused by ongoing neuronal cell death, available evidence suggests that loss of neurons during normal aging is actually limited. Instead, brain cells shrink and the brain becomes more compact.[2,3] Recent studies focusing on the effects of normal aging on the human cerebral cortex suggest that there is a small overall loss of neurons from the neocortex.[4] This decrease in neuron number is nowhere near as massive as older studies had indicated. In fact, some neocortical areas do not lose any neurons with aging. Aging increases intracranial cerebrospinal fluid volume and creates, in effect, nonpathological low-pressure hydrocephalus.

It is controversial whether the aging process alters the number of synapses present in the cortex. However, data from primates suggest significant regional reduction in the neurotransmitters dopamine, acetylcholine, norepinephrine, and serotonin with aging.[4] Glutamate levels, the primary neurotransmitter in the cortex, do not appear to be affected. Neurotransmitter deficiencies are clearly related to Alzheimer's dementia and parkinsonism, and are undoubtedly involved in many other disorders prevalent in the geriatric population. Altered neurotransmitter activity has also been implicated as a factor associated with alterations in sensitivity to anesthetic agents.

Coupling of cerebral electrical activity, cerebral metabolic rate, and cerebral blood flow remains intact in the elderly. However, cerebral blood flow and oxygen consumption is decreased in old compared to young subjects.[5] The lower cerebral metabolic activity may be a result of decreased synaptic activity and neurotransmitters.

Although biochemical and anatomical changes have been described in the aging brain, the exact mechanisms causing changes in functional reserve are unclear. Decreases in brain reserve are manifested by decreases in functional activities of daily living, increased sensitivity to anesthetic medications, and increased risk for perioperative cognitive dysfunction. Symptoms and signs of neurologic dysfunction are common among the elderly. The major changes are impairment of memory and intellect, deterioration of gait and motility, altered sleep patterns, decrements in vision, hearing, taste, and smell, diminished vibratory sensation, and changes in reflexes. Since it is now known that neurologic deterioration with aging is not necessarily a result of neuronal loss, one contributing factor may be changes in nerve fibers. Some myelin sheaths in the CNS exhibit degenerative changes with aging.[6] It is possible that such degenerative changes lead to cognitive decline through changes in conduction velocity, which cause disruption of the normal timing of neuronal circuits. There is also loss of nerve fibers from cerebral white matter. This may contribute to cognitive decline by decreasing connections between neurons.[6] Memory decline occurs in more than 40% of people older than 60 years.[7] However, studies have suggested that memory decline in aging is not inevitable. Age-related memory decline is important because it can dramatically affect the activities of daily living. Senile dementia, the progressive loss of intellectual capacity with gradual physical and mental deterioration, occurs in 2.5% of the population over the age of 65. The incidence rises to approximately 14% in those aged 75 or more.

▶ Spinal cord

Aging is associated with neuronal loss and reactive gliosis in the spinal cord. Degeneration and shrinkage of nerve fibers and loss of cell bodies are most significant in the ventral horn, in the dorsal columns of the cervical spine, and in the intermediate gray matter of the thoracic segments.[8] Atrophy is most pronounced at the cephalic and least obvious at the caudal extremity of the spinal cord. The transverse area of the cervical spinal cord, as measured by magnetic resonance imaging (MRI), decreases with age. The ratio of the anteroposterior diameter to the transverse diameter remains unchanged. This means that the cervical spinal cord decreases in size with aging while maintaining its shape. The bony spinal canal becomes narrower with age. However, with normal aging, the spinal cord area and the shape of the spinal cord are independent of the spinal canal diameter.[9]

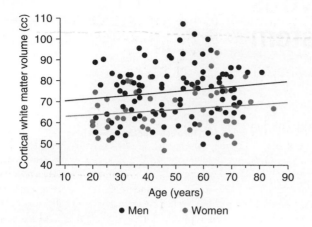

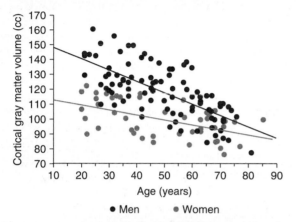

FIGURE 3-1 Volumes of cortical gray and white matter plotted as a function of age in 48 women and 95 men. Cortical gray matter volumes were significantly correlated with age in both men and women. Cortical white matter volume was not associated with age in either men or women. *(From Sullivan EV, Rosenbloom M, Serventi KL, et al. Neurobiol Aging. 2004;25:185.)*

CHANGES WHICH OCCUR IN THE PERIPHERAL NERVOUS SYSTEM WITH AGING

▶ Somatic nervous system

Peripheral nerves of all mammals deteriorate during aging. Morphologic studies have shown that aging primarily affects the myelinated nerves. In particular, large myelinated fibers undergo atrophy and the myelin sheaths undergo degenerative changes. Also, the number of myelinated nerve fibers decreases with aging (Table 3-1).

Aging affects the constitutive levels of expression of key genes encoding for major protein components of the myelin sheath. The maintenance of myelin sheath integrity involves the sustained expression of genes specifically associated with the myelin sheath. The major myelin proteins are myelin-basic protein (MBP) and proteolipid protein (PLP). Remyelination, the restoration of new myelin sheaths to demyelinated axons, is a spontaneous regenerative process that occurs within the adult mammalian CNS. Aging has a detrimental effect on remyelination. Remyelination is slowed as shown by a slowing of the rate of reappearance of transcripts for the major myelin proteins MBP and PLP, and their putative regulatory factor, Gtx. The age-related decline in remyelination is associated with an impairment of oligodendrocyte progenitor recruitment and

Table 3-1

Age-Related Changes in Composition of the Sural Nerve (M ± SD)

Nerve Fiber	Age (years)	Density Value
Myelinated	10–39	9228 ± 1036
	40–59	7663 ± 0525
	60–69	6246 ± 1378
	70–79	5270 ± 1496
Unmyelinated	20–39	27447 ± 7437
	40–59	26657 ± 6821
	60–69	28747 ± 4617
	70–79	26062 ± 5933
	80–89	27180 ± 5666

Source: Adapted from Verdu E, Ceballos D, Vilches JJ, Navarro X Influence of aging on peripheral **nerve** function and regeneration. *J Peripher Nerve Syst.* 2000;5:191.

differentiation. In addition, there may be alterations in the inflammatory response involving macrophages, which contribute to the decline in remyelination.[10]

Aging also induces functional changes. Aging decreases nerve conduction velocity of peripheral myelinated fibers. For instance, the conduction velocity of the efferent motor fibers is decreased by approximately 10–30% in elderly humans[11–14] (Table 3-2). In aged humans, the conduction of the efferent motor fibers of the ulnar nerve decreases from 58.4 to 51.5 m/s.[15] It has been proposed that in this nerve, after the 30th year, the loss of conduction velocity amounts to 0.2 m/s for each year of age.[11] On the contrary, the conduction velocity of unmyelinated fibers seems to be unaffected by the aging process.[14]

Table 3-2

Age-Related Changes in Nerve Conduction Velocity of Peripheral Nerves (M ± SD)

Nerve	Component	Age (years)	Nerve Conduction Velocity (M/S)
Ulnar	Sensory	16–36	45.7 ± 5.7
		67–91	37.3 ± 6.8
Median	Sensory	21–29	47.8 ± 4.3
		60–80	42.7 ± 6.0
		81–103	42.0 ± 7.8
Sural	Sensory	21–29	43.0 ± 4.3
		60–80	39.7 ± 6.4
		81–103	37.6 ± 5.2
Median	Motor	21–29	61.0 ± 2.9
		60–80	54.7 ± 4.0
		81–103	53.0 ± 5.6

Source: Adapted from Verdu E, et al. *J Peripher Nerve Syst.* 2000;5:191.

In patients older than 65 years, mild pure sensory or pure motor symptoms, slight and pure sensory signs confined to the feet (including absent vibratory sensation in the big toe), or absent ankle reflexes can be considered as normal aging manifestations.[16] The biceps, triceps, and knee jerks are usually retained after the age of 65 years. Some investigators have asserted that the ankle reflex should also be retained after the age of 65 years.

With aging, changes in the five senses occur. Touch is affected by poor circulation in late life. Although it is speculated that pain sensitivity declines with age, to date there is no evidence to that effect. Smell is not seriously affected with age. There is some decline in taste sensitivity late in life. Almost all older individuals show some degree of hearing loss and 13% of the population over the age of 65 has advanced signs of presbycusis. Color vision and dark adaptation are affected by aging of the eye.

▶ Autonomic nervous system

The autonomic nervous system (ANS) is comprised of nerves and their ganglia and plexuses that direct most involuntary physiologic activities through the sympathetic and parasympathetic divisions. The aging of the ANS is characterized by progressively limited capacity to adapt to stresses and changes. Reduced autonomic abilities could influence the elderly person's response to anesthesia.

Human aging is associated with a net activation of the sympathetic nervous system (SNS). The increase in SNS activity appears to be organ system specific, with the skeletal muscle and the gut being primary targets. The increased sympathetic tone of the heart is not a result of increased SNS activity, but rather a function of reduced neuronal noradrenergic reuptake. As opposed to the SNS, basal adrenal secretion and adrenal adrenergic secretion in response to stress are attenuated with aging.[17]

There is evidence to suggest that basal activity of the parasympathetic nervous system (PSNS) decreases with age. Aging results in a reduction in respiratory vagal modulation of the heart rate at rest.[18] As a result, there is loss of beat-to-beat variability during respiration. Baroreflex sensitivity decreases with aging. Current evidence suggests that this finding is not the result of aging associated alterations in the ANS. Rather, in normal individuals, depression of the baroreceptor reflex with aging is more a function of increased arterial stiffness.[19,20]

The main concern of the anesthesia provider is the responses to acute hemodynamic challenges in which the ANS and its effectors may play an important role. Advancing age results in weakening and slowing of homeostatic mechanisms, including the ANS. ANS competence can be tested by numerous methods. While taking the history, the patient should be specifically questioned concerning signs and symptoms of exercise intolerance, orthostatic hypotension, temperature intolerance, and unusual patterns of sweating (especially increased upper body sweating). During the physical examination, resting heart rate and its variability (normal variation in heart rate during the respiratory cycle) should be noted. Further examination of the ANS involves the delineation of changes in systolic blood pressure and heart rate variability on changing from supine to standing position, as well as heart rate response to Valsalva maneuver. A "how to" discussion of performance of these tests is outlined in Chap. 6 in the diabetes section under neuropathy. If preoperative ANS responses are attenuated, one has good reason to suspect that blood pressure lability will occur perioperatively.

HOW IS FUNCTIONAL RESERVE OF THE CENTRAL/PERIPHERAL NERVOUS SYSTEM AFFECTED BY AGING AND ITS ANESTHETIC RAMIFICATIONS

The rise in human life expectancy, due in part to advances in medical treatment of the sick individual, has also resulted in more and more elderly patients requiring complicated surgical procedures as part of their routine or emergency medical management. An additional complicating factor to the preoperative evaluation is the increased incidence of cognitive impairment in the elderly. Geriatric patient evaluation for any surgery should be conducted as a multidisciplinary team approach with the intent of formulating a comprehensive plan for therapy and long-term follow-up. Age-related changes in the CNS, whether normal or pathologic, have to be considered in the choice and use of anesthetics in the elderly. This is because aging decreases functional reserve of the nervous system. Changes in functional reserve are reflected in altered pharmacodynamics, and an increased susceptibility to postoperative cognitive dysfunction, delirium, and stroke.

▶ Altered pharmacodynamics

Brain sensitivity to most anesthetic agents increases with age (see Chaps. 8 and 9). This necessitates decreasing the drug dose in the elderly. The art of clinical pharmacology in anesthesia involves both maintaining adequate anesthetic depth intraoperatively, while finding a combination of drugs that results in rapid emergence at the conclusion of the anesthetic. We can increase the drug concentration and maintain it easily; however, we have little or no control on immediately decreasing the drug concentration.

Some components of the elderly drug response can be explained by pharmacokinetic changes associated with aging, and are unique to each drug. The underlying mechanism to explain altered brain pharmacodynamics is unclear at present. Altered brain pharmacodynamics may result from age-related changes in the receptors, signal transduction, or homeostatic mechanisms. Within the CNS, aging is associated with decreases in dopaminergic and cholinergic neurons and receptors as well as decreased numbers of synapses. There are also alterations in brain phospholipid chemistry associated with changes in second messengers such as diacylglycerol.[21] However, a definitive association between these changes and age-related brain pharmacodynamics has yet to be established. The increased sensitivity to benzodiazepines with aging has been the best-studied example. In animal models, no change in the benzodiazepine-binding properties of the γ-aminobutyric acid type a (GABAa) receptors has been found with aging.[22] However, the ability of midazolam to modulate GABAa receptor function has been shown to vary with age,[23] hinting that alterations in signal transduction may explain altered pharmacodynamics with this drug. The basis for changes in pharmacodynamics with other anesthetic drug classes is even murkier, and a great deal of work is yet to be done in this area.

▶ Altered pain perception (see Chap. 26)

Despite ongoing degeneration of the CNS and PNS with age, the clinical effects on pain perception are unclear and controversial. However, there is an age-related decrease in the visceral pain threshold.[24] Presently it is unclear whether this observation is linked to age-related changes in the ANS.

▶ Postoperative cognitive dysfunction and delirium

Postoperative cognitive dysfunction and delirium are discussed in Chap. 22. It is important to note that the mechanisms of postoperative stroke and neurobehavioral deficits may differ. Perioperative stroke is more the result of microemboli or ischemic levels of cerebral blood flow, whereas neurocognitive deficits immediately following anesthesia are more related to ongoing and lingering effects of anesthesia.[25]

▶ Perioperative stroke

Advanced age is an independent predictor of postoperative stroke, especially following coronary artery bypass grafting.[26] It is controversial whether this relationship is the result of increasing incidence of atherosclerosis or an increased susceptibility to ischemia secondary to the aging process. Predictive stroke risk indices incorporate advanced age as one of the important mediating factors for 5-year stroke risk. However, other factors are equally important such as systolic hypertension and atrial fibrillation.[27] How age increases stroke risk is unclear at this time.

Type of procedure is an important factor in defining perioperative stroke risk in the elderly. Following general surgery, the risk of stroke has been reported from 0.08% to 0.2%. This risk increases to 2.9% with a prior history of stroke.[28] As a general rule, cardiac, vascular, neurosurgical, and orthopedic procedures have a higher incidence of both microemboli and perioperative stroke.

PREOPERATIVE EVALUATION

Given the changes which occur in the neurologic system with aging, an important task of the preoperative examination in the elderly patient is to determine the amount of brain reserve present. Determining brain reserve allows one to plan the anesthetic in an attempt to prevent neurologic complications during the perioperative period. Brain imaging is the best means of anatomically defining brain reserve, but it is expensive, time consuming, and the importance of the information obtained is unclear. This is especially true given recent data from the Framingham study showing that brain infarction is common after age 50.[29] In addition, location of abnormalities may be more important than absolute size. Instead, the anesthesiologist must take the approach of assessing brain reserve via indirect means. In addition to the preoperative history and physical examination, preoperative neurologic assessment of specific importance to the elderly patient includes: assessment of dementia and level of cognitive functioning including ongoing delirium (see Chaps. 22 and 27), assessment of stroke risk, and assessment of ANS function as described previously. Activities of daily living and instrumental activities of daily living may also be used as indirect means of determining cognitive function by assessing one's ability to live independently (see Chap. 12). In addition, as discussed below, medical history is important to determine the presence of commonly encountered neurologic diseases of old age.

Level of cognitive functioning and stroke risk go hand in hand as higher levels of cognitive function are associated with lower risk of stroke.[30] The stroke risk index[27] is easily performed using information obtained in a routine preoperative history and physical (Table 3-3). There is no universal perioperative stroke risk index. However, this information gives the anesthesiologist a good idea of ongoing cerebrovascular disease risk prior to taking into account the stroke risk of the surgical procedure itself.

▶ Common comorbid disease states and their evaluation

Cervical spondylotic myelopathy

Cervical spondylotic myelopathy is the most common cause of spinal cord dysfunction in older persons. The aging process results in degenerative changes in the cervical spine that, in advanced stages, can cause compression of the spinal cord. With aging, the intervertebral discs dry out resulting in loss of disc height. In addition, osteophytic overgrowth occurs and the ligamentum flavum may stiffen and buckle into the spinal cord dorsally. Buckling of the ligamentum flavum into the spinal cord may occur especially during extension of the neck.[31] All these factors act to cause direct compression of the spinal cord resulting in myelopathy (clinically evident spinal cord dysfunction, Fig. 3-2). Symptoms often develop insidiously and are characterized by neck stiffness, arm pain, numbness in the hands, and weakness of the hands and legs (Table 3-4). Symptoms are believed to develop when the spinal cord has been compressed by at least 30%.[32]

The differential diagnosis includes other disease processes which cause cervical myelopathy either through cord compression or intrinsic damage to spinal cord neurons (Table 3-5). Characteristic signs and symptoms with confirmatory imaging studies (Table 3-6) diagnose the condition.

There are several anesthetic concerns in elderly patients with myelopathy. Geriatric patients are fragile, particularly their neck and spinal cord. Examination of the airway with careful attention to symptoms elicited during flexion and extension is of utmost importance (Fig. 3-2). Extension of the neck is one of the maneuvers performed during intubation for general anesthesia. Passive or active forceful movement of the neck can result in severe injury of the spinal cord.

It is important to document preexisting neurologic deficits, whether due to the myelopathy or comorbid disease, during the preoperative examination. The degree of disability secondary to myelopathy can be quantitated and followed using the European myelopathy score (Table 3-7). This allows one to characterize degree of disability pre- and postoperatively in order to determine surgical results and long-term follow-up. Anesthesiologists may use this score when following patients in the immediate postoperative period. Polypharmacy can be an issue in these patients, and many drug classes can affect the anesthetic plan. Maintenance of blood pressure during the perioperative period is important to provide adequate perfusion of the spinal cord. The fragile elderly are more susceptible to cardiovascular instability during surgery. It is important to carefully assess the need for invasive monitoring and the use of cardiovascular drugs in these patients.

Cerebrovascular disease

Cerebrovascular disease encompasses a broad range of presentations from asymptotic carotid artery disease to transient ischemic attacks to overt stroke and multi-infarct dementia. Carotid or vertebrobasilar circulation can be affected with advancing age with consequences ranging from subclinical to catastrophic.

There are several considerations for anesthetic management which are specifically important in the elderly population. Symptomatic vertebrobasilar disease is associated with a 6% incidence of perioperative stroke.[28] In these patients, neck positioning may have an important role in exacerbating ischemic injury as neck extension is associated with a reduction in flow. Cerebrovascular disease is endemic in the elderly population. However, one must always remain cognizant of commonly associated comorbidities (e.g., diabetes, coronary artery

Table 3-3

The Cardiovascular Health Study Risk Score

	Risk Points	5-Year Stroke Risk		
		Total Risk Score	Men	Women
Systolic pressure < 125 mm Hg	0	1–5	2.5%	3.5%
125–134	2			
135–144	4	6–10	3.5%	2.4%
145–154	6			
155–164	8	11–15	5.2%	3.6%
165–174	10			
175–184	12	15–20	7.9%	5.6%
185+	14			
		21–25	12%	9.2%
15 ft walk time:	1/s (max 20)			
LVH by ECG	6	26–30	19%	14%
Creatinine > 1.25 mg/dL	2			
Diabetes: definite	6	31–35	27%	21%
Impaired fasting glucose	4			
	Men Women	36–40	42%	29%
Age: 70 and under	0 0			
71–77	3 5	41–45	59%	39%
78–84	6 10			
85–91	9 15			
92+	12 20			
Atrial fibrillation by ECG	16 5			
History of heart disease	5 1			

Source: Reprinted with permission from Ref. 27.

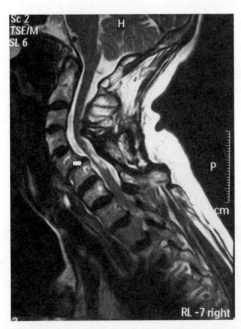

FIGURE 3-2 Magnetic resonance image of sagittal section in an elderly patient with cervical myelopathy. Arrow shows the direct compression of the spinal cord with the patient in extension.

disease), and strive to optimize their perioperative management. Careful assessment of current medications that may affect anesthetic management is crucial. Anticoagulant and antiplatelet drugs should be specifically sought for; agents causing orthostasis or which might be associated with intraoperative hypotension are also important to note.

Cardiovascular instability is common in these patients as many have underlying hypertension. Underlying cardiovascular disease processes should be optimally managed and may require more intensive intraoperative monitoring. The anesthesiologist must be continuously aware of the interactions which may occur between cardiovascular disease and cerebrovascular disease. In particular, rhythm disturbances in association with decreased cardiac output can have disastrous effects on the brain. In addition, prior stroke is a strong predictor of postoperative cardiovascular instability (odds ratio [OR] 4.5; 95% confidence interval [CI] 1.2–16.2).[33]

Stroke, or underlying cerebrovascular disease, may present in the elderly as altered mental status or delirium. Similarly, on emergence from general anesthesia, underlying cerebrovascular disease or subclinical stroke may present as a transient ischemic attack or delirium in the recovery room.

Parkinson's disease

Mankind has known Parkinson's disease across cultures for thousands of years. James Parkinson described the syndrome *the shaking palsy* in the nineteenth century. Charcot described the autonomic dysfunction in Parkinson's disease in 1887. The involvement of substantia nigra in Parkinson's disease was discovered in 1893. The neuropathological and neurochemical characteristics of the disease were described and treatment strategies devised in the twentieth century.[34,35]

Parkinson's disease occurs worldwide and affects all ethnic groups. Risk factors include family history of Parkinson's disease, very slight male preponderance,[36] head injury, and exposure to pesticides. Parkinson's disease affects approximately 3% of the population over 65 years of age.[37] In the United States, Parkinson's disease affects more than 1 million people. The etiology of Parkinson's disease is unknown in approximately 75% of the cases, the rest of the cases result from genetic etiologies and other causes include neurodegenerative disorders, cerebrovascular disease, and drugs. The lowest reported incidence is among Asians and African Blacks and the highest is among Whites.[36] Advanced age, male gender, functional and cognitive impairment, and the diagnosis of pneumonia or congestive heart failure are the strongest predictors of death. Minorities have a reduced risk of death relative to Caucasian Parkinson's disease nursing home residents.[38]

CLINICAL DIAGNOSIS The characteristic features of Parkinson's disease are shown in Table 3-8. Parkinson's disease is an important cause of perioperative morbidity and, with an increasingly elderly population, it will be encountered with greater frequency in surgical patients.

Drugs used in anesthesia may interact with antiparkinsonian medication and there is controversy about the optimal anesthetic management of patients with Parkinson's disease. Parkinson's disease is characterized by a loss of dopaminergic neurons in the substantia nigra of the basal ganglia. Loss of pigmented cells in the substantia nigra is the most consistent finding in Parkinson's disease. Normally, the quantity of nigral cells diminishes from 425,000 to 200,000 at 80 years. In Parkinson's disease, the substantia nigra shows marked depletion of cells (<100,000). The pattern of nigral cell loss in Parkinson's disease differs from that due to normal aging. In Parkinson's disease, cell loss is predominantly from the ventrolateral side of the substantia nigra, but this region is relatively spared in normal subjects.

TREATMENT OF PARKINSON'S DISEASE The goals of treatment of Parkinson's disease are to maintain patient's level of function and to institute neuroprotective therapies to halt or delay the progression of the disease process (this is where the current research is directed).

Table 3-4

Clinical Presentation of Cervical Spondylotic Myelopathy

Common Symptoms	Common Signs
Clumsy or weak hands	Atrophy of the hand musculature
Leg weakness or stiffness	Hyperreflexia
Neck stiffness	Lhermitte's sign (electric shock-like sensation down the center of the back following flexion of the neck)
Pain in shoulders or arms	
Sensory loss	
Unsteady gait	

Table 3-5

Conditions that Mimic Cervical Spondylotic Myelopathy on presentation

Amyotrophic lateral sclerosis

Extrinsic neoplasia (metastatic tumors)

Hereditary spastic paraplegia

Intrinsic neoplasia (tumors of spinal cord parenchyma)

Multiple sclerosis

Normal pressure hydrocephalus

Spinal cord infarction

Syringomyelia

Vitamin B12 deficiency

DRUG THERAPY

l-Dopa and dopamine agonists The availability of dopamine in the basal ganglia is reduced in Parkinson's disease. l-Dopa, a prodrug, is converted to dopamine in the brain. l-Dopa is administered in combination with a peripheral dopa decarboxylase inhibitor to minimize peripheral dopamine side effects.

Dopamine agonists include the nonergot alkaloids ropinirole and pramipexole and the ergot alkaloids pergolide and bromocriptine. Apomorphine is a short-acting dopamine agonist that can be administered subcutaneously, sublingually, or intranasally. An important side effect is severe nausea and vomiting, but with the concurrent use of domperidone, it may be well tolerated.

Monoamine oxide inhibitors Selegiline is an irreversible monoamine oxidase (MAO) inhibitor, also used to treat Parkinson's disease. It prolongs the action of dopamine in the striatum. Selegiline or desmethylselegiline may have a potential neuroprotective role[39] which is controversial.

Anticholinergics and amantadine These medications work by changing the balance of dopaminergic and cholinergic neurotransmitters. Because their central actions may aggravate confusion and psychosis in older patients,[40,41] use is limited.

SURGICAL TREATMENT Prior to the introduction of l-dopa in the 1960s, surgical treatment (pallidotomy and thalamotomy) of Parkinson's disease was widely used. Recently, new surgical approaches are being used like deep brain stimulation (DBS), subthalamotomy, and neurotransplantation of fetal cells. DBS of the globus pallidus interna or subthalamic nucleus improves many features of advanced Parkinson's disease.[42] DBS has the advantage that it is reversible and adjustable.

Table 3-6

Diagnostic Criteria for Cervical Spondylotic Myelopathy

Characteristic symptoms (leg stiffness, hand weakness)

Characteristic signs (hyperreflexia, atrophy of hands)

MRI or CT (showing spinal stenosis and cord compression as a result of osteophyte overgrowth, disc herniation, ligamentum hypertrophy)

MRI = magnetic resonance imaging; CT = computed tomography

Table 3-7

European Myelopathy Score

	Score
Upper motor neuron function (gait)	
1. Unable to walk, wheelchair	1
2. Walking on flat ground only with cane or aid	2
3. Climbing stairs only with aid	3
4. Gait clumsy, but no aid necessary	4
5. Normal walking and climbing stairs	5
Lower motor neuron function (hand function)	
1. Handwriting and eating with knife and fork impossible	1
2. Handwriting and eating with fork impaired	2
3. Handwriting, tying shoelaces, or a tie clumsy	3
4. Normal handwriting	4
Posterior column function (proprioception and coordination)	
1. Getting dressed only with aid	1
2 . Getting dressed clumsily and slowly	2
3. Getting dressed normally	3
Upper motor neuron function (bladder and bowel function)	
1. Retention, no control over bladder and/or bowel functions	1
2. Inadequate micturition and urinary frequency	2
3. Normal bladder and bowel function	3
Posterior cervical roots (paresthesias and dysesthesia)	
1. Disabling sensations disturbing all activities	1
2. Tolerable sensations	2
3. No paresthesia or dysesthesia	3

Note: A combined score of 18–17 = normal status; 16–13 = mild impediment (European Myelopathy Score (EMS II); 12–9 = distinct disablement (EMS II); 8–5 = severe handicap (EMS III)

Table 3-8

Characteristic Features of Parkinson's Disease

Motor Dysfunction	Nonmotor Dysfunction
Bradykinesia (slowness of voluntary movement)	Depression and anxiety
Tremor at rest (pill rolling)	Cognitive impairment
Cogwheel rigidity	Sleep disturbances
Shuffling gait	Anosmia (loss of smell)
Flexed posture with walking	Autonomic dysfunction
Retropulsion (tendency to fall back) and expressionless face (mask face) Reduced blinking Hypophonic voice	(Orthostatic hypotension syncope, constipation, urinary urgency, excessive sweating, seborrhea)
Drooling	
Micrographia	

ANESTHESIA IN THE PATIENTS WITH PARKINSON'S DISEASE

Elderly patients with Parkinson's disease most often require ophthalmologic, urologic, and orthopedic procedures. Patients with Parkinson's disease are at increased risk of specific complications and prolonged hospital stay after elective bowel resection, cholecystectomy, or radical prostatectomy. Parkinson's patients have a higher in-hospital mortality than nonParkinson's patients (7.3% vs. 3.8%, $P = 0.006$).[43]

In addition to routine history, physical examination, and preoperative testing, these patients require additional evaluation looking for specific conditions in the following systems.

Respiratory system These patients will have glottic and supraglottic musculature involved in involuntary movements characteristic of Parkinson's disease.[44,45] Excessive secretions and a dysfunctional upper airway are a cause of retained secretions, atelectasis, aspiration, and respiratory infection. Aspiration pneumonia is the most common cause of death in patients with Parkinson's disease. The anesthesiologist should be prepared for laryngospasm and postoperative respiratory failure. The use of antimuscarinic drugs for the reversal of neuromuscular blocking agents increases the viscosity of saliva, and with existing pharyngeal muscle dysfunction may worsen dysphagia and increase the risk of aspiration. Laryngospasm may be a result of poor clearance of saliva causing laryngeal irritation.

Cardiovascular system Myocardial irritability, cardiac arrhythmias, and dependent edema may occur, but the most disabling symptom is orthostatic hypotension. Orthostatic hypotension and syncope are only seen in advanced cases of Parkinson's disease and may be related to medical management of the disease. l-Dopa acting through a central mechanism similar to alpha-methyl dopa causes postural hypotension. The use of decarboxylase decreases peripheral conversion to dopamine and thus its hypotensive effects. Direct-acting dopamine agonists, such as bromocriptine and lisuride, may precipitate hypotension by causing peripheral vasodilation. Use of older antidepressants, such as amitriptyline and other tricyclic antidepressants, may cause orthostatic hypotension.

General considerations Patients should continue their antiparkinsonian medication on the day of surgery. l-Dopa has a short half-life (1–3 h) and only the enteral route of administration should be used as close to surgery as possible. l-Dopa cannot be given as a suppository as it is absorbed from the proximal small bowel only. l-Dopa can be taken either with sips of water or administered via nasogastric tube. It is important that patients do not miss medication doses postoperatively as upper airway dysfunction and obstruction secondary to Parkinson's disease contribute to the postoperative respiratory distress and failure.[46] If necessary apomorphine can be administered subcutaneously along with domperidone as an antiemetic.

Regional anesthesia has obvious advantages over general anesthesia as it avoids the effects of general anesthetics and neuromuscular blocking drugs, which may mask tremor. If sedation is required, the central anticholinergic activity of diphenhydramine is advantageous for patients with Parkinson's disease in whom tremor can render surgery difficult. Diphenhydramine has been useful particularly for ophthalmic procedures.[47] A combined regional and general anesthesia should be used where appropriate. With regional anesthesia, postoperative nausea and vomiting, which may prevent resumption of oral intake, is also avoided. If general anesthesia is required and the case is prolonged, it is worth noting that l-dopa can be administered intraoperatively via a nasogastric tube.[48] Emergence from anesthesia, even in healthy patients, is often marked by the transient appearance of a variety of pathological neurological reflexes, including hyperreactive stretch reflexes, ankle clonus, the Babinski reflex, and decerebrate posturing.[49] At emergence, Parkinson's patients can have rigid extension of the extremities, which can progress to total body rigidity.[48] Shivering is common after general anesthesia and regional analgesia will help to distinguish it from Parkinsonian symptoms.

Patients with Parkinson's disease are more prone to postoperative confusion and hallucinations. Drugs that precipitate or exacerbate Parkinson's disease should be avoided, including phenothiazines, butyrophenones (including droperidol), and metoclopramide. The latter may cause drug-induced Parkinson's disease. This is treated simply by drug withdrawal, but may lead to misdiagnosis of idiopathic Parkinson's disease and administration of l-dopa. Potential drug interactions must also be considered. Patients on MAO inhibitors have long been of specific concern to the anesthesiologist, but with the widespread use of selegiline, an MAO B type inhibitor, the likelihood of having to anesthetize a patient receiving a MAO A type inhibitor is decreased. However, there are reports of agitation, muscle rigidity, and hyperthermia in patients receiving meperidine and selegiline, so this combination should be avoided. The use of potent nonsteroidal anti-inflammatory agents has avoided the need for narcotic analgesics in patients on MAO inhibitors undergoing relatively minor procedures.

Inhalational anesthetics Inhalational anesthetic agents have complex effects on brain dopamine concentrations, inhibiting synaptic reuptake of dopamine, thereby increasing its extracellular concentration[50] and affecting both spontaneous and depolarization-evoked dopamine release.[46] These changes occur at clinically relevant concentrations of anesthetic agents. For patients taking l-dopa, anesthetic agents such as halothane, which sensitizes the heart to the action of catecholamines, should be avoided. The newer inhalational agents, isoflurane and sevoflurane, are less arrhythmogenic, but hypotension is still a concern due to hypovolemia, norepinephrine depletion, autonomic dysfunction, and the coadministration of other medications. Patients taking bromocriptine or pergolide are prone to excessive vasodilation and thus hypotension. Of historical interest, chronic trichloroethylene exposure has been implicated in the development of parkinsonism.[51]

Intravenous induction agents Previous case reports have described parkinsonian episodes in patients receiving thiopental. In animal studies thiopental decreased dopamine release from striatal synaptosomes.[46] The clinical significance of this is unclear and thiopental has not been directly implicated in exacerbating parkinsonian symptoms. Ketamine is theoretically contraindicated in Parkinson's disease because of an exaggerated sympathetic response,[52] but it has been used in these patients without harm. Recent interest has focused on the use of propofol in patients with Parkinson's disease. Functional stereotactic surgery is performed with local anesthesia, using computed tomography for the mapping of specific trigger points, where electric stimulation must be applied to achieve the therapeutic goals. Patients need sedation for this long and sometimes uncomfortable procedure, but they also need to awaken rapidly for electrocorticography or neuropsychiatric testing. Since this is an intracranial surgical procedure, access to the head and airway is very limited. In this setting, respiratory depression can quickly become an emergency and thus sedation must be carefully titrated to avoid oversedation with respiratory depression. Theoretically, propofol is an ideal agent to use while attaching the stereotactic frame because of its pharmacokinetics and pharmacodyamics, rapid return of orientation, and decreased incidence of nausea and vomiting. Again, there is a paucity of evidence about its effects in patients with Parkinson's disease but case reports have described both dyskinetic effects and abolition of tremor, in patients scheduled for stereotactic procedures leading to cancellation of surgery. As patients presenting for stereotactic surgery have their antiparkinsonian medication stopped for 12–24 h preoperatively, so that their symptoms may be observed and then seen to be abolished, some authors have recommended that propofol should not be used for these procedures because of its unpredictable effects.

Neuromuscular blocking agents There are no reported cases of nondepolarizing neuromuscular blocking drugs worsening the symptoms of Parkinson's disease. Succinylcholine has been reported to cause hyperkalemia in a patient with Parkinson's disease,[53] although the case was complicated by other factors. A later case series looked at seven patients with Parkinson's disease, who received succinylcholine as part of their anesthetic management and found no signs of succinylcholine-induced hyperkalemia.

Opioids It is well known that use of fentanyl in normal patients causes muscle rigidity, and it has been reported in patients with an established diagnosis of Parkinson's disease. Opioid-induced muscle rigidity responds to neuromuscular block and is postulated to result from presynaptic inhibition of dopamine release.[54] Acute dystonia after morphine and alfentanil have been described.[55]

It is clear that there is no simple anesthetic regimen for patients with Parkinson's disease. Much of the evidence about the safety of various anesthetic drugs or techniques is based on single case reports or small case series. The absence of randomized controlled trials evaluating various anesthetic techniques or drugs means that advice can only be based on data that have obvious limitations. What is apparent from these reports is that most patients with Parkinson's disease are elderly with coexisting medical conditions as well as the complications of the disease and its treatment. Meticulous preoperative assessment, maintenance of drug therapy up to the time of anesthesia and afterwards, avoiding known precipitating agents, and intraoperative administration of L-dopa if required, are key factors in the reduction of postoperative morbidity.

KEY POINTS

▶ The volume of the cortical gray matter and thalamus decreases with age. In comparison, the white matter volume of the cerebrum, cerebellum, corpus callosum, and pons remains fairly intact across all ages. Although in the past it was generally believed that loss of gray matter volume was caused by ongoing neuronal cell death, available evidence suggests that loss of neurons during normal aging is actually limited. Instead, brain cells shrink and the brain becomes more compact.

▶ Memory decline occurs in more than 40% of people older than 60 years. However, studies have suggested that memory decline in aging is not inevitable.

▶ Morphologic studies have shown that aging primarily affects the myelinated nerves. In particular, large myelinated fibers undergo atrophy and the myelin sheaths undergo degenerative changes. Also, the number of myelinated nerve fibers decreases with aging.

▶ The aging of the ANS is characterized by progressively limited capacity to adapt to stresses and changes. Human aging is associated with a net activation of the SNS. There is evidence to suggest that basal activity of the PSNS decreases with age.

▶ The main concern of the anesthesia provider is the responses to acute hemodynamic challenges in which the ANS and its effectors may play an important role. Advancing age results in weakening and slowing of homeostatic mechanisms, including the ANS.

- Changes in functional reserve of the CNS are reflected in altered pharmacodynamics, and an increased susceptibility to postoperative cognitive dysfunction, delirium, and stroke.

- Indirect means of assessing brain reserve in elderly patients, in addition to the preoperative history and physical examination, includes: assessment of dementia and level of cognitive functioning including ongoing delirium, assessment of stroke risk, and assessment of ANS function.

- There are several anesthetic concerns in elderly patients with cervical spondylotic myelopathy. Passive or active forceful movement of the neck can result in severe injury of the spinal cord. Maintenance of blood pressure during the perioperative period is important to provide adequate perfusion of the spinal cord.

- There are several considerations for anesthetic management of cerebrovascular disease which are specifically important in the elderly population. In patients with symptomatic vertebrobasilar disease, neck positioning may have an important role in exacerbating ischemic injury as neck extension is associated with a reduction in flow. Cardiovascular instability is common in these patients as many have underlying hypertension. Stroke, or underlying cerebrovascular disease, may present in the elderly as altered mental status or delirium.

- In patients with Parkinson's disease, the anesthesiologist should be prepared for laryngospasm and postoperative respiratory failure. The most disabling cardiovascular symptom is orthostatic hypotension.

- Patients should continue their antiparkinsonian medication on the day of surgery. It is important that patients do not miss medication doses postoperatively as upper airway dysfunction and obstruction secondary to Parkinson's disease contribute to the postoperative respiratory distress and failure.

- Drugs that precipitate or exacerbate Parkinson's disease should be avoided, including phenothiazines, butyrophenones (including droperidol), and metoclopramide.

KEY REFERENCES

- Sullivan EV, Rosenbloom M, Serventi KL, et al. Effects of age and sex on volumes of the thalamus, pons, and cortex. *Neurobiol Aging*. 2004;25:185–192.
- Seals DR, Esler MD. Human ageing and the sympathoadrenal system. *J Physiol*. 2000;528:407–417.
- Young WF. Cervical spondylotic myelopathy: a common cause of spinal cord dysfunction in older persons. *Am Fam Physician*. 2000;62:1064–1070, 1073.
- Pepper PV, Goldstein MK. Postoperative complications in Parkinson's disease. *J Am Geriatr Soc*. 1999;47:967–972.

REFERENCES

1. Sullivan EV, Rosenbloom M, Serventi KL, et al. Effects of age and sex on volumes of the thalamus, pons, and cortex. *Neurobiol Aging*. 2004;25:185–192.
2. Long JM, Mouton PR, Jucker M, et al. What counts in brain aging? design-based stereological analysis of cell number. *J Gerontol A Biol Sci Med Sci*. 1999;54:B407–B417.
3. Turlejski K, Djavadian R. Life-long stability of neurons: a century of research on neurogenesis, neuronal death, and neuron quantification in adult CNS. *Prog Brain Res*. 2002;136:39–65.
4. Peters A. Structural changes in the normally aging cerebral cortex of primates. *Prog Brain Res*. 2002;136:455–465.
5. Kamper AM, Spilt A, de Craen AJ, et al. Basal cerebral blood flow is dependent on the nitric oxide pathway in elderly but not in young healthy men. *Exp Gerontol*. 2004;39:1245–1248.
6. Peters A. The effects of normal aging on myelin and nerve fibers: a review. *J Neurocytol*. 2002;31:581–593.
7. Scott AS. Age-related memory decline. *Arch Neurol*. 2001;58:360–364.
8. Mufson EJ, Stein DG. Degeneration in the spinal cord of old rats. *Exp Neurol*. 1980;70:179–186.
9. Ishikawa M, Matsumoto M, Fujimura Y, et al. Changes of cervical spinal cord and cervical spinal canal with age in asymptomatic subjects. *Spinal Cord*. 2003;41:159–163.
10. Ibanez C, Shields SA, El-Etr M, et al. Steroids and the reversal of age-associated changes in myelination and remyelination. *Prog Neurobiol*. 2003;71:49–56.
11. Norris AH, Shock NW, Wagman IH. Age changes in the maximum conduction velocity of motor fibers of human ulnar nerves. *J Appl Physiol*. 1953;5:589–593.
12. Wayner MJ, Jr, Emmers R. Spinal synaptic delay in young and aged rats. *Am J Physiol*. 1958;194:403–405.
13. Burke D, Skuse NF, Lethlean AK. Sensory conduction of the sural nerve in polyneuropathy. *J Neurol Neurosurg Psychiatry*. 1974;37:647–652.
14. Sato A, Sato Y, Suzuki H. Aging effects on conduction velocities of myelinated and unmyelinated fibers of peripheral nerves. *Neurosci Lett*. 1985;53:15–20.
15. Wagman IH, Lesse H. Maximum conduction velocities of motor fibers of ulnar nerve in human subjects of various ages and sizes. *J Neurophysiol*. 1952;15:235–244.
16. Vrancken AF, Franssen H, Wokke JH, et al. Chronic idiopathic axonal polyneuropathy and successful aging of the peripheral nervous system in elderly people. *Arch Neurol*. 2002;59:533–540.
17. Seals DR, Esler MD. Human ageing and the sympathoadrenal system. *J Physiol*. 2000;528:407–417.
18. Tulppo MP, Makikallio TH, Seppanen T, et al. Vagal modulation of heart rate during exercise: effects of age and physical fitness. *Am J Physiol*. 1998;274:H424–H429.
19. O'Mahony D, Bennett C, Green A, et al. Reduced baroreflex sensitivity in elderly humans is not due to efferent autonomic dysfunction. *Clin Sci (Lond)*. 2000;98:103–110.
10. Brown CM, Hecht MJ, Weih A, et al. Effects of age on the cardiac and vascular limbs of the arterial baroreflex. *Eur J Clin Invest*. 2003;33:10–16.
21. Turnheim K. When drug therapy gets old: pharmacokinetics and pharmacodynamics in the elderly. *Exp Gerontol*. 2003;38:843–853.
22. Ruano D, Araujo F, Bentareha R, et al. Age-related modifications on the GABAA receptor binding properties from Wistar rat prefrontal cortex. *Brain Res*. 1996;738:103–108.
23. Bickford PC, Breiderick L. Benzodiazepine modulation of GABAergic responses is intact in the cerebellum of aged F344 rats. *Neurosci Lett*. 2000;291:187–190.
24. Lasch H, Castell DO, Castell JA. Evidence for diminished visceral pain with aging: studies using graded intraesophageal balloon distension. *Am J Physiol*. 1997;272:G1–G3.
25. Culley DJ, Baxter MG, Yukhananov R, et al. Long-term impairment of acquisition of a spatial memory task following isoflurane-nitrous oxide anesthesia in rats. *Anesthesiology*. 2004;100:309–314.
26. Zangrillo A, Crescenzi G, Landoni G, et al. Off-pump coronary artery bypass grafting reduces postoperative neurologic complications. *J Cardiothorac Vasc Anesthesiol*. 2005;19:193–196.
27. Lumley T, Kronmal RA, Cushman M, et al. A stroke prediction score in the elderly: validation and web-based application. *J Clin Epidemiol*. 2002;55:129–136.
28. Blacker DJ, Flemming KD, Wijdicks EF. Risk of ischemic stroke in patients with symptomatic vertebrobasilar stenosis undergoing surgical procedures. *Stroke*. 2003;34:2659–2663.
29. DeCarli C, Massaro J, Harvey D, et al. Measures of brain morphology and infarction in the Framingham heart study: establishing what is normal. *Neurobiol Aging*. 2005;26:491–510.
30. Elkins JS, O'Meara ES, Longstreth WT, Jr, et al. Stroke risk factors and loss of high cognitive function. *Neurology*. 2004;63:793–799.
31. Young WF. Cervical spondylotic myelopathy: a common cause of spinal cord dysfunction in older persons. *Am Fam Physician*. 2000;62:1064–1070,1073.

32. Penning L, Wilmink JT, van Woerden HH, et al. CT myelographic findings in degenerative disorders of the cervical spine: clinical significance. *AJR Am J Roentgenol.* 1986;146:793–801.

33. Posner SR, Boxer L, Proctor M, et al. Uncomplicated carotid endarterectomy: factors contributing to blood pressure instability precluding safe early discharge. *Vascular.* 2004;12:278–284.

34. Redfern RM. History of stereotactic surgery for Parkinson's disease. *Br J Neurosurg.* 1989;3:271–304.

35. Cotzias GC, Van Woert MH, Schiffer LM. Aromatic amino acids and modification of parkinsonism. *N Engl J Med.* 1967;276:374–379.

36. Zhang ZX, Roman GC. Worldwide occurrence of Parkinson's disease: an updated review. *Neuroepidemiology.* 1993;12:195–208.

37. Moghal S, Rajput AH, D'Arcy C, et al. Prevalence of movement disorders in elderly community residents. *Neuroepidemiology.* 1994;13:175–178.

38. Fernandez HH, Lapane KL. Predictors of mortality among nursing home residents with a diagnosis of Parkinson's disease. *Med Sci Monit.* 2002;8:CR241–CR246.

39. LeWitt PA. Clinical trials of neuroprotection for Parkinson's disease. *Neurology.* 2004;63:S23–S31.

40. Funakawa I, Jinnai K. Tactile hallucinations induced by trihexyphenidyl in a patient with Parkinson's disease. *Rinsho Shinkeigaku.* 2005;45:125–127.

41. Riederer P, Lange KW, Kornhuber J, et al. Pharmacotoxic psychosis after memantine in Parkinson's disease. *Lancet.* 1991;338:1022–1023.

42. Anderson VC, Burchiel KJ, Hogarth P, et al. Pallidal vs subthalamic nucleus deep brain stimulation in Parkinson's disease. *Arch Neurol.* 2005;62:554–560.

43. Pepper PV, Goldstein MK. Postoperative complications in Parkinson's disease. *J Am Geriatr Soc.* 1999;47:967–972.

44. de Bruin PF, de Bruin VM, Lees AJ, et al. Effects of treatment on airway dynamics and respiratory muscle strength in Parkinson's disease. *Am Rev Respir Dis.* 1993;148:1576–1580.

45. Easdown LJ, Tessler MJ, Minuk J. Upper airway involvement in Parkinson's disease resulting in postoperative respiratory failure. *Can J Anaesthesiol.* 1995;42:344–347.

46. Mantz J, Varlet C, Lecharny JB, et al. Effects of volatile anesthetics, thiopental, and ketamine on spontaneous and depolarization-evoked dopamine release from striatal synaptosomes in the rat. *Anesthesiology.* 1994;80:352–363.

47. Stone DJ, DiFazio CA. Sedation for patients with Parkinson's disease undergoing ophthalmologic surgery. *Anesthesiology.* 1988;68:821.

48. Furuya R, Hirai A, Andoh T, et al. Successful perioperative management of a patient with Parkinson's disease by enteral levodopa administration under propofol anesthesia. *Anesthesiology.* 1998;89:261–263.

49. Rosenberg H, Clofine R, Bialik O. Neurologic changes during awakening from anesthesia. *Anesthesiology.* 1981;54:125–130.

50. el-Maghrabi EA, Eckenhoff RG. Inhibition of dopamine transport in rat brain synaptosomes by volatile anesthetics. *Anesthesiology.* 1993;78:750–756.

51. Guehl D, Bezard E, Dovero S, et al. Trichloroethylene and parkinsonism: a human and experimental observation. *Eur J Neurol.* 1999;6:609–611.

52. Hetherington A, Rosenblatt RM. Ketamine and paralysis agitans. *Anesthesiology.* 1980;52:527.

53. Gravlee GP. Succinylcholine-induced hyperkalemia in a patient with Parkinson's disease. *Anesthesiol Analg.* 1980;59:444–446.

54. Wand P, Kuschinsky K, Sontag KH. Morphine-induced muscular rigidity in rats. *Eur J Pharmacol.* 1973;24:189–193.

55. Berg D, Becker G, Reiners K. Reduction of dyskinesia and induction of akinesia induced by morphine in two parkinsonian patients with severe sciatica. *J Neural Transm.* 1999;106:725–728.

Cardiovascular System

A.D. John

INTRODUCTION

Cardiovascular disease remains the leading cause of death and heart disease tends to affect the elderly disproportionately. Enormous effort has been focused on the various aspects of cardiovascular disease in order to gain a better understanding of the pathophysiology underlying the disease, to translate this understanding to effective clinical strategies to fight the disease, and to develop consensus guidelines to ensure optimal therapy for patients. In this chapter, consensus guidelines for optimal therapy are discussed as they apply to anesthesia personnel when caring for the elderly surgical patient. Most of the focus is on preoperative management. The following common issues in cardiovascular disease management are addressed: acute myocardial infarction, heart failure, atrial fibrillation, operative considerations in patients with pacemakers or implantable cardioverter defibrillators (ICDs), and the preoperative cardiac evaluation.

MYOCARDIAL INFARCTION

▶ Definition of myocardial infarction

The American College of Cardiology (ACC) and the Joint European Society of Cardiology have redefined myocardial infarction.[1] The past definition of myocardial infarction as used by the World Health Organization was based on the presence of two of three characteristics: typical symptoms such as chest pain and enzyme rise, and a typical electrocardiogram (ECG) including the development of Q waves. Through the use of different techniques characteristics of myocardial infarction have been elucidated. Pathologically, there is myocardial cell death and there are biochemical markers of cell death, which may be found in blood samples. Electrocardiographically, there is evidence of myocardial ischemia as revealed in ST-T wave changes or loss of myocardial tissue in Q waves. The use of various imaging studies including echocardiography, single-photon emission computed tomography (SPECT) imaging, nuclear medicine, angiography, positron emission tomography (PET), and computed tomography (CT) scan may reveal loss of tissue perfusion or cardiac wall motion abnormalities. Thus, myocardial infarction involves the loss of myocytes due to ischemia resulting from an imbalance between myocardial supply and demand due to a change in perfusion. The following sections review characteristics of myocardial infarction and then apply these characteristics to the redefinition of

myocardial infarction by the ACC and the Joint European Society of Cardiology.

Clinical symptoms of myocardial infarction[1] may include chest discomfort. The discomfort may radiate to the neck, jaw, arm, or to the back and be associated with nausea, vomiting, diaphoresis, or dyspnea. Atypical presentations of chest pain may also occur with pain duration usually lasting for at least 20 min and not affected by position or inspiration. Occasionally in patients without chest discomfort, the symptom presentation of myocardial infarction may be dizziness, syncope, nausea, vomiting, fatigue, weakness, or shortness of breath. The clinical symptoms of myocardial infarction may be varied or even absent so a high index of suspicion and vigilance must be maintained with an examination of the patient, and their electrical and biochemical markers.[1]

In order to determine presence or absence of electrocardiographic changes it is necessary to perform a 12-lead ECG. When examining multiple ECGs, the abnormality noted must be present on two consecutive ECGs to be considered significant. The ST segment and the T wave often are useful to note ischemic changes. The QRS change is a component used to define the presence of myocardial necrosis. If present, a bundle branch block, left ventricular hypertrophy, or Wolff-Parkinson-White Syndrome may interfere with an accurate diagnosis of myocardial ischemia or infarction. Left bundle branch block can obscure the diagnosis of Q waves whereas right bundle branch block does not. If a new Q wave becomes present in a patient with left bundle branch block, then it is usually pathognomonic. Left bundle branch block, whether new onset, or old, may make the diagnosis of ST segment elevation difficult. Tall or peaked T waves are seen in the early phases of an acute myocardial infarction. ST depression in leads V1 through V3 without ST segment elevation elsewhere may indicate posterior ischemia or infarction.

The first differential in myocardial ischemia as observed on an ECG is the presence or absence of ST segment elevation. For ST segment elevation to be significant, it must be ≥0.2 mV in leads V1, V2, and V3 and ≥0.1 mV in other leads. The ST segment elevation must occur in two or more contiguous leads with frontal plane contiguity being defined by the sequence of AVL, I, AVR, II, AVF, and III. For non-ST segment elevation, ST segment depression, T-wave changes, or both should be noted in two or more contiguous leads. Symmetric T-wave inversions should be greater than 1 mm. Q waves indicative of a myocardial infarction should be ≥30 ms, ≥1 mm in depth in all leads other than V1, V2, and V3, and present in two or more contiguous leads.[1]

When myocardial cell death occurs, the damaged myocytes release various proteins such as myoglobin, cardiac troponins, creatinine kinase, and lactate dehydrogenase.[1] The cardiac troponins and the creatinine kinase (CK) MB fraction are most reflective of myocardial cell damage with cardiac troponins being both highly specific and sensitive for even microscopic areas of myocardial necrosis. Cardiac troponins peak about 2 days after an acute myocardial infarction, but the CK-MB isoform tends to peak at 24 h after an acute myocardial infarction. It is recommended that patients have initial blood work, followed by subsequent blood work at 6–9 h and again between 12 and 24 h if samples are negative while the clinical suspicion is high.[1] The maximal troponin concentration, either troponin T or I, should exceed the decision limit (that is the 99th percentile for a control group) during the first 24 h after the suspected ischemic event. If CK-MBs are used, then the maximal value of CK-MB must exceed twice the upper limit of normal for the institution or the maximal CK-MB value exceeds the 99th percentile value for a control group on two successive samples. It is not recommended that other biomarkers such as lactate dehydrogenase (LDH) isoforms or total CKs be used when troponins and CK-MBs are available.[1]

Pathologically, myocardial necrosis[1] takes between 4 and 6 h to occur after onset of myocardial ischemia and this is chiefly dependent on the amount of collateral blood flow to the ischemia area. Myocardial infarctions are classified by location—anterior, lateral, inferior, posterior, or septal; and by size—microscopic with a focal area of necrosis, small involving less than 10% of the ventricle, medium which involves 10–30% of the ventricle, or large which involves more than 30% of the ventricle. Acute infarctions are usually less than a week old and are characterized by the presence of polymorphonuclear leukocytes. Healing infarctions are between 1 and 4 weeks old and are characterized by mononuclear cells and fibroblasts. The healed infarction is characterized by scar formation and usually develops after 5–6 weeks.[1]

With the above in mind, the Consensus Committee has redefined myocardial infarction in the following manner.[1] The criteria for an acute resolving or recent myocardial infarction should include either a characteristic change in the biochemical markers (a rapid rise and fall of the CK-MB or characteristic rise and gradual fall of troponins), along with one or more specific indicators such as symptoms characteristic of ischemia; ECG changes (either ST segment elevation or ST segment depression indicative of ischemia); the ECG showing the presence of pathologic Q waves; an acute coronary intervention such as angioplasty; or there should be pathological findings characteristic of an acute myocardial infarction. Whereas, the criteria for an established myocardial infarction depend on the presence of either pathological changes, characteristic of a healing or healed myocardial infarction, or the presence of pathological Q waves on serial ECGs, because the time elapsed is such that biochemical markers are no longer present and the patient may or may not remember any symptoms.[1]

▶ ST-T elevation myocardial infarction

The ACC and the American Heart Association (AHA)[2,3] have recently updated the guidelines for the management of patients with an ST segment elevation myocardial infarction. Since the majority of deaths occur within the first 2 h after the onset of symptoms, the concept of the golden hours and minimizing the time to initiating reperfusion is paramount.[2,3] With the onset of symptoms, it is recommended that a sublingual nitroglycerin be taken and the personnel involved in the decision-making process concerning reperfusion

therapy be notified. Although many forms of aspirin are available, a chewable aspirin of 325 mg should be administered if possible. If appropriate, the goal for an ST elevation myocardial infarction is to achieve a door to needle time for fibrinolysis of 30 min and door to balloon time for percutaneous coronary intervention of 90 min.[2,3]

▶ Evaluation

As part of the history it should be determined whether the patient has had any prior episodes of myocardial ischemia, other angina, or myocardial infarction, and if the patient has undergone any prior coronary interventions such as fibrinolysis, angioplasty, stenting, or coronary artery bypass grafting. The patient's current medications and allergies should be obtained. The severity of the chest discomfort should be rated on a scale of 1–10 with 1 being mild to none and 10 being the most severe pain experienced. The description of the discomfort may range from crushing, vice-like to large weight on the chest, or even heartburn. There may be radiation to the neck, jaw, shoulders, upper extremities, or even epigastrium. The duration of the discomfort, whether it is waxing and waning, and the degree of similarity to any prior episodes should be noted. Any type of associated symptoms such as nausea, vomiting, weakness, fatigue, dizziness, light-headedness, syncope, and diaphoresis with loss of color of the complexion should be elicited. Half of diabetics with type 2 diabetes for more than 10 years will have autonomic dysfunction. Impaired pain sensation and a tendency to misinterpret fatigue, dyspnea, nausea, vomiting, and diaphoresis as a blood glucose abnormality are more common among diabetics. Risk factors for bleeding disorders should be obtained, as well as the use of any medications, which may increase the bleeding risk. In the elderly, especially hypertensive elderly patients, severe tearing pain radiating to the back or shoulders with ST segment elevation should alert one to the possibility of an acute aortic dissection, along with pericardial tamponade and acute coronary artery disruption. In elderly patients, any history of mental decline or dementia may be indicative of amyloid angiopathy with concomitant increased risk of intracerebral hemorrhage. It is important to ascertain if elderly patients have had a transient ischemic attack (TIA), ischemic stroke, or hemorrhagic stroke and also determine if they have had an episode of facial or limb numbness, weakness or loss of sensation, ataxia, or vertigo, which may be a manifestation of cerebrovascular disease. Since atherosclerosis is a diffuse disease, the elderly, the diabetic, and the hypertensive are at increased risk.[2,3]

In order to properly evaluate the patient for appropriate therapy the following information must also be obtained. How long has the patient been experiencing the chest discomfort—has it been longer than 15 min, but less than 12 h? Are there contraindications to fibrinolysis? Absolute contraindications include prior intracerebral hemorrhage, structural cerebral vascular lesions like arteriovascular malformations, malignant intracranial neoplasms, an ischemic stroke within 3 months unless it is a new-onset ischemic stroke occurring within 3 h of the acute coronary event, suspected aortic dissection, active bleeding or a bleeding diathesis, and significant closed head injury or facial trauma within 3 months. Relative contraindications include chronic, severe, poorly controlled hypertension; severe hypertension on presentation with systolic blood pressure greater than 180 mm Hg or diastolic blood pressure greater than 110 mm Hg; dementia or any unknown intracranial pathology; major surgery within 3 weeks, even laser eye surgery; noncompressible vascular puncture sites; high international normalized ratio (INR) from concurrent use of anticoagulants; any gastrointestinal or genitourinary bleeding, especially active peptic ulcer bleeding; advanced cancer; severe liver or kidney disease; serious systemic disease; or cardiopulmonary resuscitation (CPR) lasting more than 10 min.

When diagnosing an acute ST segment elevation myocardial infarction, the differential diagnosis of life-threatening and non-life-threatening conditions must be considered and excluded in order to avoid serious complications for the patient.[2,3] Life-threatening conditions include the following: aortic dissection which can present with chest pain that may be searing, ripping in quality with radiation to the back or lower extremities, and the pain may last for hours with absent pulses or an aortic regurgitant murmur. A pulmonary embolus or infarction may present with chest discomfort similar to a myocardial infarction or may present with pleuritic chest pain, hemoptysis, or dyspnea. A tension pneumothorax may present with pleuritic pain, dyspnea, and decreased breath sounds with hyperresonance. Boerhaave's syndrome with esophageal rupture and mediastinitis may reveal free air under the diaphragm on chest x-ray. A perforating ulcer may also present with free air under the diaphragm, chest pain, and occasionally posterior radiation, along with syncope, hematemesis, or melena. Non-life-threatening conditions include bundle branch block, left ventricular hypertrophy with strain, Wolff-Parkinson-White syndrome, early repolarization, cerebral T-wave inversion, hypertrophic cardiomyopathy, myocarditis, atypical angina, vasospastic angina, Brugada syndrome, pericarditis, pleurisy, peptic ulcer disease, biliary colic, pancreatitis, gastroesophageal reflux, esophageal spasm, and panic attack.[2,3]

The physical examination[2,3] should be focused on the airway, breathing, and circulation. A general assessment with vital signs, the determination of jugular venous distention, peripheral pulses, systemic perfusion, along with cardiac and pulmonary auscultation and a focused neurological assessment is requisite. An acute myocardial event often reveals a restless, agitated, anguished patient with clenched fists, ashen or pale with cool, clammy skin. A low-grade fever may be a nonspecific sign of myocardial necrosis. Anterior myocardial infarctions often are tachycardic, hypertensive, and characterized by high sympathetic tone. Inferior or posterior myocardial infarctions are characterized by a high vagal tone and present with bradycardia and hypotension. Fast, slow, or irregular pulses indicate arrhythmias or heart block. Low cardiac output may be revealed as small volume pulses. An anterior myocardial infarction may present with a paradoxical systolic impulse indicating a ventricular aneurysm or left ventricular dyskinesis. An inferior myocardial infarction may have a soft S1 indicative of decreased left ventricular contractility or first degree arteriovenous (A-V) block. A paradoxical splitting of S2 may arise from left bundle branch block or severe left ventricular dysfunction. Congestive heart failure may manifest as pulsus alternans, pulmonary crackles, and an S3 gallop. A right ventricular infarction may present with jugular venous distention, hypotension, and right ventricular S3 and S4 gallops. Whereas, an S4 gallop often indicates a decrease in ventricular compliance. A thrill at the left sternal border with a harsh holosystolic murmur, S3, pulmonary edema, and cardiogenic shock is characteristic of ventricular septal rupture. Cardiogenic shock and pulmonary edema without a thrill, but with the murmur of mitral regurgitation (MR) is seen with papillary muscle rupture. Whereas, left ventricular free wall rupture presents as electromechanical dislocation with cardiac tamponade or cardiogenic shock. Aortic dissection may present with absent pulses and the murmur of aortic regurgitation. A neurological assessment is important, and should encompass cognitive function with the presence of dysarthria, aphasia, or hemispatial defect. Motor assessment should look for facial asymmetry, pronator drift, reflex symmetry, and limb

dysmetria. A sensory examination searching for loss of pinprick is also warranted.[2,3]

The ACC and the AHA Task Force[2,3] emphasize the importance of obtaining a 12-lead ECG within 10 min of contact between the patient with symptoms of an acute myocardial infarction or angina and the hospital medical staff, and continuous cardiac monitoring should then also be instituted. For those patients whose ECG is not diagnostic, but who remain symptomatic, serial ECGs should be done at 5–10 min intervals, and right sided ECG should be done to evaluate the right ventricle in those patients with an inferior ST elevation myocardial infarction. The initial laboratory evaluation should include: complete blood count (CBC) with platelet count, INR, a partial thromboplastin time (PTT), electrolytes, magnesium, blood urea nitrogen (BUN), creatinine, glucose, serum lipid profile, and cardiac biomarkers for myocardial damage. CK-MB takes 3–12 h for initial elevation, will peak at 24 h after damage, and returns to normal between 48 and 72 h after an infarction. Cardiac troponin I (cTn-I) takes 3–12 h for initial elevation, will peak at 24 h after damage, and takes 5–10 days to return to normal. Cardiac troponin T (cTn-T) takes 3–12 h for initial elevation, will peak between 12 and 48 h after damage, and takes 5–14 days to return to normal. Myoglobin, though infrequently used, takes 1–4 h for initial elevations, will peak within 6–7 h after damage, and returns to normal within 24 h. Of the cardiac specific markers, cardiac troponins are considered the optimal markers for diagnosis of myocardial damage and following serial markers is beneficial in evaluating reperfusion therapy; but for at least 18 h after the onset of an acute ST segment elevation myocardial infarction, they cannot be relied on to diagnose a reinfarction. A portable chest x-ray should be done and if the diagnosis of aortic dissection is likely, then either a contrast chest CT or magnetic resonance imaging (MRI) should be done. An echocardiograph is useful in providing information as to cardiac structure and function and may be of benefit in guiding therapy.[2,3]

▶ Therapy

The ACC and the AHA Task Force[2,3] emphasize the importance of prompt diagnosis and initiation of therapy. Often results of cardiac specific biomarkers will not be available immediately, but treatment should not be delayed. Based on the history and physical, clinical signs and symptoms, ECG findings, and echocardiographical findings, if available, appropriate therapy should be instituted. Supplemental oxygen is beneficial acutely and for at least 6 h after an uncomplicated ST elevation myocardial infarction. In patients with ischemic discomfort, sublingual nitroglycerin (0.4 mg) should be administered every 5 min for a total of three doses and if symptoms are persisting, then intravenous nitroglycerin is recommended to control ongoing ischemia, control hypertension, and help in the management of pulmonary congestion. Contraindications to the use of nitroglycerin include avoiding in patients who have used a phosphodiesterase inhibitor within the past 24 h (48 h for tadalafil), hypotension with systolic blood pressure less than 90 mm Hg, severe bradycardia, or in those in whom a right ventricular infarction is suspected. Analgesia should be provided with morphine sulfate 2–4 mg IV with increments of 2–8 mg IV every 5–15 min. The goal is to allow the patient to be pain free by addressing all components that affect the myocardial supply-demand relationship that are contributing to ongoing ischemia. A chewable aspirin 325 mg should be given unless the patient has already received one. If a patient has severe nausea and vomiting or upper gastrointestinal disorder, a 300 mg aspirin suppository may be given and for patients with genuine aspirin allergy, manifested by hives, bronchospasm, or anaphylaxis, substitution with clopidogrel or ticlidopine is acceptable. The prompt initiation of beta-blocker therapy in patients without contraindication is markedly beneficial in reducing the magnitude of the infarction and incidence of complications from the infarction, in reducing the rate of reinfarction, and also in reducing the frequency of life-threatening ventricular arrhythmias. Beta-blockers are able to achieve this effect through the decrease in myocardial oxygen demand by reducing the heart rate, systemic arterial pressure, myocardial contractility, and by increasing myocardial supply by prolonging diastole and thereby increasing the perfusion to the subendocardium and ischemic myocardium.[2,3]

Once therapy has been started, if appropriate, the treating physician or cardiologist must determine the choice of reperfusion—fibrinolysis versus percutaneous coronary intervention.[2,3] Guidelines to this decision-making process are illustrated in Fig. 4-1. Patients who have undergone fibrinolysis, but continue having symptoms or worsening of their myocardial infarction, should have percutaneous coronary intervention unless contraindicated.[2,3] Emergent coronary artery bypass grafting is indicated for those patients who have failed percutaneous coronary intervention with persistent pain or hemodynamic instability and whose coronary anatomy is amenable to surgical intervention. Coronary artery bypass grafting is recommended for those who are not candidates for fibrinolytic therapy or percutaneous coronary intervention with persistent or recurrent ischemia that is refractory to medical therapy with a large area of myocardium at risk and have coronary anatomy amenable to surgery. Patients who have been in cardiogenic shock for less than 18 h or who develop cardiogenic shock within 26 h of having an ST segment elevation myocardial infarction and have left main disease or severe multivessel disease are candidates for coronary artery bypass grafting. Patients who develop life-threatening ventricular arrhythmias and have triple vessel disease or significant left main disease are candidates for bypass grafting. Patients undergoing repair of postinfarction ventricular septal rupture or mitral valve repair should have coronary artery bypass grafting to the affected vessels at the same time.[2,3]

Ancillary medications are of benefit according to the ACC and the AHA Task Force.[2,3] Unfractionated heparin should be used for patients undergoing angioplasty or surgical revascularization with coronary artery bypass grafting. For patients undergoing fibrinolysis with nonspecific fibrinolytics (streptokinase, urokinase, and anistreplase), the recommendation is still to use unfractionated heparin as an adjuvant especially in those with a large infarction, anterior infarction, or left ventricular thrombus. But, for patients undergoing fibrinolysis with fibrin specific fibrinolytics (alteplase, reteplase, and tenecteplase) the recommendation is to use unfractionated heparin on a weight-based regimen with specific goal-directed therapy aimed at maintaining the activated PTT at 1.5–2 times control. When unfractionated heparin is being administered, daily platelet counts should be done. Although low molecular weight heparin may not assist in early reperfusion, it does however prevent reocclusion and reinfarction and so may be an acceptable alternative for unfractionated heparin in those who are under 76 years and have no significant evidence of renal dysfunction. For elderly patients, those who are older than 75 years, low molecular weight heparin is not recommended as a substitute for unfractionated heparin. According to the Task Force, for patients with heparin-induced thrombocytopenia, bivaliruden may be used as an alternative to unfractionated heparin. Preliminary studies indicate that a highly specific factor Xa antagonist (fonda parinux) may be of use if further studies are confirmatory, but is not currently recommended. Aspirin doses between 75 and 162 mg are recommended to be continued indefinitely. The only exception to continued aspirin use is a true aspirin allergy as manifested by hives, bronchospasm, or anaphylaxis. The thienopyridines, ticlopidine, and clopidogrel are adenosine diphosphate (ADP) receptor antagonists, but ticlopidine may cause neutropenia and thrombolic thrombocytopenia, and so clopidogrel is recommended after cardiac catheterization and stenting. If cardiac surgery is planned, the use of thienopyridines may result in excessive bleeding. The early use of glycoprotein 2b/3a inhibitors such as abciximab, tirofiban, and eptifibatide is recommended for patients presenting with an acute ST segment myocardial infarction.[2,3]

The ACC and AHA Task Force[2,3] recommend several other measures and medications to optimize therapy and improve mortality. During an acute ST segment elevation myocardial infarction, there is a significant increase in circulating catecholamines along with increases in cortisol and glucagon levels and a decreased sensitivity to insulin. The Task Force advocates tight glucose control for diabetics with the institution of insulin therapy as necessary to normalize blood glucose levels. Metformin should be withheld for 48 h after an intravenous contrast injection and should not be given to patients in congestive heart failure or who are in renal failure. The prophylactic administration of magnesium is discouraged; and the recommendation is to only administer magnesium to correct

---

Fibrinolysis is generally preferred if:
- *Early presentation (3 h or less from symptom onset and delay to invasive strategy: see below)*

- *Invasive strategy is not an option*
  Catheterization laboratory occupied/not available
  Vascular access difficulties
  Lack of access to a skilled PCI laboratory

- *Delay to invasive strategy*
  Prolonged transport
  (Door-to-balloon)–(door-to-needle) time is greater than 1h
  Medical contact-to-balloon or door-to-balloon time is greater than 90 min

An invasive strategy is generally preferred if:
- *Skilled PCI laboratory available with surgical backup*
  Medical contact-to-balloon or door-to-balloon time less than 90 min (Door-to-balloon)–(door-to-needle) is less than 1h
- *High risk from STEMI*
  Cardiogenic shock
  Killip class greater than or equal to 3

- *Contraindications to fibrinolysis, including increased risk of bleeding and ICH*

- *Late presentation*
  Symptom onset was more than 3 h ago

- *Diagnosis of STEMI is in doubt*

FIGURE 4-1 Assessment of reperfusion options for patients with ST elevation myocardial infarction (STEMI). PCI = percutaneous coronary intervention, ICH = intracranial hemorrhage. (Adapted from Antman EM, Anbe DT, Armstrong PW, et al. ACC/AHA guidelines for the management of patients with ST-elevation myocardial infarction:executive summary:a report of the ACC/AHA Task Force on Practice Guidelines (Committee to revise the 1999 guidelines on the management of patients with acute myocardial infarction). J Am Coll Cardiol. 2004;44:671–719.)

documented magnesium deficits especially in the presence of diuretic use, and to treat torsade de pointes. The oral ingestion of an angiotensin-converting enzyme (ACE) inhibitor within the first 24 h of an ST segment myocardial infarction, especially for patients who have a left ventricular ejection fraction less than 0.40, or have pulmonary congestion, or have an anterior infarction, is encouraged as long as there are no contraindications to ACE inhibitor therapy and the systolic blood pressure is greater than 100 mm Hg. It is recommended that a lower starting dose be initiated with gradual titration to recommended dosage levels. Intravenous administration should be avoided due to significant hypotension. If there is intolerance to ACE inhibitors then angiotensin receptor blockers (ARBs) may be instituted instead, with valsartan and candesartan being the ARBs suggested by the Task Force, but with it being noted by the Task Force that the data is not as exhaustive on ARBs as on ACE inhibitors. The calcium channel blockers verapamil or diltiazem may be used if beta-blockers are contraindicated or ineffective in treating rapid ventricular response due to atrial fibrillation or flutter, but are contraindicated in the presence of congestive heart failure, left ventricular dysfunction, or atrioventricular block.[2,3]

▶ Complications

The complications of an acute ST segment elevation myocardial infarction include cardiogenic shock, right ventricular infarction, muscular rupture, and arrhythmias. The ACC and AHA Task Force have established treatment guidelines for these complications.[2,3] Cardiogenic shock may present with clinical signs of congestive heart failure, shock, hypoperfusion, or acute pulmonary edema. In the presence of low output cardiogenic shock, treatment is guided by an assessment of blood pressure (Fig. 4-2). In patients with systolic blood pressure greater than 100 mm Hg, therapy should be initiated with IV nitroglycerin. If the systolic blood pressure is between 70 and 100 mm Hg and signs and symptoms of shock are not present, then dobutamine IV with a dosage range of 2–20 mcg/kg/min is recommended. If, however, the systolic blood pressure is between 70 and 100 mm Hg and signs and symptoms of shock are present, then the preferred agent is dopamine IV at a dosage of 5–15 mcg/kg/min. When the systolic blood pressure is less than 70 mm Hg and signs and symptoms of shock are present, the pharmacological agent of choice is norepinephrine IV with recommended dosage range of 0.5–30 mcg/min with further therapeutic consideration being guided by echocardiographic findings, angiographic findings, or pulmonary artery findings. The principle therapeutic interventions being intraaortic balloon counterpulsation and reperfusion or revascularization. If a patient with an acute ST segment myocardial infarction presents with hypovolemia or has hypovolemia complicating the myocardial infarction, the cause should be determined, but fluid, blood, and/or vasopressors administered until the underlying cause is corrected. For those patients whose myocardial infarction is complicated with pulmonary edema, oxygen should be administered, furosemide at a dosage of 0.5–1 mg/kg IV be given, along with IV morphine at least 2–4 mg IV. If the systolic blood pressure is greater than 100 mm Hg, then IV nitroglycerin should be administered or sublingual nitroglycerin until the IV nitroglycerin is started. If symptoms of shock are present with systolic blood pressures below 100 mm Hg, dopamine at a dose of 5–15 mcg/kg/min should be started. The key to guiding therapy is rapid and accurate diagnosis and echocardiography is a useful tool in this regard.[2,3]

Right ventricular infarction or ischemia[2,3] in the setting of an ST segment elevation myocardial infarction identifies a subset with significantly increased morbidity and mortality. In patients with inferior ischemia, evidence for a right ventricular infarction should be sought. The most predictive ECG findings are those of an elevation of 1 mm or more of the ST segment in lead V1, and in the right precordial lead V4R. A common clinical scenario is profound hypotension after the administration of sublingual nitroglycerin in the setting of an acute myocardial infarction. Clinically there is hypotension, clear lung fields, and jugular venous distention on inspiration. Echocardiography will often show right ventricular (RV) dilatation and asynergy. Occasionally in those with patent foramen ovale with right to left shunting, there may be persistent hypoxia unresponsive to oxygen therapy. Treatment of a right ventricular infarction should include volume loading with normal saline to correct hypotension, maintenance of atrioventricular synchrony with prompt cardioversion of atrial fibrillation, and atrioventricular sequential pacing if necessary. In those patients with significant left ventricular dysfunction, the use of an intra-aortic balloon pump helps unload the left ventricle and thus assist the right ventricle. It is important to establish reperfusion early within 6 h, which is the optimal time window for both percutaneous coronary intervention and coronary artery bypass grafting, and if surgery cannot be done within this time window, the recommendation is to wait for 4 weeks to allow the right ventricle to recover and improve function. Often inotropic support will be necessary in addition to the above measures to sustain cardiac performance.[2,3]

In the setting of an acute ST segment elevation, the presence of severe MR and cardiogenic shock correlates[2,3] with poor prognosis and significant mortality, approximately 70% when managed medically versus 40% with surgical correction. Significant MR in the setting of an extensive myocardial infarction with severe left ventricular dysfunction is difficult to manage and will require afterload reduction and often an intraaortic balloon pump to help with afterload reduction and maintain cardiac function. The mortality of these patients is increased, especially the elderly. Severe MR due to papillary muscle dysfunction carries better prognosis, since the area of infarction is often less. The posteromedial papillary muscle is more commonly involved rather than the anterolateral papillary muscle. Papillary muscle rupture has a bimodal onset with initial presentation occurring with the first 24 h of an acute myocardial infarction and the second peak occurring between the third and fifth day. Clinically the presentation is that of abrupt onset of shortness of breath, pulmonary edema, and hypotension with a murmur of MR. Echocardiography will reveal the degree of MR, the torn papillary muscle, or chordae tendinea with an assessment of left ventricular function. At the time of repair, whether annuloplasty, papillary muscle repair, or mitral valve replacement, appropriate coronary artery bypass grafting should be done if warranted.[2,3]

The incidence of ventricular septal rupture[2,3] after an acute myocardial infarction is declining, especially with prompt reperfusion therapy, and now occurs in only about 1% of patients with an acute ST segment myocardial infarction. Ventricular septal rupture may occur within 24 h after an infarction or about 3–5 days later. It often presents with hypotension, shortness of breath, chest pain with a harsh holosystolic murmur, and a thrill at the left sternal border. A pulmonary artery catheter will reveal an increase in oxygen saturation from the right atrium to the right ventricle and also the presence of large V waves. An echocardiograph will show right ventricular overload and left to right flow on color Doppler with the presence of the ventricular septal rupture. These patients require the prompt insertion of an intraaortic balloon pump, along with inotropes and vasodilators with nitroprusside being the vasodilator

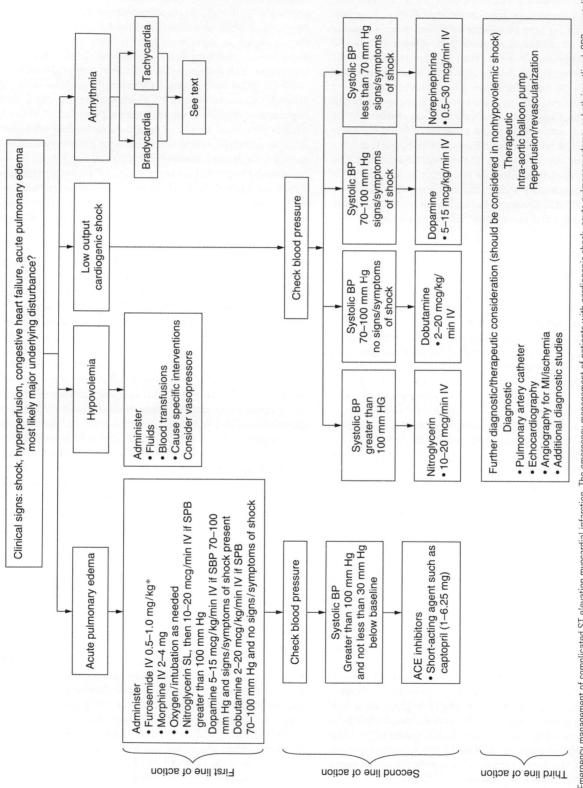

FIGURE 4-2 Emergency management of complicated ST elevation myocardial infarction. The emergency management of patients with cardiogenic shock, acute pulmonary edema, or both is outlined. SBP = systolic blood pressure, IV = intravenous, BP = blood pressure, ACE = angiotensin-converting enzyme, MI = myocardial infarction. *Furosemide less than 0.5 mg/kg for new-onset acute pulmonary edema without hypovolemia; 1mg/kg for acute or chronic volume overload, renal insufficiency. (*Reprinted with permission from Antman EM, Anbe DT, Armstrong PW, et al. ACC/AHA guidelines for the management of patients with ST elevation myocardial infarction:executive summary:a report of the ACC/AHA Task Force on Practice Guidelines (Committee to revise the 1999 guidelines of the management of patients with acute myocardial infarction). J Am Coll Cardiol. 2004;44:671–719.)*

of choice, in order to maintain hemodynamics until emergent surgical repair can be performed. Unfortunately, surgical mortality is significant and can range from 20% to 50%. For patients in cardiogenic shock, the mortality approaches 90%. Recent efforts at transcatheter closure of ventricular septal rupture have been successful, but the current recommendation remains surgical repair with excision of necrotic tissue and concomitant coronary artery bypass grafting.[2,3]

Cardiac rupture of the left ventricular free wall[2,3] occurs in about 1–6% of patients with an acute ST segment elevation myocardial infarction. It also exhibits a bimodal incidence with the early peak occurring during the first 24 h after an infarction, which represents the evolution of the infarction, and a later peak at 3–5 days after an infarction representing an expansion of the infarction-related ventricular wall. Cardiac rupture occurs more commonly in the elderly, those with an anterior infarction, women, and those experiencing their first myocardial infarction. Corticosteroid use, nonsteroidal anti-inflammatory drugs (NSAIDs), Q waves on the ECG, lack of a prior history of angina or myocardial infarction, and hypertension during the acute phase of an ST segment myocardial infarction along with the use of fibrinolytic therapy more than 14 h after the onset of the myocardial infarction are also risk factors for myocardial rupture. The key to preventing cardiac rupture is early reperfusion and the presence of collateral circulation. Clinically patients often have anginal, pleuritic, or pericardial chest pain with syncope, hypotension, nausea, restlessness, arrhythmias, and/or sudden death. Cardiac rupture presents with shock, cardiac tamponade, and electromechanical dissociation. Echocardiography is useful in diagnosing cardiac rupture, pseudoaneurysm, and pericardial tamponade, and also in visualizing the site of rupture and assessing cardiac function. The number of patients with cardiac rupture that are able to make it to the operating room is small and the mortality even with surgery is over 50%.[2,3]

Patients with an ST segment elevation myocardial infarction are at risk for developing cardiac arrhythmias.[2,3] Ventricular tachyarrhythmias occur with foci of enhanced automaticity, loss of transmembrane resting potential, and the development of reentrant rhythms in border zones between ischemic and nonischemic myocardium. Atrial arrhythmias are caused by atrial infarction, increased atrial stretch, and excessive sympathetic stimulation. On the other hand, vagal stimulation and ischemia to the conduction system can cause bradyarrhythmias. With the onset of reperfusion[2,3] accelerated idioventricular rhythms characterized by a wide QRS complex occurring at a rate of less than 100 bpm, but faster than the regular atrial rate may be seen; most frequently during the first 12 h of the infarction. Since these rhythms are often indicative of reperfusion, treatment is not necessary. In fact, treatment of these rhythms may lead to hemodynamic deterioration. In inferior ST segment elevation myocardial infarctions, accelerated junctional rhythms with narrow QRS complex and rates above 60 bpm not preceded by atrial activity may also be noted; usually treatment is not necessary unless the rhythm is indicative of digitalis toxicity. In the setting of an acute myocardial infarction, ectopic ventricular activity may be seen including isolated ventricular premature beats and couplets. Suppression of these rhythms with antiarrhythmic treatment is detrimental, rather electrolytes such as potassium and magnesium should be checked and replenished and acid base status corrected.[2,3]

Ventricular fibrillation is an ominous rhythm in the setting of an acute ST segment elevation myocardial infarction. Ventricular fibrillation is more common among elderly patients over the age of 75, especially in the period of an acute myocardial infarction. Ventricular

fibrillation is characterized as either primary ventricular fibrillation or secondary ventricular fibrillation based on the time course of occurrence relative to the onset of the myocardial infarction. Primary ventricular fibrillation encompasses the first 24–48 h after a myocardial infarction, whereas secondary ventricular fibrillation occurs 48 h after the infarction. The peak incidence of primary ventricular fibrillation is in the first 4 h of an ST segment elevation myocardial infarction and then gradually declines, but remains an important contributor to the risk of mortality during the first 24 h. Although primary ventricular fibrillation is associated with higher in-hospital mortality, especially if occurring within the first 4 h, patients that survive to discharge have the same overall prognosis as those who did not experience primary ventricular fibrillation. Secondary ventricular fibrillation not only occurs 48 h after the onset of an acute myocardial infarction, but also usually occurs in the presence of severe congestive heart failure and cardiogenic shock, and thus carries with it an overall worse prognosis and increased mortality. Arrhythmogenic risk factors for ventricular fibrillation include hypokalemia and hypomagnesemia. The goals of prevention or decreasing the risk for ventricular fibrillation include maintaining serum potassium at a level greater than 4.0 mEq/L and magnesium at a level greater than 2.0 mEq/L in the setting of an acute myocardial infarction. The verified presence of ventricular fibrillation necessitates immediate cardioversion. The recommended initial monophasic dose is 200 J, the second shock at 300 J, and if necessary the third shock at 360 J. If one is using a biphasic defibrillator, then the recommended dosage is halved. Once instituting advanced cardiac life support (ACLS) and encountering difficult to convert ventricular fibrillation, vasopressin 40 U IV may be substituted for 1 mg of epinephrine. For refractory ventricular fibrillation, amiodarone is the drug of choice with a dose of 300 mg IV or 5 mg/kg IV along with continued unsynchronized electric shock. Amiodarone is superior to lidocaine. Lidocaine and bretylium have similar efficacy with little to no benefit, and procainamide IV may or may not be of any benefit in refractory ventricular fibrillation. Current recommendations focus on the beneficial effects of correcting hypokalemia and hypomagnesemia, along with correction of acid base abnormalities, and the prompt institution of beta-blocker therapy (as long as no contraindications exist to decrease sympathetic tone), and the prompt discontinuation of antiarrhythmic medications for ventricular fibrillation within 6–24 h, as long as there has been no recurrence of the arrhythmia.[2,3]

Ventricular tachycardia,[2,3] when occurring in the setting of an acute ST segment elevation myocardial infarction, is classified as being monomorphic or polymorphic and either sustained or nonsustained. Sustained ventricular tachycardia lasts longer than 30 s and causes hemodynamic compromise. Ventricular tachycardia that occurs late, that is, after 48 h from a myocardial infarction, warrants electrophysiological studies. Monomorphic ventricular tachycardia at a rate of less than 170 bpm that occurs early in the setting of an acute myocardial infarction is an unusual rhythm and also warrants electrophysiological studies. Ventricular tachycardia at rates of less than 150 bpm does not necessarily need emergency cardioversion, as long as there is no hemodynamic compromise. These rhythms may be treated with amiodarone, preferably, or procainamide. In the setting of a low ejection fraction 4 or more days after an acute myocardial infarction, the presence of nonsustained ventricular tachycardia may presage sudden death. Rapid polymorphic ventricular tachycardia should be treated with unsynchronized cardioversion beginning with a monophasic energy level of 200 J; if unsuccessful in converting, then increasing to 300 J and if still unsuccessful, then increasing the energy level to 360 J. Sustained monomorphic ventricular tachycardia at a rate greater than 150 bpm associated with angina, pulmonary edema, or hypotension should be treated with synchronized electric shock starting at 100 J for monophasic shock and increasing as necessary and required to achieve conversion. If monomorphic ventricular tachycardia is not associated with angina, pulmonary edema, or hypotension, then the recommended therapy is amiodarone 150 mg over 10 min or 5 mg/kg with a repetition of the dose every 15 min as necessary, or an infusion at 1 mg/min for 6 h, followed by an infusion at 0.5 mg/min over the next 18 h. The maximum recommended dosage for amiodarone is 2.2 g over a 24-h period. Synchronized cardioversion beginning at a monophasic energy level of 50 J may be necessary. Rarely, episodes of sustained drug refractory polymorphic ventricular tachycardia may occur in the setting of an acute ST segment elevation myocardial infarction. In this circumstance, aggressive efforts including intravenous beta-blockade, intravenous amiodarone, intra-aortic balloon pump, and prompt revascularization with either percutaneous coronary intervention or coronary artery bypass grafting; as well as aggressive intravenous efforts to normalize serum potassium to a level greater than 4 mEq/L and magnesium at a level of 2 mEq/dL, should be undertaken. The routine use of antiarrhythmic drugs such as lidocaine should not be instituted in an attempt to prevent ventricular arrhythmias, rather the focus must be on reestablishing perfusion, stopping the ischemia, ensuring optimal acid base status, and normalizing electrolytes.[2,3] As long as ventricular fibrillation or ventricular tachycardia is not transient or due to reversible ischemia or reinfarction,[2,3] placement of an ICD should be considered using the Task Force recommendations.

The supraventricular tachycardias[2,3] of importance in the setting of an acute ST segment elevation myocardial infarction include paroxysmal supraventricular tachycardia, atrial flutter, and the most frequent, atrial fibrillation. Over 20% of patients who are at least 65 years of age or older will experience atrial fibrillation in the setting of an acute ST segment elevation myocardial infarction. The development of atrial fibrillation in this setting is associated with worse in hospital and overall prognosis, and is also associated with an increased mortality as well as stroke. In the post-myocardial-infarction setting, atrial fibrillation may be due to excessive sympathetic outflow, atrial stretch due to ventricular dysfunction, atrial infarction, chronic lung disease, hypoxia, and hypokalemia; and it is associated with larger infarctions, anterior infarctions, advanced heart block, congestive heart failure, and pericarditis. Atrial fibrillation may also occur with inferior infarctions due to right coronary artery occlusion with loss of the sinoatrial (SA) nodal artery. In unstable patients with rapid heart rate and hypotension, heart failure, or ischemia, once the underlying cause has been addressed, electrical cardioversion may be necessary. Synchronized cardioversion is performed beginning with 200 J of monophasic current and then increasing to 100-J increments to a maximum of 400 J with at least a 1-min interval between consecutive shocks in order to avoid myocardial damage. For atrial flutter, the initial energy level is much lower at 50 J of monophasic current. Atrial overdrive pacing may be effective in terminating atrial flutter and supraventricular tachycardia. Beta-blockers are effective medications to slow the ventricular response in atrial fibrillation. If beta-blockers are contraindicated because of severe pulmonary disease or congestive heart failure, then intravenous diltiazem at 0.25 mg/kg or a 20-mg bolus followed by an infusion may be used. Verapamil at a dose of 2.5–10 mg IV over 2 min with a repeat of 5–10 mg after 15–30 min may also be used. The problem with calcium channel blockers lies in their negative inotropic effects and their association with increased mortality with oral use after an ST segment elevation myocardial infarction. Intravenous amiodarone for rate control is a drug of choice in the critically ill patient and studies have shown that in postmyocardial infarction with arrhythmia there is a reduction in mortality due to a decrease in arrhythmic deaths.[2,3]

In the setting of an acute myocardial infarction, bradyarrhythmias[2,3] account for almost one-third of cardiac arrhythmias. They are especially common with inferior ST segment myocardial infarction and with reperfusion of the right coronary artery. Heart block develops in about 10% of patients with an acute infarction and intraventricular conduction delays occur in about 10–20% of acute infarctions. Patients presenting to the hospital with a bundle branch block, though this accounts for less than 5% of those with acute myocardial infarction, have a significantly increased mortality rate in hospital. Atrioventricular block also predicted a higher in-hospital mortality rate, but for those patients that did survive to discharge was not predictive of long-term outcome. During an acute ST segment myocardial infarction, the development of atrioventricular and intraventricular blocks tended to reflect the extent of the infarcted region. If the location of the atrioventricular conduction block was intranodal, the site of the infarction was usually infero-posterior with the right coronary artery being involved in 90% of the cases and the left circumflex coronary artery being involved in the remaining 10%. The type of block tends to be first-degree block or Mobitz type I second-degree block. These blocks are usually transient lasting 2–3 days and tend to have a low mortality rate unless associated with hypotension and/or congestive heart failure. Permanent pacing is rarely necessary, but occasionally temporary pacing may be necessary if the bradycardia is associated with syncope, angina, or inadequate left ventricular systolic function. If, on the other hand, the atrioventricular conduction delay is more distal, that is, infranodal, the site of the infarction tends to be anteroseptal with the septal perforators of the left anterior descending artery being in the involved arterial supply. The type of block tends to be second-degree Mobitz type II and third degree block. These blocks tend to be associated with a high degree of mortality because of the extensive infarcted area, loss of ventricular function, and the presence of ventricular arrhythmias. Pacing—both temporary and often permanent pacing—is necessary for these infranodal blocks. For sinus pauses more than 3 s, sinus bradycardia with a heart rate less than 40 bpm associated with hypotension or signs of hemodynamic insufficiency or symptomatic sinus bradycardia, atropine 0.6–1 mg IV should be given with a maximum dose of 2 mg or 0.04 mg/kg. If unsuccessful then temporary pacing, either transcutaneous or transvenous, is necessary. In the setting of an acute myocardial infarction, isoproterenol is not recommended because of an excessive increase in myocardial oxygen demand. Glucagon in presence of excessive beta-blockade, or beta and calcium channel blockage, may be considered.[2,3] Placement of a permanent pacemaker should be considered using the recommended guidelines of the Task Force for permanent pacing and in consultation with a cardiologist.[2,3]

Non-ST segment elevation myocardial infarction

The majority of patients with unstable angina or non-ST segment elevation myocardial infarction are elderly and these conditions are associated with an increased risk of death or reinfarction within 30 days.[4] The ACC and AHA Task Force emphasize the importance of an early invasive study for patients who have recurrent angina or ischemia at rest or with minimum activity, an elevated troponin T or I, new ST segment depression, depressed left ventricular ejection fraction, hemodynamic instability, heart failure, an S3 gallop, pulmonary edema, sustained-ventricular tachycardia, a percutaneous coronary intervention with 6 months, or a history of prior myocardial infarction. Treatment according to the Task Force should include anticoagulation with heparin (when appropriate), an aspirin, a thienopyradine, as well as a glycoprotein 2b/3a antagonist.[4]

HEART FAILURE

Heart failure[5–11] is a disease that becomes more common as aging occurs. According to the AHA, heart failure is a major health problem with at least 5 million patients currently diagnosed and with at least half a million people who will be newly diagnosed each year.[12] Heart failure is the most common Medicare diagnosis-related group[13] with the cost of heart failure being well over 25 billion dollars[12] and the majority of patients, over 75%, being 65 years of age or older.[14] In order to assist physicians in the diagnosis and management of heart failure, the ACC and the AHA in 2005 updated their guidelines for chronic heart failure.

▶ Definition

Heart failure[10,11] is a complex clinical syndrome that impairs the quality of life and functional capacity of the affected person. As defined by the ACC and the AHA Task Force, heart failure represents a clinical syndrome that cannot be delineated by a specific diagnostic test, but is dependent on diagnosis by history and physical examination. The chief clinical components of heart failure are dyspnea and fatigue, and fluid retention. The mechanics of heart failure are not understood fully, but integral to the progression of heart failure is the process of cardiac remodeling, which often precedes the clinical development of heart failure symptoms. The neuroendocrine system through the release of a variety of hormones including angiotensin, aldosterone, norepinephrine, vasopressin, and endothelin, along with a variety of cytokines affects the underlying process of cardiac remodeling and plays a fundamental role in the development and progression of heart failure.[10,11]

According to the ACC/AHA Task Force on heart failure[10,11] the evaluation, definitions, and diagnosis of heart failure are dependent on a detailed history and physical examination to evaluate disorders or behaviors that may participate in the development or progression of heart failure. The patient's current level of function, as well as the ability to perform routine activities and activities of daily living must be determined. This assessment of level of function is a basic component of all subsequent evaluations, as is the determination of volume status. In assessing volume status, the patient's weight, height, body mass index, as well as orthostatic vital signs should be followed. The initial laboratory assessment should include a CBC, serum electrolytes, calcium, magnesium, BUN, serum creatinine, fasting blood glucose, Hg A1C, lipid profile, liver function tests, thyroid-stimulating hormone, B type naturietic peptide, and urinalysis. A 12-lead ECG and a posteroanterior (PA) and lateral chest x-ray should also be obtained. Further testing should be done based on clinical indications.[10,11]

▶ Treatment

The ACC/AHA Task Force[10,11] classifies heart failure into four stages with recommendations for the diagnoses and treatment of each of the stages (Fig. 4-3). Stage A consists of patients at high risk for heart failure, but who do not have structural disease or symptoms of heart failure. Stage A patients tend to be hypertensive patients, diabetics, patients with obesity, or metabolic syndrome, and also patients with atherosclerotic disease, or those who have a family history of cardiomyopathy, or a history of exposure to cardiotoxins. The therapeutic goals for these patients are to encourage smoking cessation, encourage the cessation of alcoholic intake and illicit drug use, along with treating hypertension in accordance to Joint National Commission 7 guidelines, aggressive treatment of diabetes to current American Diabetes Association and American College of Endocrinology guidelines with a goal of Hg A1C below 7, and control of metabolic syndrome. The uses of ACE inhibitors and ARBs have been shown to be beneficial for diabetics and those with vascular disease.[10,11]

Once patients develop structural heart disease[10,11] they advance to Stage B heart failure, which is characterized by structural heart disease, but without signs or symptoms of heart failure. Patients who are typically in Stage B heart failure are those who have had a previous myocardial infarction, patients who have signs of left ventricular remodeling such as left ventricular hypertrophy, or those with depressed left ventricular ejection fraction; patients with asymptomatic valvular disease are also included in this category. All the recommendations for therapy for Stage A patients should be utilized for Stage B patients. Beta-blockers and ACE inhibitors should be used in all patients with a history of myocardial infarction. If patients are intolerant of ACE inhibitors, then ARBs should be used instead. For appropriate patients coronary revascularization should be considered, and for those with valvular disease either valvular replacement or repair. Those patients who have an ejection fraction of below 30%, 40 days after a myocardial infarction, should be considered for an ICD.[10,11]

Once patients develop symptoms of heart failure, they have progressed to Stage C heart failure.[10,11] Stage C patients have structural heart disease and either prior or current symptoms of heart failure where symptoms include shortness of breath and fatigue, along with reduced exercise tolerance. The therapeutic recommendations include all of those for Stages A and B, along with dietary salt restriction. Medications that should be routinely used include beta-blockers with the preference being bisoprolol, carvedilol, or sustained release metoprolol, ACE inhibitors, and diuretics for fluid reduction. In patients with moderate to severe symptoms, aldosterone antagonists should be used. The addition of ARBs and digitalis may be beneficial for certain patients, and for those patients who continue to be symptomatic the addition of nitrate and hydralazine may be beneficial. For patients with an ejection fraction less than 30%, the implantation of an ICD may be warranted. In those patients with cardiac dysynchrony, cardiac resynchronization therapy should be considered.[10,11]

The last stage is Stage D[10,11] and consists of patients who have marked symptoms despite maximal medical therapy and undergo frequent recurrent hospitalizations for the management of heart failure. Efforts must be undertaken to ensure that all the recommendations for Stages A, B, and C are being instituted. In selected patients, heart transplantation may be an option. Other treatment modalities that may be tried include continuous intravenous inotropic support or the surgical implantation of a ventricular assist device. If the above are not viable options, then compassionate care and hospice should be considered.[10,11]

ATRIAL FIBRILLATION

In the adult population, atrial fibrillation is the most common sustained cardiac arrhythmia and the prevalence of atrial fibrillation

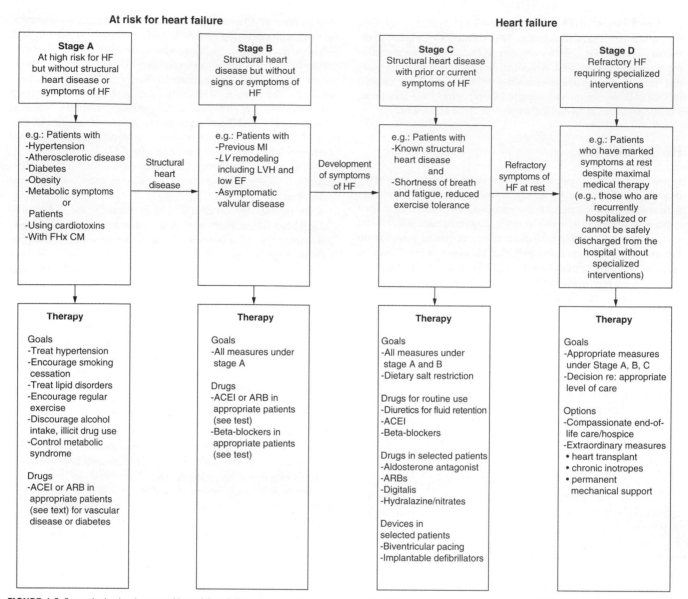

FIGURE 4-3 Stages in the development of heart failure (HF)/recommended therapy by stage. FHx CM = family history of cardiomyopathy, ACEI = angiotensin-converting enzyme inhibitors, ARB = angiotensin receptor blocker. *(Reprinted from Hunt SA, Abraham WT, Chin MH, et al. ACC/AHA 2005 guideline update for the diagnosis and management of chronic heart failure in the adult: a report of the American College of Cardiology/American Heart Association Task Force on Practice Guidelines. (Writing Committee to update the 2001 guidelines for the evaluation and management of heart failure). Am Coll Cardiol. Web site: http://www.acc.org/clinical/guidelines/failure/index.pdf.*

increases with age.[15,16] Atrial fibrillation is often associated with heart disease, thromboembolism, and hemodynamic instability that result in increased morbidity and mortality. The ACC/AHA/and European Society of Cardiology (ESC) Task Force on atrial fibrillation[15] define atrial fibrillation as a supraventricular tachyarrhythmia with uncoordinated atrial activation and subsequent impairment of atrial mechanical function, which manifests on the ECG as loss of P wave and the presence of irregular fibrillatory waves of varying sizes, shape, and timing, and variable ventricular response. An irregular, rapid, wide complex QRS tachycardia in the presence of atrial fibrillation often indicates an accessory pathway or bundle branch block. Atrial fibrillation is considered paroxysmal if it terminates, persistent if it is sustained, and recurrent when there are two or more episodes. With atrial fibrillation, there is a concomitant 5% increase per year in ischemic strokes as well as an increase in mortality for elderly patients with atrial fibrillation compared to age-matched patients in normal sinus rhythm.[15]

Atrial fibrillation[15] is often associated with valvular disease, coronary artery disease, and hypertension, especially in patients with left ventricular hypertrophy. Acute causes of atrial fibrillation include early postoperative complication of myocardial infarction and postoperative complication of cardiac or thoracic surgery. Other acute causes include acute alcohol ingestion, myocarditis, pulmonary embolism or pulmonary disease, along with hyperthyroidism. Fluctuations in autonomic nervous system control may trigger atrial fibrillation in susceptible patients. Symptoms of atrial fibrillation include palpitations, light-headedness, fatigue, dyspnea, and chest pain. In patients with persistent atrial fibrillation, they may develop a tachycardia-related cardiomyopathy, and polyuria is often associated with the release of atrial natriuretic peptide. If the patient with atrial fibrillation develops syncope, the possibility of aortic stenosis, sinus node dysfunction, hypertrophic cardiomyopathy, or an accessory pathway must be explored. An evaluation of atrial fibrillation should include a history and physical focusing on the nature of the symptoms, the clinical type of atrial fibrillation, the time from onset of symptoms to the delineation of atrial fibrillation, along with response to pharmacological treatments and a determination of intrinsic cardiac disease or other acute causes. An ECG should be analyzed to verify rhythm, determine preexcitation, bundle branch block, left ventricular hypertrophy, presence of myocardial infarction, and to measure the various intervals including RR, QRS, and QT intervals. A chest x-ray will exclude a pulmonic cause for the atrial fibrillation. An echocardiogram can assess cardiac size, function, valvular morphology, atrial thrombus, peak pulmonary pressures, and pericardial disease. Laboratory testing should assess basic electrolytes, renal function, and thyroid disease. Additional testing may include Holter monitoring and electrophysiological studies if necessary.[15]

In analyzing the changes in the atria, which facilitate the development of atrial fibrillation, Kistler et al[17] found that with aging there is regional conduction slowing, anatomic conduction delay at the aorta, and structural changes with areas of low voltage. In addition, there is both sinus node dysfunction and an increase in effective refractory period with aging. These changes may lead to an increased propensity toward atrial fibrillation.

According to the ACC/AHA/ESC Task Force[15] the recommendation is for immediate electrical cardioversion in patients with paroxysmal atrial fibrillation and rapid ventricular response who are having evidence of an acute myocardial infarction, symptomatic hypotension, angina, or heart failure unresponsive to pharmacological intervention. The Affirm Study[18] showed that there is no benefit to rhythm control over rate control for patients with atrial fibrillation. In fact, rate control was associated with lower adverse drug risks. In their follow-up, the Affirm Study group[19] showed that for older patients and those without heart failure, there is a survival benefit to rate control. Integral to this is the use of warfarin to prevent thromboembolism and improve survival.[20] Recent work such as PAPA BEAR[21] has shown that amiodarone may be both safe and effective in prophylactic prevention of atrial fibrillation after high-risk cardiac surgery.

CARDIAC RHYTHM DEVICES

A significant number of elderly patients may have a cardiac rhythm management device such as a pacemaker or ICD. In order to assist in the appropriate management of patients with such devices, the American Society of Anesthesiologists (ASA) has recently issued a Practice Advisory for the Perioperative Management of Patients with Cardiac Rhythm Management Devices: Pacemakers and Implantable Cardioverter Defibrillators.[22] What follows is a summary of the information contained in the advisory. The ASA Task Force consisted of anesthesiologists and cardiologists who examined the available literature, and the response from ASA members and Heart Rhythm Society members in order to define the key issues and develop a consensus advisory on the appropriate management of patients with a cardiac rhythm management device. For the purpose of the following discussion, the reader is referred to Fig. 4-4, which provides a stepwise approach to the perioperative management of the patient with a cardiac rhythm device.

Pacemaker nomenclature[22] is based on a five-position letter coded designation. Position 1 indicates the chamber paced with letter

designation: O—no chamber paced; A—atrium paced; V—ventricle paced; D—both atrium and ventricle paced. Position 2 indicates the chamber sensed with letter designation: O—no chamber sensed; A—atrium sensed; V—ventricle sensed; D—both atrium and ventricle sensed. Position 3 indicates the response to sensing: O—no response to sensing; I—inhibited in response to sensing; T—triggered in response to sensing; D—both triggered and inhibited by sensing. Position 4 indicates pacemaker programmability: O—no programmability; R—rate modulation. Position 5 indicates multiside pacing: O—none; A—atrium; V—ventricle; and D—both atrium and ventricle. Examples of various modes are as follows: AOO—asynchronous atrial pacing regardless of the underlying rhythm. AAI—atrially paced, atrially sensed, and inhibits when the atrium fails to produce an impulse within a preset time frame. The device will generate an atrial impulse, and there is no ventricular sensing in this mode. This is an atrial antibradycardia pacing mode. VOO—asynchronous ventricular pacing regardless of the underlying cardiac rhythm. VVI—ventricular paced, ventricular sensed, and inhibited. When the ventricle fails to produce an impulse within a preset time period, the pacemaker will generate a ventricular impulse. There is no atrial sensing or atria-ventricular synchrony. It is antibradycardiac ventricular only pacing. DDI—both chambers are paced, both atria and ventricle are sensed, and it is inhibited. The ventricle is paced when there is no intrinsic ventricular activity. The atrium is paced when atrial activity does not occur within the preset time period. DDD is dual chamber atria-ventricular sequential pacing. The atria will be paced if there is no atrial activity and the ventricle will be paced if there is no ventricular activity after any atrial activity paced or sensed within a preset A-V time period.[22]

ICDs[22] are also characterized by letter designations in various positions. Position 1 indicates the chamber that is shocked: O—no chamber, A—atrium, V—ventricle, D—both atrium and ventricle are shocked. Position 2 indicates the antitachycardia pacing chamber: O—none, A—atrium, V—ventricle, D—both the atrium and the ventricle. Position 3 indicates the tachycardia detection means: E—electrocardiogram, H—hemodynamic, although no hemodynamic sensors have been approved for clinical tachycardiac detection. Position 4 indicates the pacemaker function of the ICD and has the five-position letter designation as discussed above for pacemakers.[22]

The need to address the management of patients with either pacemakers or ICDs has been done by the Task Force.[22] The perioperative period has been further subdivided into the preoperative period, the intraoperative period, and the postoperative period; and finally the need for emergent cardioversion in a patient with a cardiac rhythm management device is addressed.

▶ Preoperative evaluation

There are four key elements in the preoperative evaluation.[22] Does the patient have a cardiac rhythm management device, a pacemaker, or ICD? If the patient has such a device, what type of device is it? Is the patient dependent on the cardiac rhythm management device for antibradycardiac pacing? How well does the device function? These are the essential questions that must be successfully answered in order to assure an appropriate preoperative evaluation according to the ASA's Task Force.[22]

As part of the determination[22] of the presence of a cardiac rhythm management device, there should be a focused history from the patient with regards to the type of device, the reason for the device, the most recent evaluation of the device, and other pertinent information that the patient may have. A thorough review of the medical

Example of a stepwise approach to the perioperative treatment of the patient with Cardia Rhythm Management Device (CRMD)

Perioperative period	Patient/CRMD condition	Intervention
Preoperative evaluation	Patient has CRMD	• Focused history • Focused physical examination
	Determine CRMD type (pacemaker, ICD, CRT)	• Manufacturer's CRMD identification card • Chest x-ray studies (no data available) • Supplemental resources[a]
	Determine whether patient is CRMD-dependent for pacing function	• Verbal history • Bradyarrhythmia symptoms • Atrioventricular node ablation • No spontaneous ventricular activity[b]
	Determine CRMD function	• Comprehensive CRMD evaluation[c] • Determine whether pacing pulses are present and create paced beats
Preoperative preparation	EMI unlikely during procedure	• If EMI unlikely, special precautions are not needed
	EMI likely: CRMD is pacemaker	• Reprogram to asynchronous mode when indicated • Suspend rate-adaptive functions[d]
	EMI likely: CRMD is ICD	• Suspend antitachyarrhythmia functions • If patient is dependent on pacing function, alter pacing functions as above
	EMI likely: all CRMD	• Use bipolar cauter; ultrasonic scalpel • Temporary pacing and external cardioversion-defibrillation available
	Intraoperative physiologic changes likely (e.g., bradycardia, ischemia)	• Plan for possible adverse CRMD-patient interaction
Intraoperative management	Monitoring	• Electrocardiographic monitoring per ASA standard • Peripheral pulse monitoring
	Electrocautery interference	• CT/CRP-no current through PG/leads • Avoid proximity of CT to PG/leads • Short bursts at lowest possible energy • Use bipolar cautery; ultrasonic scalpel
	Radiofrequency catheter ablation	• Avoid contact of radiofrequency catheter with PG/leads • Radiofrequency current path far away from PG/leads • Discuss these concerns with operator
	Lithotripsy	• Do not focus lithotripsy beam near PG • R wave triggers lithotripsy? Disable atrial pacing
	MRI	• Generally contraindicated • If required, consult ordering physician, cardiologist, radiologist and manufacturer
	RT	• PG/leads must be outside of RT field • Possible surgical relocation of PG • Verify PG function during/after RT course
	ECT	• Consult with ordering physician, patient's cardiologist, a CRMD service, or CRMD manufacturer
Emergency defibrillation-cardioversion	ICD: Magnet disabled	• Terminate all EMI sources • Remove magnet to reenable therapies • Observe for appropriate therapies
	ICD: Programming disabled	• Programming to reenable therapies or proceed directly with external cardioversion-defibrillation
	ICD: Either of above	• Minimize current flow through PG/leads • PP as far as possible from PG • PP perpendicular to major axis PG/leads • To extend possible, PP in anterior-posterior location
	Regardless of CRMD type	• Use clinically appropriate cardioversion/defibrillation energy
Postoperative Management	Immediate postoperative period	• Monitor cardiac R&R continuously • Backup pacing and cardioversion/defibrillation capability
	Postoperative interrogation and restoration of CRMD function	• Interrogation to assess function • Settings appropriate ?[e] • Is CRMD an ICD?[f] • Use cardiology/pacemaker-ICD service if needed

FIGURE 4-4 Example of a stepwise approach to the perioperative treatment of the patient with a cardiac rhythm management device. CRP = current return pad, CRT = cardiac resynchronization therapy, CT = cautery tool, ECT = electroconvulsive therapy, EMI = electromagnetic interference, ICD = internal cadioverter defibrillator, MRI = magnetic resonance imaging, PG = pulse generator, PP = external cardioversion-defibrillation pads. R&R = rhythm and rate, RT = radiation therapy. [a]Manufacturer's database, pacemaker clinic records, cardiology consultation. [b]With CRMD-programmed VVI at lowest programmable rate. [c]Ideally CRMD function assessed by interrogation, with function altered by reprogramming if required. [d]Most times this will be necessary; when in doubt, assume so. [e]If necessary, reprogram appropriate settings. [f]Restore all antitachycardia therapies. *(Reprinted from Zaidan JR, Atlee JL, Belott P, et al. Practice advisory for perioperative management of patients with cardiac rhythm management devices:pacemakers and implantable cardioverter defibrillators: a report by the American Society of Anesthesiologist Task Force on Perioperative Management of Patients with Cardiac Rhythm Management Devices. Anesthesiology. 2005;103:186–198.)*

records, ECGs, rhythm strips, and chest x-ray should be done, and a palpation of the device and examination for scars should be included in the physical examination of the patient. Next, the type of device must be determined. Obtaining the manufacturer identifi-

cation card from the patient, or the patient's cardiologist, or pacemaker clinic records usually does this. If these efforts are unsuccessful, a chest x-ray may be done since most current cardiac rhythm management devices have an x-ray code, which can be used to identify the manufacturer of the device and then further information can be obtained from the manufacturers database. The third point is determining whether the patient is dependent on the cardiac rhythm management device for antibradycardiac pacing. History or medical record indicating a symptomatic bradycardia event that necessitated the implantation of the cardiac rhythm management device often does this. It is also possible that the patient had a nodal ablation that necessitated the implantation of the device. If there is no indication of either of the above, then it may be necessary to convert the device to the lowest rate VVI mode and examine the ECG for spontaneous ventricular activity. Lastly, the cardiac rhythm management device function should be assessed by a comprehensive evaluation. If this is not done, the minimum acceptable is an evaluation of the device, with the help of a cardiologist or pacing service, to determine if the device is capable of pacing and generating a paced beat.[22]

▶ Preoperative preparation

In order to be properly prepared for any possible adverse occurrences that may occur during the perioperative period, certain issues should be thought of and planned for in order to optimize patient safety.[22] The first is to determine if there is going to be electromagnetic interference during the procedure. Next, should the cardiac rhythm management device be reprogrammed so that special algorithms are disabled and the device is converted to an asynchronous pacing mode? If the cardiac rhythm management device has antitachycardiac functions, should these be suspended so that they are not inadvertently triggered? Since surgical procedures entail the use of electrocautery, recommending the use of bipolar cautery and ensuring the placement of return currents and generating currents away from the pulse generator and leads of the cardiac rhythm management device; making sure that both emergent pacing and defibrillating capabilities are present and available. Finally, planning for a smooth induction and stable anesthetic so that the limits set on the cardiac rhythm management device are not reached and the device is not activated.[22]

There are several situations in which there may be an increase in likelihood of electromagnetic interference.[22] These include the use of electrocautery, radio frequency ablation, during MRI, during radiation therapy, during electroconvulsive therapy (ECT), and during lithotripsy. In pacemaker-dependent patients, special algorithms such as rate adaptive functions should be suspended and the pacemaker converted into an asynchronous pacing mode. Placing a magnet over a pacemaker usually converts the pacemaker into an asynchronous pacing mode at a fixed rate without rate responsiveness. Some pacemakers may not have a magnet response and the magnet response may vary depending on the manufacturer and the pacemaker battery life. For some patients the magnet response rate may be excessive, and in others the placement of magnet over the pacemaker may alter the pacemaker's function, programming, and battery life. Placing a magnet over an ICD usually suspends the device's tachyarrhythmia therapy without altering the device's ability to pace for bradyarrhythmias. Some ICDs may not have a magnet response and often there is no reliable means to detect a magnet response. Certain ICDs may be permanently disabled by magnet application, and in others program function and settings may be changed. It is for these reasons that the Task Force recommends that cardiac rhythm devices be assessed and adjusted prior to and after the proposed procedure by a cardiologist or pacemaking service.[22]

Intraoperative monitoring

The Task Force's[22] recommendation is that ASA standards are followed, and that there should be continuous monitoring of the ECG from the start of the anesthetic procedure, throughout the procedure or operating course, until transferred out of the postanesthetic area location. It is also the Task Force's recommendation that the peripheral pulse be also continuously monitored during this period. A variety of techniques may be employed in order to achieve this and include: manual palpation of the pulse, monitoring intraarterial pressure, ultrasound monitoring of peripheral pulse, using pulse oximetry, or using pulse plethesmography, and auscultation of heart sounds. It is the Task Force's recommendation that the ASA standards be followed and that both the ECG and peripheral pulse be continuously monitored for the entire period in all patients who undergo anesthetic care regardless of whether that patient receives monitored anesthetic care, sedation, regional, or general anesthesia.[22]

▶ Intraoperative management of sources of electromagnetic interference

The main sources of electromagnetic interference intraoperatively that the Task Force[22] addresses are electrocautery, radio frequency ablation, lithotripsy, MRI, radiation therapy, and electroconvulsive therapy. When using electrocautery, bipolar electrocautery should be used whenever possible. The electrocautery return pad should be positioned so that it is as far away from the cardiac rhythm management device and wires as possible. When using the electrosurgical instrument, it is important not only to avoid the leads and cardiac rhythm management device, but also to avoid waving the activated electrode over the pulse generator or leads because an active electrode of electrocautery may have an inhibitory effect on the cardiac rhythm management device. When using the electrocautery, the lowest possible energy level should be chosen and the electrocautery used in short, irregular, and intermittent bursts. The ASA's position on harmonic scalpels is that when using the above suggestions they are relatively safe and preferred over unipolar electrocautery. The Heart Rhythm Society's position was more equivocal on the use of harmonic scalpels, but the Task Force took the overall position in favor of harmonic scalpel use, bearing in mind the above mentioned other recommendations on the use of electrosurgical instruments.[22]

When using radio frequency ablation,[22] direct contact between the radio frequency ablation catheter and the cardiac rhythm management device and its leads is to be avoided. In addition, the electrical path of the radio frequency ablation catheter to electrical current return pad should be kept as far away from the cardiac rhythm management device and its leads as possible. When undergoing lithotripsy it is the Task Force's recommendation that the lithotripsy beam be focused away from the cardiac rhythm management device and its leads, and if the lithotripsy system triggers in the R wave to disable the atrial pacing system prior to performing lithotripsy. According to the Task Force, radiation therapy may be safely done on patients with cardiac rhythm management devices as long as the device is outside the field of radiation. In certain instances, this may require surgical movement of the device prior to beginning radiation therapy. One of the potential problems that may be encountered is a runaway pacemaker where there is multiple internal component failure resulting in potentially lethal rapid erratic pacing. To avoid such a situation and also to avoid device failure, it is usually the manufacturer recommendation that the cardiac rhythm management device be checked prior to, during, and after the completion of therapy.[22]

The Task Force's recommendation[22] on MRI for patients with cardiac rhythm management devices is that the MRI should be avoided. If an MRI is needed, then the ordering physician should consult the cardiologist, the diagnostic radiologist, and the device manufacturer in order to determine what the most appropriate course is. The Task Force's position on ECT for patients with cardiac rhythm management devices is that it may be safely performed as long as the cardiac rhythm management device has been disabled. ICDs should be disabled, but the ability to treat malignant arrhythmias that may be induced by ECT should be present and prepared for. Patients who are pacemaker dependent may need temporary pacing and a change to an asynchronous mode in order to avoid any potential inhibition of the pacemaker. Thus, the devices should be evaluated prior to the ECT shock therapy and then once again after the ECT shock therapy.[22]

Postoperative

During the postoperative period[22] ASA standards should be followed and maintained. In addition, the Task Force recommends continuous monitoring of the cardiac rate and rhythm with ECG and peripheral pulse monitoring. The cardiac rhythm management device should be interrogated and restored to appropriate settings by the cardiologist or pacemaker service. Once this has been done, and the patient has met discharge criteria, the patient may then be safely discharged from the postoperative monitoring setting.[22]

Emergency defibrillation and cardioversion

The ability to successfully institute emergent cardioversion or defibrillation must be possible throughout the entire perioperative period, for patients with cardiac rhythm management devices. The Task Force recommendation[22] is that emergency and ACLS guidelines are followed. If a patient has an ICD that has been magnet disabled, all sources of electromagnetic interference should be terminated and the magnet removed in order to reenable the antitachycardic therapy of the device. The successful restoration of the cardiac rhythm management device's antitachycardic function must be observed and verified. If the device function is not restored or is not immediately reenabled by programming, then emergent external defibrillation or cardioversion must be done in accordance to ACLS guidelines. The cardioversion pads should be placed in an anterior-posterior position, which will minimize the current flowing through the generator and leads of the cardiac rhythm management device and be in a direction perpendicular to the long axis of the device's generator and leads. The energy level chosen should be at an appropriate level to restore cardiac function.[22]

CARDIOVASCULAR PREOPERATIVE EVALUATION

Many elderly patients with preexisting cardiac disease have already undergone cardiac evaluations and prior cardiac procedures such as stress tests, echocardiograms, ECGs, revascularization procedures such as coronary artery bypass grafting or cardiovascular stenting. Thus, the ability to further optimize a patient may be limited. The ACC and the AHA have developed detailed guidelines for perioperative cardiovascular evaluation[23,24] and it is their guidelines that serve as the basis of cardiovascular evaluation in all populations at risk who are to undergo a perioperative evaluation.[25,26]

In the elderly, the key component of risk assessment is determination of current functional assessment as defined by metabolic equivalents (METs) for common daily activities, and this should be assessed as part of the history. Activities designated as between one and four METs[23,24] include the ability to maintain basic hygiene, the ability to take care of oneself, to eat, drink, and use the bathroom, the ability to walk around the house, and the ability to dress oneself. An energy expenditure of four METs includes daily activities such as light housework, doing the dishes, dusting, and the ability to walk about a block on level ground. An energy expenditure of 4–10 METs includes activities such as climbing a flight of stairs, walking up hill, a brisk walk on level ground, the ability to do heavy housework such as scrubbing floors, lifting, or moving heavy furniture. The ability to participate in sporting activities such as golf, swimming, or tennis and the ability to climb three or more flights of stairs without difficulty reflects a higher level of physical activity and metabolic energy expenditure and thus a better functional status.[23,24]

The nature and type of surgical procedure has a significant impact on risk assessment for the elderly. In older patients undergoing noncardiac surgery, emergency surgery is an independent predictor of adverse postoperative outcomes.[27–29] According to the ACC/AHA Task Force, surgical risk can be designated as high-risk procedures, intermediate-risk procedures, and low-risk procedures.[23,24] High-risk surgical procedures have a perioperative incidence of death and/or myocardial infarction of greater than 5% and this category includes major emergency procedures and operations, aortic and major vascular surgery, peripheral vascular surgery, and prolonged surgical procedures with large fluid shifts and/or blood loss. Intermediate-risk procedures have a perioperative risk of death and/or myocardial infarction of less than 5% and include the following: thoracic and abdominal surgery, orthopedic surgery, prostate surgery, head and neck surgery, and carotid surgery. Low-risk surgical procedures are those that have a risk for death and/or myocardial infarction of less than 1% and include such procedures as endoscopies, cataracts, breast surgery, and superficial procedures.

The ACC/AHA Task Force recommends an eight-step approach to perioperative cardiovascular risk assessment. This approach takes into consideration the history, physical, the nature and type of surgery, an assessment of the patients functional exercise capacity, and objective data such as ECGs, laboratory values, echocardiogram reports, exercise stress test evaluation results, and reports of cardiovascular examinations and procedures.[23,24] A summary of this stepwise approach follows[23–25]:

▶ Step 1: Assessment of whether the surgical procedure is emergent or nonemergent, because if the surgery is emergent, then there is usually no time for a detailed preoperative cardiac evaluation. This does not exclude the possibility of a detailed cardiovascular evaluation postoperatively.

▶ Step 2: Determine if the patient has undergone a coronary revascularization procedure within the last 5 years and whether the patient has been stable without any signs or symptoms of recurrent ischemia. If the patient has been symptom free, then further cardiac workup is not usually necessary.

▶ Step 3: Determine if the patient has had a detailed cardiac evaluation within the past 2 years. Unless, there were adverse findings or the patient has developed signs and symptoms of new or unstable angina, there is no need to repeat the workup.

▶ Step 4: If the patient has a major clinical predictor of cardiac risk and the surgery is nonemergent, then the surgery should be delayed until an appropriate cardiac workup has been done. The major predictors of cardiac risk include unstable coronary syndromes, decompensated heart failure, significant arrythmias, or severe valvular disease.

▶ Step 5: Assess those patients with intermediate clinical predictors of cardiovascular risk in terms of surgical risk and exercise capacity to determine what further cardiovascular workup is appropriate. The intermediate predictors of cardiac risk include mild angina, prior myocardial infarction, compensated or prior congestive heart failure, or diabetes mellitus.

▶ Step 6: In patients with intermediate clinical predictors of cardiovascular morbidity and mortality, determine if they have good exercise capacity. If such patients have good exercise capacity, a functional capacity of four METs or greater, and they are undergoing an intermediate-risk surgical procedure, then there is no need for further cardiac evaluation. On the other hand, if they have poor exercise capacity, a functional capacity of less than four METs, or they are undergoing a high-risk surgical procedure, then further noninvasive cardiac workup is recommended.

▶ Step 7: Involves the analysis of patients with low clinical predictors of cardiac risk. Unless a patient has multiple risk factors, a functional capacity less than four METs, and/or is going to undergo high-risk surgery, no further workup is necessary.

▶ Step 8: Involves the assessment of patients with known coronary artery disease in order to determine if further invasive testing and correction of coronary disease is appropriate or will improve the overall prognosis for the patient. If it is not possible to improve the prognosis, then further testing is not needed.

KEY POINTS

▶ The criteria for an acute resolving or recent myocardial infarction should include either a characteristic change in the CK-MB or troponins along with one or more specific indicators such as symptoms characteristic of ischemia; ECG changes; the ECG showing the presence of pathologic Q waves; an acute coronary intervention such as angioplasty; or there should be pathological findings characteristic of an acute myocardial infarction.

▶ The criteria for an established myocardial infarction depend on the presence of either pathological changes, characteristic of a healing or healed myocardial infarction, or the presence of pathological Q waves on serial ECGs.

▶ Since the majority of deaths occur within the first 2 h after the onset of symptoms, the concept of the golden hours and minimizing the time to initiating reperfusion is paramount.

▶ When diagnosing an acute ST segment elevation myocardial infarction, the differential diagnosis of life-threatening and non-life-threatening conditions must be considered and excluded in order to avoid serious complications for the patient.

▶ The complications of an acute ST segment elevation myocardial infarction include cardiogenic shock, right ventricular infarction, muscular rupture, and arrhythmias.

▶ Heart failure represents a clinical syndrome that cannot be delineated by a specific diagnostic test, but is dependent on diagnosis by history and physical examination. The chief clinical components of heart failure are dyspnea and fatigue, and fluid retention.

▶ Heart failure is classified into four stages with recommendations for the diagnoses and treatment of each of the stages.

▶ In the adult population, atrial fibrillation is the most common sustained cardiac arrhythmia and the prevalence of atrial fibrillation increases with age.

▶ There is no benefit to rhythm control over rate control for patients with atrial fibrillation.

▶ There are four key elements in the preoperative evaluation of cardiac rhythm devices. Does the patient have a cardiac rhythm management device, a pacemaker, or ICD? If the patient has such a device, what type of device is it? Is the patient dependent on the cardiac rhythm management device for antibradycardiac pacing? How well does the device function?

▶ The important issues for perioperative management of cardiac rhythm devices are to determine if there is going to be electromagnetic interference during the procedure; to determine if the device should be reprogrammed; recommending the use of bipolar cautery and ensuring the placement of return currents and generating currents away from the pulse generator and leads of the cardiac rhythm management device; making sure that both emergent pacing and defibrillating capabilities are present and available; planning for a smooth induction and stable anesthetic so that the limits set on the cardiac rhythm management device are not reached and the device is not activated; and continuous monitoring of ECG and peripheral pulse.

▶ In the elderly, the key component of cardiac risk assessment is determination of current functional assessment as defined by metabolic equivalents (METs) for common daily activities.

▶ The nature and type of surgical procedure has a significant impact on cardiac risk assessment for the elderly.

KEY ARTICLES

▶ Antman EM, Anbe DT, Armstrong PW, et al. ACC/AHA guidelines for the management of patients with ST-elevation myocardial infarction: executive summary: a report of the ACC/AHA Task Force on Practice Guidelines (Committee to revise the 1999 guidelines on the management of patients with acute myocardial infarction). *J Am Coll Cardiol.* 2004;44:671–719.

▶ Hunt SA, Abraham WT, Chin MH, et al. ACC/AHA 2005 guideline update for the management of chronic heart failure in the adult: summary article: a report of the American College of Cardiology/American Heart Association Task Force on Practice Guidelines (Writing Committee to update the 2001 guidelines for the evaluation and management of heart failure). *J Am Coll Cardiol.* 2005;46:1116–1143.

▶ Affirm Writing Group. A comparison of rate control and rhythm control in patients with atrial fibrillation. *N Engl J Med.* 2002;347:1825–1833.

▶ Zaidan JR, Atlee JL, Belott P, et al. Practice advisory for perioperative management of patients with cardiac rhythm management devices: pacemakers and implantable cardioverter defibrillators: a report by the American Society of Anesthesiologist Task Force on Perioperative Management of Patients with Cardiac Rhythm Management Devices. *Anesthesiology.* 2005;103:186–198.

▶ Eagle KA, Berger PB, Calkins H, et al. ACC/AHA guideline update for perioperative cardiovascular evaluation for noncardiac surgery: executive summary: a report of the American College of Cardiology/American Heart Association Task Force on practice guidelines (Committee to update the 1996 guidelines on perioperative cardiovascular evaluation for noncardiac surgery). *Circulation.* 2002;105:1257–1267.

REFERENCES

1. Alpert JS, Thygesen K, Antman E, et al. Myocardial infarction redefined—a consensus document of the Joint European Society of Cardiology/American College of Cardiology Committee for the redefinition of myocardial infarction. *J Am Coll Cardiol.* 2000;36:959–969.
2. Antman EM, Anbe DT, Armstrong PW, et al. ACC/AHA guidelines for the management of patients with ST-elevation myocardial infarction: executive summary: a report of the ACC/AHA Task Force on Practice Guidelines (Committee to revise the 1999 guidelines on the management of patients with acute myocardial infarction). *J Am Coll Cardiol.* 2004; 44:671–719.
3. Antman EM, Anbe DT, Armstrong PW, et al. ACC/AHA guidelines for the management of patients with ST-elevation myocardial infarction: a report of the American College of Cardiology/American Heart Association Task Force on Practice Guidelines (Committee to revise the 1999 guidelines for the management of patients with acute myocardial infarction). *Circulation.* 2004;110:e82–e293.
4. Brunwald E, Antman EM, Beasley JW. ACC/AHA 2002 Guideline update for the management of patients with unstable angina and non-ST segment elevation myocardial infarction—summary article: a report of the American College of Cardiology/American Heart Association Task Force on Practice Guidelines (Committee on the Management of Patients With Unstable Angina). *J Am Coll Cardiol.* 2002;40:1366–1374.
5. Rich MW. Office management of heart failure in the elderly. *Am J Med.* 2005;118:342–348.
6. Martinez-Selles M, Robles JAG, Prieto L, et al. Heart failure in the elderly; age-related differences in clinical profile and mortality. *Int J Cardiol.* 2005;102:55–60.
7. Ceia F, Fonseca C, Mota T, et al. Etiology, comorbidity, and drug therapy of chronic heart failure in the real world: the EPICA substudy. *Eur J Heart Fail.* 2004;6:801–806.
8. Lainscak M. Implementation of guidelines for management of heart failure in heart failure clinic: effects beyond pharmacological treatment. *Int J Cardiol.* 2004;97:411–416.
9. Alehagen U, Lindstedt G, Levin LA, et al. The risk of cardiovascular death in elderly patients with possible heart failure: results of a 6-year followup of a Swedish primary care population. *Int J Cardiol.* 2005;100: 17–27.
10. Hunt SA, Abraham WT, Chin MH, et al. ACC/AHA 2005 guideline update for the management of chronic heart failure in the Adult: summary article: a report of the American College of Cardiology/American Heart Association Task Force on Practice Guidelines (Writing Committee to update the 2001 guidelines for the evaluation and management of heart failure). *J Am Coll Cardiol.* 2005;46:1116–1143.
11. Hunt SA, Abraham WT, Chin MH, et al. ACC/AHA 2005 guideline update for the diagnosis and management of chronic heart failure in the adult: a report of the American College of Cardiology/American Heart Association Task Force on Practice Guidelines (Writing Committee to update the 2001 guidelines for the evaluation and management of heart failure). *Am Coll Cardiol.* Web site: http://www.acc.org/clinical/guidelines/failure/index.pdf.
12. American Heart Association. *Heart Disease and Stroke Statistics: 2005 Update.* Dallas, TX: American Heart Association; 2005.
13. Massie BM, Shah NB. Evolving trends in the epidemiologic factors of heart failure: rationale for preventive strategies and comprehensive disease management. *Am Heart J.* 1997;133:703–712.
14. Masoudi FA, Havranek EP, Krumholz HM. The burden of chronic congestive heart failure in older persons: magnitude and implications for policy and research. *Heart Fail Rev.* 2002;7:9–16.
15. Fuster V, Ruden LF, Asinger RW, et al. ACC/AHA/ESC guidelines for the management of patients with atrial fibrillation: executive summary: a report of the American College of Cardiology/American Heart Association Task Force on Practice Guidelines and the European Society of Cardiology Committee for Practice Guidelines and Policy Conferences (Committee to develop guidelines for the management of patients with atrial fibrillation). *J Am Coll Cardiol.* 2001;38:1231–1265.
16. Go AS, Hylek EM, Philips KA, et al. Prevalence of diagnosed atrial fibrillation in adults: national implications for rhythm management and stroke prevention: the Anticoagulation and Risk Factors in Atrial Fibrillation (ATRIA) study. *JAMA.* 2001;285:2370–2375.
17. Kistler PM, Sanders P, Fynn SP, et al. Electrophysiologic and electroanatomic changes in the human atrium associated with age. *J Am Coll Cardiol.* 2004;44:109–116.
18. Affirm Writing Group. A comparison of rate control and rhythm control in patients with atrial fibrillation. *N Engl J Med.* 2002;347:1825–1833.
19. Affirm Investigators: Curtis AB, Gersh BJ, Corley SD, et al Clinical factors influence response to treatment strategies in atrial fibrillation: the Atrial Fibrillation Followup Investigation of Rhythm Management (AFFIRM) study. *Am Heart J.* 2005;149:645–649.
20. Affirm Investigators: Relationship between sinus rhythm, treatment, and survival in atrial fibrillation: Followup Investigation of Rhythm Management (AFFIRM) study. *Circulation.* 2004;109:1509–1513.
21. Mitchell LB, Exner DV, Wyse DG, et al. Prophylactic and amiodarone for the prevention of arrhythmias that begin after revascularization, valve replacement, or repair. PAPA BEAR: a randomized controlled trial. *JAMA.* 2004;294:3093–3100.
22. Zaidan JR, Atlee JL, Belott P, et al. Practice advisory for perioperative management of patients with cardiac rhythm management devices: pacemakers and implantable cardioverter defibrillators: a report by the American Society of Anesthesiologist Task Force on Perioperative Management of Patients with Cardiac Rhythm Management Devices. *Anesthesiology.* 2005;103:186–198.
23. Eagle KA, Brundage BH, Chatman BR, et al. Guidelines for perioperative cardiovascular evaluation for noncardiac surgery. Report of the American College of Cardiology/American Heart Association Task Force in practice guidelines: Committee on perioperative cardiovascular evaluation for noncardiac surgery. *Circulation.* 1996;93:1278–1317.
24. Eagle KA, Berger PB, Calkins H, et al. ACC/AHA guideline update for perioperative cardiovascular evaluation for noncardiac surgery: executive summary: a report of the American College of Cardiology/American Heart Association Task Force on practice guidelines (Committee to update the 1996 guidelines on perioperative cardiovascular evaluation for noncardiac surgery). *Circulation.* 2002;105:1257–1267.
25. John AD, Sieber FE. Age-associated issues: geriatrics. *Anesthesiol Clin N Am.* 2004;22:45–58.
26. Fleicher LA. Preoperative cardiac evaluation. *Anesthesiol Clin N Am.* 2004; 22:59–75.
27. Leung JM, Dzambic. Relative importance of preoperative health status versus intraoperative factors in predicting postoperative adverse outcomes in geriatric surgical patients. *J Am Geriatr Soc.* 2002;49:1080–1085.
28. Hosberg MP, Warner MA, Lobdell CM, et al. Outcomes of surgery in patients 90 years of age and older. *JAMA.* 1989;261:1909–1915.
29. Jin F, Cheung F. Minimizing perioperative adverse events in the elderly. *Br J Anesth.* 2001;877:608–624.

Respiratory System

CHAPTER

5

Weili Weng

INTRODUCTION

A substantial proportion of the perioperative risk among elderly patients is attributable to respiratory complications. The excess risk is explained in part by structural and functional changes in the respiratory system associated with aging. This chapter discusses what changes occur in the respiratory system with aging, and how these changes affect anesthetic management.

STRUCTURAL AND FUNCTIONAL CHANGES OF THE RESPIRATORY SYSTEM WITH AGING

▶ Conducting airways

The conducting airways include the air passages from the mouth and nose to the level of the respiratory bronchioles. In the upper airway, minor changes occur in the cartilaginous and muscular support of the nose and pharynx. Cartilage continues to grow throughout life, accounting in part for the apparently large ears and nose of the elderly. There is also a slow, but continuous loss of dermal collagen, elastin, and water content, along with some muscle atrophy. This may allow for the collapse of the exterior nose with inspiratory flow, and contribute to snoring, dry mouth, propensity to mucosal injury, and bleeding.[1] The loss of muscular pharyngeal support predisposes the elderly to upper airway obstruction and affects tracheobronchial structural integrity.[2]

Increased diameters of trachea and central airways

The large cartilaginous airways show a modest increase in size with age. The diameters of the trachea and bronchi increase about 10% from youth to old age,[3] resulting in a functionally insignificant increase in anatomic dead space.[4] Although calcification of cartilage in the wall of the central airways[5] and hypertrophy of bronchial mucous glands occur with advanced age,[6] these and other changes in the extraparenchymal conducting airways have little clinical significance. It has been proposed that compliance of both the large and small airways increases with age. These airways may be more prone to compression in the elderly during forced maximum exhalation,[7] resulting in decreased maximum expiratory flow rates and increased residual volume (RV).

Decreased upper airway reflexes

Protection of the airway is the most essential function of the upper airway reflexes. The upper airway reflexes consist of many different types of responses such as sneezing, apnea, swallowing, laryngeal closure, coughing, expiration reflex, and negative pressure reflex. Depression of the upper airway reflexes increases the chance of pulmonary aspiration and compromises the ability to maintain the airway.[8] The upper airway protection reflex is preserved in the elderly. However, the reflex requires greater stimulation to trigger than in younger people. In addition, the laryngo-upper esophageal sphincter contractile reflex is decreased secondary to the deleterious effect of aging on the afferent arm of this reflex.[9] Other factors contributing to the progressive loss of the ability to maintain airway protection include decreased cough reflex and decreased number and activity of respiratory cilia.[10] Neurologic disorders commonly seen in the elderly, such as cerebrovascular disease and Parkinson's, are associated with dysphagia and impairment of both the motor and sensory components of the coughing reflex.[11]

▶ Lung parenchyma

Reduced total alveolar surface area and elastic recoil

The lung parenchyma includes gas-exchange airways distal to the terminal bronchioles, the pulmonary capillary, and interstitial structure of the lung. The number of alveoli remains essentially the same in healthy elderly adults as in younger adults; however, the respiratory bronchioles and alveolar ducts undergo progressive enlargement with age. The proportion of lung made up of alveolar ducts increases, and the alveolar septa become shortened, leading to the flattened appearance of the alveoli (Fig. 5–1).[12] The proportion of alveolar air decreases as the volume of air in alveolar ducts increases. Overall, the alveolar surface area decreases 15% by age 70.[13]

Studies in monkeys using electron microscopy have shown that aging is associated with an increase in the number of alveolar pores of Kohn per alveolus. In addition, there may be impaired pulmonary surfactant production with aging, as suggested by alterations in the alveolar type II cells of older animals. Both the increased number of alveolar pores of Kohn and the postulated decrease of surfactant production could play a role in the pathogenesis of *aging lung*.[14] Recent studies reveal that surfactant production also decreases in humans.[15]

The morphological changes in the lung associated with aging are similar to those observed in mild pulmonary emphysema. However, different mechanisms are responsible for the pathological changes observed in these distinct disease entities. Aging by itself does not produce the septa destruction or inflammation usually seen with pulmonary emphysema. Cumulative oxidative

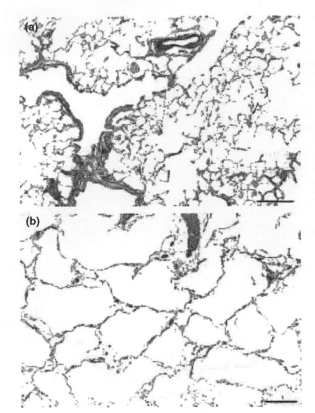

FIGURE 5–1 Lung parenchyma from (a) a nonsmoking 29-year-old subject and (b) a 100-year-old nonsmoking patient who died from pneumonia. Note marked enlargement of alveoli without any inflammatory infiltrate. *(Reproduced with permission from Ref. 18.)*

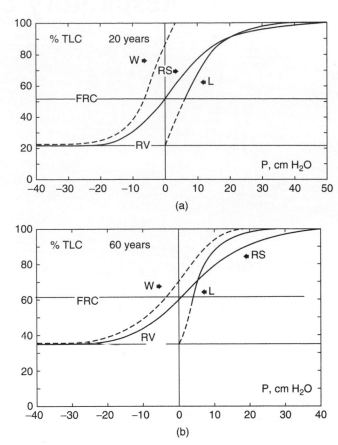

FIGURE 5–2 Static pressure–volume curve of the lung. (L = lungs; W = chest wall; RS = respiratory system) FRC: functional residual capacity; TLC: total lung capacity. (a) A 20-year-old man. (b.) A 60-year-old man. Note that the static compliance of the chest wall is substantially decreased in the older man, while FRC increases. *(Adapted from Refs. 19 and 21.)*

damage by industrial and environmental factors—namely reactive oxygen species, including the superoxide anion, hydrogen peroxide, and hydroxyl radical—is thought to be responsible for the structural deterioration and functional decline of the lung in aging.

In order to permit a clear distinction between the process of aging and the unique anatomical aspects of emphysema, the changes associated with aging have been termed *ductectasia*.[16] This structural term conveys the concept of an aging-related shift of intrapulmonary gas volume from the alveoli to the alveolar duct and respiratory bronchioles. To avoid confusion and simplify the nomenclature, the National Heart, Lung, and Blood Institute recommends use of the term *aging lung* to apply to the uniform airspace enlargement.[17]

Aging affects the elastic properties of the lung tissue and thoracic wall. The elastic recoil forces in lung parenchyma depend on surface tension at the small airway and alveoli, as well as contraction of the lung elastic fibers.[18] The lung parenchyma loses elastic recoil and becomes more compliant and the volume-pressure curve of the lung undergoes a shift to the left. In contrast, because of calcification of the ribs and vertebral joints, the chest wall becomes stiffer. This results in a shift to the right of the volume-pressure curve of the thorax (Fig. 5–2).[19] The volume-pressure curve of the aged total system (lung and thorax) is flatter and shows less compliance. These effects are attributed to changes in lung connective tissue. Of interest, the total lung content of collagen and elastin does not change with aging. In addition, the ratio of lung weight to body weight does not decrease with aging, suggesting little or no lung destruction.

Impairment of lung defense functions

Lung defenses consist of two components: local and humoral defenses. Local defenses include cough and pulmonary clearance by mucocilia; as mentioned previously, both are functionally decreased. Humoral defenses include cellular and immune responses. There are age-related changes in T-cell regeneration which produce a progressive decrease in T-cell function. Failure of T-cell homeostasis appears to result from cumulative defects of T-cell generation.[20] By the end of the seventh decade of life, T-cell homeostasis is no longer guaranteed.

▶ Pulmonary mechanics

Chest wall stiffens and compliance decreases

Chest wall compliance decreases progressively with age.[19,21–23] The rigidity has been attributed to calcification and other structural changes within the rib cage and its articulations including calcification of costal cartilage, sternum and rib, vertebral articulations, and narrowing of intervertebral disk spaces.[24] Age-associated changes in the chest wall also occur as a result of osteoporosis resulting in partial (wedge) or complete (crush) vertebral fractures. These modifications of the chest wall not only alter its compliance but also modify the curvature of the diaphragm, negatively affecting its force-generating capabilities.[18,25] As a consequence, the respiratory work requirement to

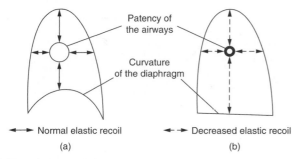

FIGURE 5-3 Decreased elastic recoil leads to enlargement of thorax and flattening of the diaphragm. The flatter diaphragm requires more muscle power and, consequently, more energy to develop the same transdiaphragmatic pressure (increased work of breathing). *(Reproduced with permission from Ref. 22.)*

move the thoracic bellow increases with age. For an equivalent level of ventilation, the effort required may be 30% greater for a 60-year-old than for a 20-year-old (Fig. 5–3).[19]

Decreased respiratory muscle strength

The speed and strength of contraction of skeletal muscle decline with age. Between the ages of 20 and 80 years, the strength of muscular contraction is gradually reduced by 15–35%.[26] The decrease in muscle strength is due to a decrease in muscle mass (cross-sectional fiber area); a decrease in the number of muscle fibers, especially type II *fast-twitch* fibers and motor units; alterations in neuromuscular junctions; and loss of peripheral motor neurons with selective denervation of type II muscle fibers.[27,28] Activation at the neuromuscular junction remains unchanged for a given fiber, but aging is generally associated with motor neuron loss. Data obtained from adult and aged rats suggest that an impairment of the sarcoplasmic reticulum Ca^{2+} pump may contribute to a slowing of contraction (reduced maximal shortening velocity) and relaxation.[29] Decreased synthesis of muscle myosin heavy chain (i.e., decreased "repair" ability)[30] and a decline in mitochondrial respiratory chain function may also contribute to reduced skeletal muscle performance.[31] Respiratory muscle strength is also related to nutritional status. Malnutrition reduces respiratory muscle strength and may impair respiratory muscle capacity to handle increased ventilatory loads in thoracopulmonary disease.[32]

Measurements of respiratory muscle strength reveal a decreasing trend with age. However, the relative contribution of the diaphragm or the intercostal muscles to this decrease is not well characterized. In two relatively small studies, the maximal inspiratory pressure (Pimax) and maximal expiratory pressure (Pemax) decrease with age, especially in women older than 55 years.[33,34] In a more recent and larger study of 65–85-year-old healthy subjects, a decline was noted in Pimax and Pemax with age, although the age-related decline was greater in men. These investigators were able to derive reference equations for both Pimax and Pemax based on this group of healthy elderly men and women.[35] In general, diaphragm strength is reduced by about 25% in healthy elderly individuals compared with young adults.[36]

Extrinsic factors alter respiratory muscle mechanics. As the functional residual capacity (FRC) increases and the total lung capacity (TLC) remains nearly constant, the rest length of inspiratory muscles is shortened. This shortening decreases the contractility of the inspiratory muscles. The radiographic hallmarks of this shortening include elevated end-expiratory rib position, increased anterior-posterior diameter, and a flattened diaphragmatic dome at rest.[3] This results in an increased oxygen cost of breathing when ventilation must be increased during physical activity.[37]

Increased pulmonary arterial pressure and pulmonary vascular resistance

There is no increase in the pulmonary capillary wedge pressure with age. However, pulmonary arterial pressure and pulmonary vascular resistance are increased in the elderly. These changes are not attributable to coronary disease or left ventricular systolic dysfunction. A decline in the volume of the pulmonary capillary bed results in an increase of the mean pulmonary artery pressure by 30%, and an increase of the pulmonary vascular resistance by up to 80%.[38] In a study of 134 patients (inclusion criterion included presence of a sinus rhythm, absence of chronic obstructive pulmonary disease (COPD) or pulmonary embolism, normal global or segmental wall motion, no right or left ventricular hypertrophy or dilatation, no significant valvular disease, no pericarditis), echocardiography revealed a significant correlation between systolic pulmonary artery pressure (SPAP) and age. SPAP increased from 23 ± 5 mm Hg between 20 and 29 years old to 32 ± 6 mm Hg at 80 years or older.[39]

▶ Lung volumes and capacities

Decreased VC, increased RV, minimal change in FRC

As illustrated in Fig. 5–4, the relationship of age to respiratory function is reflected in lung volume changes. The four primary lung volumes are tidal volume (TV), RV, expiratory reserve volume (ERV), and inspiratory reserve volume (IRV). Lung capacities are derived by combining two or more primary lung volumes. The four lung capacities are TLC, FRC, vital capacity (VC), and inspiratory capacity (IC). TLC is the sum of all four primary volumes.

The physiologic reasons for the decrease in VC are complex. Since VC represents the difference between TLC and RV, VC may be diminished either by increasing RV or decreasing TLC. TLC is relatively unaffected by aging. Although the lung is more distensible (reduced static recoil), the reduced muscle strength and more rigid chest wall of the aged prohibit an increase in maximum volume of the thorax. Therefore, the reduction in VC results from an increase in RV. With aging, VC falls approximately 20 mL/year while RV increases approximately 20 mL.[40,41] RV increases with age secondary to increased chest wall stiffness, loss of lung elastic recoil, and decreased force generation by respiratory muscles (Fig. 5–5). Increased chest wall rigidity prevents the chest wall from decreasing intrathoracic volume. In individuals younger than 40 years of age, RV is primarily determined by the amount of "squeezing" force that can be applied by chest wall and respiratory muscles.[42]

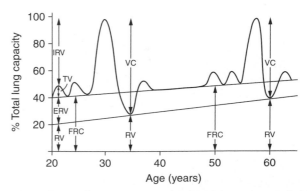

FIGURE 5-4 Diagram representing the effects of aging on lung volumes and capacities. *(Reproduced with permission from Gracey DR, ed. Pulmonary Disease in the Adult. c 1981 St. Louis, Mo: Mosby; c1981.)*

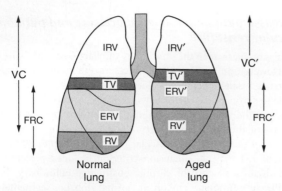

FIGURE 5–5 Schematic representation of lung volume changes with aging. *(Reproduced with permission from Ref. 41.)*

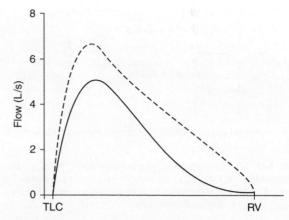

FIGURE 5–7 Changes in the expiratory flow–volume curve with aging. Data from 10 older subjects (mean age 71 years; solid line) and 10 younger subjects (mean age 24 years; broken line). TLC: total lung capacity; RV: residudal volume. *(Adapted from Ref. 50.)*

FRC also increases with age, although to a lesser degree because this increase is counteracted slightly by stiffening of the chest wall.[37] FRC is the volume in which the outward forces of the chest wall are balanced by the inward lung recoil force. FRC increases as the lung recoil forces diminish.[43]

Reduction in maximum expiratory flow with aging

The decrease in maximum expiratory flow rate in the elderly results from the decrease in elastic recoil pressure associated with aging. The decrease in elastic pressure will affect both the site of airflow limitation as well as the driving pressure to limit maximum expiratory flow. Forced expiratory volume in one second (FEV$_1$) decreases by approximately 30 mL/year in healthy nonsmokers (Fig. 5–6).[40,44] All the parameters of flow, including peak flow and flow at the middle portion of vital capacity, decrease in a similar manner. In a study of over 400 subjects aged 70 years or older living at home in a nonmining town in South Wales, Burr et al. showed that there was a progressive decline in FEV$_1$ with age, independent of smoking or environmental exposure.[45] It has been estimated that FEV$_1$ decreases 30 mL/year in men and 23 mL/year in women who are nonsmokers. The rate of decline increases after age 65.[46] In grain elevator workers, the annual decline of lung function was greatest in persons above 50 years of age, regardless of smoking history.[47] Oxidants may have a role in mediating the decline in lung function with age. In a survey of 178 men and

women aged 70–96 years, intake of the antioxidant vitamin E was associated with a significantly higher FEV$_1$.[48] This suggests that cumulative exposure to oxidants may provide a mechanism for age-associated decline in lung function.[49]

The interaction between the elastic properties of the lung and thorax are illustrated by the flow-volume curve (Fig. 5–7). The characteristic changes in the flow-volume curve with aging suggest the presence of an obstructive pattern, even in lifetime nonsmokers.[50]

▶ Gas exchange

Decreased diffusing capacity of carbon monoxide and oxygen

Ventilation-perfusion (V/Q) mismatch and the loss of functional alveolar surface area significantly decrease the diffusing capacity with age.[51–53] The decrease in oxygen diffusing capacity is greater in men than women (0.24 mL oxygen/mm Hg/year vs. 0.16 mL oxygen/mm Hg/year in men and women, respectively).[54] Changes in diffusing capacity of the lung for carbon monoxide (DLCO) have also been studied by several groups. A progressive reduction of maximal carbon monoxide capacity has been seen in elderly patients of both sexes (Fig. 5-8).

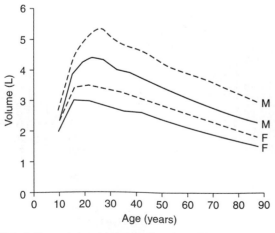

FIGURE 5–6 Changes in forced expiratory volume in 1 s (FEV$_1$, solid line) and forced vital capacity (FVC, broken line) with aging. Data have been averaged from 746 healthy, nonsmoking subjects. M: males, F: females. *(Adapted from Ref. 46.)*

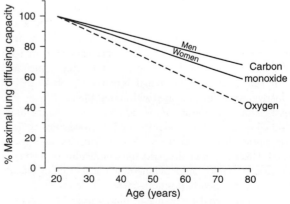

FIGURE 5–8 Maximal diffusing capacities for carbon monoxide and oxygen decline with aging. *(Adapted from Refs. 52 and 53.)*

Impaired ventilation-perfusion matching and increased alveolar-arterial oxygen gradient

In the aged, lung airway closure at lung bases begins to occur in the tidal volume range. Inspired gas is preferentially distributed to the apexes rather than the bases.[55] As a result, a reduction in capillary oxygen tension occurs in the basilar lung regions with low ventilation and high perfusion ratios. Therefore, while the mean alveolar oxygen tension remains unchanged, the arterial oxygen tension decreases by approximately 4 mm Hg/decade after age 20.[56] In the recumbent position, the abnormal distribution of ventilation is exaggerated causing the decrease in arterial oxygen tension to become more pronounced.

Closing volume (CV) is the lung volume when small airways start to close during exhalation. The site at which the small airways begin to close during expiration may shift more distally in the airways. As a consequence, the airways close at a smaller exhaled tidal volume, thus increasing the CV. Closing capacity (CC) is defined as sum of RV and CV. CC represents the lung volume at which the elastic recoil of the lungs becomes insufficient to support small bronchioles without cartilaginous support (<1 mm). When CV exceeds FRC, airway closure occurs and distribution of ventilation changes. This change produces a mismatching of ventilation to perfusion that widens the alveolar-to-arterial gradient for oxygen by approximately 4 mm Hg/decade of life. As a result, arterial oxygen tension becomes progressively lower in the elderly. The equation mean arterial $PO_2 = 102 - 0.33 \times$ age in years (mm Hg) describes the progressive decrease in arterial PO_2 with age.[56] At about 44 years of age, closing capacity reaches FRC in the supine position (Fig. 5–9).[57] By age 66, closing capacity equals FRC in the erect position.

The relative V/Q mismatching with aging leads to increases in physiological dead space.[58] However, because carbon dioxide production is decreased in the elderly, arterial carbon dioxide does not increase.

▶ Control of ventilation

Decreased ventilatory response to hypercapnia and hypoxia

The central nervous system regulates ventilation via both central and peripheral chemoreceptors. With aging decrements occur in both mechanisms: the chemosensitive cells of the brain stem respiratory center become less responsive and the peripheral chemoreceptors

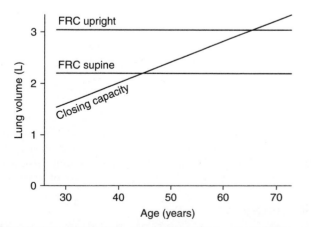

FIGURE 5–9 Functional residual capacity (FRC) and closing capacity (CC) as a function of age. *(Reprinted with permission from Ref. 57.)*

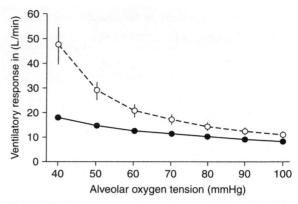

FIGURE 5–10 Ventilatory response to isocapnic progressive hypoxia in eight young normal men (broken line) and eight elderly normal men aged 64–73 (solid line). Values are mean ± SEM. *(Adapted from Ref. 60.)*

in the carotid and aortic bodies become less sensitive to oxygen.[59] This decreased sensitivity to fluctuating oxygen and carbon dioxide levels causes elderly patients to experience more apnea and hypoxemia during sleep.

The elderly have a diminished ventilatory response to hypercapnia, measured as the slope of the relation between ventilation and $PaCO_2$.[60] The elderly also display a diminished ventilatory response to hypoxia (Fig. 5–10).

HOW IS FUNCTIONAL RESERVE OF THE PULMONARY SYSTEM AFFECTED BY AGING AND ITS ANESTHETIC IMPLICATIONS

The effects of aging on the lung include progressive major structural and functional changes (Table 5–1). These changes act to decrease pulmonary reserve. Overall, the effects of aging result in little functional change in the older individual when unstressed. But these changes become readily evident during stress. For instance, the decrease in respiratory muscle strength is likely to be relevant in elderly patients when an additional load is placed on the respiratory muscles, such as pneumonia or left ventricular failure. As another example, increased alveolar-arterial oxygen gradient may be reflected in a decreased resting oxygen tension and result in impairment of preoxygenation. The elderly are also less adept at meeting the respiratory demands induced by hypoxemia or hypercarbia. They may not increase minute ventilation appropriately when the stress of illness provokes an increase in carbon dioxide production. More important, a much greater decrease in arterial oxygen tension is required to increase minute ventilation in the elderly.[61]

There are significant changes in respiratory function resulting from anesthesia and surgery that are superimposed on the age-related changes. Understanding these decreased pulmonary capacities and the effects of the anesthetic process provide a guide in selecting supportive and prophylactic measures.

▶ Impaired respiratory function with general anesthesia

The combination of the supine position, general anesthesia, and abdominal incision leads to a further reduction in FRC. General anesthesia decreases FRC by 15–20%.[62] Surgical maneuvers (retractors, position change, pack, and abdominal gas insufflations) may cause

Table 5–1

The Major Changes in Respiratory System with Aging

Airway and Lung Parenchyma

Increased trachea, central airways diameter, and anatomic dead space

Decreased upper airway reflexes

Decreased effective cough

Decreased effective ciliary cleaning

Reduced total alveolar surface area

Reduced elastic recoil

Impaired lung defense functions

Pulmonary Mechanics

Decreased chest wall compliance

Decreased respiratory muscle strength

Increased lung compliance, but minimal change in total pulmonary compliance

Increased work of maximal breathing

Decreased maximum inspiratory and expiratory flow

Decreased maximal breathing capacity

Increased pulmonary arterial pressure and pulmonary vascular resistance

Lung Volumes

Increased reserve volume

Decreased vital capacity

Decreased FEV_1

Minimal changes in functional residual capacity

Increased small airway closure and closing volume

Relatively unaffected total lung capacity

Gas Exchange

Impaired ventilation–perfusion matching

Increased alveolar–arterial oxygen gradient

Increased dead space fraction

Decreased maximal diffusing capacities for carbon monoxide and oxygen

Control of Ventilation

Decreased ventilatory response to hypercapnia

Decreased ventilatory response to hypoxia

Increased sleep–related disruption of ventilation

Increased sensitivity to narcotic–induced ventilatory depression

---

additional reductions in FRC. FRC reduction is associated with impairment of V/Q matching, decreased efficiency of gas exchange, and increased $P(A\text{-}a)O_2$.[63] The combination of a reduced FRC and an age-associated increase in closing volume predispose patients to atelectasis. In addition, vital capacity can be decreased as much as 25–50%, especially after upper abdominal incisions. Postoperative pain and analgesics both contribute to a reduction in tidal volume and impaired clearing of secretions through normal cough mechanisms.

▶ Blunted hypoxic pulmonary vasoconstriction

Hypoxic pulmonary vasoconstriction (HPV) is a mechanism for the control of blood distribution within the lungs. HPV automatically

increases pulmonary vascular resistance in poorly aerated regions of the lungs, thereby redirecting pulmonary blood flow to regions richer in oxygen content.[64] HPV provides regional pulmonary vascular adjustment to maintain V/Q matching and may be abolished during inhalational anesthesia. HPV is blunted in the elderly during anesthesia. This causes a greater propensity toward intraoperative V/Q mismatch and increased $P(A\text{-}a)O_2$ in the elderly during anesthesia.[57]

▶ Increased sensitivity to narcotic-induced ventilatory depression

As discussed previously, ventilatory responses to hypoxia and hypercarbia are impaired in the elderly. Anesthetic agents such as benzodiazepines, opioids, and inhalation anesthetics further exaggerate these impairments.[65] These changes compromise the usual protective responses against hypoxemia and hypercapnia during the perioperative period.

PREOPERATIVE EVALUATION

The major consideration in evaluating the elderly surgical candidate is whether or not the patient's pulmonary function is adequate to tolerate the operation, the stress of the postoperative period, and the long-term functional demands. When the planned operation will result in loss of functioning pulmonary tissue (lobectomy, pneumonectomy), there is a risk of postoperative respiratory insufficiency if the patient's preoperative pulmonary function is already compromised.[66] For those with preexisting pulmonary impairment, this additional loss of pulmonary reserve may result in serious postoperative problems unless the patient is carefully evaluated preoperatively in order to give the surgeon reliable guidelines about how much pulmonary tissue the patient can safely lose. Based on the majority of reports, age >70 years represents an independent risk factor for lung resection, but this increased risk is mainly due to comorbidity in this age group.[67, 68]

▶ Preoperative pulmonary testing

History and physical examination

Besides a thorough history and physical examination, preoperative evaluation of the respiratory system should include examination of the dentition. Good dental hygiene has been shown to be a reliable marker of good respiratory function in the elderly.[69]

Chest x-ray

Preoperative chest x-ray is helpful in elderly patients with suspected cardiac or pulmonary disease. Seymour et al. examined the value of the preoperative chest x-ray in 223 patients aged 65 years and older undergoing general surgery. Forty percent of patients had an abnormality regarded as clinically significant, although in only 5% of the patients did the chest x-rays affect the course of treatment.[70] Most studies demonstrate that the incidence of significant lung field abnormalities increases in patients aged 60 years and above with no history of chronic obstructive airway disease. Routine preoperative chest x-ray is recommended in patients over the age of 60 years.[71-73]

Spirometry

Spirometry is frequently used for the diagnosis of respiratory diseases in the elderly. Unfortunately, reliable predictive values for the spirometric variables in the elderly population are lacking. VC is a useful determination if its limitations are understood. The predicted value decreases with age, and its measurement requires full cooperation from the patient. The VC is an indicator of the volume of air that a patient is able to move. The VC is near normal in patients with moderately severe obstructive airway disease, but is reduced in individuals with restrictive pulmonary disease and those weakened by neuromuscular disease.

The ability to clear postoperative secretions is closely related to the velocity of forced air movement. FEV_1 is a dynamic measurement of a patient's ability to move air volume over time. The FEV_1 is reported both as a percentage of the VC (FEV_1/VC) as well as an actual volume. Both values are important in determining lung function. If the VC is significantly reduced by restrictive lung disease, the FEV_1/VC ratio may be satisfactory, whereas the actual volume exhaled can be abnormal. The FEV_1 is reduced in obstructive airway disease, but the degree of reduction can be influenced by medications and aggressive pulmonary toilet. The FEV_1 is a useful test to monitor patients with marginal pulmonary function undergoing preoperative therapy to optimize pulmonary function.

The value of routine preoperative pulmonary function testing remains controversial in circumstances where the surgical procedure does not involve the lung. In this situation, preoperative spirometry is recommended if a patient has poorly characterized dyspnea or exercise intolerance. In addition, spirometry may be useful in patients with obstructive lung disease or asthma, if it is not clear from the clinical evaluation whether the patients are at their optimal baseline status.

Preoperative spirometry has an established role in lung resection surgery. FEV_1 has shown good correlation when predicting morbidity in thoracic surgery patients. An FEV_1 >1.5 L predicts positive outcomes in patients older than 70 years.[74,75] Haraguchi and colleagues showed that a predicted postoperative FEV_1 <55% was the strongest independent predictor of pulmonary complications after pulmonary resection. Subsequently, using this predictor as exclusion criteria, they decreased their pulmonary morbidity rate from 33% to 9.8% and mortality rate from 10% to 0% for elderly patients undergoing resection for lung cancer.[68] For more detail on preoperative evaluation of the lung resection, refer to the guidelines published by the American College of Chest Physicians.[76]

Blood gas determination

Arterial blood gas determination is routine in the preoperative evaluation of a candidate for thoracic surgery. Measurement of $PaCO_2$ provides an indication of the patient's alveolar ventilation; any value above 46 mm Hg is a sign of hypoventilation. There are multiple causes for this, and the specific reason should be sought in each patient. The measurement of PaO_2 must be viewed with a consideration of the possibilities for error in its measurement. At sea level, normal PaO_2 is greater than 85 mm Hg. The majority of patients with COPD have a PaO_2 of 80 mm Hg or below, and values in the range of 70–80 mm Hg are not associated with significant postoperative problems. If the PaO_2 is less than 70 mm Hg, an attempt should be made to determine the cause and to improve the patient's gas exchange preoperatively. The most frequent cause is uneven distribution of V/Q mismatch, but other possibilities include right-to-left shunting as a result of underlying thoracic disease (e.g., shunting through a lung cancer or a nonfunctional lobe). More sophisticated pulmonary function tests may be required, including determination of alveolar-arterial oxygen difference, calculation of right-to-left shunt fraction, and split pulmonary function (V/Q scanning).

Carbon monoxide diffusion capacity

The DLCO is an important parameter of pulmonary reserve. The DLCO is decreased by severe chronic obstructive and restrictive pulmonary disease. It also can be decreased by some chemotherapy drugs (e.g., bleomycin, mitomycin, and perhaps paclitaxel) and occasionally by radiation. This makes measurement of the DLCO particularly important in cancer patients who have received chemotherapy or radiation preoperatively. Predicted postoperative diffusing capacity percent is a strong predictor of complications and mortality after lung resection. A DLCO of less than 50% of the predicted number is associated with high risk of postoperative pulmonary complications, and a DLCO of less than 30% of predicted generally precludes consideration of thoracotomy and pulmonary resection. There is little interrelationship between predicted postoperative diffusing capacity percent and predicted postoperative FEV_1, indicating that these values should be assessed independently in estimating operative risk.[77]

Exercise testing

Exercise tolerance predicts morbidity in elderly patients. Exercise testing may include (1) exercise capacity, (2) exercise oximetry, (3) treadmill walking, and (4) stair climbing.[78] Measurement of exercise capacity by supine bicycle ergometry appears to be of value in establishing preoperative pulmonary risk stratification in elderly patients prior to major elective abdominal and noncardiac surgery.[79] A quantified measurement of exercise capacity is the maximal oxygen consumption per kilogram body weight ($VO_{2\ max}$). A $VO_{2\ max}$ <50% of predicted value is an independent risk factor for cardiopulmonary morbidity and mortality after pulmonary resection.[80,81] Simply having the patient walk flights of stairs can give a valuable functional assessment in the clinic. Brunelli and colleagues[82] studied 109 patients over 70 years undergoing lobectomy for cancer. Patients who could climb more than four flights of stairs had <20% cardiopulmonary complication rate, whereas those who could not climb at least three flights of stairs had a 57% complication rate.

Split pulmonary function studies

The split pulmonary function test is a scintigraphic technique which can measure the relative contribution of the parenchyma to be resected to the total lung function. The postoperative VC and FEV_1 can be predicted for a patient who may require resection of a portion of lung neoplasm (predicted postoperative FEV_1 = preoperative FEV_1 minus the percentage perfusion in the involved lung). Patients with impaired ventilatory function (preoperative FEV_1 <2.0 L) are considered acceptable candidates for a pneumonectomy if the predicted postoperative FEV_1 exceeds 800 mL. Patients with borderline pulmonary function can undergo resection safely if they have an FEV_1 equal to or greater than 1.6 L or 40% of its predicted value, a predicted postoperative FEV_1 of 700 mL or more, a maximum oxygen consumption of 10 mL × kg (−1) × min (−1) or greater, or stair climbing of three flights or more.[82]

Maximum voluntary ventilation

Maximum voluntary ventilation (MVV) reflects the status of the respiratory muscles, compliance of the thorax-lung complex, and airway resistance. MVV is a quick and easy way to assess the strength of the patient's pulmonary musculature prior to surgery. The test is performed by having the patient inhale as deeply and rapidly as possible for up to 15 s. The total volume of air moved during the test is expressed as L/s or L/min. One major drawback is that the test is effort dependent. Patients with an MVV of less than 50% of the predicted amount experience a prohibitively high operative mortality after pneumonectomy.

COMMON COMORBID STATES SEEN IN THE ELDERLY

▶ Chronic obstructive pulmonary disease

COPD continues to cause a heavy health and economic burden both in the United States and around the world. Some important risk factors for COPD include smoking, occupational exposure, air pollution, airway hyperresponsiveness, asthma, and certain genetic variations. COPD is the primary diagnosis in 18% of all hospital admissions in patients older than 65. It is the fourth leading cause of death in the United States.[83] With COPD education, early diagnosis, and aggressive preoperative pulmonary treatment, complication rates in the elderly with COPD can be minimized.

▶ Obesity

Increases in body fat percentage and abdominal body fat occur with increasing age.[84] Obesity is commonly considered a surgical risk factor, but the degree of risk has been imprecisely quantified. Obesity is often associated with abnormal cardiorespiratory and metabolic function, which may predispose a patient to morbidity and mortality after surgery. For instance, obese patients have lower ERV, functional RV, TLC, and DLCO compared with age-matched normal subjects.[85] However, there is little evidence that excessive body weight in itself should contraindicate general surgery. Obesity does not appear to be a risk factor for postoperative pulmonary complications. In a large series of 2964 patients undergoing elective noncardiac surgery, obese patients (body mass index >30) had no increase in the risk of pneumonia or respiratory failure when compared with nonobese patients.[86] The incidence of pulmonary complications for obese patients across pooled studies is approximately 12% (relative risk = 1.3) compared with nonobese patients. These data indicate that obesity should not necessarily influence the decision to proceed with surgery.[87]

▶ Sleep apnea

Sleep apnea increases with age, although the severity of the disorder may actually decrease in the elderly.[88] The prevalence of sleep apnea syndrome in the elderly is reportedly as high as 60% in men over 65 years of age.[89] A greater number of episodes of desaturation and apnea occur in men during sleep than in women, until women reach menopause. Following menopause, men and women begin to have approximately equal numbers of episodes of nocturnal desaturation.[90] Sleep-disordered breathing may also be associated with impairment in cognitive function, and is reported to be more frequent in Alzheimer's disease.[91] Risk factors for sleep apnea include obesity, anatomical abnormalities, aging, and family history. It has been associated with hypertension, cardiovascular and pulmonary diseases, and increased mortality. The elderly patient with sleep apnea is at risk for partial or total airway obstruction.

▶ Pulmonary malignancies

The leading cause of cancer death in the United States is lung cancer.[92] Metastatic disease involving the lungs is observed in a vast number of additional malignancies. Most primary lung cancers can be classified into two major groups: non-small-cell lung cancer, for which surgery remains a major component of therapy, and small-cell lung cancer which is primarily a nonsurgical disease. Histology and stage at presentation are the two most significant factors affecting the patient survival rate. Nearly 70% of all lung cancers are inoperable, because of extensive mediastinal or distant metastatic disease.

▶ Adult respiratory distress syndrome

There is a progressive decline in survival from adult respiratory distress syndrome (ARDS) with age. For example, mortality from ARDS at 28 days hospitalization was 25.4% in patients less than 70 years and 50.3% in those older than 70 years.[93] Approaches to treatment do not differ among age groups and should focus on identification of the underlying causes of ARDS combined with ventilator management based on low tidal volume protective strategies to minimize ongoing ventilator-induced lung injury.

PERIOPERATIVE ANESTHESIA MANAGEMENT

Clinicians can institute strategies to reduce the risk of pulmonary morbidity during the perioperative period.

▶ Smoking cessation

Smoking cessation, including brief counseling and pharmacotherapy, should occur at least 4–8 weeks preoperatively to maximize the reduction of postoperative respiratory complications.[94,95] Smoking produces some potentially reversible effects that may be relevant to perioperative morbidity. Although the reversal of many effects requires long-term (weeks to months) smoking cessation, based on the physiology of carbon monoxide elimination, a short abstinence period (12–72 h) is sufficient to normalize several important cardiovascular parameters.[96] Anesthesia providers and surgeons have an obligation to instruct patients not to smoke before surgery.

▶ Aspiration prophylaxis

Because aspiration pneumonia in the elderly is related to certain risk factors, including dysphagia and aspiration, preventive measures involve approaches such as pharmacological therapy, swallowing training, dietary management, oral hygiene, and positioning. Another important preoperative management is to provide the patient with whatever physical and mental preparation is needed.

▶ Optimizing pulmonary conditions (asthma and COPD treatment)

Every effort should be made to treat and correct, as much as possible, the underlying pulmonary pathophysiology of elderly patients with evidence of acute or chronic lung disease at the time of preoperative assessment.[97] Despite earlier studies suggesting that patients with asthma were at risk for postoperative pulmonary complications,[98] studies in the modern era have found no increase in risk of clinically important complications. Warner and colleagues reviewed the records of 703 patients with asthma undergoing surgery.[99] Perioperative bronchospasm occurred in only 1.7% of patients. Respiratory failure occurred in one patient and laryngospasm occurred in two patients. There were no other clinically significant postoperative pulmonary complications or deaths in the entire group. Thus, asthmatic patients can undergo anesthesia and surgery safely, and clinicians should strive to optimize the asthmatic patient's pulmonary status preoperatively. In particular, a 1-week course of systemic corticosteroids (e.g., prednisone 40–60 mg daily) can be safely used as needed without an increase in the risk of respiratory infection or wound complications. The goal of treatment is to render the patient wheeze-free and asymptomatic if possible, and to achieve a peak flow rate of greater than 80% of predicted or personal best.

▶ Choose regional techniques

Regional anesthesia is frequently used in elderly patients undergoing surgery. Many studies have shown that the type of anesthesia has no substantial effect on perioperative morbidity and mortality in any age group. However, it intuitively makes sense that elderly patients would benefit from regional anesthesia because they remain minimally sedated throughout the procedures, airway manipulation is avoided, and excellent postoperative pain control is initially provided. However, a multitude of factors influence the outcome. These factors make it difficult to decide if and when one technique is unequivocally better than another. Regional anesthesia appears to be safe and beneficial in elderly patients. The decision to provide a regional anesthetic must be assessed on a case-by-case basis, and particular consideration should be given to the health status of the patient, the operation being performed, and the expertise of the anesthesiologist.[100]

▶ Hypoxia prevention

Methods to prevent perioperative hypoxemic episodes in elderly patients include reduction of preoperative medication, a 3-min period of preoxygenation prior to induction of general anesthesia, increased inspired oxygen content postoperatively, early postoperative respiratory therapy, and adequate hydration to allow mobilization of secretions. Intraoperatively, anesthesiologists should strive to prevent silent aspiration by avoiding deep sedation when the airway is unprotected and applying gentle, as opposed to vigorous ventilation, when higher ventilatory pressures are required to provide sufficient ventilation with the unprotected airway.[22]

▶ Adequate ventilator setting

The loss of lung elastic recoil means that passive expiration during anesthesia and paralysis is slowed. Care must be taken to select appropriate ventilator settings to avoid trauma to the lungs. Air trapping (auto positive end-expiratory pressure [PEEP]) can occur if the expiration time is not sufficient to allow passive emptying of the lung. This results in a slow increase in lung volume and pulmonary pressure.[101] In some cases, the ventilator I/E ratio must be adjusted to eliminate air entrapment.

▶ Postoperative pain control

Clinicians should carefully titrate analgesic doses and frequently assess patients for adequacy of pain control and adverse side effects of pain medication. Thoracic or lumbar epidural analgesic techniques may benefit patients undergoing thoracic or upper abdominal surgery. These techniques quickly allow restoration of pulmonary function with minimal morbidity, thereby decreasing hospital stay and health care costs.[102]

PREDICTORS OF PULMONARY COMPLICATIONS IN THE ELDERLY

Pulmonary complications in the elderly are a significant source of morbidity, mortality, and prolonged length of hospitalization. The incidence of postoperative pulmonary complications in elderly patients has been reported to range from 7% to 33%.[103] Multiple studies have identified predictors of pulmonary complications in the elderly. The National Veterans Affairs Surgical Quality Improvement Program examined 160,805 patients undergoing major noncardiac surgery with the objective of developing a preoperative risk index for predicting postoperative pneumonia (postoperative pneumonia was defined using the Centers for Disease Control and Prevention definition of nosocomial pneumonia). As shown in Table 5–2, the postoperative pneumonia risk index takes into account various risk factors such as type of surgery, age, functional status, emergency surgery, type of anesthetic, and drug use; and assigns point values to each using a logistic regression statistical model. In Table 5–2 it is demonstrated that five risk classes were identified, each giving different rates of postoperative pneumonia which varied in incidence from 0.24% to 15.9%.[104]

In the Veterans Affairs Medical Centers study, type of surgical procedure dominates the analysis. Age is also a bigger risk factor than previously suggested by the literature. Since veterans who receive care at the Veterans Affairs Medical Centers often have greater comorbid illness, this predictive model may not be representative of other, healthier populations. Only 3.2% of study patients were female. Patient-specific factors such as age and functional status are likely to be risk factors in women, but their associated odds ratios may differ from those obtained in the VA study. Additional research is needed to validate the VA model in other groups, including women.

While the National Veterans Affairs Surgical Quality Improvement Program examined only postoperative pneumonia, other investigators have looked at a wider spectrum of postoperative pulmonary complications. Brooks-Braun examined predictors of postoperative pulmonary complications in a cohort of 400 patients undergoing elective abdominal surgery.[105] In this study, the definition of postoperative pulmonary complications was not as rigid as the VA study and relied more on the clinical findings of atelectasis and pneumonia. The incidence of pulmonary complications was reported to be 22.5%. Six independent risk factors were identified including age ≥60 years, impaired preoperative cognitive function, smoking history within the past 8 weeks, body mass index ≥27, history of cancer, and upper abdominal incision. Of interest, many of the preoperative risk factors identified by Brooks-Braun were similar to the VA study (see Table 5–2 for comparison). However, on further testing, the six-factor model of Brooks-Braun was only able to predict 55% of patients who developed postoperative pulmonary complications. The negative predictive value of the model was stronger at 81% and the mean predictive value was 68%. Thus, the six-factor model for prediction of postoperative pulmonary complications after abdominal surgery is not ready for use in the clinical setting to guide patient care.[103]

In assessing the data of both Brooks-Braun and the VA study, the two most important risk factors for postoperative pulmonary complications appear to be age and type of surgery. Until better data become available, the postoperative pneumonia risk index is probably the best means of identifying patients at risk for postoperative pneumonia and may be useful in guiding perioperative respiratory care.

Table 5-2

Arozullah Multifactorial Risk Index for Predicting Postoperative Pneumonia

Variable	Odds Ratio (95% CI)	Point Value
Type of surgery		
Abdominal aortic aneurysm repair	4.29 (3.34–5.50)	15
Thoracic	3.92 (3.36–4.57)	14
Upper abdominal	2.68 (2.38–3.03)	10
Neck	2.30 (1.73–3.05)	8
Neurosurgery	2.14 (1.66–2.75)	8
Vascular	1.29 (1.10–1.52)	3
Age		
≥80 years	5.63 (4.62–6.84)	17
70–79 years	3.58 (2.97–4.33)	13
60–69 years	2.38 (1.98–2.87)	9
50–59 years	1.49 (1.23–1.81)	4
Functional status		
Totally dependent	2.83 (2.33–3.43)	10
Partially dependent	1.83 (1.63–2.06)	6
Weight loss >10% in last 6 months	1.92 (1.68–2.18)	7
History of COPD	1.72 (1.55–1.91)	5
General anesthesia	1.56 (1.36–1.80)	4
Impaired sensorium	1.51 (1.26–1.82)	4
History of cerebrovascular accident	1.47 (1.28–1.68)	4
Blood urea nitrogen level		
<2.86 mmol/L (<8 mg/dL)	1.47 (1.26–1.72)	4
7.85–10.7 mmol/L (22–30 mg/dL)	1.24 (1.11–1.39)	2
≥10.7 mmol/L (≥30 mg/dL)	1.41 (1.22–1.64)	3
Transfusion >4 units	1.35 (1.07–1.72)	3
Emergency surgery	1.33 (1.16–1.54)	3
Steroid use for chronic condition	1.33 (1.12–1.58)	3
Current smoker within 1 year	1.28 (1.17–1.42)	3
Alcohol intake >2 drinks/day in past 2 weeks	1.24 (1.08–1.42)	2

Class	Point Totals	Postoperative Pneumonia Rates (Validation Cohort)
1	<15	0.24%
2	16–25	1.18%
3	26–40	4.6%
4	41–55	10.8%
5	>55	15.9%

Source: Adapted from Ref. 104.

SUMMARY

A substantial proportion of the perioperative risk among elderly patients is attributable to respiratory complications. The excess risk is explained in part by structural and functional changes associated with aging which act to decrease the reserve of the respiratory system. The respiratory system changes may be accelerated or decelerated by lifestyle but are usually evident by the fourth or fifth decade. Overall, the effects of aging result in little change in function when the older individual is assessed in the unstressed state, but these age-related changes become readily evident during times of stress, such as the perioperative period. In addition to these changes, there are many intraoperative manipulations performed by anesthesia providers which alter the respiratory system. An awareness of the age-related changes in the respiratory system, combined with an understanding of changes in pulmonary physiology which occur with anesthesia and surgery, will help the anesthesiologist to anticipate and treat perioperative respiratory complications in aged patients.

KEY POINTS

▶ The effects of aging on the lung act to decrease pulmonary reserve. Some important changes with aging include an age-related shift of intrapulmonary gas volume from the alveoli to the alveolar duct and respiratory bronchioles; measurements of respiratory muscle strength reveal a decreasing trend with age; with aging, closing volume will exceed FRC leading to increased V/Q mismatching and widening of the alveolar-to-arterial gradient.

▶ There are significant changes in respiratory function resulting from anesthesia and surgery that are superimposed on the age-related changes to further decrease pulmonary reserve.

▶ The major consideration in evaluating pulmonary function of the elderly surgical candidate is whether or not the patient has sufficient pulmonary reserve to tolerate the operation, the stress of the postoperative period, and the long-term functional demands.

▶ Clinicians can institute strategies to reduce the risk of pulmonary morbidity during the perioperative period including smoking cessation, aspiration prophylaxis, optimizing pulmonary conditions and ventilator settings, prevention of hypoxia, and postoperative pain control.

▶ Pulmonary complications in the elderly are a significant source of morbidity, mortality, and prolonged length of hospitalization. The two most important risk factors for postoperative pulmonary complications appear to be age and type of surgery.

KEY ARTICLES

▶ Janssens JP, Pache JC, Nicod LP. Physiological changes in respiratory function associated with ageing. *Eur Respir J.* 1999;13(1):197–205.

▶ Zaugg M, Lucchinetti E. Respiratory function in the elderly. *Anesthesiol Clin N Am.* 2000;18(1):47–58, vi.

▶ Smetana GW. Preoperative pulmonary assessment of the older adult. *Clin Geriatr Med.* 2003;19(1):35–55.

▶ Smetana GW. Preoperative pulmonary evaluation. *N Engl J Med.* 1999;340(12):937–944.

▶ Arozullah AM, Khuri SF, Henderson WG, et al. Development and validation of a multifactorial risk index for predicting postoperative pneumonia after major noncardiac surgery. *Ann Intern Med.* 2001;135(10):847–857.

REFERENCES

1. Close LG, Woodson GE. Common upper airway disorders in the elderly and their management. *Geriatrics*. 1989;44(1):67–68, 71–62.
2. Berry DT, Phillips BA, Cook YR, et al. Sleep-disordered breathing in healthy aged persons: possible daytime sequelae. *J Gerontol*. 1987;42(6):620–626.
3. Mihara F, Fukuya T, Nakata H, et al. Normal age-related alterations on chest radiography. A longitudinal investigation. *Acta Radiol*. 1993;34(1):53–58.
4. Gibellino F, Osmanliev DP, Watson A, et al. Increase in tracheal size with age. Implications for maximal expiratory flow. *Am Rev Respir Dis*. 1985;132(4):784–787.
5. Liebow A. *Biochemical and structural changes in the aging lung: summary*. New York: Grune & Stratton; 1964.
6. Hernandez JA, Anderson AE, Jr., Holmes WL, et al. The Bronchial Glands In Aging. *J Am Geriatr Soc*. 1965;13:799–804.
7. Knudson RJ, Clark DF, Kennedy TC, et al. Effect of aging alone on mechanical properties of the normal adult human lung. *J Appl Physiol*. 1977;43(6):1054–1062.
8. Shaker R, Ren J, Bardan E, et al. Pharyngoglottal closure reflex: characterization in healthy young, elderly, and dysphagic patients with predeglutitive aspiration. *Gerontology*. 2003;49(1):12–20.
9. Kawamura O, Easterling C, Aslam M, et al. Laryngo-upper esophageal sphincter contractile reflex in humans deteriorates with age. *Gastroenterology*. 2004;127(1):57–64.
10. Brandstetter RD, Kazemi H. Aging and the respiratory system. *Med Clin N Am*. 1983;67(2):419–431.
11. Ebihara S, Saito H, Kanda A, et al. Impaired efficacy of cough in patients with Parkinson's disease. *Chest*. 2003;124(3):1009–1015.
12. Verbeken EK, Cauberghs M, Mertens I, et al. The senile lung. Comparison with normal and emphysematous lungs. 1. Structural aspects. *Chest*. 1992;101(3):793–799.
13. Thurlbeck WM, Angus GE. Growth and aging of the normal human lung. *Chest*. 1975;67(2 Suppl.):3S–6S.
14. Shimura S, Boatman ES, Martin CJ. Effects of ageing on the alveolar pores of Kohn and on the cytoplasmic components of alveolar type II cells in monkey lungs. *J Pathol*. 1986;148(1):1–11.
15. Betsuyaku T, Kuroki Y, Nagai K, et al. Effects of ageing and smoking on SP-A and SP-D levels in bronchoalveolar lavage fluid. *Eur Respir J*. 2004;24(6):964–970.
16. Ryan SF, Vincent TN, Mitchell RS, et al. Ductectasia; an asymptomatic pulmonary change related to age. *Med Thorac*. 1965;22:181–187.
17. The definition of emphysema. Report of a National Heart, Lung, and Blood Institute, Division of Lung Diseases workshop. *Am Rev Respir Dis*. 1985;132(1):182–185.
18. Janssens JP, Pache JC, Nicod LP. Physiological changes in respiratory function associated with ageing. *Eur Respir J*. 1999;13(1):197–205.
19. Turner JM, Mead J, Wohl ME. Elasticity of human lungs in relation to age. *J Appl Physiol*. 1968;25(6):664–671.
20. Goronzy JJ, Weyand CM. T cell development and receptor diversity during aging. *Curr Opin Immunol*. 2005.
21. Mittman C, Edelman N, Norris A, et al. Relationship between chest wall and pulmonary compliance and age. *J Appl Physiol*. 1965;20:1211–1216.
22. Zaugg M, Lucchinetti E. Respiratory function in the elderly. *Anesthesiol Clin N Am*. 2000;18(1):47–58, review.
23. Wahba WM. Influence of aging on lung function—clinical significance of changes from age twenty. *Anesth Analg*. 1983;62(8):764–776.
24. Crapo R. The aging lung. In: Mahler DA, ed. *Pulmonary Disease in the Elderly Patient*. New York: Marcel Dekker; 1993:1–21.
25. Kammoun S, Rekik WK, Ayoub A. The aging lung: structural and functional modifications related to aging. *Tunis Med*. 2001;79(1):10–14.
26. Robinson S. Physical fitness in relation to age. In: *Aging of the Lung: Perspectives*. New York: Grune & Stratton; 1964.
27. Tolep K, Kelsen SG. Effect of aging on respiratory skeletal muscles. *Clin Chest Med*. 1993;14(3):363–378.
28. Brown M, Hasser EM. Complexity of age-related change in skeletal muscle. *J Gerontol A Biol Sci Med Sci*. 1996;51(2):B117–B123.
29. Narayanan N, Jones DL, Xu A, et al. Effects of aging on sarcoplasmic reticulum function and contraction duration in skeletal muscles of the rat. *Am J Physiol*. 1996;271(4 Pt. 1):C1032–C1040.
30. Balagopal P, Rooyackers OE, Adey DB, et al. Effects of aging on in vivo synthesis of skeletal muscle myosin heavy-chain and sarcoplasmic protein in humans. *Am J Physiol*. 1997;273(4 Pt. 1):E790–E800.
31. Taylor DJ, Kemp GJ, Thompson CH, et al. Ageing: effects on oxidative function of skeletal muscle in vivo. *Mol Cell Biochem*. 1997;174(1–2):321–324.
32. Arora NS, Rochester DF. Respiratory muscle strength and maximal voluntary ventilation in undernourished patients. *Am Rev Respir Dis*. 1982;126(1):5–8.
33. Black LF, Hyatt RE. Maximal respiratory pressures: normal values and relationship to age and sex. *Am Rev Respir Dis*. 1969;99(5):696–702.
34. McElvaney G, Blackie S, Morrison NJ, et al. Maximal static respiratory pressures in the normal elderly. *Am Rev Respir Dis*. 1989;139(1):277–281.
35. Bassey EJ, Harries UJ. Normal values for handgrip strength in 920 men and women aged over 65 years, and longitudinal changes over 4 years in 620 survivors. *Clin Sci (Lond)*. 1993;84(3):331–337.
36. Tolep K, Higgins N, Muza S, et al. Comparison of diaphragm strength between healthy adult elderly and young men. *Am J Respir Crit Care Med*. 1995;152(2):677–682.
37. Johnson BD, Reddan WG, Pegelow DF, et al. Flow limitation and regulation of functional residual capacity during exercise in a physically active aging population. *Am Rev Respir Dis*. 1991;143(5 Pt. 1):960–967.
38. Davidson WR, Jr., Fee EC. Influence of aging on pulmonary hemodynamics in a population free of coronary artery disease. *Am J Cardiol*. 1990;65(22):1454–1458.
39. Dib JC, Abergel E, Rovani C, et al. The age of the patient should be taken into account when interpreting Doppler assessed pulmonary artery pressures. *J Am Soc Echocardiogr*. 1997;10(1):72–73.
40. Muiesan G, Sorbini CA, Grassi V. Respiratory function in the aged. *Bull Physiopathol Respir (Nancy)*. 1971;7(5):973–1009.
41. Chan ED, Welsh CH. Geriatric respiratory medicine. *Chest*. 1998;114(6):1704–1733.
42. Leith DE, Mead J. Mechanisms determining residual volume of the lungs in normal subjects. *J Appl Physiol*. 1967;23(2):221–227.
43. Muravchick S. Anesthesia for the elderly. In: Miller RD, ed. *Miller's Anesthesia*. 5th ed. Philadelphia: Churchill Livingstone; 2000:2210–2228.
44. Knudson RJ, Slatin RC, Lebowitz MD, et al. The maximal expiratory flow-volume curve. Normal standards, variability, and effects of age. *Am Rev Respir Dis*. 1976;113(5):587–600.
45. Burr ML, Phillips KM, Hurst DN. Lung function in the elderly. *Thorax*. 1985;40(1):54–59.
46. Knudson RJ, Lebowitz MD, Holberg CJ, et al. Changes in the normal maximal expiratory flow–volume curve with growth and aging. *Am Rev Respir Dis*. 1983;127(6):725–734.
47. Tabona M, Chan–Yeung M, Enarson D, et al. Host factors affecting longitudinal decline in lung spirometry among grain elevator workers. *Chest*. 1984;85(6):782–786.
48. Dow L, Tracey M, Villar A, et al. Does dietary intake of vitamins C and E influence lung function in older people? *Am J Respir Crit Care Med*. 1996;154(5):1401–1404.
49. Schunemann HJ, McCann S, Grant BJ, et al. Lung function in relation to intake of carotenoids and other antioxidant vitamins in a population–based study. *Am J Epidemiol*. 2002;155(5):463–471.
50. Fowler RW, Pluck RA, Hetzel MR. Maximal expiratory flow–volume curves in Londoners aged 60 years and over. *Thorax*. 1987;42(3):173–182.
51. Stam H, Hrachovina V, Stijnen T, et al. Diffusing capacity dependent on lung volume and age in normal subjects. *J Appl Physiol*. 1994;76(6):2356–2363.
52. Cohn JE, Carroll DG, Armstrong BW, et al. Maximal diffusing capacity of the lung in normal male subjects of different ages. *J Appl Physiol*. 1954;6(10):588–597.
53. Crapo RO, Morris AH. Standardized single breath normal values for carbon monoxide diffusing capacity. *Am Rev Respir Dis*. 1981;123(2):185–189.
54. Neas LM, Schwartz J. The determinants of pulmonary diffusing capacity in a national sample of U.S. adults. *Am J Respir Crit Care Med*. 1996;153(2):656–664.
55. Wagner PD, Laravuso RB, Uhl RR, et al. Continuous distributions of ventilation–perfusion ratios in normal subjects breathing air and 100 percent O2. *J Clin Invest*. 1974;54(1):54–68.
56. Sorbini CA, Grassi V, Solinas E, et al. Arterial oxygen tension in relation to age in healthy subjects. *Respiration*. 1968;25(1):3–13.

57. Lumb A. *Nunn's Applied Respiratory Physiology.* Vol Pt. I. 5th ed. Oxford: Butterworth–Heinemann; 2000:53.

58. Miller RM, Tenney SM. Dead space ventilation in old age. *J Appl Physiol.* 1956;9(3):321–327.

59. Carskadon MA, Dement WC. Respiration during sleep in the aged human. *J Gerontol.* 1981;36(4):420–423.

60. Kronenberg RS, Drage CW. Attenuation of the ventilatory and heart rate responses to hypoxia and hypercapnia with aging in normal men. *J Clin Invest.* 1973;52(8):1812–1819.

61. Peterson DD, Pack AI, Silage DA, et al. Effects of aging on ventilatory and occlusion pressure responses to hypoxia and hypercapnia. *Am Rev Respir Dis.* 1981;124(4):387–391.

62. Don HF, Wahba M, Cuadrado L, et al. The effects of anesthesia and 100 percent oxygen on the functional residual capacity of the lungs. *Anesthesiology.* 1970;32(6):521–529.

63. Rehder K. Mechanics of the lung and chest wall. *Acta Anaesthesiol Scand Suppl.* 1990;94:32–36.

64. Fishman AP. Acute hypoxia and pulmonary vasoconstriction in humans: uncovering the mechanism of the pressor response. *Am J Physiol Lung Cell Mol Physiol.* 2004;287(5):L893–L894.

65. Arunasalam K, Davenport HT, Painter S, et al. Ventilatory response to morphine in young and old subjects. *Anaesthesia.* 1983;38(6):529–533.

66. Haraguchi S, Koizumi K, Hatori N, et al. Prediction of the postoperative pulmonary function and complication rate in elderly patients. *Surg Today.* 2001;31(10):860–865.

67. Okada M, Nishio W, Sakamoto T, et al. Long–term survival and prognostic factors of five–year survivors with complete resection of non–small cell lung carcinoma. *J Thorac Cardiovasc Surg.* 2003;126(2):558–562.

68. Birim O, Zuydendorp HM, Maat AP, et al. Lung resection for non–small–cell lung cancer in patients older than 70: mortality, morbidity, and late survival compared with the general population. *Ann Thorac Surg.* 2003;76(6):1796–1801.

69. Osterberg T, Era P, Gause–Nilsson I, et al. Dental state and functional capacity in 75–year–olds in three Nordic localities. *J Oral Rehabil.* 1995;22(8):653–660.

70. Seymour DG, Pringle R, Shaw JW. The role of the routine pre–operative chest x–ray in the elderly general surgical patient. *Postgrad Med J.* 1982;58(686):741–745.

71. Ishaq M, Kamal RS, Aqil M. Value of routine pre–operative chest x–ray in patients over the age of 40 years. *J Pak Med Assoc.* 1997;47 (11):279–281.

72. Silvestri L, Maffessanti M, Gregori D, et al. Usefulness of routine preoperative chest radiography for anaesthetic management: a prospective multicentre pilot study. *Eur J Anaesthesiol.* 1999;16(11):749–760.

73. Tornebrandt K, Fletcher R. Pre–operative chest x–rays in elderly patients. *Anaesthesia.* 1982;37(9):901–902.

74. Kearney DJ, Lee TH, Reilly JJ, et al. Assessment of operative risk in patients undergoing lung resection. Importance of predicted pulmonary function. *Chest.* 1994;105(3):753–759.

75. Ribas J, Diaz O, Barbera JA, et al. Invasive exercise testing in the evaluation of patients at high–risk for lung resection. *Eur Respir J.* 1998;12(6):1429–1435.

76. Beckles MA, Spiro SG, Colice GL, et al. The physiologic evaluation of patients with lung cancer being considered for resectional surgery. *Chest.* 2003;123(1 Suppl.):105S–114S.

77. Ferguson MK, Reeder LB, Mick R. Optimizing selection of patients for major lung resection. *J Thorac Cardiovasc Surg.* 1995;109(2):275–281; discussion 281–273.

78. Mazzone PJ, Arroliga AC. Lung cancer: preoperative pulmonary evaluation of the lung resection candidate. *Am J Med.* 2005;118(6): 578–583.

79. Gerson MC, Hurst JM, Hertzberg VS, et al. Prediction of cardiac and pulmonary complications related to elective abdominal and noncardiac thoracic surgery in geriatric patients. *Am J Med.* 1990;88(2): 101–107.

80. Richter Larsen K, Svendsen UG, Milman N, et al. Exercise testing in the preoperative evaluation of patients with bronchogenic carcinoma. *Eur Respir J.* 1997;10(7):1559–1565.

81. Villani F, Busia A. Preoperative evaluation of patients submitted to pneumonectomy for lung carcinoma: role of exercise testing. *Tumori.* 2004;90(4):405–409.

82. Brunelli A, Monteverde M, Al Refai M, et al. Stair climbing test as a predictor of cardiopulmonary complications after pulmonary lobectomy in the elderly. *Ann Thorac Surg.* 2004;77(1):266–270.

83. Hurd S. The impact of COPD on lung health worldwide: epidemiology and incidence. *Chest.* 2000;117(2 Suppl.):1S–4S.

84. Dehn MM, Bruce RA. Longitudinal variations in maximal oxygen intake with age and activity. *J Appl Physiol.* 1972;33(6):805–807.

85. Pelosi P, Croci M, Ravagnan I, et al. Total respiratory system, lung, and chest wall mechanics in sedated–paralyzed postoperative morbidly obese patients. *Chest.* 1996;109(1):144–151.

86. Thomas EJ, Goldman L, Mangione CM, et al. Body mass index as a correlate of postoperative complications and resource utilization. *Am J Med.* 1997;102(3):277–283.

87. Smetana GW. Preoperative pulmonary evaluation. *N Engl J Med.* 1999; 340(12):937–944.

88. Shochat T, Pillar G. Sleep apnea in the older adult: pathophysiology, epidemiology, consequences, and management. *Drugs Aging.* 2003;20(8): 551–560.

89. Pack AI, Millman RP. Changes in control of ventilation, awake, and asleep, in the elderly. *J Am Geriatr Soc.* 1986;34(7):533–544.

90. Krieger J, Sforza E, Boudewijns A, et al. Respiratory effort during obstructive sleep apnea: role of age and sleep state. *Chest.* 1997;112(4): 875–884.

91. Dealberto MJ, Pajot N, Courbon D, et al. Breathing disorders during sleep and cognitive performance in an older community sample: the EVA Study. *J Am Geriatr Soc.* 1996;44(11):1287–1294.

92. Jemal A, Murray T, Ward E, et al. Cancer statistics, 2005. *CA Cancer J Clin.* 2005;55(1):10–30.

93. Ely EW, Wheeler AP, Thompson BT, et al. Recovery rate and prognosis in older persons who develop acute lung injury and the acute respiratory distress syndrome. *Ann Intern Med.* 2002;136(1):25–36.

94. Anderson ME, Belani KG. Short–term preoperative smoking abstinence. *Am Fam Physician.* 1990;41(4):1191–1194.

95. Lindstrom D, Wladis A, Linder S, et al. Preoperative cessation of smoking seems to reduce the frequency of complications. *Lakartidningen.* 2004;101(21–22):1920–1922.

96. Gracey DR, Divertie MB, Didier EP. Preoperative pulmonary preparation of patients with chronic obstructive pulmonary disease: a prospective study. *Chest.* 1979;76(2):123–129.

97. Pien LC, Grammer LC, Patterson R. Minimal complications in a surgical population with severe asthma receiving prophylactic corticosteroids. *J Allergy Clin Immunol.* 1988;82(4):696–700.

98. Gold MI, Helrich M. A study of complications related to anesthesia in asthmatic patients. *Anesth Analg.* 1963;42:238–293.

99. Warner DO, Warner MA, Barnes RD, et al. Perioperative respiratory complications in patients with asthma. *Anesthesiology.* 1996;85(3): 460–467.

100. Tsui BC, Wagner A, Finucane B. Regional anaesthesia in the elderly: a clinical guide. Drugs Aging. 2004;21(14):895–910.

101. Joyne M. Aging: physiology and anesthetic implications. In: Faust R, ed. *Anesthesiology Review.* 2nd ed. Philadelphia: Churchill Livingstone; 1994:194–195.

102. Gruber EM, Tschernko EM. Anaesthesia and postoperative analgesia in older patients with chronic obstructive pulmonary disease: special considerations. *Drugs Aging.* 2003;20(5):347–360.

103. Brooks–Brunn JA. Validation of a predictive model for postoperative pulmonary complications. *Heart Lung.* 1998;27(3):151–158.

104. Arozullah AM, Khuri SF, Henderson WG, et al. Development and validation of a multifactorial risk index for predicting postoperative pneumonia after major noncardiac surgery. *Ann Intern Med.* 2001;135(10):847–857.

105. Brooks–Braun J. Predictors of postoperative pulmonary complications following abdominal surgery. *Chest.* 1997;111:564–571.

Endocrine System

A.D. John

With aging, alterations occur in the endocrine system, which have implications for geriatric anesthesia. This chapter summarizes the changes in the aging endocrine system which have important bearing on management of the elderly surgical patient.

THYROID

There are minimal changes in thyroid physiology, which occur with normal aging. In older persons, there is a lower thyroid-stimulating hormone (TSH) response to thyrotropin-releasing hormone (TRH) stimulation. In addition, total T_3 is decreased. In older men, there is an increase in baseline TSH levels and a decrease in free T_3 and free T_4 levels. Although thyroid physiology is not significantly altered with age, abnormalities in thyroid function are common in the elderly. Hypothyroidism occurs in 10% of females and 2% of males older than 60 years.[1] Hyperthyroidism is less common in the aged than hypothyroidism.

Numerous drugs can affect thyroid function (Table 6–1). This is important, as polypharmacy is common in the elderly. Of note is amiodarone. Amiodarone may cause thyroid abnormalities, which range from changes in thyroid function tests to thyrotoxicosis or hypothyroidism.

▶ Hyperthyroidism

Hyperthyroidism[1–3] is a hypermetabolic state with characteristic signs and symptoms including tremor, tachycardia, weakness, fatigability, palpitations, exopthalmos, sweating, heat intolerance, diarrhea, weight loss, and goiter. In the elderly, manifestations of hyperthyroidism[1–3] are often atypical and it is necessary to have a high index of suspicion. Symptoms can mimic other diseases of the elderly or be erroneously attributed to aging. Myopathy is often the most common sign and symptom of hyperthyroidism, but the need to exclude it as a side effect of cholesterol-lowering medications, or as a result of rheumatological disease, or deconditioning is imperative. Cardiovascular symptoms may include angina, heart failure, and atrial fibrillation. Changes from baseline in an elderly patient such as agitation, confusion, dementia, depression, lethargy, fatigue, or weakness may also be a manifestation of hyperthyroidism in the elderly. Another common problem in the elderly is that medications can mask the classic signs and symptoms of hyperthyroidism. For instance, beta-blockers decrease the heart rate, lower blood pressure, and suppress tremors. The signs and symptoms in the elderly are thus more subtle and hyperthyroidism should be borne in mind when there is atrial fibrillation, heart failure, lethargy, weakness, changes in mental status, moods, or baseline level of functioning.[1–4]

Most cases of hyperthyroidism in the elderly are accounted for by Graves' disease and toxic multinodular goiter. Hyperfunctioning thyroid nodule, adenoma, subacute thyroiditis, follicular carcinoma, excess thyroid hormone ingestion, and secondary causes such as a TSH-secreting pituitary tumor are less common. Diagnosis is made by a markedly suppressed TSH (<0.05 mcU/mL) and an elevated FT4 (free T4) (Table 6-2).

In the elderly, toxic multinodular goiter[1,2] is more common and often has been present for a period of time with subclinical hyperthyroidism being the presentation. Multinodular goiter is associated with both venous obstruction and tracheal compression. These should be excluded by examination and radiographical study with computed tomography (CT) scan or magnetic resonance imaging (MRI). Therapy for multinodular goiter consists of antithyroid medications and beta-blockers to decrease the symptoms of hyperthyroidism, radioactive iodine (I 131) to make the patient euthyroid, and surgery if compression or obstruction exists.[1,2]

Graves' disease[2,5] is caused by TSH receptor antibodies, which stimulate the thyroid and are associated with other autoimmune manifestations such as pernicious anemia, Addison's disease, Graves' dermatopathy, and ophthalmopathy.

Solitary hyperfunctioning adenoma are diagnosed clinically or by ultrasound and confirmed by radionuclide scan. Solitary hyperfunctioning adenoma responds well to radioactive iodine.[2,6] Subacute thyroiditis may be associated with pain and tenderness and results from leakage of thyroid hormones from the thyroid gland after a viral infection. The radionuclide uptake is reduced, but serum thyroglobulins are elevated, and antithyroid antibodies may be transiently present. Treatment involves symptomatic relief with aspirin, nonsteroidal anti-inflammatory drugs, beta-blockers, and glucocorticoid for patients nonresponsive to aspirin and nonsteroidal anti-inflammatory drugs (NSAIDs). Hyperthyroidism may also be caused by exogenous iodine administration, which can occur in a variety of ways including foods, vitamins, herbals, radiocontrast materials, and medications especially amiodarone (see Table 6–1).[1–3,7]

Subclinical hyperthyroidism[8] is a laboratory diagnosis with a suppressed TSH and a normal free thyroxine (FT4) and free triiodothyronine (FT3). The causes of persistent subclinical hyperthyroidism include multinodular goiter, Graves' disease, thyroid adenoma, and either excessive thyroid replacement therapy or intentional thyroid suppressive therapy. Manifestations in the elderly may include

Table 6.1

Drugs Affecting Thyroid*

Drugs Causing Hypothyroidism

A. Inhibition of thyroid hormone synthesis and/or release

   1. Lithium (acts like iodine)

   2. Amiodarone

   3. Iodine (expectorants, potassium iodine solutions—SSKI,* Radiocontrast material, betadine douches, topical antiseptics)

   4. Aminogluthimide

   5. Interferon-α

   6. Interleukin-2

   7. Thionamides

   8. Perchlorate

B. Decreased absorption of T4 due to hormone binding in the intestine

   1. Cholestyramine

   2. Colistipol

   3. Aluminum hydroxide

   4. Calcium carbonate

   5. Sucralfate

   6. Iron sulfate

Drugs Causing Hyperthyroidism

   1. Amiodarone (due to its iodine contents)

   2. Iodine ingestion

   3. Radiographic contrast media

   4. Interferon-α

*SSKI, saturated solution of potassium iodine.
Source: Reprinted with permission from Ref. 1.

Table 6-2

Thyroid-Stimulating Hormone Abnormalities

A. Causes of High TSH (thyroid-stimulating hormone)

   1. Hypothyroidism

   2. Recovery from severe illness

   3. Pituitary excess due to pituitary tumors causing secondary hyperthyroidism (very rare)

B. Causes of Low TSH (thyroid-stimulating hormone)

   1. Hyperthyroid state

     a. Both T3 and T4 elevated

       1. Graves' disease

       2. Toxic multinodular goiter

     b. Only T3 elevated with normal T4

       1. T3 toxicosis (Graves' disease)

       2. Exogenous T3 ingestion (cytomel)

     c. Only T4 elevated with normal T3

       1. Hyperthyroidism patient with nausea, vomiting, and starvation causing decreased conversion of T4 to T3.

   2. Hypothyroid state

     1. Pituitary or hypothalamic disease (both T4 and T3 low)

   3. Euthyroid rate

     1. Sick euthyroid (both T3, T4 low, rT3* elevated)

     2. Drugs such as glucocorticoids, octreatide, and dopamine

*rT3, reverse T3 (triiodothyronine).
Source: Adapted from Ref. 1.

palpitations, tremor, heat intolerance, anxiety, fear, and inability to concentrate. There may be an increased risk of Alzheimer's or dementia.[8,9] Cardiovascular complications[8] of subclinical hyperthyroidism include sinus tachycardia, atrial premature beats, atrial fibrillation, and over time the increased cardiac workload leads to an increase in ventricular mass with resulting diastolic and systolic dysfunction. In older patients, the increased cardiac dysfunction may contribute to an increased mortality in patients with subclinical hyperthyroidism.[8,10,11] Hyperthyroidism is associated with an increased risk of osteoporosis and fractures,[8,12] but whether this holds for subclinical hyperthyroidism as well is not quite clear. However, subclinical hyperthyroidism does lead to increased markers of bone turnover and may play a role in contributing to increased risk for osteoporosis and fractures.[8]

Patients with hyperthyroidism should not undergo elective surgery until a euthyroid state is achieved. However, occasionally surgical stress may precipitate thyrotoxicosis. In particular, with the elderly, it is important to recognize and manage thyroid storm. Thyroid storm is a life-threatening complication of Graves' manifested by tachycardia, hyperthermia, heart failure, neurological changes, and hepatic dysfunction and is often precipitated by trauma, infection, an iodine load, or surgery. The treatment of thyroid storm is outlined in Table 6–3.[2,5]

▶ Hypothyroidism

Hypothyroidism[1–3,13] is characterized by a generalized slowing of the metabolic state. Its symptoms include fatigue, lethargy, weakness, cold intolerance, slow speech with hoarseness, hypoactive reflexes, thickening, drying, and coarsening of the skin, a generalized slowing of mental processes, and memory impairment. Weight gain, constipation, nonpitting edema, hypercholesterolemia, hypertriglyceridemia, hyponatremia, and macrocytic anemia may also be found. Cardiovascular signs and symptoms include bradycardia, atrial fibrillation, and heart failure. There are often musculoskeletal signs and symptoms including carpal tunnel syndrome, weakness and difficulty moving, cerebellar dysfunction, and neuropathy. It is important to note that the manifestations of hypothyroidism in the elderly are not quite as clear as those in younger people, and symptoms of coexisting disease may cloud the clinical picture.[1,2,4,14]

Failure of the thyroid gland is the principle cause of hypothyroidism, with secondary hypothyroidism due to failure of the hypothalamus-pituitary axis occurring less frequently. Primary causes of hypothyroidism include autoimmune lymphocytic thyroiditis (Hashimoto's thyroiditis and atrophic thyroiditis, postablative); subacute thyroiditis; drug-induced resulting from amiodarone, cytokines, lithium, and interferon; iodine-associated including both iodine deficiency and iodine-induced; and subclinical hypothyroidism. Testing for hypothyroidism includes both TSH and free thyroxine (FT4) (Table 6–2). If TSH is high and FT4 is low, then the cause is most likely primary hypothyroidism. If TSH is high and FT4 is normal, then most likely there is subclinical hypothyroidism. If TSH is high and FT4 is

Table 6-3

Treatment of Thyroid Storm

Treatment	Dose and Route	Action
β-Blockers		
Propranolol	▷ 1 mg/min IV (as required) and 60–80 mg every 4 h po or by NG tube	Antagonizes effects of increased adrenergic tone, blocks T4-to-T3 conversion
Esmolol (alternative)	▷ 250–500 ug/kg IV followed by IV infusion 50–100 ug/kg/min	
Thionamides		
Propylthiouracil	▷ 800–1000 mg po immediately, then 200 mg every 4 h po or by NG tube	Blocks new thyroid hormone synthesis,
Methimazole (alternative)	▷ 30 mg po immediately, then 30 mg every 6 h po or by NG tube	blocks T4-to-T3 conversion (propylthiouracil only)
Iodinated contrast agents*		
Iopanoic acid or ipodate	▷ 0.5–1.0 g/d po or by NG tube	Blocks T4-to-T3 conversion, blocks thyroid hormone release (via iodine release)
Iodine		
Lugol's solution	▷ 10 drops tid po or by NG tube	Blocks thyroid hormone release
or SSKI	▷ 5 drops every 6 h po or by NG tube	
or Sodium iodide	▷ 0.5–1.0 g IV every 12 h	
Glucocorticoids		
Hydrocortisone	▷ 100 mg IV every 8 h	Blocks T4-to-T3 conversion, immunosuppression
or Dexamethasone	▷ 2 mg IV every 6 h	

Note: IV = intravenously, po = by mouth, NG = nasogastric, T4 = thyroxine, T3 = triiodothyronine, SSKI = saturated solution of potassium iodide, tid = three times a day. ˙Limited availability.
Source: Reprinted with permission from Ref. 5.

high, there is the possibility of pituitary dysfunction, resistance to thyroid hormone, or testing artifact.[1–3,13]

To optimize surgical outcome it is best to obtain a euthyroid state prior to surgery. However, subclinical cases of hypothyroidism have not been shown to significantly increase surgical risk. Current recommendations include continuing thyroid replacement on the day of surgery. In elderly patients predisposed to hypothyroidism, it is important to promptly recognize and treat myxedema coma. Myxedema coma[1,14] is a severe life-threatening, but very rare complication of hypothyroidism. According to Rehman et al.,[1] myxedema coma is more common in persons over 75 years old. An altered mental status,[1,14] which may present as confusion, disorientation, or lethargy, is one of the essential elements in the diagnosis of myxedema coma. The next important element in the diagnosis is defective temperature regulation with hypothermia. However, according to Fliers and Wiersinga[14] the temperature may be normal in a hypothermic patient with an infection. The third key element in the diagnosis of myxedema coma is the presence of a precipitating event, stress, or illness such as cold exposure or infection. Patients in myxedema coma are not only hypothermic, but frequently have altered sensorium and bradycardia. Treatment is outlined in Table 6–4. According to Fliers,[14] there appears to be a high mortality associated with myxedema coma.

Table 6-4

Characteristics and Treatment of Myxedema Coma

Hypothyroxinemia	Large doses of intravenous thyroxine
Hypothermia	Blankets, no active rewarming
Hypoventilation	Mechanical ventilation
Hypotension	Cautious use of volume expanders, vasopressors
Hyponatremia	Mild fluid restoration, hypertonic saline if necessary
Hypoglycemia	Glucose administration
Hypocortisolemia	Glucocorticoid administration
Precipitating event (e.g., infection, trauma, stroke, hypothermia, hemorrhage, diuretics, sedatives, burns, hypoglycemia)	Identification and elimination by specific treatment

Source: Reprinted with permission from Ref. 14.

PARATHYROID

There is an age-related increase in serum parathyroid hormone (PTH). In addition, there is age-related impairment in PTH receptor-mediated signaling, particularly in intestinal cells. However, the biologic relevance of these changes is unclear.

▶ Hyperparathyroidism

Primary hyperparathyroidism[15–17] tends to affect people over the age of 50 and postmenopausal women three times more frequently than men. Primary hyperparathyroidism tends to be a laboratory diagnosis with the following general criteria: serum calcium at least 1 mg/dL above normal, PTH elevation, serum phosphorous being either low/normal or low, and serum alkaline phosphatase possibly elevated. Once hypercalcemia is confirmed, diagnostic algorithms, as recommended in several endocrinology textbooks, may be followed to assess the etiology.[18]

The classic presentation of primary hyperparathyroidism, osteitis fibrosa cystica, is rarely seen. Most patients present with fairly well preserved central bone density. Although there is cortical thinning, trabecular plates are preserved both in number and connectivity. Primary hyperparathyroidism is associated with calcium phosphate deposition in the renal parenchyma along with an increase in nephrolithiasis. Creatinine clearance is often decreased, even without other causes. Hypertension, left ventricular hypertrophy, valvular and myocardial calcification, along with endothelial dysfunction and changes in vascular compliance or reactivity can be due to hyperparathyroidism. Although the classic muscle atrophy is rarely seen, most patients with primary hyperparathyroidism complain of weakness, fatigue, anxiety, and depression. With mild hyperparathyroidism pancreatitis is rarely observed but peptic ulcer disease may be present. In mild hyperparathyroidism, problems with dentition, anemia, and keratopathy are rarely seen, but both gout and pseudogout may occasionally be present although the mechanism for this remains unknown.[15]

Once the diagnosis of primary hyperparathyroidism is made, bone densitometry should be performed. According to the 2002 National Institutes of Health (NIH) Workshop guidelines,[15,19] surgery is recommended if serum calcium is greater than 1 mg/dL above normal, 24 h urinary calcium excretion exceeds 400 mg/day, creatinine clearance is reduced by 30%, and the T-score for bone density is less than 2.5, or age is less than 50. If surgery is not undertaken, medical therapy should include hydration, ambulation, the avoidance of thiazide diuretics, as well as the avoidance of high calcium diets (Table 6–5). There is a lack of safe and effective drug therapy. Oral phosphates may cause ectopic calcification and increases in PTH levels. Raloxifene lowers serum calcium and reduces bone turnover markers, but does not affect PTH levels. Alendronate may increase bone mineral density, but does not reduce calcium or PTH levels. Cinacalcet is a calcium mimetic that reduces serum calcium, but does not improve bone density.

▶ Hypoparathyroidism

The most common cause of hypoparathyroidism[18,20] is postsurgical (usually following thyroid surgery), and then autoimmune destruction of the parathyroid is the next most common cause. Hypocalcemia is often the presenting manifestation of hypoparathyroidism. The symptoms of hypocalcemia most commonly observed include perioral numbness and tingling, as well as numbness and tingling of the hand and feet. Abdominal cramping, bronchospasm, and laryngospasm may occur. Chvostek's sign (facial spasm as a result of tapping on the facial nerve) and Trousseau's sign (carpal spasm after inflation of the blood pressure cuff 20 mm Hg above systolic pressure) indicate significant hypocalcemia. Anxiety, confusion, psychosis, seizure may also occur along with arrhythmias and congestive heart failure. Diagnostic algorithms are well described for determining the cause of hypocalcemia.[18] Treatment usually includes calcium, vitamin D, correction of hypomagnesemia, and exclusion and correction of hypoalbuminemia. If renal failure is a cause, then there should be reduction of hyperphosphatemia with phosphate binders (Table 6–5).

The important anesthetic issues concerning parathyroid disease in the elderly focus on the effects of alterations in plasma calcium concentration. Hypocalcemia may cause prolongation of ST segments and QT interval. The effects of hypercalcemia on the electrocardiogram (ECG) are less specific. Hypercalcemia enhances digitalis toxicity.

Table 6-5

Treatments for Hyperparathyroidism and Hypoparathyroidism

Process Affected by Treatment	Treatment for Hyperparathyroidism	Treatment for Hypoparathyroidism
Secretion of parathyroid hormone by parathyroid gland	Parathyroidectomy Calcium-sensing-receptor agonist*	Parathyroid autograft
Activation of receptor for parathyroid hormone	Blocker or type 1 receptor*	Parathyroid hormone (1–34)*
Release of calcium from bone	Bisphosphonates Estrogen	
Uptake of calcium from gut	Blocker of vitamin D receptor*	Vitamin D analogue Calcium salts
Excretion of calcium in urine	Forced natriuresis	Thiazide
Exchange with extracorporeal calcium pool	Dialysis	Intravenous calcium

*This treatment is not currently available.
Source: Reprinted with permission from Ref. 20.

PAGET'S DISEASE

Paget's disease[21–23] affects older individuals, and is the second most common bone disorder after osteoporosis. It tends to affect men more than women. Patients with Paget's have a dull achy pain that is constant, worse with rest, weight bearing, and warmth. Less than 1% will have malignant transformation to osteosarcoma. Headaches, hearing loss, entrapment neuropathies, increased size of the head, hip or joint pain, bowing of the limbs, and kidney stones are possible. High-output cardiac failure and valvular calcification may occur. Many patients are initially asymptomatic and present with elevations of their alkaline phosphatase or have radiographic findings characteristic of the disease. Radioisotope bone scan and CT scan of the head and neck should be done, as well as analysis of alkaline phosphatase, liver function tests, and vitamin D. There appears to be a genetic component to the disease since one-fifth of patients with Paget's disease have had first-degree relatives with the disease. Although Paget's disease is not curable, the use of bisphosphonates such as pamidronate, alendronate, and risedronate along with vitamin D and calcitonin may halt progression and even cause remission of Paget's disease. The major anesthetic concern with Paget's disease is the technical difficulties, which may occur with performance of spinal and epidural anesthesia.

OSTEOPOROSIS

Osteoporosis[24,25] is the most common bone disorder and increasingly affects people as they continue to age. Osteoporosis is characterized by a net loss in bone, not a decrease in ratio of mineral to matrix as in osteomalacia. This leads to decreased strength and increased susceptibility to fractures with lower applied force. Osteoporotic fractures have a characteristic age-dependent pattern—wrist fractures tend to occur in the late fifties and early sixties, vertebral fractures in the sixties and seventies, and hip fractures in the seventies and eighties.[24,25]

Key to assessment of osteoporosis[24,25] is an assessment of risk factors (Table 6–6). The most prominent risk factor is age; as one ages the likelihood of osteoporosis increases, as does the likelihood of an osteoporotic fracture. The clinical presentation[24,25] of osteoporosis is pain, fracture, and subsequent deformity. Acute pain from a fracture usually does not last more than 3 months, but mechanical changes associated with the results of the fracture may lead to persistent discomfort. Valsalva maneuvers, straining, prolonged sitting or standing, and bending aggravate vertebral pain associated with osteoporotic fractures; whereas lying with knees and hips flexed on the side or rising from a lateral position tends to relieve vertebral osteoporotic fracture pain. Nerve rest pain, sciatica, diffuse generalized bone pain are not characteristic of osteoporotic pain. Malignancy and other causes must be excluded. Osteoporotic fractures are sudden and associated with minimally traumatic events or daily activities such as opening a window, coughing, lifting, a sudden movement, or a slight slip and fall. Osteoporotic fractures tend to be in the mid-lower thoracic vertebrae or lumbar vertebra and result in the kyphosis associated with elderly women. The presence of a fracture in the cervical or high thoracic (above T6/T7) region should prompt a search for malignancy or other pathology.[24,25]

Treatment for osteoporosis[24,26] includes weight resistance exercise to increase bone strength, physical therapy to improve strength, coordination to prevent falls, and medications. The use of estrogens as the mainstay for therapy has been curtailed after the release of the results from the Women's Health Initiative.[27] This study showed that

Table 6-6
Osteoporosis
Risk Factors for Osteoporosis
Advanced age
Female Gender
Asian, white, or Hispanic ethnicity
Small body size/weight <127 lb (57.7 kg)
Positive family history in first-degree relative(s)
Premature natural or surgical menopause
History of prolonged amenorrhea
Low calcium intake
Low vitamin D intake or exposure
Immobilization/sedentary lifestyle
Smoking
Alcoholism
Eating disorders (especially anorexia nervosa)
Hyperthyroidism (endogenous or exogenous)
Hyperparathyroidism
Malabsorption syndromes
Renal or liver disease
Rheumatoid arthritis
Medications Associated with Osteoporosis
Glucocorticoids
Excess thyroid hormone
Anticonvulsants (phenytoin, carbamazepine, phenobarbital)
Heparin
Cyclosporin A
Gonadotropin-releasing hormone analogues
Highly active antiretroviral therapy for AIDS
Chemotherapeutic agents causing hypogonadism
Excess vitamin A or D
Methotrexate
Loop diuretics
Neuroleptics, metoclopramide, and other drugs that raise prolactin

Source: Adapted from Ref. 25.

use of estrogens was associated with an increase in heart disease, stroke, deep vein thrombosis, pulmonary embolism, and breast and uterine cancer. Raloxifene is a selective estrogen receptor modulator that increases bone mass and decreases the risk of vertebral fractures. Whether raloxifene has all the adverse effects of estrogen is unknown. Calcitonin increases bone mass, but may not affect the rate of hip fractures and has side effects of nausea and flushing. The bisphosphonates—alendronate, risedronate, and pamidronate—inhibit osteoclast activity and may improve bone mass. Recombinant PTH, teriparatide, in small doses may stimulate bone formation and improve bone density. In Europe, strontium ranelate has been approved for the treatment of osteoporosis and reportedly decreases the risk of vertebral fracture, but side effects include headache, nausea, diarrhea, and venous thromboembolism. Calcium and vitamin D supplementation continue to be relatively safe as long as serum calcium levels are monitored, and care is taken when administered to patients with a history of nephrolithiasis.[24,26]

ADRENAL

The adrenal gland consists of the adrenal cortex with its three layers covering the adrenal medulla. The outer layer of the adrenal cortex, the zona glomerulosa, produces the mineral corticoid aldosterone. The middle layer of the adrenal cortex, the zona fasciculata, secretes the glucocorticoid cortisol. The innermost cortical layer, the zona reticularis, produces dihydroepiandrosterone sulfate (DHEA[S]). The function of DHEA(S) is not known. The adrenal medulla contains chromaffin cells, which principally secrete epinephrine and also a small amount of norepinephrine. The major age-related change in the adrenal cortex is a large decrease in biosynthesis of DHEA(S) associated with a reduction in size of the zona reticularis. Basal adrenaline secretion from the adrenal medulla is markedly reduced with aging. However, corresponding plasma levels of epinephrine do not change because of age-related decreases in plasma clearance.

Adrenal disorders are rare. In addition, adrenal conditions involving changes in hormone production are generally considered diseases of the younger age groups. As a result, the following comments will be confined to those of pertinence to the elderly.

▶ Hyperaldosteronism

Excess aldosterone production is classified as either primary (associated with suppressed renin production) or secondary (associated with increased renin production and activation of the renin-aldosterone system).[28] The causes of primary hyperaldosteronism are shown in Table 6–7. Causes of secondary hyperaldosteronism include hypovolemia, diuretic use, renal artery stenosis, and malignant hypertension.

Hyperaldosteronism affects older individuals, and as pointed out by Lim et al.[29] may be the cause of hypertension in about 10% of hypertensives. Mosso et al.[30] note that the more severe the hypertension, the greater the likelihood that hyperaldosteronism is a cause. In addition to hypertension, the adverse effects of hyperaldosteronism include ventricular hypertrophy, smooth muscle hypertrophy, endothelial dysfunction, fibrosis, and vascular damage.[31–33] Hyperaldosteronism is also associated with an increased rate of cardiovascular events.[34]

Hypertension caused by primary hyperaldosteronism due to an aldosteronoma may be surgically curable.[35] The key is to correctly diagnose the patient. Historically hyperaldosteronism[35,36] is associated with hypertension, hypokalemia, hypernatremia, alkalosis, and muscle weakness. The lack of hypokalemia is often taken as a false sense of reassurance that primary aldosteronism can be excluded. However, as Conn[37] noted, hyperaldosteronism may be present for years before hypokalemia becomes apparent. As recommended by Fehaily and Duh,[28] indications for hyperaldosteronism screening include hypertensive patients who are hypokalemic, difficult to control hypertensives who require multiple medications, and hypertensives who have left ventricular hypertrophy. Screening includes determination of a morning plasma aldosterone concentration and plasma renin activity measurement.[28] If the ratio of plasma aldosterone to plasma renin activity is greater than 30 with a plasma aldosterone concentration greater than or equal to 15 ng/L and plasma renin activity is less than or equal to 1 ng/mL/h, then the diagnosis of primary hyperaldosteronism can be made. Once the diagnosis of primary hyperaldosteronism is made, the next step is to determine whether it is an aldosterone producing adenoma (the primary cause) or whether it is idiopathic hyperaldosteronism (the next most frequent cause) (Table 6–8). The current recommendations for treatment are unilateral laparoscopic adrenalectomy for aldosterone-producing adenomas and pharmacotherapy with spironolactone for idiopathic hyperaldosteronism.[28,36] Anesthetic issues of concern in management of patients with hyperaldosteronism include hypertension and chronic hypokalemia. Chronic hypokalemia is associated with abnormal glucose tolerance and may suppress baroreceptor tone. Hypovolemia should be aggressively managed.

▶ Hypercortisolism

In the elderly patient presenting with Cushing's syndrome, treatment should focus on addressing the marked metabolic complications of Cushing's syndrome with its attendant increase in cardiovascular risk due to obesity, hypertension, diabetes, lipid disorders, hypercoagulability, and impaired fibrinolysis.[38,39] During anesthesia, the important management issues include hypertension, diabetic states, and fluid and electrolyte balance. In addition to increasing morbidity and mortality for the elderly, there are also the concomitant consequences of osteoporosis,[38] cognitive impairment,[40] and a decrease in brain volume that is only partially reversible after treatment of Cushing's syndrome.[41] There is now increasing evidence that sustained hypercortisol states are associated with cognitive dysfunction.[42] The interaction, if any, between hypercortisol states, anesthesia, and cognitive dysfunction is unclear at this time.

DIABETES

The American Diabetes Association[43] defines diabetes with reference to abnormal glucose tests, which have been confirmed with repeat testing on a different day. The three principle criteria used to define diabetes are contained in Table 6–9. Symptoms of diabetes include polyuria, polydipsia, weight loss, fatigue, weakness, blurred vision, poor wound healing, and increased frequency of infections. Risk factors for diabetes include age over 45 years; body mass index (BMI) >27; high risk ethnic group such as Native American, African American, Hispanic, and Asian; gestational diabetes or delivery of a large infant over 9 lb; impaired glucose tolerance; hypertension; high-density lipoprotein (HDL) less than 35 mg/dL, or triglycerides greater than 250 mg/dL.[43]

The American Diabetes Association[43] classifies diabetes as type I, type II, other specific types, and gestational diabetes (Table 6–10).

Table 6-7

Causes of Primary Hyperaldosteronism

Aldosterone-producing adenoma (APA), 60%*

Idiopathic hyperaldosteronism (IHA), 34%*

Angiotensin-II responsive adenoma, 5%

Unilateral primary adrenal hyperplasia (PAH), <1%

Glucocorticoid-remediable aldosteronism (GRA), <1%

Aldosterone-producing adrenocortical carcinoma, <1%

Familial hyperaldosteronism, type II, (FH-II), very rare

*Recent reports suggest that the frequency of APA is lower and the frequency of IHA is higher in populations screened for primary hyperaldosteronism.
Source: Reprinted with permission from Ref. 28.

Table 6-8

Differentiating between Aldosterone-Producing Adenomas (APA) and Idiopathic Hyperaldosteronism (IHA)

	APA, aldosteronoma	IHA
Frequency	60% (decreasing)	30% (increasing)
Age and sex	Young age (<50 years)	Older than APA
	More women	More men
Clinical features and severity of hypertension	Nonspecific features, high blood pressure that is more pronounced than IHA	Nonspecific features, high blood pressure
Biochemical features	▸ Severe hypokalemia (<3.0 mmol/L)	▸ Lesser degree of hypokalemia
	▸ Postural test: plasma aldosterone concentration does not change (unresponsive to angiotensin II)	▸ Postural test: plasma aldosterone concentration is increased
	▸ Salt loading does not affect aldosterone level	▸ Salt loading decreases aldosterone level
	▸ Angiotensin-converting enzyme inhibitor does not affect aldosterone level	▸ Angiotensin-converting enzyme inhibitor decreases aldosterone level
	▸ Aldosterone secretion is influenced by ACTH (circadian rhythm)	▸ Normal plasma levels or cortisol, 18-oxocortisol and 18-hydroxy cortisol
	▸ Higher plasma aldosterone concentrations (>25 ng/dL or 700 pmol/l), and aldosterone excretion (>30 mcg/24 h) than IHA	
	▸ Increased plasma levels of cortisol, 18-oxocortisol and 18-hydroxy cortisol	
Imaging	CT scan: solitary adrenal tumor, usually <2 cm	CT scan: normal or bilateral enlargement
	NP-59; unilateral uptake	NP-59; negative or bilateral uptake
Treatment	Unilateral laparoscopic adrenalectomy	Medical treatment with mineralocorticoid receptor antagonists

Source: Reprinted with permission from Ref. 28.

Type I diabetes is characterized by an insulin deficiency usually due to beta-cell destruction. This may be idiopathic without associated autoimmunity or specific human leukocyte antigen (HLA) type. Immune-mediated is, however, the more common version of type I diabetes. It is associated with one or more antibodies to islet cells,

Table 6-9

Criteria for the Diagnosis of Diabetes Mellitus

1. Symptoms of diabetes plus casual plasma glucose concentration >200 mg/dL (11.1 mmol/L). Casual is defined as any time of day without regard to time since last meal. The classic symptoms of diabetes include polyuria, polydipsia, and unexplained weight loss.

or

2. Fasting plasma glucose >126 mg/dL (7.0 mmol/L). Fasting is defined as no caloric intake for at least 8 h.

or

3. 2-h postload glucose >200 mg/dL (11.1 mmol/L) during an oral glucose tolerance test (OGTT). The test should be performed as described by the World Health Organization, using a glucose load containing the equivalent of 75 g anhydrous glucose dissolved in water.

Note: In the absence of unequivocal hyperglycemia, these criteria should be confirmed by repeat testing on a different day. The third measure (OGTT) is not recommended for routine clinical use.
Source: Reprinted with permission from Ref. 43.

insulin, tyrosine phosphatases, and glutamic acid decarboxylase[44] and there is a higher incidence of HLA types DR3 and DR4. Viral infections such as coxsackie or mumps may also lead to beta-cell destruction and type I diabetes. Type II has a hereditary concordance greater than 80% between identical twins. However, type II is also more difficult to define because it encompasses a progression from decreased insulin and glucose sensitivity, to increased insulin production, to progressive beta-cell desensitization to glucose, and ultimately to decreased insulin production. Gestational diabetes is both a specific entity and a risk factor for type II diabetes. Other specific types of diabetes include genetic diseases, pancreatic diseases, endocrine diseases, and drugs.[43]

Not only are there many causes of diabetes, but also there are numerous types of complications that arise from it because of the multiplicity of systems affected by the disease.[43,45–47] Major complications can involve the cardiovascular, renal, gastrointestinal, neurological, and ophthalmologic systems as well as the occurrence of an increased incidence of infection and foot ulcers.

▸ Diabetes-related complications and treatment goals

Assessment

As with all aspects of medicine, the evaluation of diabetes begins with a complete history and physical, with an analysis of laboratory results and records of prior evaluations and referrals. Current

Table 6-10

Etiologic Classification of Diabetes Mellitus

I. Type 1 diabetes (β-cell destruction, usually leading to absolute insulin deficiency)

   A. Immune-mediated

   B. Idiopathic

II. Type 2 diabetes (may range from predominantly insulin resistance with relative Insulin deficiency to a predominantly secretory defect with insulin resistance)

III. Other specific types

   A. Genetic defects of β-cell function

     1. Chromosome 12, HNF-1α (MODY3)

     2. Chromosome 7, glucokinase (MODY2)

     3. Chromosome 20, HNF-4α (MODY1)

     4. Chromosome 13, insulin promoter factor-1 (IPF-1; MODY4)

     5. Chromosome 17, HNF-1β (MODY5)

     6. Chromosome 2, NeuroD1 (MODY6)

     7. Mitochondrial DNA

     8. Others

   B. Genetic defects in insulin action

     1. Type A insulin resistance

     2. Leprechaunism

     3. Rabson-Mendenhall syndrome

     4. Lipoatrophic diabetes

     5. Others

   C. Diseases of the exocrine pancreas

     1. Pancreatitis

     2. Trauma/pancreatectomy

     3. Neoplasia

     4. Cystic fibrosis

     5. Hemochromatosis

     6. Fibrocalculous pancreatopathy

     7. Others

   D. Endocrinopathies

     1. Acromegaly

     2. Cushing's syndrome

     3. Glucagonoma

     4. Pheochromocytoma

     5. Hyperthyroidism

     6. Somatostatinoma

     7. Aldosteronoma

     8. Others

   E. Drug- or chemical-induced

     1. Vacor

     2. Pentamidine

     3. Nicotinic acid

     4. Glucocorticoids

     5. Thyroid hormone

     6. Diazoxide

     7. β-adrenergic agonists

     8. Thiazides

     9. Dilantin

     10. α-Interferon

     11. Others

   F. Infections

     1. Congenital rubella

     2. Cytomegalovirus

     3. Others

   G. Uncommon forms of immune-mediated diabetes

     1. "Stiff-man" syndrome

     2. Anti-insulin receptor antibodies

     3. Others

   H. Other genetic syndromes sometimes associated with diabetes

     1. Down syndrome

     2. Klinefelter's syndrome

     3. Turner's syndrome

     4. Wolfram syndrome

     5. Friedreich's ataxia

     6. Huntington's chorea

     7. Laurence-Moon-Biedl syndrome

     8. Myotonic dystrophy

     9. Porphyria

     10. Prader-Willi syndrome

     11. Others

IV. Gestational diabetes mellitus (GDM)

Source: Reprinted with permission from Ref. 43.

medications, treatments, and compliance with prior treatments and medications provide insight as to both the severity of the disease process and efficacy of the therapeutic modalities. Nutritional status, eating habits, health beliefs, exercise patterns, and the use of tobacco, alcohol, and other substances provide important information. Assessment for risk factors of atherosclerotic disease such as smoking, hypertension, obesity, lipid disorders, and family history should be done. A history of infections as well as episodes of hypoglycemia and ketoacidosis should be sought. During the review of systems, emphasis should be placed on eliciting information concerning ongoing cardiac, neurological, peripheral vascular, cerebrovascular, ophthalmologic, and infectious disease processes. In analyzing the medication list, emphasis should be placed on the potential for medications to affect blood glucose levels and also to avoid possible drug-drug interactions. This requires significant effort because in the elderly, polypharmacy tends to be the rule rather than the exception.

The physical examination should be comprehensive and also focused in order to obtain the maximal amount of information with reference to the patient's current state of diabetic control and potential anesthetic and operative issues. Information on height and weight with a calculation of BMI is useful in determining whether there is coexisting obesity and also the degree of obesity. Blood pressure and heart rate values should be examined along with orthostatic values. Many patients, especially the elderly and the hospitalized, have abnormal intravascular volume status. An accurate assessment of volume status is essential for proper intraoperative and postoperative fluid management. Not only is the combination of blood pressure and heart rate informative as to hemodynamic and fluid status, but also the heart rate alone provides useful information. If a patient is tachycardic, it is important to ascertain why. One must ask: Is the patient in pain? Is the patient about to be septic? Is the patient's metabolic demand exceeding the body's ability to compensate? Is the patient hypoglycemic? Is the patient undergoing stress with a catechol response? Is the patient inadequately beta-blocked? Similarly, if a patient is bradycardic, one must ask: Is the patient septic? Has the patient's metabolic demand exceeded the body's ability to compensate? Is the patient catechol depleted? Is the patient overly beta-blocked? A working differential must be in place prior to induction of anesthesia in order to ensure optimal patient care.

The oral examination is very revealing not only in terms of airway examination, but also in terms of overall health. Poor oral hygiene tends to be reflective of poor overall health care and a lack of attention to health maintenance. In examining the neck, range of motion should be assessed since diabetics tend to have stiff joints and a decreased range of motion. The carotids should be auscultated for bruits and the potential for cerebrovascular disease. The cardiac examination should include rate, rhythm, murmurs, clicks, radiation, point of maximal impulse, and thrills. This allows one to evaluate the cardiac function and physical findings and determine both a baseline prior to an operative procedure and if any interval changes have occurred. An examination of the extremities for signs of peripheral vascular disease including the presence, absence, and strength of peripheral pulsations should be done, along with an assessment for unrecognized infection. The abdominal examination should focus on the presence or absence of organomegaly, masses, infection, bruits, and bowel sounds. The neurological examination should include an evaluation of the mental status, motor strength, reflexes, coordination, and sensory deficits. The lungs should be auscultated to exclude pulmonic processes.

Since elderly diabetic patients tend to be on multiple medications, obtaining a metabolic profile may be worthwhile. The levels of key electrolytes, sodium, and potassium should be determined. Current glucose levels both in reference to a patient's baseline and as a baseline for subsequent comparisons are useful. A Hg A1c is useful to indicate overall glycemic control with the current American Diabetes Association recommendation being below 7 and values above 10 corresponding to poor control.[47] A fasting lipid profile provides information as to concomitant cardiovascular risk rather than acute glycemic issues. The serum creatinine along with blood urea nitrogen (BUN) helps to provide information on volume status and renal function. However, it must be borne in mind that as patients age, their muscle mass diminishes as does the creatinine that one measures. Since urinary tract infections tend to be common among diabetics, a urinalysis can provide insight as to the presence of infection, ketones, protein, and sediment. Ideally, tests for microalbuminuria provide the earliest indications of renal disease in diabetics. The ECG should be analyzed for rate, rhythm, presence of atrial hypertrophy, ventricular enlargement, ectopy, and signs of prior myocardial infarction. Any interval change since the prior ECG should bear in mind the higher incidence of silent myocardial infarctions among diabetics. In examining the chest films, the lung characteristics, the size and position of the heart and great vessels, the degree of calcification of the bony structures and vertebrae, the presence or absence of fluid collections, and characteristics of the diaphragm should be noted.

Cardiovascular disease and diabetes

There is a higher incidence of cardiovascular disease in patients with diabetes.[48–50] Diabetics are at increased risk not only for myocardial infarction, but also for death prior to reaching the hospital with a myocardial infarction.[51] The National Cholesterol Education Program has defined diabetes as a coronary heart disease risk equivalent because of the high risk of developing coronary artery disease within a decade of being diagnosed with diabetes and the higher mortality associated with diabetes and coronary artery disease.[52] With the current intensive focus on cardiovascular disease, the risk of cardiovascular death has decreased, but there has not been a decrease in cardiovascular death in patients with diabetes.[53] Thus, risk factor modification assumes greater significance in diabetics since aggressive risk factor modification has proven beneficial in terms of nondiabetics and cardiovascular disease. The American Diabetes Association has taken this into consideration in the strong advocacy for risk factor modification for diabetics with special emphasis on hypertension, hyperlipidemia, antiplatelet therapy, smoking cessation, and coronary heart disease screenings.[47]

With regard to hypertension, the two key studies are UK Prospective Diabetes Study (UKPDS) and the Hypertension Optimal Treatment (HOT) trial.[54–56] The UKPDS found that although intensive glucose therapy was beneficial in reducing cardiovascular events, there was an even more significant effect with reducing blood pressures for both cardiovascular and cerebrovascular events. The HOT study demonstrated that aggressive diastolic blood pressure reduction reduced cardiovascular mortality. These findings have been incorporated into the current Joint National Committee (JNC) on prevention, detection, evaluation, and treatment of high blood pressure (JNC-7) guidelines.[57] JNC-7 acknowledges that gaining control of blood pressure may be difficult and that most patients will require more than one medication for blood pressure control. In high-risk cardiovascular patients, angiotensin-converting enzyme

(ACE) inhibitors have been shown to improve cardiovascular morbidity and mortality.[58,59] Both the American Diabetes Association[47] and the American Geriatric Society[60] recommend close monitoring of renal function, electrolytes, and orthostatic vitals when employing ACE inhibitors and diuretics to control blood pressure especially in the elderly who may require more than one medication in order to achieve desired blood pressure goals. Despite all the recommendations and the higher prevalence of hypertension among diabetics, hypertension remains for the large part uncontrolled.[61]

Dyslipidemias are widely prevalent among diabetics and are part of the complex relationship between diabetes and associated cardiovascular and cerebrovascular events leading to increased morbidity and mortality. Multiple studies have shown the clear benefit of aggressive lipid management. The Heart Protection Study[62] noted a decrease in cardiovascular mortality of over 20% with the use of simvastatin. This was in keeping with the prior findings of the Scandinavian Simvastatin Survival Study,[63] which showed that use of simvastatin led to both a decrease in mortality and also a decrease in the need for further revascularizations. Since triglycerides tend to be one of the major lipid abnormalities for diabetics, it has been shown that the reduction of triglycerides can also beneficially affect mortality.[64] Further work from the British Heart Protection Study provides clear data that for patients with diabetes, cholesterol-lowering therapy with a statin is beneficial in reducing major vascular events even if the patient only has diabetes, but does not have coronary artery disease or high cholesterol.[65] The American Diabetes Association has utilized this information to help establish its recommendations for lipid goals.[47] To achieve these goals combination therapy with statins, fibrates, and niacin may be necessary. But as both the number of medications used and the dosage of the medications are increased, the likelihood of associated drug toxicities increases, and great care must be taken to prevent side effects and toxic reactions.[47] In keeping with this are the findings of the Lescol Intervention Prevention Study (LIPS) group, which note that diabetics have a worse outcome after coronary interventions, but the use of a statin—fluvastatin—led to a morbid reduction of over 50% in major adverse cardiac events.[66]

Diabetes is associated with prothrombotic state that contributes to the increased risk of higher mortality from cardiovascular disease.[67,68] Diabetics are at increased risk for both atherosclerosis and vascular thrombosis, partly due to changes in the coagulation and fibrinolytic systems and also platelet abnormalities. Platelets are hypersensitive to aggregating agents and there is increased production of thromboxane which leads to both vasoconstriction and platelet aggregation. One of the early studies showing the benefits of aspirin was the Physicians Health Study,[69] which noted a marked reduction in myocardial infarctions among diabetic physicians on aspirin. Subsequent work such as the HOT trial[56] has continued to show both a significant reduction in cardiovascular events, as well as a marked decrease in myocardial infarction for patients on aspirin. Colwell[67] presents information as to the beneficial effect of aspirin plus clopidogrel in acute coronary syndromes and also the beneficial effect of aspirin plus glycoprotein 2b/3a inhibitors on decreasing mortality in patients with acute coronary syndromes; although there is an increase in the likelihood of bleeding with this combination. However, the beneficial effects on mortality justify the use of this combination therapy.

Recent studies[70] have indicated that current assessment guidelines may miss a number of patients with silent ischemia. However, there are still no well-established data in asymptomatic patients that advanced testing with nuclear stress tests or stress echocardiography leads to better outcomes. Rather, the emphasis should be on risk reduction and encouraging the adoption of proven beneficial therapy such as lipid reduction, blood pressure control, smoking cessation, weight reduction, increased physical activity, and aspirin therapy. Following this, a detailed history and physical examination with laboratory and ECG analysis, determination of exercise capacity, and adherence to the American Heart Association/American College of Cardiology (AHA/ACC) preoperative assessment guidelines lead to optimal patient care.

Diabetic neuropathy

Seventy-five to ninety percent of all diabetics have diabetic neuropathy with the elderly having more pronounced effects. The American Diabetes Association[71] classifies neuropathies as sensory neuropathies—acute sensory neuropathy and chronic distal symmetric polyneuropathy, focal and multifocal neurophthisis, and autonomic neuropathy.

Autonomic neuropathy[71–75] has many clinical manifestations and it may be difficult to determine which neuropathies are not attributable to diabetes and to correctly diagnose and exclude them. Cardiovascular manifestations include resting tachycardia, exercise intolerance, orthostatic hypotension, cardiac degeneration and silent myocardial infarction, alterations in blood flow to skin and extremities, and temperature intolerance. The gastrointestinal system is affected with a variety of changes ranging from and including esophageal dysmotility, diarrhea, constipation, incontinence, and diabetic gastroparesis. Genitourinary syndromes include cystopathy, neurogenic bladder, and sexual dysfunction in women and erectile dysfunction in men. Besides temperature intolerance, there are abnormalities of sweating with increased upper body sweating and increased gustatory sweating in response to certain foods such as cheese and spicy foods. Decreased lower body sweating with resulting skin dryness and cracking can contribute to increased infections and ulcerations of the diabetic foot. Autonomic neuropathy affects metabolic response to glucose regulation with both a decreased ability to detect and respond to hypoglycemia. Ocular manifestations of autonomic neuropathy include Argyll Robertson-like pupil and a decreased diameter of a dark-adapted pupil.[71–75]

As pointed out by Luukinen and Airaksinen,[76] orthostatic hypotension for older diabetics is predictive of a higher risk of vascular death. This increase in morbidity and mortality associated with autonomic neuropathy is one of the reasons the American Diabetes Association[71] advocates the performance of standard examinations for the diagnosis of cardiovascular autonomic neuropathy (Table 6-11).

Other clinical manifestations of diabetic neuropathy include impaired vibratory perception and position sense. There is depression of the deep tendon reflexes, sensory ataxia, and a deep-seated dull aching pain in the feet. There is a shortening of the Achilles tendon and wasting of the small muscles of the feet with hammertoes, and subsequent weakening of the hands and feet. Distal muscle weakness can be seen as an inability to stand on the heels or toes. Allodynia with burning superficial pain is characteristic; but later there is hypoalgesia. There is a decreased thermal sensation with impaired vasomotor and blood flow and decreased autonomic function leading to decreased sweating and dry skin and increased risk for foot ulceration and gangrene. In the elderly there is an increase in proximal muscle neuropathy. These can present as pain in the buttocks, thighs, and hips that can have a variable initiation. Proximal muscle neuropathy can have either abrupt or gradual

Table 6-11

Diagnostic Tests of CAN

▸ Resting heart rate >100 bpm is abnormal.

▸ Beat-to-beat HRV
With the patient at rest and supine (not having had coffee or a hypoglycemic episode the night before), heart rate is monitored by ECG or autonomic instrument while the patient breathes in and out at six breaths per minute, paced by a metronome or similar device. A difference in heart rate of >15 bpm in normal, <10 bpm is abnormal. The lowest normal value for the expiration-to-inspiration ratio of the R-R interval is 1.17 in people 20–24 years of age. There is a decline in the value with age.

▸ Heart rate response to standing
During continuous ECG monitoring, the R-R interval is measured at beats 15 and 30 after standing. Normally, a tachycardia is followed by reflex bradycardia. The 30:15 ratio is >1.03.

▸ Heart rate response to the Valsalva maneuver
The subject forcibly exhales into the mouthpiece of a manometer to 40 mm Hg for 15 s during ECG monitoring. Healthy subjects develop tachycardia and peripheral vasoconstriction during strain and an overshoot bradycardia and rise in blood pressure with release. The ratio of longest R-R to shortest R-R should be >1.2.

▸ Systolic blood pressure response to standing
Systolic blood pressure is measured in the supine subject. The patient stands, and the systolic blood pressure is measured after 2 min. Normal response is a fall of <10 mm Hg, borderline is a fall of 10–29 mm Hg, and abnormal is a fall of >30 mm Hg with symptoms.

▸ ECG QT/QTc intervals
The QTc should be <440 ms.

Abbreviation: CAN = cardiovascular autonomic neuropathy.
Source: Adapted from Ref. 71.

onset, progressing to weakness with inability to get up from a sitting position. It can coexist with distal symmetric polyneuropathy and may have fasciculations that may be provoked by percussion or may occur spontaneously with electrophysiological studies indicating a lumbosacral plexopathy. The elderly are also at greater risk for mononeuropathies, which tend to occur spontaneously, acutely, and with pain. These tend to affect the ulnar, median, peroneal, and cranial nerves 3, 6, and 7, and are characterized by a spontaneous remission and lack progression. These mononeuropathies must be distinguished from the nerve entrapment syndromes such as carpal tunnel, which are more frequent in diabetics, but which tend to be gradual in onset and progressive in nature.[71–75]

In addressing the pain and discomfort associated with diabetic neuropathy, the American Diabetes Association[71] recommends a stepwise approach beginning with an exclusion of nondiabetic causes, stabilizing the blood sugar, and then attempting to achieve an Hg A1c of less than 7. Pain control is initiated with tricyclics, then anticonvulsants, and finally utilizing opiates. However, Gilron et al.[77] recently demonstrated that a lower dose combination of opiates and anticonvulsants achieves better analgesia than higher doses of either drug alone.

Diabetes and the urological system

Diabetic effects on the urological system encompass diabetic nephropathy, urological cystopathy, erectile dysfunction, and infective

processes. Diabetic nephropathy affects over 40% of type I diabetics and over 20% of type II diabetics.[47,78] The National Kidney Foundation[79] defines diabetes as a risk factor for chronic kidney disease and recommends screening and risk factor reduction. The effects of diabetes in leading to end-stage renal disease are worse for certain ethnic groups namely Native Americans, Hispanics, and African Americans.[47] Since it appears that aggressive risk factor reduction and tight blood pressure and glucose control as revealed in the Diabetes Control and Complications Trial (DCCT) and UKPDS study, as well as follow-up of DCCT in the Epidemiology of Diabetes Interventions and Complications (EDIC) study[80] can decrease both the rate of progression to end-stage kidney disease and the renal complications of diabetes, the American Diabetes Association recommends the early diagnosis and treatment of microalbuminuria along with aggressive risk factor reduction and blood glucose control. ACE inhibitors have been shown to be beneficial[55,58] as have angiotensin receptor blockers,[81–83] but the attention should be paid to both serum potassium and serum creatinine when these antihypertensives are being used.

Diabetic cystopathy affects almost 50% of diabetics and increases with age.[84] In diabetic cystopathy there is impaired sensation of bladder fullness, an increase in bladder capacity, a reduction in bladder contractility, and a resulting increase in residual urine. This residual urine increases the risk for urinary tract infections, urethral reflux, hydronephrosis, pyelonephritis, and urosepsis. Both cystopathy and erectile dysfunction result from microvascular changes of diabetes and the polyneuropathy associated with diabetes.[84]

Diabetic retinopathy

Diabetic retinopathy is a significant complication of diabetes and a leading contributor to visual impairment in the elderly.[47,85] As was shown in the DCCT and the UKPDS, aggressive glycemia control along with blood pressure control can markedly reduce the progression of diabetic eye complications.

Metabolic complications

In the elderly there is increasing morbidity and mortality from hyperglycemia especially as patients age.[86,87] This holds true for both diabetic ketoacidosis and hyperglycemic hyperosmolar syndrome.[86] Causes of hyperglycemia in the elderly most commonly include infection and pancreatitis. Elderly diabetics are more likely to present without a prior diagnosis of diabetes and are at greater risk for having omitted their medication even if diagnosed. Cerebrovascular events, subdural hematoma, myocardial infarction, pulmonary embolism, intestinal obstruction or ischemia, along with heat stroke, trauma, burns, and alcohol intoxication are also precipitating causes. Among medications diuretics, beta-blockers and steroids have a contributing effect. Diabetic ketoacidosis tends to evolve rapidly over hours whereas hyperglycemia hyperosmolar syndrome may occur more gradually over days. Patients tend to be volume-depleted, hypotensive, and tachycardic with the mental state ranging from confusion to coma. Treatment consists of replacement of fluids, insulin, and electrolytes, and thus gradually correcting the deficits that are present. Mortality and morbidity tend to increase with age because of a more severe precipitating event, decreased insulin reserve and sensitivity, and diminishing physiological reserve.[86,87] This places elderly diabetics at greater overall risk.

Although hypoglycemia is not a new problem, the pronounced efforts by physicians to achieve euglycemia have led to an increased awareness of the problem[88,89] and an attempt by the American

Diabetes Association to define the problem.[90] Normally, as the body senses a decrease in glucose there is a decrease in the release of insulin and an increase in the release of the counter regulatory hormone glucagon and epinephrine. This counter regulatory mechanism is compromised in diabetics and the degree of compromise worsens with time. There may be a defect in glucose counter regulation and also hypoglycemic unawareness. With hypoglycemic unawareness, the warning signs of hypoglycemia such as palpitations, anxiety, diaphoresis, and hunger are lost over time, and the ability to recognize hypoglycemia is reduced. A functional disorder called hypoglycemia-associated autonomic failure can also occur where prior episodes of hypoglycemia lessen the body's response to subsequent episodes of hypoglycemia. Avoiding hypoglycemia for a period of several weeks can reverse this. There is also an exercise-induced hypoglycemia-associated autonomic failure in that exercise reduces the release of epinephrine in response to hypoglycemia in muscles. Finally, there is the sleep-related hypoglycemia-associated autonomic failure in that sleep reduces the sympathoadrenal response to hypoglycemia leading to unawareness of hypoglycemia and reduced arousal from sleep. It is the combination of these mechanisms that worsens the result of iatrogenic hypoglycemia[88,89] and increases the severity of the consequences of hypoglycemia among the elderly, including the potential for mortality.

Diabetes and aging

The effects of diabetes on aging are multiple. As pointed out by Olshansky and colleagues,[91] continued growth in life expectancy cannot be assumed especially in light of the increasing prevalence of obesity and the earlier onset of diabetes with its assortment of medical complications. The impact of diabetes extends beyond the comorbidities of hypertension, hyperinsulinemia, and lipid abnormalities. The Comparison of Longitudinal European Studies of Aging (CLESA) project (cross-national determinants of quality of life and health services for the elderly) which examined the results of aging studies from six different countries found that the strongest risk factors for mortality were disability, age greater than 80, cancer, and being male, with the other health-related variables being diabetes, heart disease, respiratory disease.[92]

Evans[93] points out that aging is associated with marked changes in body composition, the principle one being sarcopenia (i.e., the loss of skeletal muscle), along with continuing gains in both total body fat and visceral fat with aging. These changes are attributed to decreasing physical activity, decreasing endocrine function, increasing insulin resistance, and increasing dietary protein requirement. Since diabetes has a higher rate of occurrence with aging, Goodpaster et al.[94] was able to demonstrate that changes in body composition despite lowering of normal weight may place elderly individuals, both male and female, at greater risk for abnormal glucose tolerance and diabetes, especially if they have an increased amount of muscle fat or abdominal visceral fat. As one ages and is hyperglycemic, there is a progressive decrease in both insulin secretion and insulin responsiveness. Gertow et al.[95] has demonstrated that one of the possible sources of increased insulin resistance is an abnormality of fatty acid metabolism, which is manifested by abnormalities in fatty acid-handling proteins. Sengstock et al.[96] has recently demonstrated that with aging there is increased insulin resistance and that this increased insulin resistance is associated with increasing arterial stiffness.

Diabetes affects brain aging, impairing cognition and playing a role in dementia.[97] Richerson et al.[98] examined the question of whether diabetes with its effect on cognition, peripheral nerves, and psychomotor responses has an increased effect in addition to aging on speed of reflexes. They demonstrated that diabetics (mean age ≈ 60 years) had slower reflexes than their age-matched controls and had slower reflexes than young adults (mean age = 22 years).

Optimizing diabetic control

To manage the complications of diabetes, the results of multiple studies including DCCT, UKPDS, along with the work of Van Den Berghe et al.[99] and Umpierrez et al.[100] have led both the American College of Endocrinology and the American Diabetes Association to advocate tight control of in-hospital glucose with a fasting blood sugar goal of 110 mg/dL and a maximal level of 180 mg/dL.[46,47] The goal of long-term glucose control is to achieve an Hg A1c of less than 7.

In order to achieve these goals there are currently available five classes of oral glucose-lowering agents[101,102] in addition to insulin with a variety of formulations[103–105] (Fig. 6–1). The *sulfonylureas* act on the pancreas to increase insulin secretion from the beta cells, reduce serum glucagon, and increase insulin binding to the insulin receptors on target tissues. They are protein bound, metabolized by the liver, and excreted by the liver and kidney. The currently used sulfonylureas tend to be glyburide, glipizide, and glimepiride. These second-generation sulfonylureas have a peak action between 1 and 6 h and half-lives varying between 4 and 10 h depending on the formulation. In the elderly these effects are more pronounced, because of reduced metabolism and elimination putting them at greater risk of hypoglycemia. The next class is the *biguanides*, which decrease hepatic glucose production, and also reduce low-density lipoprotein (LDL) and very low-density lipoprotein (VLDL) concentrations, and inhibit intestinal glucose absorption. They have a half-life of over 12 h, are not metabolized, and are excreted in the urine. Metformin is the currently used biguanide. It may cause a lactic acidosis, decrease vitamin B_{12} absorption, and occasionally diarrhea. The third class of oral hypoglycemics is the *alpha-glucosidase inhibitors*. Acarbose and miglitol are agents of this class that act by inhibiting alpha-glucosidase in the brush borders of the small intestine decreasing the breakdown of oligosaccharides and disaccharides to glucose, thereby decreasing the amount of postprandial glucose. These drugs are metabolized within the gastrointestinal tract, have a half-life of 2 h, and are excreted in the urine. These agents cause abdominal discomfort, flatulence, and diarrhea as the main side effects rather than hypoglycemia. The fourth class of agents is the *thiazolidinediones* of which troglitazone, rosiglitazone, pioglitazone are currently used. These agents decrease hepatic glucose production, enhance insulin's action in the liver and skeletal muscle, and decrease insulin resistance. They do this by binding to nuclear receptors and subsequently activating or suppressing genes. These agents are metabolized in the liver and excreted by the kidney. Although liver function needs to be closely followed, the dosages are not affected by aging. The last class of oral agents is the *meglitinides* of which repaglinide and nateglinide are examples. These agents are rapid acting with short half-lives and work by slowing adenosine triphosphate (ATP)-dependent potassium channels leading to an increase in insulin secretion. These agents are highly protein bound to albumin and are metabolized in the liver by cytochrome P450 CYP 3A4. They are affected by drugs, which affect this system such as inhibitors like erythromycin and ketokonazole and inducers such as barbiturates, carbamazepine, rifampin, and troglitazone. The meglitinides are insulin secretogogues and as such they have been associated with hypoglycemia.

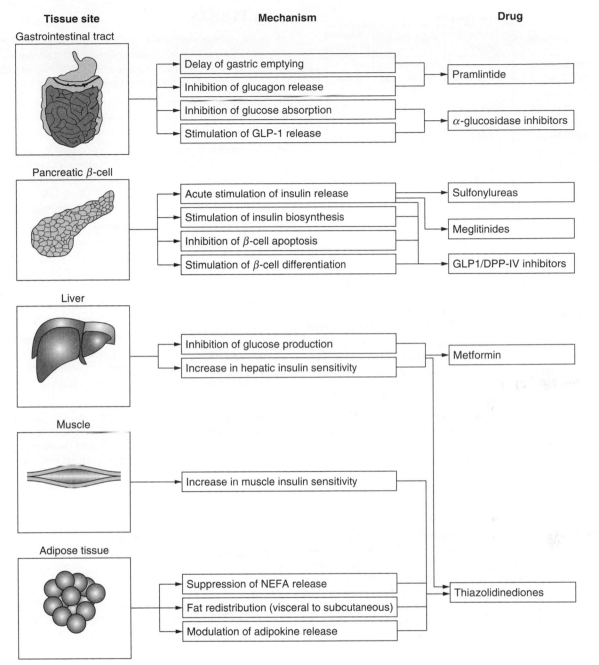

FIGURE 6-1 Pharmacologic treatment of hyperglycemia according to site of action GLP 1 = glucagon-like peptide 1, DPP-IV = dipeptidyl peptidase IV. *(Reprinted with permission from Stumvoll M, Goldstein BJ, van Haeften TW. Type 2 diabetes; principles of pathogenesis and therapy. Lancet. 2005;365:1333–1346.)*

Insulin preparations are classified by the speed of action. The principal categories are rapid-acting, short-acting, intermediate-acting, and long-acting (Fig. 6–2). Recent work by Linkeschova et al.[105] has advocated the use of continuous insulin infusion in order to achieve better glycemic and metabolic control.

Even with multiple classes of oral hypoglycemics and a variety of insulin preparations, the ability to achieve tight glycemic control as advocated by the American Diabetes Association and the American College of Endocrinology remains elusive, and so the search continues for other agents without the various side effects of current hypoglycemics, and current insulin preparations. Takei and Kasatani[106] reviewed the current foci of research and clinical trials. The first possible agent is glucagon-like peptide, GLP-1, which is secreted by L-cells in the small intestine in response to oral glucose. Carbohydrates, fat, hormones, and the nervous system also modulate secretion. GLP-1 promotes insulin secretion and sensitivity and increases insulin gene transcription and insulin synthesis. It also stimulates the formation of new pancreatic islet cells, slows beta-cell death, inhibits glucagon secretion, delays gastric emptying, reduces food intake, and decreases appetite.[106–109] The problem with GLP-1 is its extremely short half-life of 2–5 min secondary to degradation by dipeptidyl peptidase IV (DPP IV).[110] Synthetic analogs of Excodin–4, a naturally occurring GLP-1 analog that is DDP IV resistant, are under clinical trials. Other sites being targeted for investigation include protein kinase C, glycation and lipoxidation end products, nuclear factor kappa,[110] and delaying the mitochondrial decay associated

Insulin types			
Type of Insulin	Onset of Action	Peak Effect	Duration of Action
Rapid-acting Lispro/aspart	15–30 min	30–90 min	3–4 h
Short-acting Regular insulin	30–60min	2–4 h	6–10 h
Intermediate-acting NPH lente	1–4 h	4–12 h	12–24 h
Long-acting Ultralente Glargine	1–2 h 1h	8–20 h 3–20 h	24–30 h 24 h

FIGURE 6-2 Insulin types. *(Reprinted with permission from Ref. 118.)*

with aging.[111] Lastly, there is a continuing search for alternative routes for insulin delivery; nasal—which has problems with low bioavailability and dose-to-dose variation; pulmonary—which appears to be fairly effective, the principle problems being concomitant respiratory disease, smoking, and problems with inhaler usage; oral—such as hexyl-insulin monoconjugate 2 (HIM2) preparations which are resistant to gastrointestinal degradation, have long half-lives, and cause significant decrease in postprandial glucose.[112,113]

In writing for the Steno-2 study group, Gaede and Pederson[114] recommend an approach targeting a variety of risk factors when managing diabetes on an outpatient basis. Hyperglycemia should be tightly controlled to achieve the target goals already discussed with one of the early agents being metformin as long as no contraindications exist. Blood pressure control is often difficult to achieve and more than one medication class is required. However, the beneficial affects of beta-blockers and ACE inhibitors should be utilized. Dyslipidemias are both common and detrimental, and statins have shown positive effects. The utilization of aspirin to prevent cardiovascular mortality is advocated as long as bleeding contraindications are not present. The most beneficial change of behavior is smoking cessation along with an increase in exercise; but since most people have a limited ability or willingness to increase their exercise or change their behavior, an increase in fish consumption may be beneficial. Ultimately, through individualized risk assessment, education, close monitoring, persistent follow-up, attempts to achieve defined endpoints, and an understanding that polypharmacy and multimodel treatment will be necessary, it is possible to markedly improve microvascular and macrovascular complications with a resulting 50% reduction of cardiovascular mortality, myocardial infarctions, coronary interventions, strokes, leg revascularizations, and amputations.[114] These findings are in keeping with the recent treatment guidelines of the American College of Geriatrics.[60]

Recent work such as Lazar et al.[115] and Carvalho et al.[116] continue to demonstrate the benefits derived from tight glycemic control and the maintenance of normoglycemia during cardiac surgery. The degree of monitoring and control during cardiac surgery, however, is not always available during routine anesthetic care. There is a need for further data from general surgical, trauma, transplant, and neurosurgical patients as well as a better understanding of what the adverse effects of strict glucose control are, and if one threshold value is appropriate for all patients.[117] Several recent reviews on intraoperative glucose management provide clinical guidelines and treatment algorithms for diabetic patients.[118]

KEY POINTS

▶ In the elderly, manifestations of hyperthyroidism are often atypical. Patients with hyperthyroidism should not undergo elective surgery until a euthyroid state is achieved. However, occasionally surgical stress may precipitate thyrotoxicosis.

▶ Subclinical cases of hypothyroidism have not been shown to significantly increase surgical risk. However, current recommendations include continuing thyroid replacement on the day of surgery.

▶ The important anesthetic issues concerning parathyroid disease in the elderly focus on the effects of alterations in plasma calcium concentration. Hypocalcemia may cause prolongation of ST segments and QT interval. The effects of hypercalcemia on the ECG are less specific. Hypercalcemia enhances digitalis toxicity.

▶ Anesthetic issues of concern in management of patients with hyperaldosteronism include hypertension and chronic hypokalemia. Chronic hypokalemia is associated with abnormal glucose tolerance and may suppress baroreceptor tone. Hypovolemia should be aggressively managed.

▶ During anesthesia, the important management issues with Cushing's syndrome include hypertension, diabetic states, and fluid and electrolyte balance.

▶ Major complications of diabetes can involve the cardiovascular, renal, gastrointestinal, neurological, and ophthalmologic systems as well as the occurrence of an increased incidence of infection and foot ulcers.

▶ There is a higher incidence of cardiovascular disease in patients with diabetes. Diabetics are at increased risk for myocardial infarction. Recent studies have indicated that current assessment guidelines may miss a number of patients with silent ischemia. However, there is still no well-established data in asymptomatic patients that advanced testing with nuclear stress tests or stress echocardiography leads to better outcomes.

▶ In the elderly there is increasing morbidity and mortality from hyperglycemia especially as patients age. This holds true for both diabetic ketoacidosis and hyperglycemic hyperosmolar syndrome.

▶ The pronounced efforts by physicians to achieve euglycemia have led to an increased awareness of the problem of hypoglycemia.

▶ To manage the complications of diabetes, both the American College of Endocrinology and the American Diabetes Association advocate tight control of in-hospital glucose with a fasting blood sugar goal of 110 mg/dL and a maximal level of 180 mg/dL. The goal of long-term glucose control is to achieve an Hg A1c of less than 7.

▶ Recent work demonstrates the benefits derived from tight glycemic control and the maintenance of normoglycemia during cardiac surgery. There is a need for further data from general surgical, trauma, transplant, and neurosurgical patients, as well as a better understanding of what the adverse effects of strict glucose control are, and if one threshold value is appropriate for all patients.

KEY REFERENCES

▶ Rehman SU, Cope DW, Senseney AD, et al. Thyroid disorders in elderly patients. *South Med J.* 2005;98:543–549.

▶ Fehaily MA, Duh QY. Clinical manifestations of aldosteronism. *Surg Clin N Am.* 2004;88:887–905.

▶ American Diabetes Association. Standards of medical care in diabetes. *Diabetes Care.* 2005;28(Suppl.):S4–S36.

▶ Willett LL, Albright ES. Achieving glycemic control in type 2 diabetes: a practical guide for clinicians on oral hypoglycemics. *South Med J.* 2004;97:1088–1092.

▶ Edelman SV, Morello CM. Strategies for insulin therapy in type 2 diabetes. *South Med J.* 2005;98:363–371.

▶ Lazar HL, Chipken SR, Fitzgerald CA, et al. Tight glycemic control in diabetic coronary artery bypass graft patients improves perioperative outcomes and decrease recurrent ischemic events. *Circulation.* 2004;109:1497–1502.

▶ Carvalho G, Moore A, Qizilbash B, et al. Maintenance of normoglycemia during cardiac surgery. *Anesth Analg.* 2004;99:319–324.

▶ Coursin DB, Connery LE, Ketzler JT. Perioperative diabetic and hyperglycemic management issues. *Crit Care Med.* 2004;32 (Suppl.):S116–S125.

REFERENCES

1. Rehman SU, Cope DW, Senseney AD, et al. Thyroid disorders in elderly patients. *South Med J.* 2005;98:543–549.
2. Topliss DJ, Eastman CJ. Diagnosis and management of hyperthyroidism and hypothyroidism. *Med J Aust.* 2004;180:186–193.
3. Demers LM. Thyroid disease: pathophysiology and diagnosis. *Clin Lab Med.* 2004;24:19–28.
4. U.S. Preventive Services Task Force Screening for Thyroid Disease: Recommendation Statement. *Am Fam Physician.* 2004;69: 2415–2418.
5. Ginsberg J. Diagnosis and management of Graves' disease. *CMAJ.* 2003;168:575–585.
6. Erdogan ME, Kueuk NO, Anil C, et al. Effect of radioiodine therapy on thyroid nodule size and function in patients with toxic adenomas. *Nuc Med Commun.* 2004;25:1083–1087.
7. Martino E, Bartalena L, Bogazzi F, et al. Effects of Amiodarone on the thyroid. *Endocr Rev.* 2001;22:240–254.
8. Biondi B, Palmieri EA, Klain M, et al. Subclinical hyperthyroidism: clinical features and treatment options. *Eur J Endocrinol.* 2005;152:1–9.
9. Kalmijn S, Mehta KM, Pols HA, et al. Subclinical hyperthyroidism and the risk of dementia. The Rotterdam study. *Clin Endocrinol.* 2000;53:733–737.
10. Pearle JV, Maissonneuve P, Shepperd MC, et al. Prediction of all cardiovascular mortality in elderly people from one low serum thyrotropin result: a 10 year cohort study. *Lancet.* 2001;58:861–865.
11. Biondi B, Fazio S, Palmieri EA, et al. Mortality in elderly patients with subclinical hyperthyroidism. *Lancet.* 2002;359:799–800.
12. Vestergaard P, Rejnmark L, Weeke J et al. Fracture risk in patients treated for hyperthyroidism. *Thyroid.* 2000;10:341–348.
13. Laurberg P, Andersen S, Pedersen IB, et al. Hypothyroidism in the elderly: pathophysiology, diagnosis, and treatment. *Drugs Aging.* 2005;22:23–28.
14. Fliers E, Wiersinga WM. Myxedema coma. *Rev Endocr Metab Disord.* 2003;4:137–141.
15. Silverberg SJ, Bilezikian JP. Asymptomatic primary hyperparathyroidism: a medical perspective. *Surg Clin N Am.* 2004;84:787–801.
16. Ferris RL, Simental AA. Molecular biology of primary hyperparathyroidism. *Otolaryngol Clin N Am.* 2004;37:819–831.
17. Akerstrom G, Hellman P. Primary hyperparathyroidism. *Curr Opin Oncol.* 2004;16:1–7.
18. Heller H. Calcium homeostasis. In: Griffen JE, Ojeda SR, eds. *Textbook of Endocrine Physiology.* 5th ed. New York: Oxford University Press; 2004.
19. Bilezikian JP, Potts JT, El-Hajj Fuleihan G, et al. Summary statement from a workshop on asymptomatic primary hyperparathyroidism: a perspective for the 21st century. *J Clin Endocrinol Metab.* 2002;87: 5353–5361.
20. Marx SJ. Hyperparathyroid and hypoparathyroid disorders. *N Engl J Med.* 2000;343:1863–1875.
21. Roodman GD, Windle JJ. Paget's disease of bone. *J Clin Invest.* 2005;115:200–208.
22. Walsh JP. Paget's disease of bone. *Med J Aust.* 2004;181:262–265.
23. Schneider D, Hoffman MT, Peterson JA. Diagnosis and treatment of Paget's disease of bone. *Am Fam Physician.* 2002;65:2069–2072.
24. Simon LS. Osteoporosis. *Clin Geriatr Med.* 2005;21:603–629.
25. Becker C. Clinical evaluation for osteoporosis. *Clin Geriatr Med.* 2003;19:299–320.
26. Seeman E, Eckman JA. Treatment of osteoporosis: why, whom, when, and how to treat. *Med J Aust.* 2004;180:298–303.
27. Rossouw JE, Anderson GL, Prentice RL, et al. Risks and benefits of estrogen plus progestin in healthy postmenopausal women: principal results from the Women's Health Initiative randomized controlled trial. *JAMA.* 2002;288:321–333.
28. Fehaily MA, Duh QY. Clinical manifestations of aldosteronism. *Surg Clin N Am.* 2004;88:887–905.
29. Lim PD, Rodgers P, Cardale K, et al. Potentially high prevalence of primary aldosteronism in a primary care—population. *Lancet.* 1999;353:(9146)40.
30. Mosso L, Carvajal C, Gonzalez A, et al. Primary aldosteronism and hypertensive disease. *Hypertension.* 2003;42:161–165.
31. Fritsch Neves M, Schiffrin EL. Aldosterone: a risk factor for vascular disease. *Curr Hypertens Rep.* 2003;5:59–65.
32. Rossi GP, Sacchetto A, Pavan E, et al. Remodeling of the left ventricle on primary aldosteronism due to Conn's adenoma. *Circulation.* 1977;95: 1471–1478.
33. Pitt B, Remme W, Zennad F, et al. Eplerenone, a selective aldosterone blocker on patients with left ventricular dysfunction after myocardial infarction. *N Eng J Med.* 2003;348:1309–1321.
34. Milliez P, Girered P, Plouin PF, et al. Evidence for an increased rate of cardiovascular events in patients with primary aldosteronism. *J Am Coll Cardiol.* 2005;45:1243–1248.
35. Conn JW. Primary aldosteronism. *J Lab Clin Med.* 1955;45:6–17.
36. Vaughan ED. Disease of the adrenal gland. *Med Clin N Am.* 2004;88:443–466.
37. Conn JW, Cohen E, Rovner DR. Suppression of plasma renin activity in primary aldosteronism. *JAMA.* 1964:190:213–221.
38. Arnaldi G, Angeli A, Atkinson AB, et al. Diagnosis and complications of Cushing's syndrome: a consensus statement. *J Clin Endocrinol Metab.* 2003;88:5593–5602.
39. Pivonello R, Faggiano A, Lombardi G, et al. Metabolic syndrome and cardiovascular risk in Cushing's syndrome. *Endocrinol Metab Clin N Am.* 2005;327–339.
40. Forget H, Lacroix A, Somma M, et al. Cognitive decline in patients with Cushing's syndrome. *J Int Neuropsychol Soc.* 2000;6:20–29.
41. Bourdeau I, Bard C, Forget H, et al. Cognitive function and cerebral assessment in patients who have Cushing's syndrome. *Endocrinol Metab Clin N Am.* 2005;34:357–369.
42. Belanoff J, Gross K, Yager A, et al. Corticosteroids and cognition. *J Psychiatr Res.* 2001;35:127–145.
43. American Diabetes Association. Diagnosis and classification of diabetes mellitus. *Diabetes Care.* 2005;28(Suppl.):S37–S42.
44. Falorni A, Brozzetti A. Diabetes-related antibodies in adult diabetic patients. *Best Pract Res Clin Endocrinol Metab.* 2005;19:119–133.
45. Stratton IM, Adler AI, Neil HA, et al. Association of glycemia with macrovascular and microvascular complications of type 2 diabetes (UKPD 35); prospective observational study. *Br Med J.* 2000;321: 405–412.
46. Clemens A, Siegel E, Gallwitz B. Global risk management in type 2 diabetes: blood glucose, blood pressure, and lipids—update on the background of the current guidelines. *Exp Clin Endocrinol Diabetes.* 2004;112:493–503.
47. American Diabetes Association. Standards of medical care in diabetes. *Diabetes Care.* 2005;28(Suppl.):S4–S36.
48. Nesto RW. Correlation between cardiovascular disease and diabetes mellitus current concepts. *Am J Med.* 2004;116:11S–22S.
49. Hu FB, Stampfer MJ, Haffner SM, et al. Elevated risk of cardiovascular disease prior to clinical diagnosis of type 2 diabetes. *Diabetes Care.* 2002;25:1129–1134.
50. Norhammer A, Tenerey A, Nilsson G, et al. Glucose metabolism in patients with acute myocardial infarction and no previous diagnosis of diabetes mellitus: a prospective study. *Lancet.* 2002;359:2140–2144.

51. Miettinen H, Lehto S, Salomaa V, et al. For the Finmonica Myocardial Infarction Register Study Group. *Diabetes Care.* 1998;21:69–75.

52. Executive Summary of the Third Report of the National Cholesterol Education Program [NCEP] Expert Panel on Detection, Evaluation, and Treatment of High Blood Cholesterol in Adults. (Adult Treatment Panel III). *JAMA.* 2001;285:2486–2497.

53. Gu K, Cowie CC, Harris MI. Diabetes and decline in heart disease mortality in U.S. adults. *JAMA.* 1999;281:1291–1297.

54. UK Prospective Diabetes Study Group. Tight blood pressure control and risk of macrovascular and microvascular complications in type 2 diabetes (UKPDS 38). *Br Med J.* 1998;317:703–713.

55. UK Prospective Diabetes Study Group. Efficacy of atenolol and captopril in reducing the risk of macrovascular complications in type 2 diabetes (UKPDS 39). *Br Med J.* 1998;317:713–720.

56. Hansson L, Zanchette A, Carruthers SG, et al. Effects of intensive blood pressure lowering and low dose aspirin in patients with hypertension; principal results of the hypertension optimal treatment (HDT) randomized trial. HOT study group. *Lancet.* 1998;351:1755–1762.

57. The seventh report of the Joint National Committee on prevention, detection, evaluation, and treatment of high blood pressure. The JNC 7 Report. *JAMA.* 2003;289:2560–2572.

58. Heart outcomes prevention evaluation study investigators: effects of ramipril on cardiovascular and microvascular outcomes in people with diabetes mellitus: results of the HOPE study and MIRCO-HOPE sub-study. *Lancet.* 2000;355:253–259.

59. Progress group: randomized trial of a perindopril-based blood pressure lowering regimen among 6,105 individuals with previous stroke or transient ischemic attack. *Lancet.* 2001;358:1033–1041.

60. Olson DE, Norris S. Diabetes in older adults: overview of AGS guidelines for the treatment of diabetes mellitus in geriatric populations. *Geriatrics.* 2004;59:18–25.

61. Maahs, DM, Kinney GL, Wadwa P, et al. Hypertension prevalence, awareness, treatment, and control in an adult type 1 diabetic population and a comparable general population. *Diabetes Care.* 2005;28: 301–306.

62. Heart Protection Study Collaborative Group. MRC/BHF Heart Protection Study of cholesterol lowering with simvastatin in 20,536 high risk individuals: a randomized placebo controlled trial. *Lancet.* 2002;360:7–22.

63. Haffner SM, Alexander CM, Cook TJ, et al. Reduced coronary events in simvastatin-treated patients with coronary heart disease and diabetes or impaired fasting glucose levels: subgroup analysis in the Scandinavian Simvastatin Survival Study. *Arch Int Med.* 1999;159: 2661–2667.

64. Rubins HB, Robbins SJ, Collins D, et al. Gemfibrozil for the secondary prevention of coronary heart disease in men with low levels of high density lipoprotein cholesterol. Veterans Affairs High-Density Lipoprotein Cholesterol Intervention Trial Study Group. *N Eng J Med.* 1999;341: 410–418.

65. Collins R, Armitage J, Parish S, et al. MRC/BHF Heart Protection Study of cholesterol-lowering with simvastatin in 5,963 people with diabetes: a randomized placebo controlled trial. *Lancet.* 2003;361:2005–2016.

66. Arampatzis CA, Goodhart D, Serruys PW, et al. Fluvastatin reduces the impact of diabetes on long term outcome after coronary intervention— A Lescol Intervention Prevention Study (LIPS) sub-study. *Am Heart J.* 2005:149:329–335.

67. Colwell JA. Antiplatelet agents for the prevention of cardiovascular disease in diabetes mellitus. *Am J Cardiovasc Drugs.* 2004;4:87–106.

68. American Diabetes Association. Aspirin therapy in diabetes. *Diabetes Care.* 2004;S72–S73.

69. Final report on the aspirin component of the ongoing Physicians Health Study Research Group. *N Eng J Med.* 1989;321:129–135.

70. Wackers FJ, Young LH, Inzucchi SE, et al. Detection of silent myocardial ischemia in asymptomatic diabetic subjects: the DIAD study. *Diabetes Care.* 2004;27:1954–1961.

71. Boulton AJM, Vinik AI, Arezzo JC. Diabetic Neuropathies. A statement by the American Diabetes Association. *Diabetes Care.* 2005;28:956–962.

72. Sinnreich M, Taylor BU, Dyck PJ. Diabetic neuropathies. Classification, clinical features, and pathophysiological basis. *Neurologist.* 2005;11:63–79.

73. Freeman R. Autonomic peripheral neuropathy. *Lancet.* 2005;365:1259–1270.

74. Kelkar P. Diabetic Neuropathy. *Semin Neurol.* 2005;25:168–173.

75. Vinik AI, Mehrabyan A. Diabetic Neuropathies. *Med Clin N Am.* 2004;88:947–999.

76. Luukinen H, Airaksinen KE. Orthostatic hypotension predicts vascular death in older diabetic patients. *Diabetes Res Clin Pract.* 2005;67: 163–166.

77. Gilron I, Bailey JM, Tu D, et al. Morphine, gabapentin, or their combination for neuropathy pain. *N Eng J Med.* 2005;352:1324–1334.

78. American Diabetes Association. Nephropathy in Diabetes. *Diabetes Care.* 2004;27:(Suppl.);79S–83S.

79. National Kidney Foundation. Clinical practice guidelines for chronic kidney disease: evaluation, classification, and stratification. *Am J Kidney Dis.* 2002;2(Suppl.):S46–S75.

80. Writing Team for DCCT/EDIC Research Group. Sustained effect of intensive treatment of type 1 diabetes mellitus on development and progression of diabetic nephropathy. *JAMA.* 2003;2159–2167.

81. Lewis EJ, Hunsicker LG, Clarke WR, et al. Reno-protective effect of the angiotensin-receptor antagonist irbesartan in patients with nephropathy due to type 2 diabetes. *N Eng J Med.* 2001;345:851–860.

82. Brenner BM, Cooper ME, de Zeeuw D. Effect of losartan in renal and cardiovascular outcomes in patients with type 2 diabetes and nephropathy. *N Eng J Med.* 2001;345:861–869.

83. Parveng HH, Lehnert H, Bachner-Mortensen J, et al. The effect of irbesartan on the development of diabetic nephropathy in patients with type 2 diabetes. *N Eng J Med.* 2001;345:870–878.

84. Sasaki K, Yoshimura N, Chancellor MB. Implication of diabetes mellitus in urology. *Urol Clin N Am.* 2003:1–12.

85. Jawa A, Keomt J, Fonseca VA. Diabetic nephropathy and retinopathy. *Med Clin N Am.* 2004;1001–1036.

86. Gaglia JL, Wyckoff J, Abrahamson MJ. Acute hyperglycemia crisis in the elderly. *Med Clin N Am.* 2004;88:1063–1084.

87. Newton CA, Raskin P. Diabetic ketoacidosis in type 1 and type 2 diabetes mellitus. *Arch Intern Med.* 2004;164:1925–1931.

88. Cryer PE. Diverse causes of hypoglycemia associated autonomic failure in diabetes. *N Eng J Med.* 2004;351:2271–2279.

89. Banarer S, Cryer PE. Hypoglycemia in type 2 diabetes. *Med Clin N Am.* 2004;88:1107–1116.

90. ADA Workgroup on hypoglycemia. Defining and reporting hypoglycemia in diabetes. *Diabetes Care.* 2005;28:1245–1249.

91. Olshansky SJ, Passaro DJ, Hershow RC, et al. A potential decline in life expectancy in the United States in the 21st century. *N Eng J Med.* 2005;351:1138–1145.

92. Noale EM, Minicuci N, Bardage C, et al. Predictors of mortality: an international comparison of sociodemographic and health characteristics from six longitudinal studies on aging: the CLESA project. *Exp Gerontol.* 2005;40:89–99.

93. Evans WJ. Protein nutrition, exercise, and aging. *J Am CollNutr.* 2004;23:601S–609S.

94. Goodpaster BH, Krishnaswami S, Resnick H, et al. Association between regional adipose tissue distribution and both type 2 diabetics and impaired glucose tolerance in elderly men and women. *Diabetes Care.* 2003;26:372–379.

95. Gertow K, Pietilainen KH, Yki-Jarvinen H, et al. Expression of fatty acid handling proteins in human adipose tissue in relation to obesity and insulin resistance. *Dibetologia.* 2004;47:1118–1125.

96. Sengstock DM, Vaitkevicius PV, Supiano MA. Arterial stiffness is related to insulin resistance in nondiabetic hypertensive older adults. *J Clin Endocrinol Metab.* 2005;90(5):2823–2827.

97. Launer LJ. Diabetes and brain aging: epidemiologic evidence. *Curr Diabetes Rep.* 2005;5:59–63.

98. Richerson SJ, Robinson CJ, Shum J. A comparative study of reaction times between type II diabetics and non-diabetics. *Biomed Eng Online.* 2005;4:12.

99. Van Den Berghe G, Wouters P, Weekers F, et al. Intensive insulin therapy in critically ill patients. *N Eng J Med.* 2001;345:1359–1367.

100. Umpierrez GE, Isaacs SD, Bazargan H, et al. Hyperglycemia; an independent marker of in-hospital mortality in patients with undiagnosed diabetes. *J Clin Endocrinol Metab.* 2002;87:978–982.

101. Krentz AJ, Bailey CS. Oral antidiabetic agents: current role in type 2 diabetes mellitus drugs. 2005;65:385–411.

102. Willett LL, Albright ES. Achieving glycemic control in type 2 diabetes: a practical guide for clinicians on oral hypoglycemics. *South Med J.* 2004;97:1088–1092.

103. Vivian EM, Olarte SV, Gutierriez AM. Insulin strategies for type 2 diabetes mellitus. *Ann Pharmacother.* 2004;38:1916–1923.

104. Edelman SV, Morello CM. Strategies for insulin therapy in type 2 diabetes. *South Med J.* 2005;98:363–371.

105. Linkeschova R, Raoul M, Bott U, et al. Less severe hypoglycemia, better metabolic control, and improved quality of life in type 1 diabetes mellitus with continuous subcutaneous insulin infusion (CSII) therapy; an observational study of 100 consecutive patients followed for a mean of 2 years. *Diabetes Med.* 2002;19:746–751.

106. Takei I, Kasatani T. Future therapy of diabetes mellitus. *Biomed Pharmacother.* 2004;58:578–581.

107. Flint A, Raben A, Ersboll AK, et al. The effect of physiological levels of glucagon-like-peptide-1 on appetite, gastric emptying, energy and substrate metabolism on obesity. *Int J Obes Relat Met Disord.* 2001;25:781–792.

108. Hongxiang H, Arash N, Xiaoqning Z, et al. Glucagon-like-peptide 1 inhibits apoptosis of insulin-secreting cells via a cyclic adenosine monophosphate dependent protein kinase A and a phosphatidylinositol-3-kinase-dependent pathway. *Endocrinology.* 2003;144:1444–1455.

109. George GH, Oleg GC. Glucagon-like-peptide-1 synthetic analogs: new therapeutic agents for use in treatment of diabetes mellitus. *Curr Med Chem.* 2003;10:2471–2483.

110. Ahren B, Simonsson E, Larsson H, et al. Inhibition of dipeptidyl peptidase IV improves metabolic control over a 4-week study period in type 2 diabetes. *Diabetes Care.* 2002;25:869–875.

111. Ames BN, Liu J. Delaying mitochondrial decay of aging with acetylcarnitine. *Ann N Y Acad Sci.* 2004;1033:108–116.

112. Knipes M, Dandona P, Tripathy D, et al. Control of post-precordial glucose by an oral insulin product (HIM2) in patients with type 2 diabetes. *Diabetes Care.* 2003;26:421–466.

113. Clement S, Dandona P, Still G, et al. Oral modified insulin (HIM2) in patients with type 1 diabetes mellitus: results from a phase I/II clinical trial. *Metabolism.* 2004;53:54–58.

114. Gaede P, Pedersen O. Target intervention against multiple-risk markers to reduce cardiovascular disease in patients with type 2 diabetes. *Ann Med.* 2004;36:355–366.

115. Lazar HL, Chipken SR, Fitzgerald CA, et al. Tight glycemic control in diabetic coronary artery bypass graft patients improves perioperative outcomes and decrease recurrent ischemic events. *Circulation.* 2004;109:1497–1502.

116. Carvalho G, Moore A, Qizilbash B, et al. Maintenance of normoglycemia during cardiac surgery. *Anesth Analg.* 2004;99:319–324.

117. Coursin DB, Connery LE, Ketzler JT. Perioperative diabetic and hyperglycemic management issues. *Crit Care Med.* 2004;32(Suppl.):S116–S125.

118. Ahmed Z, Lockhart C, Weiner M, et al. Advances in diabetic management: implications for anesthesia. *Anesth Analg.* 2005;100:666–669.

Urinary and Hepatic System

Punita T. Sharma

CHAPTER

7

THE AGING LIVER

The biological aging process is associated with cellular senescence leading to a decrease in organ function. In spite of the known effects of the aging process, the influence of such changes on the pharmacokinetic and pharmacodynamic properties of most drugs is not well studied. Despite the progressive decline in cellular function with aging, the aging liver preserves its function relatively well. This may be due to its capacity to regenerate.

▶ Anatomy

Macroscopically, the liver undergoes brown atrophy with old age. This is secondary to the accumulation of lipofuscin in the hepatocytes as a by-product of lipid and protein metabolism.[1] There is a marked reduction in liver size by 60 years of age as detected by ultrasound.[2] This is probably due to the decline in the hepatic and splanchnic blood flow of the order of 40%.[3] This parallels the decrease in cardiac output which accompanies aging. The decline in the hepatocyte mass, hepatic blood flow, and age-related changes in hepatic sinusoidal endothelium has an effect on drug transfer, oxygen delivery, and reduced hepatic drug clearance.[3-5] The capacity of the liver to regenerate is more or less maintained in the elderly, although it may be delayed. This may be due to decreased responsiveness to hepatotropic growth factor. Hepatic resections for hepatocellular carcinoma can therefore be carried out in noncirrhotic elderly people without problems. Histologically, hepatocytes enlarge with aging. Some evidence suggests an increase in nuclear polyploidy and size. Aging of the liver mainly affects the sinusoids and the Kupffer cells. Pseudocapillarization, which manifests as a reduction in sinusoidal fenestration and subendothelial collagen deposition, causes a reduction in oxygen-dependent hepatocyte functions such as oxidative drug metabolism.[6] The number of mitochondria per hepatic volume decreases as the number of swollen, vacuolated mitochondria increases. The number of lysosomes and dense bodies also increases. Protein synthesis decreases with aging. Serum albumin levels decrease slightly but remain within the normal range.

▶ Hepatic function

Aging has been shown to be associated with multiple changes in hepatic function. In contrast to renal clearance, there are no reliable methods to easily estimate the hepatic drug clearance. No age-specific alterations in conventional liver biochemistry (serum bilirubin, serum aminotransferases, hepatic alkaline phosphatase, and other liver blood tests) are seen, but a number of dynamic measurements of liver function decline from early adulthood to senescence.[7] Dynamic liver function is reflected by galactose elimination, aminopyrine demethylation, or caffeine clearance and decreases with the reduction in liver volume and blood flow.[2,8] Other specific liver functions like hepatic nitrogen clearance are impaired by about 50% with advancing age. A number of studies have suggested increased susceptibility to stress insult in aged animals, but there are no comparable studies in human beings. A possible mechanism to explain impairment of liver cell proliferation may be related to an age-related decline in mitogen-activated protein kinase activity in epidermal growth factor-stimulated rat hepatocytes.[9] Key proteins are manufactured by the liver and may show changes with aging. A decrease in the level of serum albumin and an increase in α-1 acid glycoprotein are commonly seen in the elderly. Serum levels of cholesterol, high-density lipoprotein cholesterol, and triglycerides increase with age but decrease in individuals over 90 years.[10] These may contribute to the increased risk of coronary artery disease in the elderly. Plasma cholinesterase activity may be reduced in the elderly. It is the combination of impairment in liver cell proliferation and comorbid disease states (i.e., alcohol consumption, smoking, nutritional status, coexistent disease, and genetic influences), which play a significant role in age-related liver dysfunction rather than parenchymal liver changes alone.[5]

▶ Pharmacology

Physiologic changes that occur with aging have an impact on the pharmacologic response in elderly patients. These changes are well described and include (1) plasma protein binding, (2) body content, (3) drug metabolism, and (4) pharmacodynamics. In the liver, changes primarily affect the plasma protein binding and drug metabolism.

Plasma protein binding

There is a decrease in the level of serum albumin with age and an increase in α-1 acid glycoprotein concentration. This may affect drug pharmacokinetics. The main plasma-binding protein for acidic drugs (e.g., diazepam, phenytoin, warfarin, salicylic acid) is albumin and for basic drugs (e.g., lidocaine, propranolol) is α-1 acid glycoprotein. The effect of alterations in plasma-binding protein on drug effect depends on which protein the drug is bound to and the resulting change in fraction of unbound drug. In general, changes in plasma-binding protein levels are not a predominant factor in determining modifications in pharmacokinetics with aging. This is because the initial and transient effect of protein binding on free plasma concentration is rapidly counterbalanced by its effect on clearance.[5,11]

Hepatic drug metabolism

The hepatic enzyme systems are classified as those involved in phase 1 or phase 2 metabolism. Drugs are usually metabolized to a more water-soluble form in the liver. Some of the drugs may also be activated in the liver. These are referred to as prodrugs. Enalapril is one such drug which is converted to its active form enalaprilat. Biotransformation of prodrugs is impaired when hepatic congestion occurs with comorbid disease states such as severe congestive heart failure.

Phase 1 of hepatic drug metabolism leads to structural alteration of the drug by oxidation, reduction, esterification, and hydrolysis. The phase 1 reaction is primarily performed by a group of enzymes located on the endoplasmic reticulum of the liver cell referred to as the cytochrome P-450 (CYP) enzyme system (microsomal mixed-function oxidative system or CYP). Sotaniemi et al. has reported a 30% decline in hepatic drug metabolism after 70 years of age. However, other studies show that the amount of liver microsomal monoenzyme oxidase remains unaltered with aging.[12] The reduction in phase 1 metabolism in the elderly is clinically insignificant compared with the metabolic effects of tobacco, alcohol, and environmental factors on the liver.[8]

Phase 2 metabolism leads to conjugation with chemical ligands such as glucuronide, sulphate, acetate, or glutathione. This depends on the activity of specific cytosolic enzymes. There is no consensus as to whether phase 2 metabolism is affected by aging, although some studies have shown a slight decline in conjugation with aging.[2] Many drugs, including some tricyclic antidepressants and benzodiazepines, are metabolized extensively by both pathways prior to excretion in the urine or bile.

Hepatic clearance (Clhep) is defined by the equation: $Cl(hep) = Q \times E$; where Q is the hepatic blood flow and E is the hepatic extraction ratio. The extraction ratio is defined by the removal of a given drug by the liver. Drugs can be classified into three groups based on their extraction ratio (Table 7-1): high (E>0.7); those with intermediate extraction ratio (E 0.3–0.7); and finally those with low extraction ratio (E<0.3). Substances eliminated by the liver that have a high extraction ratio undergo flow-limited metabolism, because hepatic clearance will be almost equal to hepatic blood flow. This means that any reduction in liver blood flow will reduce clearance of drugs with high hepatic extraction ratio by as much as 20–40%. Drugs with a low extraction ratio on the other hand do not show a decrease in clearance with decrease in blood flow irrespective of which CYP enzymes are involved.[13] The metabolism of these drugs is influenced by intrinsic clearance (a term that describes total enzyme activity and liver mass) and/or protein binding, and is termed capacity-limited.[3]

Renal disease also influences the activity of drug-metabolizing enzymes. Animal studies in chronic renal failure (CRF) have shown a major down regulation (40–85%) of hepatic CYP-mediated metabolism. Studies have also suggested the presence of circulating uremic factors in the serum that down regulate the activity of CYP enzymes by 30–35% secondary to reduced gene expression.[14,15] Phase 2 reactions such as acetylation and glucuronidation are also involved, with the activity of some enzymes being induced and others inhibited.[16]

Table 7-1

Hepatic Extraction Ratio for Commonly Used Anesthetic Drugs

High Extraction Ratio (E > 0.7)	Intermediate Extraction Ratio (E 0.3–0.7)	Low Extraction Ratio (E < 0.3)
Amiodarone	Aspirin	Alfentanil
Amitriptyline	Codeine	Acetaminophen
Diltiazem	Morphine	Bupivacaine
Fentanyl	Triazolam	Celecoxib
Sufentanil		Carbamazepine
Lidocaine		Diazepam
Meperidine		Oxazepam
Metoprolol		Phenytoin
Ketamine		Thiopental
Labetalol		Theophylline
Propofol		Warfarin
Propranolol		
Glyceryl nitrate		
Nifedipine		
Verapamil		

PHARMACOLOGY OF SPECIFIC DRUGS WITH RESPECT TO THE LIVER

▶ Inhaled anesthetics

Splanchnic (and hepatic) blood flow is reduced with increasing doses of isoflurane, as a result of a decrease in systemic arterial pressure. Liver function tests are minimally affected and there is no described incidence of hepatic toxicity related to the use of isoflurane.

Desflurane is metabolized to a minimal extent, and more than 99% of absorbed desflurane is eliminated unchanged via the lungs. A small amount of absorbed desflurane is oxidatively metabolized by hepatic CYP enzymes. Almost no serum fluoride ions are detectable after desflurane administration. It is unlikely that desflurane will affect liver function tests or cause hepatotoxicity. However, all fluorinated anesthetics may cause acute hepatic damage under rare circumstances. Severe desflurane hepatotoxicity has been reported after colon surgery in an elderly patient.[17]

Approximately 3% of absorbed sevoflurane is biotransformed. Sevoflurane is metabolized in the liver by CYP 2E1, with the predominant product being hexafluoroisopropanol.[18] Hepatic metabolism of sevoflurane also produces inorganic fluoride. Serum fluoride concentrations reach a peak shortly after surgery and decline rapidly. Sevoflurane is not known to cause hepatotoxicity or alterations in hepatic function testing. In fact, it has been demonstrated that liver function in elderly patients is well preserved with both desflurane and sevoflurane.[19]

Nitrous oxide is not known to produce any changes in renal or hepatic function and is neither nephrotoxic nor hepatotoxic in the elderly.

▶ Induction drugs and benzodiazepines

Thiopental has a low hepatic extraction ratio, so metabolism is less important than redistribution in terminating its initial effect after

Table 7-2

Drugs Metabolized by the Liver and Its Anesthetic Implications in the Elderly

Drugs	Metabolized by Liver	Anesthetic Implications
Midazolam	Dependent on phase 1 metabolism, 1 and 4 hydroxy derivatives (active)	Cleared slowly in the elderly
Diazepam	Dependent on phase 1 metabolism, desmethyldiazepam, oxazepam, temazepam (active)	Elimination half-life increased in elderly
Lorazepam	Undergoes phase 2 metabolism, conjugation with glucuronic acid (inactive)	Elimination half-time not prolonged in elderly
Propofol	Metabolized primarily in liver; highly protein bound	Elderly show decreased rate of plasma clearance
Etomidate	Phase 1, hydrolysis in liver	Age-dependent decreased clearance
Ketamine	Demethylation to norketamine (active); E > 0.7	Decrease in liver blood flow decreases ketamine metabolism
Thiopental	Metabolized in liver strongly bound to albumin; E < 0.3	Redistribution more important than metabolism in terminating effect of initial bolus
Morphine	Undergoes phase 2 metabolism (morphine-6-glucouronide)	Decreased clearance secondary to smaller volume of distribution, not liver metabolism
Fentanyl	E > 0.7	Decreased hepatic blood flow will prolong effects
Succinylcholine	Metabolized by plasma cholinesterase	Severe liver disease prolongs action if associated with decreased plasma cholinesterase activity
Pancuronium	Yes, active metabolite	Prolonged action
Vecuronium	Yes, biliary excretion	Prolonged duration of action
Rocuronium	Yes, biliary excretion	Prolonged duration of action
Atracurium	Minimum, Hofmann degradation, ester hydrolysis	Drug of choice; clearance unchanged with age
Cisatracurium	No, Hofmann degradation and ester hydrolysis	Drug of choice; clearance unchanged with age
Mivacurium	Yes, plasma cholinesterase	Duration of action prolonged as a result of decreased plasma cholinesterase activity
Edrophonium	Yes	Prolonged duration of action
Neostigmine	No	No effect

a single bolus dose (Table 7-2). With repeated doses, plasma protein binding and metabolism may play a role and recovery can be prolonged. Barbiturates are metabolized in the liver and are strongly protein bound to albumin.[20]

Propofol is metabolized primarily in the liver to less-active metabolites that are then excreted by the kidney.[21] Propofol is highly protein bound, and its pharmacokinetics, like that of the barbiturates, may be affected by conditions that alter serum protein levels.[22] Clearance of propofol is reduced in the elderly. Extrahepatic clearance of propofol has been suggested to explain this observation because total body clearance of propofol exceeds hepatic blood flow.

Metabolism of etomidate occurs in the liver, where it is primarily hydrolyzed to inactive compounds.[23] Elimination is both renal (78%) and biliary (22%). Etomidate shows an age-dependent decreased clearance and initial volume of distribution, which accounts for the decrease in dose requirements in the elderly.[24]

Ketamine is metabolized extensively by microsomal enzyme systems to norketamine, which is further metabolized and excreted in the urine and bile. Norketamine is one-fifth to one-third as potent as ketamine and has central nervous system (CNS) excitatory activity. Protein binding is much lower with ketamine than with the other parenteral anesthetics. Ketamine has a high hepatic extraction ratio.

Therefore, a decrease in blood flow, as seen in elderly, will decrease the metabolism of ketamine.

The dose of midazolam required to produce sedation during upper gastrointestinal endoscopy is decreased approximately 75% in the aged.[25] These changes are related to both increased brain sensitivity and decreased drug clearance.[26] Benzodiazepines that depend on phase 1 metabolism, like diazepam and midazolam, are cleared slowly in the elderly. Lorazepam, which undergoes phase 2 metabolism, is not affected by age but its slow onset of action and prolonged duration limits its usefulness in the elderly.

▶ Opioids

All opioids are metabolized in the liver followed by renal and biliary excretion of the metabolites. The only exception is remifentanil which is hydrolyzed by tissue and plasma esterases. Morphine clearance is decreased in the elderly due to a smaller volume of distribution. Fentanyl and sufentanil have a high hepatic extraction ratio; hence factors leading to a decrease in hepatic blood flow tend to prolong its effects. Alfentanil has a low extraction ratio; hence hepatic blood flow does not play a role in its clearance. It appears that the increased potency of sufentanil, alfentanil, and fentanyl in the elderly is primarily related to an increase in brain sensitivity to opioids with age rather than alterations in metabolism. Brain sensitivity to remifentanil also increases with age although it is not metabolized in the liver. There is also a decrease in remifentanil clearance with age, and approximately one-third the infusion rate is required in the elderly.

▶ Muscle relaxants

In general, age does not significantly affect the pharmacodynamics of muscle relaxants. However, the duration of action may be prolonged if the drug depends on liver or renal metabolism. Recent data suggest that there may be increased sensitivity of the neuromuscular junction to neuromuscular blocking agents as a result of reduced muscle activity in the elderly.[27]

Depolarizing neuromuscular blocking agents

The action and clearance of succinylcholine are not age-dependent, although onset time is significantly delayed in the elderly patients. Severe liver disease may decrease plasma cholinesterase activity sufficiently to produce a prolonged duration of action.

Nondepolarizing neuromuscular blocking agents

Aminosteroids Pancuronium clearance decreases in the elderly because of its dependence on both hepatic metabolism and renal excretion.[28] Plasma clearance of vecuronium is lower in the elderly.[29] The age-related prolonged duration of action of vecuronium may reflect decreases in volume of distribution and hepatic clearance. Rocuronium shows a prolonged duration of action because of decrease in volume of distribution and plasma clearance.[30]

Benzylisoquinolones Atracurium depends to a small extent on hepatic metabolism and excretion, and its elimination half-life is prolonged in the elderly. However, clearance is unchanged with age, suggesting that alternative pathways of elimination (ester hydrolysis and Hofmann elimination) assume importance in the elderly.[31] Cisatracurium undergoes Hofmann degradation and is unaffected by age or liver disease. The duration of action of mivacurium is prolonged by about 30% as a result of decreased plasma cholinesterase activity in the elderly.[32]

Reversal Agents Doses of reversal agent are generally not modified for older patients with the exception of edrophonium, which has a prolonged duration of action compared with younger patients.

▶ Local anesthetic agents

In the elderly patient, the elimination half-life is increased for both lidocaine and bupivacaine. The risk of overdose is therefore increased when the local anaesthetic agent is given in repeated doses and as a continuous infusion.[33] Changes in elimination half-life for lidocaine are related to liver metabolism as the capacity to metabolize lidocaine by the liver is decreased with liver disease, such as cirrhosis.[34] Bupivacaine has a low hepatic extraction ratio, and the age-related decline in plasma clearance is most likely due to a decrease in hepatic enzyme activity and protein binding rather than alteration in liver blood flow.

COMMON LIVER DISEASES ENCOUNTERED IN THE ELDERLY

Although there are no specific age-related liver diseases, biliary tract disease, alcoholism, and chronic hepatitis (including cirrhosis) are the most common liver diseases encountered in the elderly (Table 7-3).

Table 7-3
Common Liver Diseases Encountered in the Elderly

Disease	Anesthetic Implications
Alcoholism	Liver dysfunction—mild to alcoholic cirrhosis, alcohol-induced-cardiomyopathy, altered nutritional status, high risk of postoperative pneumonia, postoperative delirium tremens
Cirrhosis (alcoholic or chronic viral hepatitis)	Liver dysfunction; portal hypertension leading to GI bleed (microcytic anemia); hyperdynamic circulatory state (increased cardiac output, increased circulating blood volume, decreased peripheral vascular resistance); reduced arterial oxygenation (intapumonary shunt); ascites; multiple coagulation abnormalities; thrombocytopenia (splenic sequestration); intraoperative considerations include replacement of third space losses, blood loss, serum glucose level, maintain hepatic blood flow and temperature; major postoperative complications include sepsis, hemorrhage, hepatorenal failure
Biliary tract disease (gallstones and malignancies)	Duration of action of vecuronium and pancuronium may be prolonged

▶ Biliary tract disease in the elderly

In the elderly, biliary tract disease is commonly associated with malignancy and gallstones. Emergency surgery is associated with increased risk in patients older than 65 years.[35] Laparoscopic procedures have the lowest morbidity in the elderly.[36] Alterations in laboratory values with biliary tract disease include an increase in the conjugated fraction of bilirubin, slight increase in transaminase, and a marked increase in alkaline phosphatase level. Drugs that are excreted through the biliary tract, like vecuronium and pancuronium, may have a prolonged duration of action.

▶ Alcoholism

Alcoholism is a common problem in the elderly that is often unrecognized. Between 2% and 10% of the community-dwelling elderly meet the criteria for alcohol abuse or dependence. Depression and solitary living conditions are the main contributors to this problem.

Alcoholism is associated with altered nutritional status. The nutritional deficiencies commonly observed include serum thiamine, folate, pyridoxine, niacin, vitamin A, zinc, and copper. Hypomagnesemia, hypocalcemia, and hypokalemia may occur with acute intoxication or withdrawal. Anemia is usually macrocytic (B_{12} deficiency), and the serum albumin is depressed.

Other alterations in laboratory values observed with alcoholism include elevations in serum aminotransferase (aspartate aminotransferase and alanine aminotransferase [AST and ALT]), serum γ-glutamyl transpeptidase (GGTP), and γ globulin levels. Either leukocytosis or leukopenia may be observed. After consuming similar amounts of alcohol, measured serum alcohol levels are higher in geriatric patients than younger individuals secondary to an age-related decrease in the activity of gastric alcohol dehydrogenase.[37]

Alcohol-related problems in the elderly often manifest themselves in the form of accidents or falls.[38] The clinical presentation can vary from asymptomatic patient with enlarged liver to critically ill patients with alcoholic cirrhosis. Anorexia, nausea with hepatosplenomegaly, and jaundice strongly suggest the diagnosis. These patients may also have alcohol-induced cardiomyopathy.

Cirrhosis

Alcoholism and chronic viral hepatitis may be associated with progression of liver disease to cirrhosis with portal hypertension and esophageal varices. The risk of anesthesia and surgery is increased in the presence of cirrhosis. Cirrhotic patients with ascites display a hyperdynamic circulatory state with decreased total peripheral vascular resistance and increased cardiac output and plasma volume. Reduced arterial oxygenation may occur secondary to intrapulmonary vasodilation, ventilation perfusion mismatch, impaired hypoxic pulmonary vasoconstriction, and mechanical factors such as ascites and pleural effusion. PaO_2 values of 60–70 mm Hg are common in patients with cirrhosis.

ANESTHETIC MANAGEMENT OF ELDERLY PATIENTS WITH RESPECT TO THE LIVER

Preoperative assessment

The two primary objectives in preoperative assessment of the elderly hepatic system are to identify liver disease processes and to determine the functional reserve of the liver.[39] Liver diseases of importance to anesthetic management include biliary obstruction and cirrhosis. Risk factors for operative mortality in patients with obstructive jaundice include hematocrit value <30%, serum bilirubin level >11 mg/dL, and biliary obstruction secondary to malignancy, azotemia, hypoalbuminemia, and cholangitis.[40] The Child-Pugh score is used to stage cirrhosis (Table 7-4). A high Child-Pugh score is an important risk factor for perioperative complications. In the cirrhotic patient, liver reserve can also be assessed via preoperative laboratory testing. In particular, elderly patients with cirrhosis displaying a preoperative aspartate transaminase level more than twice normal are at increased risk of postoperative death following liver resection.[41]

Renal assessment should be included when evaluating elderly patients with liver failure as it is an important cause of postoperative

Table 7-4

Child-Pugh Scoring System

Points	1	2	3
Ascites	None	Small or diuretic controlled	Tense
Encephalopathy	Absent	Mild	Marked
Albumin (g/L)	>3.5	2.8–3.5	<2.8
Bilirubin (mg/dL)	<2	2–3	>3
PT (sec above control), or INR	<4 <1.7	4–6 1.7–2.3	>6 >2.3

Note: Child-Pugh Class A, 5–6 total points, abdominal surgery perioperative mortality: 10%; Child-Pugh Class B, 7–9 total points, abdominal surgery perioperative mortality: 30%; Child-Pugh Class C, 10–15 total points, abdominal surgery perioperative mortality: 82%.

mortality. Factors predisposing to postoperative hepatorenal syndrome are high bilirubin and presence of gram-negative bacterial infection.

Premedication

The degree of CNS impairment is an important consideration in the administration of sedative or narcotic premedications. These drugs may trigger or exacerbate hepatic encephalopathy in the elderly patient with liver disease.[42] Drugs that are metabolized through the phase 2 pathway, such as lorazepam, are better tolerated than those that undergo phase 1 metabolism. However, the slow onset and prolonged duration of lorazepam may limit its use for premedication.

Intraoperative management

From the standpoint of the effect of aging on the liver, there is no evidence that a specific injected or inhaled drug is preferable for induction or maintenance of anesthesia. Intraoperative measurement of serum glucose should be done frequently as elderly patients with liver dysfunction are prone to hypoglycemia. Maintaining body temperature is important as unintentional hypothermia in the elderly is associated with impaired coagulation[43,44] and may lead to delayed metabolism of drugs.

Considerations that are helpful in maintaining the hepatic blood flow should be kept in mind. In particular, controlled positive pressure ventilation (PEEP) with high mean airway pressure can compromise hepatic blood flow.[45] Hepatic blood flow is similar with regional and general anesthesia techniques, provided arterial blood pressure is maintained.[46]

THE AGING KIDNEY

With advanced age, the kidney shows both functional decline and structural damage (Table 7-5). Despite the substantial decline in renal function with age, in the unstressed state removal of waste products and regulation of volume and extracellular fluid composition is sufficient to maintain homeostasis. However, kidney function may acutely deteriorate under various stresses imposed by environment, disease, or medical therapies.[47]

Anatomy

Renal mass decreases about 20% between the ages of 30 and 80 (Table 7-5).[48] Under light microscopy, the aging human kidney is characterized by increased fibrosis, tubular atrophy, and arteriosclerosis.[49,50] There is also an age-related glomerulosclerosis which accounts for a 20–30% loss of glomeruli when comparisons are made to young adults.[51]

Some of the pathologic changes in the aging kidney may be related to ischemia. Autoregulation of renal blood flow (RBF) is not closely coupled to local or regional metabolic requirements making the renal cortex particularly vulnerable to ischemia, especially with sympathoadrenal vasoconstriction.[52]

Renal function

Glomerular filtration rate and renal blood flow (RBF)

Glomerular filtration rate (GFR) is employed to measure renal function. There is a progressive decline in the GFR with aging. RBF to the kidneys is maintained up to the fourth decade. Thereafter it is reduced approximately 10% per decade. This decline is accompanied

Table 7-5

Age-Related Changes in Renal Function

Anatomical

Decrease in

  Renal mass (especially cortical)

  Renal blood flow (especially cortical)

  Renal plasma flow

Renal Function

Decrease in

  Glomerular filtration rate

  Tubular function

  Concentrating ability

  Diluting capacity

  Drug excretion

Impairment in

  Sodium handling

  Potassium handling

  Acid load excretion

  Fluid handling

Others

Increase in plasma atrial natriuretic peptide Antidiuretic hormone (vasopressin)

Decrease in renin and aldosterone levels Erythropoietin

---

by a 50% reduction in GFR between the ages of 20 and 90, in spite of compensatory hyperfiltration and hyperfunction by the remaining nephrons.[53] Even though GFR declines, the serum creatinine level remains normal due to the decreased lean body mass in the elderly. Blood urea nitrogen gradually increases at a rate of 0.2 mg/dL/year.

The elderly are prone to disorders of sodium and water excretion.[54] The kidney's ability to maximally concentrate urine after water deprivation is decreased, and its ability to excrete maximally diluted urine after water loading is lost. This tubular dysfunction is accentuated during the night, which leads to the common symptom of nocturnal polyuria.[55]

Plasma renin and aldosterone activity

Both plasma renin activity and aldosterone levels decrease after the fourth decade. The fall in renin activity may be related to a diminished ability to activate prorenin (renin precursor). The decreased aldosterone levels are related to lower renin activity.[56] The hyporenin-hypoaldosterone state in the elderly can predispose to hyperkalemia especially with nonsteroidal anti-inflammatory drugs (NSAIDs), angiotensin-converting enzyme (ACE) inhibitors, β-blockers, and potassium sparing diuretics. Plasma atrial natriuretic peptide rises progressively with increasing age as the basal renin and aldosterone levels decline.[57]

Renal-concentrating ability

Maximum ability to concentrate urine decreases with age from 1100 to 1200mOsm/kg at age 30 to approximately 800 mOsm/kg in the octogenarian.[58] An age-related increase occurs in osmoreceptor sensitivity. For the same osmolar stimulus, the elderly release twice as much antidiuretic

hormone (ADH, vasopressin) as younger persons. Studies suggest that there is a decreased responsiveness of the collecting duct to ADH.

Renal-diluting ability

The stress of anesthesia and surgery may impair the ability of the elderly kidney to excrete dilute urine secondary to excessive ADH secretion. Aging may also cause an intrinsic impairment of renal-diluting capacity.

FLUID AND ELECTROLYTE BALANCE

It is important to evaluate and treat electrolyte imbalances in the perioperative period in the elderly. Postoperative electrolyte imbalance is a marker for frailty and a risk factor for poor outcome in elderly patients.[59]

Sodium disorders

Hyponatremia occurs in about 2.5% of all hospitalized patients and in 4% of all postoperative patients. It is about 10 times more common in the elderly, occurring in 10–20% of geriatric patients. Hyponatremia may occur as a result of diuretic-induced renal dysfunction, age-induced higher levels of ADH secretion, or impaired ability of the aging kidney to excrete free water. Inadequate dietary sodium, increased sodium loss from diarrhea or vomiting, or administration of hypotonic solutions may contribute to hyponatremia in hospitalized elderly patients. Symptoms are primarily related to the CNS and are more apparent if the onset is acute rather than gradual. Acute hyponatremia should be more aggressively treated than chronic hyponatremia as it is associated with significant morbidity and mortality.[60] Rapid correction of sodium should be avoided and may cause central pontine myelenolysis.[61,62] Overcorrection of serum sodium to a hypernatremic state (>150 meq/L) has recently been suggested to cause central pontine myelenolysis as well.[61]

An important cause of perioperative acute hyponatremia and change in mental status is transurethral resection of the prostate (TURP) syndrome. Prostatic hypertrophy also causes obstructive uropathy, water conservation, and hyponatremia.[63]

Hypernatremia in the elderly is usually due to water loss and is rarely due to excessive sodium intake. Hypernatremia rarely occurs from a decreased renal concentrating ability alone, and is usually associated with dehydration. The incidence is about 1.5% in the geriatric hospitalized patients with an associated mortality rate of 42%.[64] It has been suggested that hypernatremia be used as a marker of neglect in quality of care assessments of nursing homes.[65]

The inability to communicate thirst to the caregivers, a poorly functioning thirst mechanism, decreased fluid intake, and dehydration secondary to infection may play a role in producing hypernatremia in the elderly. Other possible etiologies might include excessive urinary loss secondary to poorly controlled diabetes mellitus, diabetes insipidus, diuretics, lithium, hypercalcemia, Addison's disease, or postobstructive diuresis. Severe hypernatremia is associated with CNS dysfunction and may lead to loss of brain volume and intracranial hemorrhage. Treatment includes frequent monitoring of electrolytes while restoring intravascular volume. The therapeutic goal is to decrease osmolarity by 1–2 mOsm/L/h.

Potassium disorders

Total body potassium level declines with age, more so in women than in men. The decline is thought to be due to the decrease in muscle mass that accompanies aging.[66] Surprisingly, hyperkalemia is more common than hypokalemia in elderly persons.

Potassium balance is intact until the glomerular filtration rate is less than 10 mL/min. However, the elderly are at increased risk of developing hyperkalemia before the onset of end-stage renal disease (ESRD). This is secondary to a decrease in renin synthesis and impairment of renin release. Elderly patients with hyperkalemia have low concentrations of plasma renin and aldosterone, perhaps secondary to reduced glomerular filtration and sympathetic insufficiency.[67]

Hypokalemia is most often due to the three Ds: drugs (β-agonists, insulin); diuretics (loop, thiazide); and diarrhea (laxative use, organic causes). Chronic hypokalemia is better tolerated than acute. Preoperative low serum potassium predicts serious postoperative arrhythmias.

▶ Metabolic acidosis

Chronic anion gap metabolic acidosis is generally seen in the elderly, and is due to an inability of the kidneys to excrete the daily acid load produced as a result of protein metabolism. The ability to compensate for metabolic acidosis by acidification of urine is reduced and excretion of acid load requires almost three times as long in the elderly.[68] An impaired ability to acutely excrete an acid load may also result in hyperkalemia.[69]

PHARMACOLOGY OF ANESTHETIC AGENTS WHICH DEPEND ON RENAL ELIMINATION

▶ Anxiolytics

Diazepam and midazolam have active metabolites dependent on kidney elimination (Table 7-6). Benzodiazepines should be avoided in the elderly with renal insufficiency.

▶ Opioids

The clearance of the major metabolite of morphine, morphine-6-glucuronide, is dependent on renal excretion. Morphine-6-glucuronide has 40 times more analgesic activity than morphine. Similarly, the main metabolite of hydromorphone, hydromorphone-3-glucuronide, accumulates in renal impairment. Hydromorphone-3-glucuronide is thought to be pharmacologically inactive, but its activity has not been fully studied. Approximately 75% of fentanyl is excreted in the urine as metabolites, with less than 10% excreted as unchanged drug. The major metabolite, nor-fentanyl, is inactive. There is considerable interpatient variability in fentanyl pharmacokinetics, but no dosage modification appears necessary in patients with renal failure when fentanyl is given as a bolus. Meperidine is metabolized to nor-meperidine, which is neuroexcitatory. The neuroexcitatory effects range from tremor to convulsions. Plasma blood levels of nor-meperidine are increased in the elderly. Regular administration of meperidine is contraindicated in patients with any degree of renal failure.[70]

▶ Choice of muscle relaxants

Plasma clearance of vecuronium[71] and pancuronium[28] are prolonged. These drugs should be avoided because of their delayed and unpredictable elimination in elderly patients with renal insufficiency. Rocuronium is primarily dependent on hepatic clearance, but prolongation of blockade has been reported in patients with severe renal impairment. Pipecuronium and doxacurium are 60–90% renally excreted. Mivacurium is minimally dependent on the kidney for elimination and is recommended for short procedures. Atracurium and cisatracurium undergo Hofmann degradation and ester hydrolysis, and are minimally affected by age or kidney disease. They are the drugs of choice for elderly patients with kidney disease.

TABLE 7-6

Drugs With Active or Toxic Metabolites Dependent on Renal Excretion and Its Anesthetic Implications in the Elderly

Drug	Metabolites	Activities	Anesthetic Implications
Fentanyl	Norfentanyl, inactive	Sedation	Drug of choice for ESRD
Hydromorphone	Hydromorphone-3-glucuronide, inactive		Dosing guidelines with renal dysfunction are sparse
Morphine	Morphine-3-glucuronide Morphine-6-glucuronide	Antianalgesic Analgesic (40 times the potency of morphine)	Metabolites accumulate with renal impairment
Meperidine	Normeperidine	Neuroexcitatory	Plasma levels of nor-meperidine increased in elderly
Diazepam	Oxazepam	Sedative	Prolonged action
Midazolam	1-hydroxy-midazolam	Sedative	Prolonged action
Sodium nitroprusside	Thiocyanate	Neurotoxic	Avoid if possible
Enflurane	Fluoride	Nephrotoxic	Avoid
Vecuronium	Desacetyl-vecuronium	Relaxant	Prolonged action
Pancuronium	3-hydroxy-pancuronium	Relaxant	Prolonged action
Procainamide	n-Acetyl-procainamide (NAPA)	Neurotoxic	Avoid/monitor NAPA levels
Neostigmine			Prolonged action
Glycopyrrolate			Less prolonged action

► Inhalational agents

The modern potent inhalational agents resist biodegradation. Both isoflurane and desflurane undergo minimal biodegradation with no reports of renal toxicity. Fluoride-induced nephrotoxicity is a possibility with sevoflurane or enflurane anesthesia. Clinical studies show no evidence of increased serum creatinine or blood urea nitrogen following sevoflurane administration.[72] The typical plasma concentration of fluoride ions incurred after routine general anesthesia with enflurane or sevoflurane may be sufficient to impair tubular responsiveness to ADH.

ANESTHETIC MANAGEMENT OF ELDERLY PATIENTS WITH REGARD TO THE KIDNEYS

► Preoperative considerations

There are no specific renal diseases which are common to the elderly. However, the anesthesiologist will often encounter the older patient with acute renal failure (ARF) or end stage renal disease (ESRD).

Acute renal failure

ARF is more common in the elderly than in younger persons. The incidence of ARF in the postoperative period and in the intensive care unit (ICU) setting ranges from 7% to 15%.[73,74] These estimates may be conservative with the aging of the population and the variable definition of ARF. ARF is associated with increased mortality, which is well documented in the cardiac[75,76] and vascular surgery[77,78] literature. Whether ARF itself is an independent predictor of poor outcome or merely another component of multisystem organ dysfunction remains controversial. Preoperative renal status is the best universal predictor of postoperative renal failure, and age is a determining factor in the extent of recovery after ARF. Acute tubular necrosis accounts for nearly 90% of cases of perioperative renal failure.[79]

The causes of ARF can be categorized into prerenal, renal, and postrenal. Prerenal failure in the elderly is mainly due to poor perfusion of the kidneys. The renal causes of ARF primarily include nephrotoxic injury secondary to drugs and a number of primary renal disorders such as acute tubular necrosis, acute glomerulonephritis, and acute interstitial nephritis. Postrenal causes include prostate carcinoma, bladder tumor, gynecological malignancies, stones, strictures, and blockage of urinary catheter. The signs and symptoms of ARF depend on the cause, the severity of renal injury, and the speed with which ARF develops. Patients may present with clinical or biochemical complications of uremia, an absent or decreased urine flow, evidence of fluid retention, or unexpected elevation in the blood urea nitrogen and serum creatinine levels. Nonoliguric renal failure is increasingly being recognized. Nonoliguric ARF carries a better prognosis than oliguric or anuric ARF.[80,81] This reflects the less severe nature of nonoliguric renal failure.[82]

Laboratory testing used in the differential diagnosis of perioperative oliguria is shown in Table 7-7. The postrenal causes are excluded by physical examination. Prior administration of diuretics makes it difficult to confirm the etiology of acute renal tubular dysfunction.

The management of ARF remains preventive and supportive. Identification and correction of risk factors such as preexisting chronic renal insufficiency, volume depletion, hypotension, sepsis, and nephrotoxin exposure reduces the threat and consequences of postoperative ARF. The principles of ARF treatment include medical management in the form of salt-water restriction, judicious use of diuretics, correction of electrolyte abnormalities, avoiding nephrotoxic drugs, and aggressively treating infections. Studies have failed to demonstrate that drugs such as low-dose dopamine,[83] atrial natriuretic peptide,[84] or diuretics[85] can prevent onset or deterioration of renal function. No drugs are currently available that hasten renal recovery once ARF has occurred, although some studies show that fenoldopam may reduce the risk of acute renal failure in patients in whom endogenous and exogenous catecholamine action may induce a renal vascular constrictive condition.[86] Other studies by Bove et al. found no difference in clinical outcome when fenoldopam was compared to dopamine in a high-risk population undergoing cardiac surgery.[87]

Chronic renal failure (CRF) and end-stage renal disease in the elderly

The incidence of patients on dialysis, 75 years or older, in the United States in 1997 was 22.7%.[88] In the elderly, the relative risk versus benefit of dialysis must be discussed with the family and the patients themselves. A study by Joly et al.[89] regarding octogenarians reaching ESRD concluded that the survival of patients treated conservatively was shorter than those on dialysis. Sixty percent of deaths in the conservative group were attributed to uremia and pulmonary edema, suggesting that dialysis would prolong life to some extent.

Patients with chronic renal failure (CRF) and ESRD are at risk of perioperative intravascular volume overload and electrolyte imbalances. These patients achieve the greatest benefit from dialysis close to operation. In emergent cases, removing heparin from the dialysis circuit is an option especially if intraoperative bleeding is likely. Elective or emergent abdominal operation eliminates the option of postoperative peritoneal dialysis. Alternative methods of dialysis may be created in these patients (e.g., central catheter access). Increased mortality is seen when serum blood urea nitrogen exceeds 75 mg/dL.

Although hemodialysis and peritoneal dialysis can prolong life, they are not as effective as the normal kidney's ability to clear solutes. Dialysis patients are at increased risk of complications such as infections, anemia, renal osteodystrophy, and malnutrition that are not necessarily caused by dialysis per se, but appear to be a consequence of ESRD. The treatment of anemia with recombinant human erythropoietin has resulted in improved exercise tolerance and quality of life in patients on dialysis.[90] The response to erythropoietin takes 2–6 weeks.[91] Although it is effective in chronic management of anemia, it is of little value in the acute management. The anemia of CRF is associated with left ventricular hypertrophy, an independent risk factor for early death.

TABLE 7-7

Differential Diagnosis of Oliguria

	Prerenal	Renal	Postrenal
Dipstick	Trace proteinuria	+/++ protein	0/+ protein
Sediment	Hyaline casts	Pig/WBC/ RBC casts	Crystals and RBC
Urinary sodium (mEq/1)	<40	>40	
Urinary osmolarity (mOsm/1)	>400	250–300	<300
Fractional excretion of sodium (FENa)	>1.0	<1.0	>1

During the last few decades, the pattern of ESRD has changed with an increasing number of elderly patients admitted for dialysis. The common modes of dialysis are hemodialysis and chronic peritoneal dialysis (CPD). CPD is underutilized in the elderly, in part because the "old-old" (those >80 years) cannot perform "self" dialysis, contrary to the "young-old" (those between 65 and 80 years).[92] Recent studies by Winkelmayer et al. compared hemodialysis to peritoneal dialysis and concluded that peritoneal dialysis appears to be associated with higher mortality among older patients, particularly among those with diabetes, even after controlling for a large number of risk factors for mortality.[93]

In patients with ESRD, preoperative evaluation should include consideration of concomitant drug therapy, complications of CRF (anemia, bleeding, encephalopathy, neuropathy), and underlying systemic disease (angina, diabetes). Dialysis should be performed the day before the surgery. Elective surgery should be avoided on the same day as hemodialysis because of problems of rebound heparinization, fluids shifts, hypokalemia, and disequilibrium. On the other hand, if surgery is delayed for more than 48 h, patients may be fluid overloaded, hyperkalemic, and acidotic. Uremia-induced delayed gastric emptying, platelet dysfunction,[94] and unexpected sensitivity to CNS depressant drugs should be taken into consideration. Blood transfusion is not indicated for patients with chronic stable anemia, especially if the hematocrit is more than 25%.[95] Correction of coagulopathy is indicated only in cases of diffuse petechiae, a history of uremic bleeding, or the need to restore normal platelet function before surgery. Dialysis, desmopressin, and cryoprecipitate are capable of stopping the bleeding.[96] Intravenous conjugated estrogen (0.6 mg/kg) is an alternative when given 4 or 5 days before surgery.[97] In elderly patients on peritoneal dialysis, preoperative drainage of peritoneal fluid decreases intra-abdominal pressure, allowing easier ventilation while decreasing the risk of aspiration.

▶ Intraoperative anesthetic concerns

Reduction in both RBF and GFR occurs during surgical level of general anesthesia. Paying close attention to intraoperative volume status, avoiding hemodynamic changes, and avoiding the use of nephrotoxic drugs are critical to minimizing postoperative renal deterioration in older adults.

Although use of succinylcholine has been associated with acute hyperkalemia in patients with CRF and ESRD,[98,99] Thapa and Brull[99] concluded that succinylcholine is not associated with a risk of hyperkalemia as long as there is no preoperative hyperkalemia or conditions that predispose to hyperkalemia like trauma, burns, or neuromuscular disorders.

Patients with chronic renal insufficiency are susceptible to the development of hyperkalemia. Hyperkalemia is mainly due to a transcellular shift of potassium that is provoked by various stimuli which may occur perioperatively such as insulin deficiency, β-blockers (which may be used for acute management of hypertension), and acidemia.

There are no unique monitors for the elderly with renal disease. Care must be taken in patients with a functioning arteriovenous fistula. The patency should be evaluated preoperatively by the presence of bruit or thrill. Intravenous access and blood pressure cuff should not be placed on the arm with the fistula. If possible, cannulation of the subclavian veins should be avoided in all patients with CRF or ESRD. The cannulation of these vessels is associated with an increased risk of late stenosis or thrombosis, preventing the use of arteriovenous access on the same side.

Patients with ESRD also have renal osteodystrophy, which increases the risk of fractures. Care in positioning and adequate padding of the

pressure points would avoid pressure damage to the fragile bones and skin. Care should be taken of the arteriovenous fistula.

Brachial plexus and axillary blocks have been used successfully for revision of arteriovenous shunts, provided there are no contraindications for regional anesthetic techniques. Spinal and epidural can be used successfully, but elderly patients with autonomic neuropathy are at an increased risk for developing hypotension induced by sympathetic blockade. The limiting factors in performing a regional technique are abnormal coagulation studies, inability to lie still, and psychological status.

▶ Postoperative concerns in elderly patients related to the kidneys

In the postoperative period, every effort should be made to diagnose ARF early, eliminate causative agents, and prevent further insults.

In elderly patients, the loss of renal reserve decreases the ability to handle acid, fluid, and electrolytes in the postoperative period, resulting in fluid overload, acidemia, and hyperkalemia. Postoperative hyperkalemia should be treated emergently, especially if ECG evidence is present. A number of uremic patients may have bleeding problems secondary to platelet dysfunction, thereby increasing the surgical morbidity and mortality. Furthermore, renal dysfunction hampers their ability to excrete anesthetic drugs and muscle relaxants, thereby prolonging anesthetic recovery. Adverse drug reactions occur more frequently in uremic patients than in people with normal GFR.

KEY POINTS

▶ In spite of the structural decline with aging, the aging liver preserves its function very well. The capacity of the liver to regenerate is more or less maintained in the elderly, although it may be delayed. The deterioration in liver function with aging is mainly the effect of tobacco, alcohol, and environmental factors rather than the effect of structural decline alone.

▶ Reduction in liver blood flow will reduce clearance of the drugs with high hepatic extraction ratio, but will not have the same impact on drugs with a low hepatic extraction ratio. The aging of the liver does affect the pharmacokinetics of commonly used anesthetic agents. This translates to longer elimination half-times and decreased dose requirements in the elderly.

▶ Alcohol-related problems are common in the elderly and often manifest themselves in the form of accidents or falls.

▶ The two primary objectives in preoperative assessment of the elderly hepatic system are to identify liver disease processes and to determine the functional reserve of the liver.

▶ From the standpoint of the effect of aging on the liver, there is no evidence that a specific injected or inhaled drug is preferable for induction or maintenance of anesthesia.

▶ Renal functional changes associated with aging are related to a decrease in the renal mass.

▶ Because of changes in renal physiology with aging, the elderly are prone to perioperative water and electrolyte imbalances which are primarily characterized by disorders of sodium and potassium metabolism.

▶ Opioids and muscle relaxants are the two classes of anesthetic drugs in which pharmacokinetics are most affected by aging of the kidney.

▶ Paying close attention to intraoperative volume status, avoiding hemodynamic changes, and avoiding the use of nephrotoxic drugs are critical to minimizing postoperative renal deterioration in older adults. In elderly patients, the loss of renal reserve decreases the ability to handle acid, fluid, and electrolyte in the postoperative period, resulting in fluid overload, acidemia, and hyperkalemia.

KEY ARTICLES

▶ Anantharaju A, Feller A, Chedid A. Aging liver. A review. *Gerontology*. 2002;48:343–353.

▶ Zeeh J. The aging liver: consequences for drug treatment in old age. *Arch Gerontol Geriatr*. 2001;32:255–263.

▶ Shafer SL. The pharmacology of anesthetic drugs in elderly patients. *Anesthesiol Clin N Am*. 2000;18:1–29.

▶ Beck LH. Changes in renal function with aging. *Clin Geriatr Med*. 1998;14:199–209.

▶ Pichette V, Leblond FA. Drug metabolism in chronic renal failure. *Curr Drug Metab*. 2003;4:91–103.

▶ Sladen RN. Anesthesia and renal considerations. *Anesthesiol Clin N Am*. 2000;18:1–19.

REFERENCES

1. Anantharaju A, Feller A, Chedid A. Aging liver. A review. *Gerontology*. 2002;48:343–353.
2. Woodhouse KW, James OF. Hepatic drug metabolism and aging. *Br Med Bull*. 1990;46:22–35.
3. Le Couteur DG, McLean AJ. The aging liver. Drug clearance and an oxygen diffusion barrier hypothesis. *Clin Pharmacokinet*. 1998;34:359–373.
4. Woodhouse K. Drugs and the liver. Part III: Aging of the liver and the metabolism of drugs. *Biopharm Drug Dispos*. 1992;13:311–320.
5. James OF. Parenchymal liver disease in the elderly. *Gut*. 1997;41:430–432.
6. Jansen PL. Liver disease in the elderly. *Best Pract Res Clin Gastroenterol*. 2002;16:149–158.
7. Kitani K. Aging and the liver. *Prog Liver Dis*. 1990;9:603–623.
8. Vestal RE. Aging and determinants of hepatic drug clearance. *Hepatology*. 1989;9:331–334.
9. Liu Y, Guyton KZ, Gorospe M, et al. Age-related decline in mitogen-activated protein kinase activity in epidermal growth factor-stimulated rat hepatocytes. *J Biol Chem*. 1996;271:3604–3607.
10. Tietz NW, Shuey DF, Wekstein DR. Laboratory values in fit aging individuals—sexagenarians through centenarians. *Clin Chem*. 1992;38:1167–1185.
11. Benet LZ, Hoener BA. Changes in plasma protein binding have little clinical relevance. *Clin Pharmacol Ther*. 2002;71:115–121.
12. Schmucker DL. Aging and the liver: an update. *J Gerontol A Biol Sci Med Sci*. 1998;53:B315–B320.
13. Turnheim K. When drug therapy gets old: pharmacokinetics and pharmacodynamics in the elderly. *Exp Gerontol*. 2003;38:843–853.
14. Guevin C, Michaud J, Naud J, et al. Down-regulation of hepatic cytochrome P450 in chronic renal failure: role of uremic mediators. *Br J Pharmacol*. 2002;137:1039–1046.
15. Pichette V, Leblond FA. Drug metabolism in chronic renal failure. *Curr Drug Metab*. 003;4:91–103.
16. Dreisbach AW, Lertora JJ. The effect of chronic renal failure on hepatic drug metabolism and drug disposition. *Semin Dial*. 2003;16:45–50.
17. Tung D, Yoshida EM, Wang CS, Steinbrecher UP. Severe desflurane hepatotoxicity after colon surgery in an elderly patient. *Can J Anaesth*. 2005;52:133–136.
18. Kharasch ED, Armstrong AS, Gunn K, et al. Clinical sevoflurane metabolism and disposition. II. The role of cytochrome P450 2E1 in fluoride and hexafluoroisopropanol formation. *Anesthesiology*. 1995;82:1379–1388.
19. Suttner SW, Schmidt CC, Boldt J, et al. Low-flow desflurane and sevoflurane anesthesia minimally affect hepatic integrity and function in elderly patients. *Anesth Analg*. 2000;91:206–212.
20. Burch PG, Stanski DR. The role of metabolism and protein binding in thiopental anesthesia. *Anesthesiology*. 1983;58:146–152.
21. Simons PJ, Cockshott ID, Douglas EJ, et al. Disposition in male volunteers of a subanaesthetic intravenous dose of an oil in water emulsion of 14C-propofol. *Xenobiotica*. 1988;18:429–440.
22. Kirkpatrick T, Cockshott ID, Douglas EJ, Nimmo WS. Pharmacokinetics of propofol (diprivan) in elderly patients. *Br J Anaesth*. 1988;60:146–150.
23. Gooding JM, Corssen G. Etomidate: an ultrashort-acting nonbarbiturate agent for anesthesia induction. *Anesth Analg*. 1976;55:286–289.
24. Arden JR, Holley FO, Stanski DR. Increased sensitivity to etomidate in the elderly: initial distribution versus altered brain response. *Anesthesiology*. 1986;65:19–27.
25. Bell GD, Spickett GP, Reeve PA, et al. Intravenous midazolam for upper gastrointestinal endoscopy: a study of 800 consecutive cases relating dose to age and sex of patient. *Br J Clin Pharmacol*. 1987;23:241–243.
26. Maitre PO, Buhrer M, Thomson D, Stanski DR. A three-step approach combining bayesian regression and NONMEM population analysis: application to midazolam. *J Pharmacokinet Biopharm*. 1991;19:377–384.
27. Beemer GH, Bjorksten AR. Pharmacodynamics of atracurium in clinical practice: effect of plasma potassium, patient demographics, and concurrent medication. *Anesth Analg*. 1993;76:1288–1295.
28. Duvaldestin P, Saada J, Berger JL, et al. Pharmacokinetics, pharmacodynamics, and dose-response relationships of pancuronium in control and elderly subjects. *Anesthesiology*. 1982;56:36–40.
29. Rupp SM, Castagnoli KP, Fisher DM, Miller RD. Pancuronium and vecuronium pharmacokinetics and pharmacodynamics in younger and elderly adults. *Anesthesiology*. 1987;67:45–49.
30. Matteo RS, Ornstein E, Schwartz AE, et al. Pharmacokinetics and pharmacodynamics of rocuronium (org 9426) in elderly surgical patients. *Anesth Analg*. 1993;77:1193–1197.
31. Fisher DM, Rosen JI. A pharmacokinetic explanation for increasing recovery time following larger or repeated doses of nondepolarizing muscle relaxants. *Anesthesiology*. 1986;65:286–291.
32. Maddineni VR, Mirakhur RK. Prolonged neuromuscular block following mivacurium. *Anesthesiology*. 1993;78:1181–1184.
33. Chauvin M. Acute toxicity of local anesthetics as a function of the patient's condition. *Ann Fr Anesth Reanim*. 1988;7:216–223.
34. Wojcicki J, Kozlowski K, Drozdzik M, Wojcicki M. Lidocaine elimination in patients with liver cirrhosis. *Acta Pol Pharm*. 2002;59:321–324.
35. Glenn F. Surgical management of acute cholecystitis in patients 65 years of age and older. *Ann Surg*. 1981;193:56–59.
36. Siegel JH, Kasmin FE. Biliary tract diseases in the elderly: management and outcomes. *Gut*. 1997;41:433–435.
37. Lucey MR, Hill EM, Young JP, et al. The influences of age and gender on blood ethanol concentrations in healthy humans. *J Stud Alcohol*. 1999;60:103–110.
38. Mulinga JD. Elderly people with alcohol-related problems: where do they go? *Int J Geriatr Psychiatry*. 1999;14:564–566.
39. Muravchick S. The aging process: anesthetic implications. *Acta Anaesthesiol Belg*. 1998;49:85–90.
40. Friedman LS. The risk of surgery in patients with liver disease. *Hepatology*. 1999;29:1617–1623.
41. Farges O, Malassagne B, Flejou JF, et al. Risk of major liver resection in patients with underlying chronic liver disease: a reappraisal. *Ann Surg*. 1999;229:210–215.
42. Bakti G, Fisch HU, Karlaganis G, et al. Mechanism of the excessive sedative response of cirrhotics to benzodiazepines: model experiments with triazolam. *Hepatology*. 1987;7:629–638.
43. Krause KR, Howells GA, Buhs CL, et al. Hypothermia-induced coagulopathy during hemorrhagic shock. *Am Surg*. 2000;66:348–354.
44. Rohrer MJ, Natale AM. Effect of hypothermia on the coagulation cascade. *Crit Care Med*. 1992;20:1402–1405.
45. Brienza N, Revelly JP, Ayuse T, Robotham JL. Effects of PEEP on liver arterial and venous blood flows. *Am J Respir Crit Care Med*. 1995;152:504–510.
46. Green NM, Brull SJ. The cardiovascular system. In: *Physiology of Spinal Anesthesia*. Greene NM, Brull SJ, eds. Baltimore: Williams & Wilkins; 1993:85–199.
47. McLean AJ, Le Couteur DG. Aging biology and geriatric clinical pharmacology. *Pharmacol Rev*. 2004;56:163–184.
48. Beck LH. Changes in renal function with aging. *Clin Geriatr Med*. 1998;14:199–209.
49. Melk A, Halloran PF. Cell senescence and its implications for nephrology. *J Am Soc Nephrol*. 2001;12:385–393.

50. Fuiano G, Sund S, Mazza G, et al. Renal hemodynamic response to maximal vasodilating stimulus in healthy older subjects. *Kidney Int.* 2001;59: 1052–1058.

51. Neugarten J, Gallo G, Silbiger S, Kasiske B. Glomerulosclerosis in aging humans is not influenced by gender. *Am J Kidney Dis.* 1999;34:884–888.

52. Thurau KW. Autoregulation of renal blood flow and glomerular filtration rate, including data on tubular and peritubular capillary pressures and vessel wall tension. *Circ Res.* 1964;15(Suppl.):132–141.

53. Lubran MM. Renal function in the elderly. *Ann Clin Lab Sci.* 1995;25: 122–133.

54. Lindeman RD. Overview: renal physiology and pathophysiology of aging. *Am J Kidney Dis.* 1990;16:275–282.

55. Ali H. Renal disease in the elderly: distinctive disorders, tailored treatments. *Postgrad Med.* 1996;100:44–48, 53–54, 57.

56. Noth RH, Lassman MN, Tan SY, et al. Age and the renin-aldosterone system. *Arch Intern Med.* 1977;137:1414–1417.

57. Ohashi M, Fujio N, Nawata H, et al. High plasma concentrations of human atrial natriuretic polypeptide in aged men. *J Clin Endocrinol Metab.* 1987; 64:81–85.

58. Rowe JW, Shock NW, DeFronzo RA. The influence of age on the renal response to water deprivation in man. *Nephron.* 1976;17:270–278.

59. Antonelli Incalzi R, Gemma A, Capparella O, et al. Post-operative electrolyte imbalance: its incidence and prognostic implications for elderly orthopaedic patients. *Age Aging.* 1993;22:325–331.

60. Cluitmans FH, Meinders AE. Management of severe hyponatremia: rapid or slow correction? *Am J Med.* 1990;88:161–166.

61. Ayus JC, Krothapalli RK, Arieff AI. Treatment of symptomatic hyponatremia and its relation to brain damage. A prospective study. *N Engl J Med.* 1987;317:1190–1195.

62. Ayus JC, Krothapalli RK, Arieff AI. Changing concepts in treatment of severe symptomatic hyponatremia. Rapid correction and possible relation to central pontine myelinolysis. *Am J Med.* 1985;78:897–902.

63. Hammerlein A, Derendorf H, Lowenthal DT. Pharmacokinetic and pharmacodynamic changes in the elderly. Clinical implications. *Clin Pharmacokinet.* 1998;35:49–64.

64. Snyder NA, Feigal DW, Arieff AI. Hypernatremia in elderly patients. A heterogeneous, morbid, and iatrogenic entity. *Ann Intern Med.* 1987;107: 309–319.

65. Himmelstein DU, Jones AA, Woolhandler S. Hypernatremic dehydration in nursing home patients: an indicator of neglect. *J Am Geriatr Soc.* 1983; 31:466–471.

66. Minaker KL, Rowe JW. Potassium homeostasis during hyperinsulinemia: effect of insulin level, beta-blockade, and age. *Am J Physiol.* 1982;242: E373–E377.

67. Kudoh A, Sakai T, Ishihara H, Matsuki A. Renin-aldosterone in elderly patients with hyperkalaemia under anaesthesia. *Eur J Anaesthesiol.* 1999;16:231–235.

68. Agarwal BN, Cabebe FG. Renal acidification in elderly subjects. *Nephron.* 1980;26:291–295.

69. Clark BA, Brown RS. Potassium homeostasis and hyperkalemic syndromes. *Endocrinol Metab Clin N Am.* 1995;24:573–591.

70. Chan K, Kendall MJ, Mitchard M, Wells WD. The effect of aging on plasma pethidine concentration. *Br J Clin Pharmacol.* 1975;2:297–302.

71. Lien CA, Matteo RS, Ornstein E, et al. Distribution, elimination, and action of vecuronium in the elderly. *Anesth Analg.* 1991;73:39–42.

72. Mazze RI, Callan CM, Galvez ST, et al. The effects of sevoflurane on serum creatinine and blood urea nitrogen concentrations: a retrospective, twenty-two-center, comparative evaluation of renal function in adult surgical patients. *Anesth Analg.* 2000;90:683–688.

73. Brivet FG, Kleinknecht DJ, Loirat P, Landais PJ. Acute renal failure in intensive care units—causes, outcome, and prognostic factors of hospital mortality; a prospective, multicenter study. French study group on acute renal failure. *Crit Care Med.* 1996;24:192–198.

74. Menashe PI, Ross SA, Gottlieb JE. Acquired renal insufficiency in critically ill patients. *Crit Care Med.* 1988;16:1106–1109.

75. Chertow GM, Levy EM, Hammermeister KE, et al. Independent association between acute renal failure and mortality following cardiac surgery. *Am J Med.* 1998;104:343–348.

76. Zanardo G, Michielon P, Paccagnella A, et al. Acute renal failure in the patient undergoing cardiac operation. Prevalence, mortality rate, and main risk factors. *J Thorac Cardiovasc Surg.* 1994;107:1489–1495.

77. Kashyap VS, Cambria RP, Davison JK, L'Italien GJ. Renal failure after thoracoabdominal aortic surgery. *J Vasc Surg.* 1997;26:949–955; discussion 955–957.

78. Walker SR, Yusuf SW, Wenham PW, Hopkinson BR. Renal complications following endovascular repair of abdominal aortic aneurysms. *J Endovasc Surg.* 1998;5:318–322.

79. Wilkes BM, Mailloux LU. Acute renal failure. Pathogenesis and prevention. *Am J Med.* 1986;80:1129–1136.

80. Anderson RJ, Linas SL, Berns AS, et al. Nonoliguric acute renal failure. *N Engl J Med.* 1977;296:1134–1138.

81. Baek SM, Makabali GG, Shoemaker WC. Clinical determinants of survival from postoperative renal failure. *Surg Gynecol Obstet.* 1975;140: 685–689.

82. Brenner BM, Lazarus JM. *Acute Renal Failure.* 4th ed. New York, Churchill Livingstone, 1993.

83. Marik PE. Low-dose dopamine: a systematic review. *Intensive Care Med.* 2002;28:877–883.

84. Sward K, Valsson F, Odencrants P, et al. Recombinant human atrial natriuretic peptide in ischemic acute renal failure: a randomized placebo-controlled trial. *Crit Care Med.* 2004;32:1310–1315.

85. Uchino S, Doig GS, Bellomo R, et al. Diuretics and mortality in acute renal failure. *Crit Care Med.* 2004;32:1669–1677.

86. Ranucci M, Soro G, Barzaghi N, et al. Fenoldopam prophylaxis of postoperative acute renal failure in high-risk cardiac surgery patients. *Ann Thorac Surg.* 2004;78:1332–1337; discussion 1337–1338.

87. Bove T, Landoni G, Calabro MG, et al. Renoprotective action of fenoldopam in high-risk patients undergoing cardiac surgery: a prospective, double-blind, randomized clinical trial. *Circulation.* 2005;111: 3230–3235.

88. Wright LF. Survival in patients with end-stage renal disease. *Am J Kidney Dis.* 1991;17:25–28.

89. Joly D, Anglicheau D, Alberti C, et al. Octogenarians reaching end-stage renal disease: cohort study of decision-making and clinical outcomes. *J Am Soc Nephrol.* 2003;14:1012–1021.

90. Soucie JM, McClellan WM. Early death in dialysis patients: risk factors and impact on incidence and mortality rates. *J Am Soc Nephrol.* 1996;7:2169–2175.

91. Maxwell AP. Novel erythropoiesis-stimulating protein in the management of the anemia of chronic renal failure. *Kidney Int.* 2002;62:720–729.

92. Dimkovic NB, Prakash S, Roscoe J, et al. Chronic peritoneal dialysis in octogenarians. *Nephrol Dial Transplant.* 2001;16:2034–2040.

93. Winkelmayer WC, Glynn RJ, Mittleman MA, et al. Comparing mortality of elderly patients on hemodialysis versus peritoneal dialysis: a propensity score approach. *J Am Soc Nephrol.* 2002;13:2353–2362.

94. Remuzzi G, Marchesi D, Livio M, et al. Altered platelet and vascular prostaglandin-generation in patients with renal failure and prolonged bleeding times. *Thromb Res.* 1978;13:1007–1015.

95. Barrett BJ, Fenton SS, Ferguson B, et al. Clinical practice guidelines for the management of anemia coexistent with chronic renal failure. Canadian Society of Nephrology. *J Am Soc Nephrol.* 1999;10(Suppl.13): S292–S296.

96. Mannucci PM, Remuzzi G, Pusineri F, et al. Deamino-8-D-arginine vasopressin shortens the bleeding time in uremia. *N Engl J Med.* 1983;308: 8–12.

97. Livio M, Mannucci PM, Vigano G, et al. Conjugated estrogens for the management of bleeding associated with renal failure. *N Engl J Med.* 1986;315:731–735.

98. Koide M, Waud BE. Serum potassium concentrations after succinylcholine in patients with renal failure. *Anesthesiology.* 1972;36:142–145.

99. Thapa S, Brull SJ. Succinylcholine-induced hyperkalemia in patients with renal failure: an old question revisited. *Anesth Analg.* 2000;91:237–241.

SECTION

3

PHARMACOLOGY

Pharmacology of Intravenous Drugs in the Elderly

CHAPTER

8

Brice Lortat-Jacob
Frédérique Servin

A national survey performed in France in 1996 showed that one person out of eight could expect to be submitted to an anesthetic every year. Over 30% of these patients were older than 60 years.[1] Perioperative complications are mainly overdosing during induction of general anesthesia, hemodynamic instability throughout the procedure, and undetected aspiration of gastric contents in the post anesthesia care unit (PACU) due to poor recovery. A thorough knowledge of the changes induced by aging on the pharmacology of anesthetic drugs will help in designing an appropriate anesthetic protocol, thus optimizing the whole course of anesthesia and recovery. This chapter reviews the major changes induced by aging on the pharmacology of drugs. The consequences of these changes on the pharmacology of individual drugs commonly used by the anesthetist are considered and guidelines for optimal use of these drugs are presented.

CHANGES INDUCED BY AGING ON THE PHARMACOLOGY OF INTRAVENOUS ANESTHETIC DRUGS

▶ Pharmacokinetics

Absorption

Digestive absorption of drugs is usually not modified by aging because the vast majority of drugs are absorbed by passive diffusion.[2] Bioavailability of drugs submitted to an hepatic first-pass effect (midazolam) may be increased by the reduction of their clearance, leading to higher plasma concentration for the same oral dose.

Distribution

Drug distribution is frequently modified by aging, specifically that of lipid soluble drugs. Indeed, in the elderly, a reduction in lean body mass and total body water and an increase in fat are observed. Those changes are more important in males than in females.[3] Thus, the volume of distribution at steady state of very lipid soluble drugs (diazepam, midazolam) is markedly increased in aged individuals.[4] This lowers their plasma concentration and delays their elimination. On the contrary, less lipid soluble drugs (morphine) have a smaller volume of distribution in the elderly, and their plasma concentration decreases quicker in this population.[5]

The so-called greater "sensitivity" of aged patients to the action of certain drugs has in some cases been related to a reduction in either the initial volume of distribution or the initial distribution clearance (thiopental,[6] etomidate,[7] propofol,[8] and so forth). In elderly patients compared to younger ones, the same dose will generate a markedly higher plasma concentration, and thus a greater pharmacologic effect.

All the anesthetic agents are more or less bound to plasma proteins. In the elderly, changes in anesthetic drug binding may lead to changes in pharmacologic effects. Plasma albumin concentration tends to decrease with age, and even if the albumin plasma concentration remains normal, structural protein changes may lead to a reduced efficiency in albumin-binding sites.[9] At the same time, many chronically administered drugs compete with the anesthetic agents on albumin-binding sites and thus increase their unbound fraction. Thus, over-the-counter drugs should carefully be recorded even if they do not seem to interact with anesthesia. On the contrary, alpha$_1$-acid-glycoprotein concentration is increased in many medical conditions frequently present in the elderly, such as inflammation or cancer.[10]

Elimination

Hepatic Metabolism The size of the adult liver decreases with age. Up to about 50 years, the liver represents a fairly constant fraction of total body weight (around 2.5%). From 50 years on, this proportion is progressively reduced to reach only 1.6% at 90 years.[11]

With age, liver blood flow decreases about 0.3–1.5% every year. Thus, at 65 years, the liver blood flow has lost on average 40% of its value at 25 years.[11] The elimination clearance of highly extracted anesthetic drugs (etomidate, ketamine, flumazenil, morphine, fentanyl, sufentanil, naloxone, lidocaine, and so forth) is thereby directly modified, leading to slower elimination in the aged population.[7]

Hepatic drug metabolism is achieved through two major processes: phase I (oxidation, reduction, hydrolysis) and phase II (acetylation, conjugation) reactions. Phase I reactions are mainly carried out by microsomal mono-oxygenases, which include the P-450 cytochromes (CYP450). Most studies agree that liver metabolizing capacities are not modified by aging when phase II reactions are activated.[12] For example, the intrinsic clearance of conjugated agents is not modified, but their elimination clearance will usually be reduced because of dependence on hepatic blood flow.

Changes over time in phase I reactions are more controversial. Antipyrine has a low hepatic extraction coefficient and low plasma protein binding. Therefore, its systemic clearance narrowly reflects the intrinsic clearance of its unbound fraction and the intrinsic clearance may be used to estimate the phase I metabolizing capacities. Some authors found antipyrine clearance to be reduced by aging.[13] However, others argue that age-independent parameters such as smoking, sedentary, or food habits have greater influence on antipyrine clearance than aging per se.[14] This progressive impact of lifestyle over time probably accounts for the great variability between individuals observed in the aged population. Age does not appear to be an independent covariate for the mean clearance value, but increases clearance variability between individuals. Table 8-1 shows the elimination of selected intravenous anesthetic agents.

Renal Excretion Most anesthetic agents are lipid soluble. As a result, they are filtered by the glomeruli and immediately undergo complete tubular reabsorption, which precludes their renal elimination. The kidneys will only excrete their more hydrosoluble metabolites. Some metabolites (morphine-6-glucuronide) are pharmacologically active, and their retention may prolong the pharmacological effect of the native compound due to decreased renal function.[15] Similarly, some muscle relaxants are eliminated at least in part through the kidneys. Their clearance will be reduced in the elderly.[16]

▶ Transfer to the effect site

Modeling studies based on the observation of differences between the time course of effect of numerous drugs and the evolution of their plasma concentration have led to the establishment of an *effect-site concentration*, which is closely related to the time course of effect. Effect-site concentration can be calculated from the plasma concentration via a transfer rate constant.[17] Estimation of transfer rate constants in the elderly has demonstrated that frequently in this population, the transfer of anesthetic drugs from the plasma to the biophase is delayed.[18–20] This factor may explain delayed onset and delayed recovery even when pharmacokinetics are not modified by aging.[21]

▶ Pharmacodynamics

Central nervous system

The central nervous system is the target of nearly all anesthetic agents, and consequently all the changes over time of this system will directly influence the handling of anesthetic drugs. The main effects of age on the central nervous system are[22]

Table 8-1

Elimination of Selected Anesthetic Agents

Agent	Clearance (mL/min)/E (%)	Dependent on Flow?	Metabolic Pathway	Protein Binding %	Protein	Active Metabolite
Thiopental	210/15	No	CYP450: oxidation ++ desulfuration	86	Albumin	Pentobarbital (3%)
Propofol	1800/100	Yes	Conjugation ++	98	Albumin	No
Etomidate	1500/100	Yes	Hydrolysis by liver esterases	94	Albumin	No
Ketamine	1260/90	Yes	CYP450	<30	?	Norketamine
Midazolam	500/41	±	CYP450	96	Albumin	α-OH midazolam + conjugate
Diazepam	30/2	No	CYP450	99	Albumin	N desmethyldiazepam
Flumazenil	1300/100	Yes	CYP450	50	Albumin	No
Morphine	1000/90	Yes	Conjugation	25	Albumin	Morphine 6 G
Fentanyl	900/50	Yes	CYP450	84	α1GPA	No
Sufentanil	900/72	Yes	CYP450	93	α1GPA	No
Alfentanil	300/40	±	CYP450	92	α1GPA	No
Remifentanil	4000/-	-	Tissue esterases	70	α1GPA	G190291: no clinical relevance
Pancuronium	Renal 65%/bile 10%/metabolism 25%	-	CYP450	30	-	3-OH pancuronium
Vecuronium	Renal 25%/bile 40%/metabolism 35%	-	CYP450	30	-	3-OH vecuronium
Rocuronium	Renal 35%/bile 60%/metabolism 5%	-	CYP450	30	-	No
Atracurium	420/-	-	Esterases + Hofmann reaction	50		Laudanosine
Cisatracurium	350/-	-	Hofmann reaction	50		Laudanosine
Succinylcholine	?/-	-	Cholinesterases			Choline

Note: The data given are indicative. They may vary from one publication to another.

▶ **an overall depletion in neurotransmitters** (catecholamines, dopamine, tyrosine, serotonin) related to both a decrease in their synthesis and an increased destruction by endogenous catalytic enzymes. The reduction in available neurotransmitters is not balanced by an increased activity of the receptors (upregulation). This underlying mechanism mediates important age-related diseases such as Alzheimer's dementia and Parkinson's disease.

▶ **a selective attrition of cortical neurons** in specific areas (thalamus, locus ceruleus, and so forth). There is also a reduction of about 30% of the cerebral mass by the age of 80. Cerebral blood flow and oxygen consumption undergo a similar reduction. Nevertheless, there is no correlation between age-related cerebral atrophy and intellectual processes, which suggests that at the time when the brain is heaviest, there is an important redundancy between the different neurons and areas. Electronic microscopy studies suggest that neuronal loss is accompanied by a progressive reduction in interneuronal connections in surviving cells.

INFLUENCE OF AGE ON THE PHARMACOLOGY OF SPECIFIC INTRAVENOUS ANESTHETIC DRUGS

▶ Hypnotics

Intravenous hypnotics have little in common as far as biochemistry or pharmacokinetics is concerned. They all interfere with the γ-aminobutyric acid (GABA) receptor albeit at different binding sites. All can be used for induction of anesthesia, but only propofol is commonly used for maintenance. Apart from etomidate, all hypnotic agents have markedly increased hemodynamic consequences in the elderly.

Thiopental

Many studies have demonstrated a reduction in thiopental requirements for induction of anesthesia in elderly patients compared with young adults.[23–26,27–29,30] This reduction has been reported to be over 60% in some studies. The altered response of the elderly to thiopental may be due to age-related changes in either pharmacokinetics or pharmacodynamics. Christensen et al.[29] found no differences in plasma thiopental concentrations associated with loss of consciousness (LOC) in young versus elderly patients, despite lower induction doses in the elderly. These results suggest an age-related change in thiopental pharmacokinetics but not pharmacodynamics.

Pharmacokinetics Thiopental is usually administered as a bolus dose for induction of anesthesia. Therefore, to explain an increased sensitivity of the elderly to thiopental on the basis of pharmacokinetic changes, one should look for an altered early drug distribution. A reduction in the rapid intercompartment clearance rather than a decrease in volume of the central compartment has been demonstrated.[31,6,29] Following an intravenous bolus, there is no difference in the thiopental peak plasma concentrations between young and elderly patients because the initial distribution volume is not altered by aging. Because the rapid intercompartment clearance is reduced in elderly patients, thiopental plasma concentrations decrease more slowly in these patients after the peak serum concentration is achieved. The higher thiopental plasma concentration which occurs in the minutes after the intravenous bolus results in more thiopental being available for distribution into the biophase and creates a greater anesthetic effect.

Nevertheless, this simplistic explanation may not provide sufficient pharmacokinetic rationale for decreasing the thiopental induction dose in the elderly. Avram et al.[6] estimated thiopental apparent volume of distribution at the time of its maximum effect and found no difference between the 20–45 years age group and the 66–80 years age group. The authors suggested that the decreased thiopental dose requirement in the elderly might instead be a result of a decrease in lean body mass with age. Subsequently, the hypothesis that the apparent relationship of thiopental induction dose requirements to age and gender was due to patient characteristics, such as lean body mass and cardiac output, which are known to be gender-related or altered with increasing age was further investigated.[30] To reach either the same clinical or electroencephalogram (EEG) end point, the dose required in the elderly was, 25% less and 40% less, respectively, than in the young. Age was found to be a more important predictor of thiopental dose requirement than body weight or lean body mass.

Other changes in thiopental pharmacokinetics that have been described in the elderly include an increased volume of the deep peripheral compartment and an increased terminal elimination half-life.[28,29,6] These changes have no clinical implications after a single bolus dose.

Pharmacodynamics The pharmacodynamics of thiopental in the elderly have been extensively studied by Homer and Stanski using an EEG end point as a measure of hypnotic effect.[26,31] The dose of thiopental required to achieve early burst suppressions on the EEG decreased linearly with increasing age. There was a 60% decrease between ages 20 and 80 (1 mg/kg per decade of age). However, the authors didn't find any age-related change in brain responsiveness. None of the pharmacodynamic parameters were correlated with age (maximum effect [Emax], concentration yielding 50% of effect [CE50], and coefficient of sigmoidicity of the Hill curve [γ]). Moreover, no relationship was found between the transfer rate constant (K_{EO}) and age.[26] These results were confirmed in a subsequent study[31] where no age-related changes in pharmacodynamics were found using the spectral edge of EEG as a measure of hypnosis. In this study, T 1/2 K_{EO} was linearly related to age. However, the correlation was poor, and not clinically relevant.

The observed decrease in thiopental dose requirement in the elderly does not seem to correlate with an age-related change in pharmacodynamics. Thiopental induction dose should be reduced in the elderly because of pharmacokinetic changes altering the initial distribution of the drug. It must be emphasized that when thiopental is injected quickly as in a bolus dose, albumin binding of this drug is overwhelmed by the high plasma concentration. This yields a high free fraction for distribution to the brain, thus increasing the effect. Therefore, thiopental should always be administered slowly in the elderly. Even when all the factors known to influence the size of the induction dose are considered, a pronounced interindividual variability still exists, which makes it necessary to adjust the dose on an individual basis according to effect. This increased variability is enhanced in the elderly for thiopental as it is for many other drugs.[27]

Propofol

Thanks to its pharmacological properties (rapid and pleasant recovery, reduction in postoperative nausea and vomiting [PONV]), propofol has become one of the most popular hypnotic agents for induction as well as for maintenance of anesthesia (TIVA: total intravenous anesthesia).

Nevertheless, in the aged population, its hemodynamic effects have limited its use. In 1986, Dundee et al.[32] reported an increased sensitivity to propofol in the elderly. The doses necessary to obtain LOC were lower, and the incidence of apnea and hypotension was increased. Induction doses in subjects under and over 60 years old were 2.25–2.5 mg/kg and 1.5–1.75 mg/kg, respectively. In the same year, Hilton and colleagues[33] made similar observations in a study involving 60 patients aged between 19 and 69 years. They found a strong negative correlation between age and maintenance dose as well as a strong positive correlation between age and decrease in systolic arterial blood pressure. These two studies provide support for the clinician's habit of decreasing doses in the elderly, but do not give any pharmacokinetic and/or pharmacodynamic explanation.

Pharmacokinetics Propofol is very lipid soluble and 98% bound to albumin. It is extensively distributed in all tissues including fat. Its elimination is dependent on hepatic blood flow (hepatic extraction ratio close to 1). Its high metabolic clearance (20–30 mL/kg/min) exceeds hepatic blood flow, and propofol extrahepatic metabolism has been demonstrated.[34]

Pharmacokinetic studies have clearly shown age-related changes, but with variable results. That variability can be partly explained by differences in methods, specifically with infusion schemes.

One of the first studies of propofol pharmacokinetics in the elderly was published in 1988 by Kirkpatrick et al.[35] The authors reported increased plasma concentrations in the elderly (aged 65–80 years) compared with younger subjects (aged 18–35 years) after a single bolus dose of propofol. The results were mainly explained by a lower initial distribution volume in the elderly (V1 = 19.6 L vs. 26.3 L), which is consistent with a decrease in cardiac output and total body water with increasing age. Besides, cardiac output was identified as an important determinant of propofol induction dose.[36] Moreover, that study reported a decreased metabolic clearance of propofol in the elderly compared with young subjects (1.43 L/min vs. 1.78 L/min); a decrease that could be attributed to an age-related decrease in hepatic blood flow.

In 1992, Dyck and Shafer[37] also reported lower dosage requirements in elderly patients, mainly because of pharmacokinetic alterations. They confirmed the decrease in V1 in the elderly but not a decrease in metabolic clearance. V3 (slow distribution volume) and Cl 3 (slow distribution clearance) also decreased with age. Finally, to achieve the same effect (3 s of EEG burst suppression), propofol doses had to be reduced by one-third in the elderly.

Schnider et al.[8] performed a pharmacokinetic/pharmacodynamic study in which the influence of age on propofol pharmacology was considered. They analyzed arterial blood samples in 24 healthy volunteers aged 21–81 years after a bolus of propofol followed 1 h later by a 60-min infusion. The authors found that age influences V2 (rapid distribution volume) and Cl 2 (rapid distribution clearance), but not other pharmacokinetic parameters. Specifically, metabolic clearance (Cl 1) was directly correlated to the weight, height, and lean body mass of the patient, but not age.

Schuttler et al.[38] has performed a population study of propofol pharmacokinetics using data collected from five research groups (4112 concentrations of 270 individuals aged 2–88 years). The elimination clearance decreased linearly in individuals older than 60 years, and the volume of the central compartment decreased with age if divided by body weight.

To summarize, age-related changes in propofol pharmacokinetics include alterations in initial distribution (decreased initial volume and/or impaired rapid intercompartment clearance) leading to

higher plasma concentration and increased effect of the same induction dose. A reduction in elimination clearance is due to a decrease in hepatic blood flow buffered by extra hepatic metabolism. As a consequence, when administering propofol as a target controlled infusion for induction and maintenance of anesthesia in the elderly (which improves propofol safety profile in this population[39]), it is important to ascertain that the model implemented in the target-controlled infusion (TCI) device includes age as a covariate (Fig. 8-1).

Pharmacodynamics Pharmacodynamic studies usually include two different aspects: (1) the transfer rate to the effect site illustrated by the rate constant K_{EO} or the time-to-peak effect and (2) the pharmacodynamic response itself represented by the concentration leading to 50% of maximum effect, CE50.

Considering three groups of 20 patients each (group 1: 20–40 years, group 2: 41–64 years, and group 3: 65 years and more) receiving a propofol infusion until an EEG preset end point (3 s of isoelectric EEG), Dyck and Shafer[37] did not demonstrate any age-related change in CE50 or K_{EO}. This result was strengthened by Kazama et al.[40] using BIS as a measure of effect. On the contrary, Schnider et al.[19] reported an increased sensitivity of the elderly to the hypnotic effect of propofol. They showed that the CE50 for LOC was nearly halved at 80 years (1.25 µg/mL vs. 2.35 µg/mL) compared with young subjects. In addition, K_{EO} was slightly decreased in the elderly but the result didn't reach significance. Schnider's methodology (a pharmacokinetic/pharmacodynamic population approach using a specific EEG parameter [semilinear canonical correlation]) is the most sensitive. It is therefore likely that sensitivity to propofol hypnotic effect is moderately enhanced in the elderly whereas the transfer time to the effect site is not modified in this population.

Hemodynamic Consequences of Propofol Administration Propofol is a potent vasodilator and numerous publications have outlined the risk of hypotension when using this drug in elderly patients.[32,33,35] Kazama et al.[40] compared the CE50 and K_{EO} for the effect of propofol on systolic blood pressure (SBP) in young and old subjects. They administered propofol in TCI mode to 41 patients aged 20–85 years, targeting four different concentrations maintained for 30 min each. BIS was used as a measure of hypnosis and systolic arterial blood pressure variations as a measure of

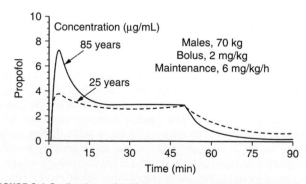

FIGURE 8-1 Predicted propofol effect site concentration after a bolus dose of 2 mg/kg followed by a continuous infusion at 6 mg/kg/h in 25- and 85-year-old subjects. Note the increased initial concentration in the elderly, the similar maintenance concentration, and the absence of delayed decrement at the end of the infusion. Simulation performed with pkpdtools excel sheet (C Minto and T Schnider, www.pkpdtools.org), using Schnider's pharmacokinetic parameters set. *(Adapted from Ref. 8.)*

hemodynamic effect. If CE50 and K_{EO} were not age-related for the hypnotic effect, they were greatly influenced by age for the hemodynamic one. Specifically, time to SBP maximum effect was dramatically delayed with increasing age: T 1/2 K_{EO} ranged from 5.68 min in the 20–39 year age group to 10.22 min in the 70–85 year age group. At the same time, the CE50 for SBP drop was more than halved between these two age brackets (4.5 (g/mL vs. 2 µg/mL). Thus, for the same hypnotic effect, the hemodynamic effect will be increased and delayed in the elderly when compared to young subjects. It is therefore particularly important to titrate propofol to effect in order to give only the required dose and no more.[41] TCI may help.[39] As far as drug interactions are concerned, the adjunct use of opioids with propofol for induction of anesthesia does not allow for any important reduction in the propofol dose, but potentates the drop in SBP and may lead to major hypotension in the absence of adrenergic stimuli.[42–44]

Etomidate

Hemodynamic stability is a major advantage of etomidate, making it popular among anesthetists for induction of anesthesia in elderly patients. Despite this fact, few studies about etomidate pharmacology in the elderly are available.

Pharmacokinetics, Pharmacodynamics Arden et al.[45] studied the pharmacokinetics and pharmacodynamics of etomidate in 21 healthy surgical subjects aged 22–82 years receiving a constant infusion rate of etomidate until achievement of a preset EEG end point. The dose of etomidate required to reach the uniform EEG end point decreased significantly with age as did the dose to produce maximal median frequency depression. None of the parameters of the pharmacodynamic model including CE50 or K_{EO} was correlated to age, suggesting that the age-related change in dose requirement was not related to increased brain sensitivity in the elderly.

The initial etomidate volume of distribution decreased significantly with increasing age (by 42% between ages 22 and 80), implying that a higher initial blood concentration in the elderly following any given dose of etomidate is part of the reason for the lower dose requirement in the elderly patient. Etomidate clearance also decreased with age, in the same order of magnitude as liver blood flow.

Thus, the basis for the decreased etomidate dose requirement in the elderly are age-dependent changes in etomidate pharmacokinetics rather than altered brain responsiveness. However, there are few dire consequences of an overdose, except during short procedures where it may lead to delayed recovery.

Midazolam

Midazolam is a benzodiazepine with an intermediate clearance dependent both on hepatic blood flow and the intrinsic clearance. It has a short elimination half-life (around 2 h).

In daily practice, the dose of a benzodiazepine required to achieve a specific sedative or hypnotic end point in most elderly patients is smaller than that required in younger patients. Bell et al.[46] found an important negative correlation between age and the intravenous dose of midazolam required for sedation during upper gastrointestinal endoscopy in patients aged between 45 and 85 years. The investigators concluded that overdosage was easy in patients aged over 70 years because the dose of midazolam necessary for endoscopy was often so small. Similarly, Kanto et al.[47] reported lower induction doses in the elderly (0.15 mg/kg) compared with young adults.

What Are the Mechanisms Responsible for This Age-Related Decrease in Midazolam Dose Requirement?

Pharmacokinetics Greenblatt et al.[48] considered the effects of age on the kinetics of a single intravenous bolus dose of midazolam in elderly healthy volunteers. Midazolam elimination half-life was significantly prolonged in elderly versus young males and total clearance was significantly reduced (about 40%). However, the total volume of distribution, the volume of the central compartment, and plasma protein binding did not differ between groups. Interestingly, among women, there were no significant differences between elderly and young volunteers. These results agree with those of Avram et al.[49] and Servin et al.[50] However, Avram et al.[49] and Servin et al.[50] reported a significantly increased distribution volume in elderly subjects of both sexes. Kanto and Albrecht[51] also failed to show major differences in midazolam pharmacokinetic parameters which were likely to explain the increased sensitivity of the elderly to the drug. The only pharmacokinetic parameter that has been shown to change with aging in all the previous studies is total body clearance, which is reportedly lower in the elderly compared with young patients.[48,50,52,53] Impaired clearance might decrease maintenance dose requirements but would not be expected to affect induction dose requirements. Interestingly, midazolam central compartment volume, plasma protein binding, and volume of distribution, factors that could influence the induction dose requirement are not affected, or only slightly affected, by the aging process. Therefore, changes in midazolam pharmacokinetics cannot explain the decreased dose requirement for induction of anesthesia in the elderly.

Pharmacodynamics Jacobs et al.[54] and Albrecht et al.[51] studied midazolam pharmacodynamics in the elderly. Jacobs used a clinical end point as a measure of the hypnotic effect of midazolam and found that the value of the CE50 for response to verbal command at 80 years was less than 25% of the value at 40 years. Albrecht et al. considered the pharmacokinetic-pharmacodynamic relationship of midazolam in nine elderly men compared with nine younger men using the EEG (median frequency of the power spectrum) as a measure of hypnotic-sedative effect. A 50% decrease in the dose required to reach the final end point was observed in the elderly. This difference could not be explained by pharmacokinetic changes. The elderly subjects only showed a significantly smaller transfer rate constant from the central compartment. Conversely, pharmacodynamic data showed large differences between young and elderly subjects. In the elderly, the CE50 was halved, the concentration-response curve was steeper, and K_{EO} was smaller. Despite different end points, these two studies report similar results: the sensitivity of the elderly to the hypnotic effect of midazolam is increased.

These results suggest that the lower doses needed in the elderly are mainly attributable to pharmacodynamic changes. Midazolam should be used with extreme caution, if at all, for anxiolysis and conscious sedation in this population where doses as low as 0.5 mg may be responsible for apnea.[46]

▶ Opioids

Ever since 1971, Belleville et al.[55] insisted on the need for reducing morphine dose with increasing age. The authors surveyed the analgesic response of postoperative patients to a dose of 10 mg intramuscular morphine in relation to age, height, weight, body surface area, operative site, and initial intensity of pain. They found that the correlation between age and analgesia was much better than any other variables examined. This led to the suggestion that age be used as the basis to determine the initial dose of morphine for postoperative pain.

Even if their study was not designed to discriminate pharmacokinetic or pharmacodynamic causes for this finding, the authors dismissed a pharmacokinetic mechanism on the basis of a lack of association between age and the incidence of side effects.

Similarly, Kaiko et al.[56] concluded that aged patients responded to morphine as though they had received three to four times the dose given to young adult patients, and that consequently, age should be used as the main criterion for choosing the initial dose of narcotic analgesic. Although these studies documented decreased dose requirements, neither a pharmacokinetic nor a pharmacodynamic explanation was proposed.

Opioids are currently used in the vast majority of surgical patients, and a poor understanding of their pharmacology may lead to serious hemodynamic or respiratory adverse events in the elderly. This review therefore considers the current knowledge of the influence of aging on the pharmacology of those opioids which are commonly used in the perioperative period.

Fentanyl

Despite the worldwide use of this agent in elderly patients, fentanyl pharmacology has not been extensively studied in this population. Fentanyl is lipid soluble with a large volume of distribution at steady state and a high clearance dependent on liver blood flow. Fentanyl pharmacokinetic studies specifically addressing the problem of aging are scarce, already rather ancient, and include small patient numbers.[20,57] Moreover, their results are conflicting. Interestingly, it seems that whatever the pharmacokinetic alterations, they do not induce important changes in fentanyl plasma concentrations.[58] This was further demonstrated in a physiological model by which Bjorkman[59] was able to estimate a difference in simulated peak concentration between a 35-year-old and a 90-year-old individual of less than 3% after a bolus dose. They also stated that the reduction in clearance (liver blood flow) with age should induce a prolonged elimination half-life in the aged.

Nevertheless, clinical studies have clearly outlined the need to reduce fentanyl doses with increasing age. As for all other opioids, this is due to an increased sensitivity to fentanyl drug effect in the elderly. Scott et al.[60] has studied whether aging decreases fentanyl dose requirements and whether this could be attributed to changes in pharmacokinetics, pharmacodynamics, or both. Fentanyl was infused to 20 patients aged 20–88 years, and EEG was used as a measure of narcotic drug effect. The pharmacokinetic parameters did not demonstrate important changes with age: only the fast intercompartmental clearance was decreased. On the contrary, the fentanyl concentration required to produce the same EEG end point showed a significant negative correlation with age, and a 50% decrease was observed from ages 20 to 89. The other pharmacodynamic parameters (maximum effect, onset time) did not show age-related changes.

Thus, using the EEG as a measure of narcotic drug effect, the decreased dose requirement in the elderly was found to have a pharmacodynamic explanation. These pharmacodynamic changes suggest that fentanyl doses should be decreased by 50% in aged patients.

Alfentanil

Alfentanil pharmacokinetics differ from other piperidine derivatives in that its rather low clearance is dependent on both liver blood flow and hepatic enzyme activity. As such, its clearance varies with the status of its metabolizing enzymes, CYP450. Thus, alfentanil clearance is reduced by coadministered drugs (i.e., erythromycin), but may be increased by enzyme inducers, and is subject to pharmacogenetic modulation and hormonal impregnation influence. All these factors will blunt the effect of aging on alfentanil pharmacokinetics, and study results will depend on the population involved, especially since the number of patients in these pharmacokinetic studies is usually low. This explains the discrepancies between the different approaches to alfentanil pharmacokinetics in the elderly.

Scott and Stanski[60] studied males ranging from 20 to 89 years old. They did not find any significant change in alfentanil pharmacokinetics with increasing age. Using the spectral edge of the EEG as a measure of narcotic drug effect, they related the significant reduction in dose requirements to pharmacodynamic changes similar to those observed with fentanyl. They reported a 50% decrease in CE50 between the ages of 20 and 85 years and no reduction in the transfer rate K_{EO}.

Lemmens and coworkers compared 14 adult women (31–52 years old) to 14 older women (56–96 years old) and could not demonstrate any influence of age on the pharmacodynamics of alfentanil.[61] Nevertheless, there were methodological problems with this older study. For one, the age groups included similar patients (what difference would one expect between 52 and 56 years old?). Obviously, a population approach would have been more appropriate. Nevertheless, the dose requirements in the older group were significantly lower than in the younger patient group. The authors related this to pharmacokinetic changes such as those reported by Helmers[62]: decreased plasma clearance (about 30%) leading to an increased elimination half-time (about 40%).

Lemmens et al.[63] subsequently observed that the pharmacokinetics of alfentanil in men (as studied exclusively by Scott and Stanski) were unaffected by age, while the pharmacokinetics in women showed a clear negative correlation between age and clearance. It should be noted that they compared pre- and postmenopause women as their cutoff age was 50 years. This suggests that hormonal status influences alfentanil clearance.

The population approach of alfentanil pharmacokinetics was undertaken by Maitre et al.[64] They found a significant reduction in alfentanil clearance with age, but also an important interindividual variability for this parameter. Raemer et al.[65] prospectively tested the population pharmacokinetic parameters reported by Maitre et al. in two groups of clinically dissimilar patients: 29 young women and 11 older men, using computer-controlled drug administration. They found that the pharmacokinetics reported by Maitre did not accurately predict the observed plasma alfentanil concentrations (bias + 53% and imprecision 53%), while the pharmacokinetics reported by Scott and Stanski accurately predicted the concentrations in both young women and elderly men (bias + 2% and imprecision 18%). To conclude, it seems that alfentanil pharmacokinetics do not depend on sex in younger patients, but that aging (menopause?) leads to a reduction in alfentanil clearance in women but not in men.

During thiopentone and alfentanil induction of anesthesia in 55 patients older than 70 years, the optimal alfentanil dose with which to obtund the hemodynamic response to tracheal intubation, while minimizing cardiovascular depression after tracheal intubation was found to be 10 µg/kg.[66] This dose is approximately half the one recommended in younger patients. These results are consistent with those obtained for fentanyl and remifentanil. Although neither a pharmacokinetic nor a pharmacodynamic explanation is given for the reduction in dose requirement in this study, one would be tempted to attribute these changes to an age-related increased sensitivity to alfentanil.

Thus, alfentanil dosing, similar to fentanyl dosing, should be reduced by about 50% in the elderly, mostly for pharmacodynamic reasons.

Sufentanil

The influence of age on sufentanil pharmacokinetics has mainly been studied in two works published in the nineties,[67,68] where high sufentanil doses (2–3 µg/kg) were administered to middle age adult and elderly patients. Both studies concluded that sufentanil pharmacokinetic parameters were not affected by aging, with the exception of a reduced initial volume of distribution leading to a higher plasma peak concentration in elderly patients.[67]

Moreover, the study of Matteo et al.[67] supports the hypothesis of an age-related change in sufentanil pharmacodynamics in the elderly. They observed that at the end of the surgery, six of the elderly patients and only one of the younger ones required naloxone to resume an adequate respiratory rate, when all the patients had received the same sufentanil dose. This cannot be accounted for by differences in the initial volume of distribution, which has no influence on the sufentanil plasma concentration several hours after a bolus dose.

The hypothesis that pharmacodynamic changes exist in the elderly for sufentanil as well as for the other µ agonists is supported by a study[69] comparing the pharmacodynamic parameters of fentanyl and sufentanil. Similar pharmacodynamic profiles were found for both drugs, with fentanyl being 12 times more potent than sufentanil. Even though data are lacking on the pharmacodynamics of sufentanil in the elderly, it seems reasonable to extrapolate from studies of fentanyl, alfentanil, and morphine and conclude that the sufentanil dose should be reduced by 50% in this population.

Remifentanil

Remifentanil is an ultrashort-acting µ opioid receptor agonist, which contains a methyl ester side chain susceptible to hydrolysis by blood and tissue esterases. Its short duration of action is due to metabolism rather than redistribution.

Remifentanil pharmacokinetics and pharmacodynamics have been described in detail by Minto et al.[18,70] In this work, the population included individuals over 80 years old, which allowed for an analysis of the changes induced by aging on remifentanil behavior. Remifentanil pharmacokinetics in elderly individuals were characterized by a decreased initial volume of distribution (with a loss of about 20% from ages 20 to 80), resulting in higher initial plasma concentrations following a bolus dose. Concurrently, remifentanil clearance, which is independent of hepatic function and renal blood flow but dependent on the number and efficiency of tissue esterases, was decreased by about 30% from ages 20 to 80.[70] Using an EEG end point as a measure of effect, pharmacodynamic differences were evident. The transfer rate from the effect site, K_{EO}, was reduced with increasing age, hinting at a delayed onset of action. Moreover, the central nervous system is more sensitive to the effect of remifentanil as the concentration required to induce 50% of EEG depression (CE50) was halved in 80-year-old patients when compared to young adults (Fig. 8-2).

Minto and colleagues[18] then performed simulations to study the influence of these pharmacological changes with age on remifentanil behavior after a bolus dose or a continuous infusion. Recovery time after a prolonged infusion was also noted. According to the simulations, after an intravenous bolus dose, initial remifentanil plasma concentrations were higher in the elderly because of a decreased V1. But the smaller K_{EO} slowed the equilibrium between blood and effect site. This resulted in an apparent peak effect-site concentration that was close in all age groups. Regardless of the lean body mass, an 80-year-old patient would require approximately half the dose of a 20-year-old to reach the same EEG peak effect. This

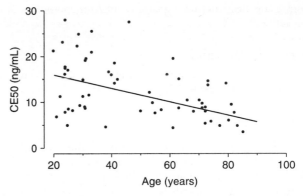

FIGURE 8-2 Progressive reduction with age of remifentanil CE50 for EEG effect. *(Adapted from Ref. 70.)*

end point would be delayed in the elderly (approximately 1 min at 20 years and 2 min at 80 years). The adjustment in initial bolus dose is due to pharmacodynamic changes (decreased CE50). The adjustment in bolus dose for age is far more important than the adjustment in bolus dose for body weight. The infusion rate required to maintain a constant EEG effect in an 80-year-old person is approximately one-third of that required in a 20-year-old. Again, the adjustment for age is far more important than the adjustment for body weight. This reduction in infusion rate is based on both pharmacokinetic (decreased clearance with age) and pharmacodynamic considerations (decreased CE50 with age).

The times required for remifentanil concentration to decrease by 50% or even 80% following prolonged infusions were rapid and hardly affected by age or duration of infusion. However, although the decrement time was rapid in all age groups, the interindividual variability was increased in the elderly.

Thus, owing to its titrability and absence of lingering effect, remifentanil appears to be a useful drug in elderly patients, provided its dosage is carefully titrated to effect. This can be optimally achieved through a target-controlled remifentanil infusion, currently available in most countries in the world. Inadequate understanding of remifentanil pharmacology in the aged patient may lead to dangerous but avoidable hemodynamic depression.[71,72]

Morphine

Owen et al.[73] studied morphine kinetics after a single intravenous bolus of 10 mg/70 kg. The volume of distribution at steady state in elderly subjects was only half that of younger patients. This difference was derived from reductions in both central and peripheral compartments. Plasma clearance was also reduced. These results are consistent with those of Baillie et al.[5] who also found a decrease in plasma clearance with increasing age (about 35%). The changes in morphine pharmacokinetics are amplified by the retention of morphine active metabolites, morphine-3- and morphine-6-glucuronide, due to the physiologic reduction in glomerular filtration rate in the aged. These two active metabolites, resulting from morphine glucuronidation in the liver, are eliminated through the kidney and their elimination is greatly impaired in renal failure patients.[15]

These findings suggest that the reported increased sensitivity of elderly subjects to the analgesic effects of morphine[55,56] may be due at least in part to altered disposition of the drug. Morphine pharmacodynamic data are lacking, but considering the results obtained with other opioids, it is prudent to reduce the amount of the first analgesic dose of morphine in the elderly, and to titrate further doses to effect.

Morphine patient-controlled analgesia (PCA) is appropriate in this population.[74]

▶ Muscle relaxants

Dosing schemes in elderly patients are often a challenge, and neuromuscular blocking agents (NMBAs) are no exception to this rule.

Clinical findings

Onset of Action The onset of action of NMBAs is usually prolonged in the elderly, whatever the study drug (succinylcholine,[75] vecuronium,[75] rocuronium,[76] pipecuronium,[77] cisatracurium,[21,78] doxacurium[79]). In studies where no difference in NMBA onset times has been found between elderly and younger patients (vecuronium,[80] rocuronium,[81] mivacurium[82]), the initial dose was two to three times the ED95, thus precluding any accurate measurement of the time to maximal effect.

Maintenance Doses/Infusion Rates The duration of action of maintenance doses of rocuronium[76] and vecuronium[83] is significantly prolonged in the elderly, whereas that of atracurium doses[83] is not. The maintenance infusion rate of mivacurium required to ensure adequate muscle relaxation is lower in elderly patients.[82,84,85] Hart et al.[86] has demonstrated a strong influence of pseudocholinesterase activity on the mivacurium infusion rates required to maintain 50% or 90% twitch depression. Similarly in Goudsouzian's study, the lowest infusion rate was observed in patients with low pseudocholinesterase activity.[85]

Recovery Recovery for muscle relaxation is usually delayed in elderly patients. Thus, the recovery index from 25% to 75% recovery of twitch height is increased by 60% (39–62 min) for pancuronium,[16] 230% (15–49 min) for vecuronium,[87] 62% (13–21 min) for rocuronium,[81] and 42% (5.5–7.8 min) for mivacurium.[82] The time to reach 25% recovery of twitch height is delayed in the elderly for doxacurium (68–97 min; 43%).[79] On the contrary, recovery from muscle relaxation is not modified by aging for atracurium,[83] cisatracurium,[78] and pipecuronium.[77]

Pharmacokinetic changes

As a result of the aging process, a number of changes occur such as deterioration in renal and hepatic function, as well as alteration in body composition with a decrease in lean body mass and in total body water. As a consequence, the pharmacokinetics of muscle relaxants are frequently modified in elderly patients.

Steroid Compounds The muscle relaxants with a steroid structure (pancuronium, vecuronium, rocuronium, pipecuronium) are mainly eliminated by the liver through metabolism and biliary excretion, and partially excreted in the urine. They are poorly bound to plasma proteins. Their large molecules are highly ionized regardless of pH, which limits their distribution to the extracellular compartment. As a consequence, their volume of distribution can be expected to remain unchanged or to slightly decrease with aging. Indeed, pancuronium and pipecuronium distribution volumes remain unchanged, whereas vecuronium and rocuronium have significantly reduced distribution volumes in the elderly.

Pancuronium is predominantly (30–70%) excreted unchanged in the urine, and approximately 20% of the drug undergoes deacetylation. Glomerular filtration rate is reduced in the elderly, and as a

consequence, so is pancuronium clearance.[16] Nevertheless, phase I metabolic reactions are not consistently modified by aging, and when urinary excretion is reduced, it is possible that some enhancement of the metabolic rate of pancuronium exists. This explains why in some studies no difference in pancuronium clearance was found between younger adults and elderly patients.[88] If this is the case, a greater proportion of active metabolite might be produced in the elderly.

Vecuronium is scarcely metabolized, with 40% excreted unchanged in the bile and 30% in the urine. A limited amount of the drug (30%) is deacetylated in the liver with one active metabolite. As both liver blood flow and glomerular filtration rate are reduced in the elderly, vecuronium clearance is reduced by approximately 30%,[88] without any modification in the volumes of distribution.[87]

The elimination of rocuronium is similar to that of vecuronium with approximately 75% eliminated in the bile and 10% in the urine. A little rocuronium undergoes deacetylation, and no significantly active metabolites are produced. Rocuronium clearance is also reduced by 30% in the elderly.[81] Both pancuronium and vecuronium have active metabolites, but their clinical significance in the anesthesia setting is negligible.

The usual pharmacokinetic parameters for steroid NMBAs are modified by aging, with a trend towards reduction in both clearance (around 30%) and distribution volumes (around 25%). These modifications have been proposed to explain prolonged duration of action, but this prolongation (at least 60%) is of a greater magnitude when compared to the kinetic changes.

Benzylisoquinoliniums The currently available benzylisoquiniliniums include atracurium, mivacurium, cisatracurium, and doxacurium. Atracurium and mivacurium are mixtures of stereoisomers with varying potencies and pharmacokinetics. Atracurium is a mixture of 10 isomers, one of them being cisatracurium. No study has yet considered the pharmacokinetics of the different atracurium isomers in young and elderly patients, and the published data have all analyzed atracurium as if it was a single compound, which is not accurate, but much less complex. Mivacurium is a mixture of three isomers. Two of them (cis-trans and trans-trans) are potent, metabolized by plasma pseudocholinesterases, and represent more than 90% of the mivacurium dose. The less potent cis-cis isomer represents less than 10% of the dose, and participates only marginally in mivacurium relaxant action.[85]

Like steroid NMBAs, benzylisoquiniliniums are big molecules which do not cross lipophilic barriers. Their distribution volumes are in the same order of magnitude as that of the steroid compounds. Distribution volumes of benzylisoquiniliniums are slightly enhanced in elderly patients. This may be due to a potential decrease in plasma protein binding in this population as these compounds are more extensively protein bound than the steroids.

Metabolism or hydrolysis of benzylisoquinolinium compounds is quite diversified. Some of them (doxacurium) are not metabolized at all but are excreted mainly in the urine and marginally in the bile. Atracurium and cisatracurium undergo spontaneous degradation through Hofmann elimination and ester hydrolysis. This process accounts for about 83% of cisatracurium elimination clearance, but only for about 40% of atracurium total elimination clearance.[89] The atracurium, which does not undergo Hofmann elimination, is probably metabolized primarily in the liver. If atracurium total elimination clearance is not modified by aging, its organ clearance is reduced. However, this reduction is counterbalanced by an enhancement of nonorgan clearance.[90]

The main mivacurium isomers are metabolized by plasma pseudo-cholinesterases. The cis-cis isomer has a much lower clearance. Maddineni, in a letter to the British Journal of Anaesthesia,[91] reported a decrease in pseudocholinesterase activity in elderly patients when compared to younger ones, though the activity remained in the normal range. This observation, which has not been confirmed by a full paper, might contribute to the reduced trans-trans and cis-trans isomer clearances.

Effect-site concentration

Muscle blood flow has been suggested as a factor which influences delivery of drugs to the end plate.[92] Regional blood flows, including muscle blood flow, are reduced in elderly people.[93] There might therefore exist a more important concentration gradient between the effect site and the plasma in elderly patients as illustrated by a lower exit rate constant, $ke0$, in the aged. The slow onset and longer duration of action of most NMBAs in elderly patients, poorly explained by the scarce changes in elimination kinetics might correspond to this phenomenon. When cisatracurium was studied, the time to maximum block was more rapid in young patients compared with elderly ones, owing to a reduction in $ke0$ with age.[21]

Pharmacodynamics

So far, all the clinical changes in NMBA behavior in elderly patients have been explained by pharmacokinetic but not pharmacodynamic alterations.[94] Plasma concentrations corresponding to a fixed degree of paralysis are not modified by aging, and the concentration response relationships remain for the most part unchanged.[16,76,79,81,88,90,95,96] This suggests that the aging process has no influence on the pharmacodynamic component of NMBA behavior.

NMBA antagonists

The use of NMBA antagonists such as neostigmine or edrophonium[97] should be widely recommended in the elderly. The onset of action of neostigmine is often delayed. Its effects are long lasting possibly due to reduced elimination with impaired renal function[98] and the dose requirements are increased.[99,100] The incidence of cardiac dysrhythmias after injection of neostigmine is increased.[101] No information is currently available on the new NMBA antagonist ORG25969 in elderly patients, but its original action sounds interesting in this population.[102]

ARE THERE ADVANTAGES TO USING TOTAL INTRAVENOUS ANESTHESIA IN THE ELDERLY OVER INHALATIONAL ANESTHESIA?

When considering the debate involving "total intravenous anesthesia versus inhalational anesthesia," it immediately appears that only hypnotic drugs are concerned, and even that the problem at the present time is propofol versus volatile anesthetic. This debate has been consistently tainted in the literature by the marketing struggle between pharmaceutical companies. Furthermore, the results of the studies are often blunted by suboptimal use of the agents. We shall try to sort out the available information relevant to two major issues in general anesthesia of the aged patients, namely hemodynamic stability during induction of anesthesia and quality of recovery. We shall not consider the problem of myocardial preconditioning which will be addressed in another part of this book.

▶ Hemodynamic stability during induction of anesthesia

The study by Nishikawa et al.[103] is a good example of an erroneous design leading to data which are impossible to construe. The authors estimated the left ventricular mechanical performance after induction of anesthesia in two groups of elderly patients: one receiving an inhalational induction with sevoflurane in the absence of opioids and the other a combination of fentanyl and propofol. All hemodynamic assessments were performed in the absence of stimulation. The authors concluded that sevoflurane was preferable in elderly patients because of a lesser effect on left ventricular performance. There are clear data in the literature[42,44] demonstrating that the addition of opioids to propofol worsens the hemodynamic consequences of induction in the absence of adrenergic stimuli. It is therefore most unfortunate that the authors did not compare propofol alone to sevoflurane. It is good clinical practice when inducing anesthesia in the elderly to ensure LOC with a slow induction with either sevoflurane or propofol and then administer a bolus dose of an opioid with rapid onset prior to any painful stimulus (i.e., tracheal intubation).

Similarly, Yamaguchi et al.[104] compared two modalities of sevoflurane administration to a bolus dose of propofol (2 mg/kg) immediately followed by 2% sevoflurane for induction of anesthesia in patients aged 70–79 years. Propofol induction was more rapid (36 s vs. 60 s), and was accompanied by a drop in mean arterial pressure (around 30 mm Hg) similar to the one obtained with the first sevoflurane group (modified vital capacity technique with sevoflurane 8% in 100% oxygen, decrease to 2% after 3 min), and greater than observed in the second sevoflurane group (initial sevoflurane concentration set initially at 8%, then decreased by 2% every minute). One might argue that the propofol bolus dose was too high for elderly patients,[32] and that it is recommended to administer propofol slowly in this population in order to minimize the hemodynamic consequences of induction.[41] Therefore, with a lower propofol dose administered slower, they might have had different results (similar induction time and good hemodynamic stability in the propofol group).

Kirkbride et al.[105] has also compared propofol induction to two techniques of sevoflurane administration. Their study design was much better and included slower propofol injection (600 mL/h), double-blind design, even if the propofol overall dose remained high (over 2 mg/kg), and N_2O administration to all patients from the start of induction. Nitrous oxide has negative inotropic properties and is often poorly tolerated in this population.[106] Their induction time was similar in all groups, and the decrease in mean arterial pressure (mainly due to a drop in SBP) was significantly greater in the propofol group. Giving propofol as a continuous infusion up to LOC always overdoses the patient due to the delayed transfer to the effect site. Schematically, the effect-site concentration which induces LOC corresponds to the plasma concentration obtained about 2 min before, and therefore all the propofol administered during those 2 min was not necessary to obtain LOC. Thus, the best way to administer propofol to elderly patients is to titrate the effect site directly using a TCI device. When this is used, the hemodynamic consequences of propofol administration are not different to what is observed with etomidate induction followed by desflurane maintenance,[39] provided the TCI system is implemented with a propofol pharmacokinetic model which includes age as a covariate. If this not the case,[107] the amount of drug delivered by the device during induction will generate a propofol concentration about twice the one expected with predictable hemodynamic consequences.

So, if propofol is to be used for induction of anesthesia in the elderly, it should be given either as a slow bolus dose of around 1 mg/kg, additional doses being given only after the drug has had the opportunity to reach its effect site, or titrated through a TCI system, provided the pharmacokinetic model includes age as a covariate. If any drop in arterial pressure is to be avoided in a given patient (i.e., severe aortic valvular stenosis), then the only choice for induction is etomidate.

▶ Recovery

Propofol has been compared to isoflurane, sevoflurane, or desflurane maintenance for speed and quality of recovery both in the ambulatory setting[108] and after a variety of inpatient surgical procedures.[109,110,111–113] The results come to a consensus: of the three volatile agents, desflurane allows the most rapid early recovery, but is no more distinguishable from sevoflurane if intermediate recovery is considered. The longest recovery is observed after isoflurane. Propofol recovery times are similar to those observed after sevoflurane anesthesia. Propofol maintenance improves early postoperative patient well-being, and reduces the incidence of PONV.[114,115] The incidence of postoperative cognitive dysfunction, greater in elderly patients than in younger adults even after minor surgery, does not seem to be influenced by the anesthetic agent administered, sevoflurane or propofol.[116] In diabetic patients receiving vecuronium, recovery from the neuromuscular block is delayed when sevoflurane is used for maintenance of anesthesia when compared to propofol.[117]

CONCLUSION

Aging induces changes in both the pharmacokinetics and the pharmacodynamics of intravenous anesthetic agents. The changes vary with the agent and its class. As aging progresses, interindividual variability increases. Therefore, it is appropriate to choose drugs with a rapid onset and a short duration of action in the aged in order to carefully titrate the doses to the desired effect and avoid unwanted side effects, mainly hemodynamic. The manner in which the drugs are handled in this population is much more important than the choice of the drug by itself, and many dosing schemes should be adapted to patient age rather than weight. Patients over 80 years may present in any surgical situation from the ambulatory setting to cardiac surgery. They are more and more intellectually alert and willing to live, but they are fragile and deserve our best care.

KEY POINTS

▶ The initial distribution of drugs is often impaired in the elderly, explaining so-called increased "sensitivity." Protein binding is less efficient. Glomerular filtration rate is reduced, slowing the excretion of water-soluble drugs or metabolites.

▶ Liver blood flow decreases with age, reducing the clearance of highly extracted drugs. The influence of age on liver enzyme activity is complex.

▶ Interindividual variability increases with age.

▶ Induction doses of thiopental, propofol, and etomidate should be reduced in elderly patients mainly due to an altered initial distribution.

▶ Midazolam doses should be dramatically reduced in the elderly, due to an increased pharmacodynamic sensitivity.

▶ Hemodynamic consequences of propofol induction are enhanced and delayed in the elderly. Propofol decrement time is not prolonged in the elderly.

▶ As a whole, opioid pharmacokinetics are hardly affected by age, and only a small part of the decreased dose requirements in the aged have a pharmacokinetic explanation. Conversely, central nervous system sensitivity to opioids is markedly increased in the elderly, which conveys the need for reducing the doses by almost 50% for an 80-year-old. The reasons for this altered central nervous system sensitivity to narcotics with aging are still unclear. The interindividual variability in opioid pharmacology is also frequently enhanced in this population. It is therefore particularly important to titrate to effect. Titration can be best achieved by choosing a short-acting drug (i.e., remifentanil) and giving it through a TCI device. In the postoperative period, morphine titration to effect can be improved by PCA.

▶ Muscle relaxant action is usually of slower onset and longer duration in elderly patients, but sensitivity to those compounds is not modified by aging. For some compounds, there is a discrepancy between the clinical profile and the pharmacokinetic changes, which might at least partially be explained by a slower transfer rate to the effect site.

▶ Atracurium and cisatracurium duration of action are not modified by aging. As for other agents, interindividual variability is increased in this population, and monitoring of neuromuscular blockade is mandatory.

▶ Elderly patients are specifically prone to silent aspiration of gastric contents in the PACU and residual blockade may participate in this complication. It is therefore recommended to favor NMBA with nonorgan elimination in this population, and to ascertain that no residual paralysis is present prior to sending the patient to the PACU.

▶ Both propofol and sevoflurane may be used for induction of anesthesia in elderly patients. If propofol is considered, a careful titration to effect, best achieved with TCI using Schnider's pharmacokinetic model, is warranted. Both propofol and sevoflurane are vasodilators, so if vasodilatation is to be avoided at all costs, etomidate induction should be the first choice. In any case, the negative inotropic effect of N_2O should be kept in mind, as well as the absence of benefit from opioid administration during the periods (i.e., up to LOC) when no painful stimuli are present.

▶ As far as recovery is concerned, the fastest clear-headed recovery is obtained with desflurane, and propofol generates a better feeling of well-being associated with less PONV.

KEY ARTICLES

▶ Avram MJ, Krejcie TC, Henthorn TK. The relationship of age to the pharmacokinetics of early drug distribution: the concurrent disposition of thiopental and indocyanine green. *Anesthesiology.* 1990;72:403–411.

▶ Sorooshian SS, Stafford MA, Eastwood NB, et al. Pharmacokinetics and pharmacodynamics of cisatracurium in young and elderly adult patients. *Anesthesiology.* 1996;84:1083–1091.

▶ Schnider TW, Minto CF, Gambus PL, et al. The influence of method of administration and covariates on the pharmacokinetics of propofol in adult volunteers. *Anesthesiology.* 1998;88:1170–1182.

▶ Jacobs JR, Reves JG, Marty J, et al. Aging increases pharmacodynamic sensitivity to the hypnotic effects of midazolam. *Anesth Analg.* 1995;80:143–148.

► Kazama T, Ikeda K, Morita K, et al. Comparison of the effect site K_{EO} of propofol for blood pressure and EEG bispectral index in elderly and younger patients. *Anesthesiology.* 1999;90:1517–1527.

► Scott JC, Stanski DR. Decreased fentanyl/alfentanil dose requirement with increasing age: a pharmacodynamic basis. *J Pharmacol Exp Ther.* 1987;240:159–166.

► Bjorkman S, Wada DR, Stanski DR. Application of physiologic models to predict the influence of changes in body composition and blood flows on the pharmacokinetics of fentanyl and alfentanil in patients. *Anesthesiology.* 1998;88:657–667.

► Minto CF, Schnider TW, Egan TD, et al. Influence of age and gender on the pharmacokinetics and pharmacodynamics of remifentanil. I. Model development. *Anesthesiology.* 1997;86:10–23.

► Kitts JB, Fisher DM, Canfell PC, et al. Pharmacokinetics and pharmacodynamics of atracurium in the elderly. *Anesthesiology.* 1990;72:272–275.

► Young WL, Matteo RS, Ornstein E. Duration of action of neostigmine and pyridostigmine in the elderly. *Anesth Analg.* 1988;67:775–778.

► Passot S, Servin F, Pascal J, et al. A comparison of target- and manually controlled infusion propofol and etomidate/desflurane anesthesia in elderly patients undergoing hip fracture surgery. *Anesth Analg.* 2005;100:1338–1342.

► Hofer CK, Zollinger A, Buchi S, et al. Patient well-being after general anaesthesia: a prospective, randomized, controlled multicentre trial comparing intravenous and inhalation anaesthesia. *Br J Anaesth.* 2003;91:631–637.

REFERENCES

1. Clergue F, Auroy Y, Pequignot F, et al. French survey of anesthesia in 1996. *Anesthesiology.* 1999;91:1509–1520.
2. Servin F. Physiologie du vieillissement. Paris DB, ed. In: Traité d'anesthésie générale. pp Section I Chapitre 16. Paris: Arnette; 2001, pp. 1–9.
3. Novak LP. Aging, total body potassium, fat-free mass, and cell mass in males and females between ages 18 and 85 years. *J Gerontol.* 1972;27:438–443.
4. Vree TB, Shimoda M, Driessen JJ, et al. Decreased plasma albumin concentration results in increased volume of distribution and decreased elimination of midazolam in intensive care patients. *Clin Pharmacol Ther.* 1989;46: 537–544.
5. Baillie SP, Bateman DN, Coates PE, Woodhouse KW. Age and the pharmacokinetics of morphine. *Age Aging.* 1989;18:258–262.
6. Avram MJ, Krejcie TC, Henthorn TK. The relationship of age to the pharmacokinetics of early drug distribution: the concurrent disposition of thiopental and indocyanine green. *Anesthesiology.* 1990;72:403–411.
7. Arden JR, Holley OF, Stanski DR. Age dependence in the pharmacokinetics and pharmacodynamics of etomidate. *Clin Pharmacol Ther.* 1985;32:179–183.
8. Schnider TW, Minto CF, Gambus PL, et al. The influence of method of administration and covariates on the pharmacokinetics of propofol in adult volunteers. *Anesthesiology.* 1998;88:1170–1182.
9. Viani A, Rizzo G, Carrai M, Pacifici GM. The effect of aging on plasma albumin and plasma protein binding of diazepam, salicylic acid, and digitoxin in healthy subjects and patients with renal impairment. *Br J Clin Pharmacol.* 1992;33:299–304.
10. Paxton JW, Briant RH. Alpha 1 acid glycoprotein concentrations and propanolol binding in elderly patients with acute illness. *Br J Clin Pharmacol.* 1984;18:806–810.
11. Iber FL, Murphy PA, Connor ES. Age-related changes in the gastrointestinal system. Effects on drug therapy. *Drugs Aging.* 1994;5:34–48.
12. Tarloff JB, Goldstein RS, Sozio RS, Hook JB. Hepatic and renal conjugation (phase II) enzyme activities in young adult, middle-aged, and senescent male Sprague-Dawley rats. *Proc Soc Exp Biol Med.* 1991;197:297–303.
13. Jorquera F, Almar M, Pozuelo M, et al. The effect of age and sex on metabolism and urinary excretion of antipyrine. *J Gerontol A Biol Sci Med Sci.* 1998;53:M14–M19.
14. Mauriz JL, Tabernero B, Garcia-Lopez J, et al. Physical exercise and improvement of liver oxidative metabolism in the elderly. *Eur J Appl Physiol.* 2000;81:62–66.
15. Chauvin M, Sandouk P, Scherrmann JM, et al. Morphine pharmacokinetics in renal failure. *Anesthesiology.* 1987;66:327–331.
16. Duvaldestin P, Saada J, Berger JL, et al. Pharmacokinetics, pharmacodynamics, and dose-response relationships of pancuronium in control and elderly subjects. *Anesthesiology.* 1982;56: 36–40.
17. Sheiner LB, Stanski DR, Voseh G, et al. Simultaneous modeling of pharmacokinetics and pharmacodynamics: application to d-tubocurarine. *Clin Pharmacol Ther.* 1979;25:358–371.
18. Minto CF, Schnider TW, Shafer SL. Pharmacokinetics and pharmacodynamics of remifentanil. 2. Model application. *Anesthesiology.* 1997;86:24–33.
19. Schnider TW, Minto CF, Shafer SL, et al. The influence of age on propofol pharmacodynamics. *Anesthesiology.* 1999;90: 1502–1516.
20. Singleton M, Rosen J, Fisher D. Pharmacokinetics of fentanyl in the elderly. *Br J Anaesth.* 1988;60:619–622.
21. Sorooshian SS, Stafford MA, Eastwood NB, et al. Pharmacokinetics and pharmacodynamics of cisatracurium in young and elderly adult patients. *Anesthesiology.* 1996;84:1083–91.
22. Muravchick S. The effects of aging on anesthetic pharmacology. *Acta Anaesthesiol Belg.* 1998;49:79–84.
23. Dundee JW, Hassard TH, McGowan WA, Henshaw J. The induction dose of pentothal: a method of study and preliminary illustrative results. *Anaesthesia.* 1982;37:1176–1184.
24. Dundee JW. The influence of body weight, sex, and age on the dosage of thiopentone. *Br J Anaesth.* 1954;26:164–173.
25. Christensen JH, Andreasen F. Individual variation in response to thiopental. *Acta Anaesthesiol Scand.* 1978;22:203–213.
26. Homer TD, Stanski DR. The effect of increasing age on thiopental disposition and anesthetic requirement. *Anesthesiology.* 1985; 62:714–724.
27. Muravchick S. Effect of age and premedication on thiopental sleep dose. *Anesthesiology.* 1984;61:333–336.
28. Christensen JH, Andreasen F, Jansen JA. Influence of age and sex on the pharmacokinetics of thiopentone. *Br J Anaesth.* 1981;53:1189–1195.
29. Christensen JH, Andreasen F, Jansen JA. Pharmacokinetics and pharmacodynamics of thiopentone: a comparison between young and elderly patients. *Anaesthesia.* 1982;37:398–404.
30. Avram MJ, Sanghvi R, Henthorn TK, et al. Determinants of thiopental induction dose requirements. *Anesth Analg.* 1993;76:10–17.
31. Stanski DR, Maitre PO. Population pharmacokinetic and pharmacodynamic of thiopental: the effect of age revisited. *Anesthesiology.* 1990;72:412–422.
32. Dundee JW, Robinson FP, McCollum JS, Patterson CC. Sensitivity to propofol in the elderly. *Anaesthesia.* 1986;41:482–485.
33. Hilton P, Dev VJ, Major E. Intravenous anaesthesia with propofol and alfentanil. The influence of age and weight. *Anaesthesia.* 1986;41:640–643.
34. Veroli P, O'Kelly B, Bertrand F, et al. Extrahepatic metabolism of propofol in man during the anhepatic phase of orthotopic liver transplantation. *Br J Anaesth.* 1992;68:183–186.
35. Kirkpatrick T, Cockshott ID, Douglas EJ, Nimmo WS. Pharmacokinetics of propofol in elderly patients. *Br J Anaesth.* 1988;60: 146–150.
36. Adachi YU, Watanabe K, Higuchi H, Satoh T. The determinants of propofol induction of anesthesia dose. *Anesth Analg.* 2001;92:656–661.
37. Dyck JB, Shafer SL. Effects of age on propofol pharmacokinetics. *Semin Anesth.* 1992;11(Suppl. 1):2–4.
38. Schuttler J, Ihmsen H. Population pharmacokinetics of propofol: a multicenter study. *Anesthesiology.* 2000;92:727–738.
39. Passot S, Servin F, Pascal J, et al. A comparison of target- and manually controlled infusion propofol and etomidate/desflurane anesthesia in elderly patients undergoing hip fracture surgery. *Anesth Analg.* 2005;100:1338–1342.
40. Kazama T, Ikeda K, Morita K, et al. Comparison of the effect site K_{EO} of propofol for blood pressure and EEG bispectral index in elderly and younger patients. *Anesthesiology.* 1999;90: 1517–1527.

41. Peacock JE, Lewis RP, Reilly CS, Nimmo WS. Effect of different rates of infusion of propofol for induction of anaesthesia in elderly patients. *Br J Anaesth.* 1990;65:346–352.

42. Billard V, Moulla F, Bourgain JL, et al. Hemodynamic response to induction and intubation. Propofol/fentanyl interaction. *Anesthesiology.* 1994; 81:1384–1393.

43. Kazama T, Ikeda K, Morita K. Reduction by fentanyl of the Cp50 values of propofol and hemodynamic responses to various noxious stimuli. *Anesthesiology.* 1997;87:213–217.

44. Vuyk J, Engbers FH, Burm AG, et al. Pharmacodynamic interaction between propofol and alfentanil when given for induction of anesthesia. *Anesthesiology.* 1996;84:288–299.

45. Arden JRA, Holley FO, Stanski DR. Increased sensitivity to etomidate in the elderly: initial distribution versus altered brain response. *Anesthesiology.* 1986;65:19–27.

46. Bell GD, Spickett GP, Reeve PA, et al. Intravenous midazolam for upper gastrointestinal endoscopy: a study of 800 consecutive cases relating dose to age and sex of patient. *Br J Clin Pharmacol.* 1987;23:241–243.

47. Kanto J, Aaltonen L, Himberg JJ. Midazolam as an intravenous induction agent in the elderly. A clinical and pharmacokinetic study. *Anesth Analg.* 1986;65:15–20.

48. Greenblatt DJ, Abernethy DR, Locniskar A, et al. Effect of age, gender, and obesity on midazolam kinetics. *Anesthesiology.* 1984;61:27–35.

49. Auram MJ, Fragen RJ, Caldwell NJ. Midazolam kinetics in women of two age groups. *Clin Pharmacol Ther.* 1983;34:505–508.

50. Servin F, Enriquez I, Fournet M, et al. Pharmacokinetics of midazolam used as an intravenous induction agent for patients over 80 years of age. *Eur J Anaesthesiol.* 1987;4:1–7.

51. Albrecht S, Ihmsen H, Hering W, et al. The effect of age on the pharmacokinetics and pharmacodynamics of midazolam. *Clin Pharmacol Ther.* 1999;65:630–639.

52. Smith MT, Heazlewood V, Eadie MJ. Pharmacokinetics of midazolam in the aged. *Eur J Clin Pharmacol.* 1984;26:381–388.

53. Avram MJ, Fragen RJ, Caldwell NJ. Midazolam kinetics in women of two age groups. *Clin Pharmacol Ther.* 1983;34:505–508.

54. Jacobs JR, Reves JG, Marty J, et al. Aging increases pharmacodynamic sensitivity to the hypnotic effects of midazolam. *Anesth Analg.* 1995;80:143–148.

55. Bellville JW, Forrest WHJ, Miller E, Brown BWJ. Influence of age on pain relief from analgesics. *JAMA.* 1971;217:1835–1841.

56. Kaiko RF, Wallenstein SL, Rogers AG, et al. Narcotics in the elderly. *Med Clin N Am.* 1982;66:1079–1089.

57. Bentley JB, Borel JD, Nenad RE, Jr, Gillespie TJ. Age and fentanyl pharmacokinetics. *Anesth Analg.* 1982;61:968–971.

58. Thompson JP, Bower S, Liddle AM, Rowbotham DJ. Perioperative pharmacokinetics of transdermal fentanyl in elderly and young adult patients. *Br J Anaesth.* 1998;81:152–154.

59. Bjorkman S, Wada DR, Stanski DR. Application of physiologic models to predict the influence of changes in body composition and blood flows on the pharmacokinetics of fentanyl and alfentanil in patients. *Anesthesiology.* 1998;88:657–667.

60. Scott JC, Stanski DR. Decreased fentanyl/alfentanil dose requirement with increasing age: a pharmacodynamic basis. *J Pharmacol Exp Ther.* 1987;240:159–166.

61. Lemmens HJ, Bovill JG, Hennis PJ, Burm AG. Age has no effect on the pharmacodynamics of alfentanil. *Anesth Analg.* 1988;67: 956–960.

62. Helmers H, Van Peer A, Woestenborghs R, et al. Alfentanil kinetics in the elderly. *Clin Pharmacol Ther.* 1984;36:239–243.

63. Lemmens HJ, Burm AG, Hennis PJ, et al. Influence of age on the pharmacokinetics of alfentanil. Gender dependence. *Clin Pharmacokinet.* 1990;19:416–422.

64. Maitre PO, Vozeh S, Heykants J, et al. Population pharmacokinetics of alfentanil: the average dose-plasma concentration relationship and interindividual variability in patients. *Anesthesiology.* 1987;66: 3–12.

65. Raemer DB, Buschman A, Varvel JR, et al. The prospective use of population pharmacokinetics in a computer-driven infusion system for alfentanil. *Anesthesiology.* 1990;73:66–72.

66. Kirby IJ, Northwood D, Dodson ME. Modification by alfentanil of the haemodynamic response to tracheal intubation in elderly patients. A dose-response study. *Br J Anaesth.* 1988;60: 384–387.

67. Matteo RS, Schwartz AE, Ornstein E, et al. Pharmacokinetics of sufentanil in the elderly surgical patient. *Can J Anaesth.* 1990;37:852–856.

68. Helmers JH, van Leeuwen L, Zuurmond WW. Sufentanil pharmacokinetics in young adult and elderly surgical patients. *Eur J Anaesthesiol.* 1994;11:181–185.

69. Scott JC, Cooke JE, Stanski DR. Electroencephalographic quantitation of opioid effect: comparative pharmacodynamics of fentanyl and sufentanil. *Anesthesiology.* 1991;74:34–42.

70. Minto CF, Schnider TW, Egan TD, et al. Influence of age and gender on the pharmacokinetics and pharmacodynamics of remifentanil. I. Model development. *Anesthesiology.* 1997;86: 10–23.

71. Elliott P, O'Hare R, Bill KM, et al. Severe cardiovascular depression with remifentanil. *Anesth Analg.* 2000;91:58–61.

72. Habib AS, Parker JL, Maguire AM, et al. Effects of remifentanil and alfentanil on the cardiovascular responses to induction of anaesthesia and tracheal intubation in the elderly. *Br J Anaesth.* 2002;88:430–433.

73. Owen JA, Sitar DS, Berger L, et al. Age-related morphine kinetics. *Clin Pharmacol Ther.* 1983;34:364–368.

74. Lavand'Homme P, De Kock M. Practical guidelines on the postoperative use of patient-controlled analgesia in the elderly. *Drugs Aging.* 1998;13:9–16.

75. Koscielniak-Nielsen ZJ, Bevan JC, Popovic V, et al. Onset of maximum neuromuscular block following succinylcholine or vecuronium in four age groups. *Anesthesiology.* 1993;79: 229–234.

76. Bevan DR, Fiset P, Balendran P, et al. Pharmacodynamic behavior of rocuronium in the elderly. *Can J Anaesth.* 1993;40: 127–132.

77. Ornstein E, Matteo RS, Schwartz AE, et al. Pharmacokinetics and pharmacodynamics of pipecuronium bromide (Arduan) in elderly surgical patients. *Anesth Analg.* 1992;74:841–844.

78. Ornstein E, Lien CA, Matteo RS, et al. Pharmacokinetics and pharmacodynamics of cistracurium in geriatric surgical patients. *Anesthesiology.* 1996;86:520–525.

79. Dresner DL, Basta SJ, Ali HH, et al. Pharmacokinetics and pharmacodynamics of doxacurium in young and elderly patients during isoflurane anesthesia. *Anesth Analg.* 1990;71:498–502.

80. McCarthy G, Elliott P, Mirakhur RK, et al. Onset and duration of action of vecuronium in the elderly: comparison with adults. *Acta Anaesthesiol Scand.* 1992;36:383–386.

81. Matteo RS, Ornstein E, Schwartz AE, et al. Pharmacokinetics and pharmacodynamics of rocuronium in elderly surgical patients. *Anesth Analg.* 1993;77:1193–1197.

82. Maddineni VR, Mirakhur RK, Mc Coy EP. Neuromuscular and haemodynamic effects of mivacurium in elderly and young adult patients. *Br J Anaesth.* 1994;73:608–612.

83. Slavov V, Khalil M, Merle JC, et al. Comparison of duration of neuromuscular blocking effect of atracurium and vecuronium in young and elderly patients. *Br J Anaesth.* 1995;74:709–711.

84. Dahaba AA, Rehak PH, List WFA. A comparison of mivacurium infusion requirements between young and elderly adults. *Eur J Anaesthesiol.* 1996;13:43–48.

85. Goudsouzian N, Chakravorti S, Denman W, et al. Prolonged mivacurium infusion in young and elderly adults. *Can J Anaesth.* 1997;44:955–962.

86. Hart PS, McCarthy GJ, Brown R, et al. The effect of plasma cholinesterase activity on mivacurium infusion rates. *Anesth Analg.* 1995;80:760–763.

87. Lien CA, Matteo RS, Ornstein E, et al. Distribution, elimination, and action of vecuronium in the elderly. *Anesth Analg.* 1991;73:39–42.

88. Rupp SM, Castagnoli KP, Fischer DM, Miller RD. Pancuronium and vecuronium pharmacokinetics and pharmacodynamics in younger and elderly subjects. *Anesthesiology.* 1987;67:45–49.

89. Fisher DM, Canfell PC, Fahey MR, et al. Elimination of atracurium in humans: contribution of Hofmann elimination and ester hydrolysis versus organ-based elimination. *Anesthesiology.* 1986;65:6–12.

90. Kitts JB, Fisher DM, Canfell PC, et al. Pharmacokinetics and pharmacodynamics of atracurium in the elderly. *Anesthesiology.* 1990;72: 272–275.

91. Maddineni VR, Mirakhur RK, McCoy EP. Plasma cholinesterase activity in elderly and young adults. *Br J Anaesth.* 1994;72:497.

92. Donati F. Onset of action of relaxants. *Can J Anaesth.* 1988;35: S52–S58.

93. Fleg JL. Alterations in cardiovascular structure and function with advancing age. *Am J Cardiol.* 1986;57:33C–44C.

94. Parker CJ, Hunter JM, Snowdon SL. Effect of age, gender, and anaesthetic technique on the pharmacodynamics of atracurium. *Br J Anaesth.* 1993;70:38–41.

95. Bell PF, Mirakhur RK, Clarke RS. Dose-response studies of atracurium, vecuronium, and pancuronium in the elderly. *Anaesthesia.* 1989;44: 925–927.

96. d'Hollander AA, Nevelsteen M, Barvais L, Baurain M. Effect of age on the establishment of muscle paralysis induced in anaesthetized adult subjects by ORG NC 45. *Acta Anaesthesiol Scand.* 1983;27:108–110.

97. Kitajima T, Ishii K, Ogata H. Edrophonium as an antagonist of vecuronium-induced neuromuscular block in the elderly. *Anaesthesia.* 1995;50:359–361.

98. Stone JG, Matteo RS, Ornstein E. Aging alters the pharmacokinetics of pyridostigmine. *Anesth Analg.* 1995;81:773–776.

99. McCarty GJ, Cooper R, Stanley JC, Mirakhur RK. Dose-response relationships for neostigmine antagonism of vecuronium-induced neuromuscular block in adults and the elderly. *Br J Anaesth.* 1992;69:281–283.

100. Young WL, Matteo RS, Ornstein E. Duration of action of neostigmine and pyridostigmine in the elderly. *Anesth Analg.* 1988;67:775–778.

101. Owens W, Waldbaum L, Stephen C. Cardiac dysrhythmias following reversal of neuromuscular blocking agents in geriatric patients. *Anesth Analg.* 1978;57:186–190.

102. Gijsenbergh F, Ramael S, Houwing N, van Iersel T. First human exposure of Org 25969, a novel agent to reverse the action of rocuronium bromide. *Anesthesiology.* 2005;103:695–703.

103. Nishikawa K, Nakayama M, Omote K, Namiki A. Recovery characteristics and postoperative delirium after long-duration laparoscope-assisted surgery in elderly patients: propofol-based vs. sevoflurane-based anesthesia. *Acta Anaesthesiol Scand.* 2004;48:162–168.

104. Yamaguchi S, Ikeda T, Wake K, et al. A sevoflurane induction of anesthesia with gradual reduction of concentration is well tolerated in elderly patients. *Can J Anaesth.* 2003;50:26–31.

105. Kirkbride DA, Parker JL, Williams GD, Buggy DJ. Induction of anesthesia in the elderly ambulatory patient: a double-blinded comparison of propofol and sevoflurane. *Anesth Analg.* 2001;93:1185–1187, table of contents.

106. McKinney MS, Fee JP. Cardiovascular effects of 50% nitrous oxide in older adult patients anaesthetized with isoflurane or halothane. *Br J Anaesth.* 1998;80:169–173.

107. Nathan N, Vial G, Benrhaiem M, et al. Induction with propofol target-concentration infusion vs. 8% sevoflurane inhalation and alfentanil in hypertensive patients. *Anaesthesia.* 2001;56:251–257.

108. Fredman B, Sheffer O, Zohar E, et al. Fast-track eligibility of geriatric patients undergoing short urologic surgery procedures. *Anesth Analg.* 2002;94:560–564, table of contents.

109. Iannuzzi E, Iannuzzi M, Viola G, et al. Desflurane and sevoflurane in elderly patients during general anesthesia: a double blind comparison. *Minerva Anestesiol.* 2005;71:147–155.

110. Juvin P, Servin F, Giraud O, Desmonts JM. Emergence of elderly patients from prolonged desflurane, isoflurane, or propofol anesthesia. *Anesth Analg.* 1997;85:647–651.

111. Chen X, Zhao M, White PF, et al. The recovery of cognitive function after general anesthesia in elderly patients: a comparison of desflurane and sevoflurane. *Anesth Analg.* 2001;93:1489–1494, table of contents.

112. Godet G, Watremez C, El Kettani C, et al. A comparison of sevoflurane, target-controlled infusion propofol, and propofol/isoflurane anesthesia in patients undergoing carotid surgery: a quality of anesthesia and recovery profile. *Anesth Analg.* 2001;93:560–565.

113. Heavner JE, Kaye AD, Lin BK, King T. Recovery of elderly patients from two or more hours of desflurane or sevoflurane anaesthesia. *Br J Anaesth.* 2003;91:502–506.

114. Hofer CK, Zollinger A, Buchi S, et al. Patient well-being after general anaesthesia: a prospective, randomized, controlled multicentre trial comparing intravenous and inhalation anaesthesia. *Br J Anaesth.* 2003;91: 631–637.

115. Luntz SP, Janitz E, Motsch J, et al. Cost-effectiveness and high patient satisfaction in the elderly: sevoflurane versus propofol anaesthesia. *Eur J Anaesthesiol.* 2004;21:115–122.

116. Rohan D, Buggy DJ, Crowley S, et al. Increased incidence of postoperative cognitive dysfunction 24 hr after minor surgery in the elderly. *Can J Anaesth.* 2005;52:137–142.

117. Saitoh Y, Hattori H, Sanbe N, et al. Delayed recovery of vecuronium neuromuscular block in diabetic patients during sevoflurane anesthesia. *Can J Anaesth.* 2005;52:467–473.

Inhalational Agents

Orion Whitaker

INTRODUCTION

Since the discovery of anesthesia it has been recognized that age may influence the response to inhalational anesthesia. In fact, the first comment that age made a difference in response to inhalational anesthetics was written in 1848 by one of the pioneers in anesthesiology, John Snow: "I have looked over my notes of cases of etherization and found that the instances in which the insensibility to the operation outlasted the unconscious state, with only one exception, occurred in subjects under 25 years of age. This peculiarity then must depend on something in which the young differ from or exceed the old."[1] Dr. Snow's observation suggests a temporary phenomena, yet many of today's concerns arise from a realization that the statement "He's never been the same since his operation" has merit and reflects a chronic phenomena.[2] Could it be that what was previously thought to be a simple, reversible process actually causes prolonged, cumulative, and possibly irreversible changes in older patients? Unfortunately, the answer may be "yes" but good human data are lacking.

While the mechanism of action of inhalational agents is still not completely understood, many patient responses are well-known.[3] For example, higher concentrations of inhalational agents can lead to hypotension, particularly in the elderly, along with untoward cardiac effects such as reduced coronary artery perfusion pressure, depressed myocardial contractility, vasodilation, electrophysiologic changes, and alterations in autonomic nervous system tone. The effects of inhalational anesthetics are complex with not only immediate biochemical and physical changes but later changes in gene expression as well as secondary changes from metabolic products. In addition, there are many actions of inhalational agents that are unclear. Alteration of gene expression seems surprising given the traditional concept that inhalational anesthetics work by a simple, reversible biochemical process.[4–6] Yet both the known and unknown effects of inhalational anesthetics have implications for geriatric anesthesia. Perhaps the most controversial idea concerning inhalational agent effects, and perhaps all agents, comes from Monk's work showing an association between greater depth of anesthesia and higher 1-year mortality.[7–10]

This chapter emphasizes the unique issues of inhalational anesthesia in the elderly. The discussion reviews the impact on the elderly patient of traditional effects, more current ideas, and a few controversial ideas dealing with the inhalation agents such as isoflurane, sevoflurane, and desflurane. Clearly there are differences between inhalation anesthetic agents, yet they share many common effects altered by aging and the concomitant loss of physiologic reserve in many body systems.

AGE-ADJUSTED DOSING: A NEED FOR DOSE REDUCTION TO PREVENT ACUTE PROBLEMS

One well-known observation for all inhalational agents is that elderly patients need less agent for a given depth of anesthesia.[11–16] Classically, MAC is defined as the minimum alveolar concentration that prevents half the patients from moving to a noxious stimulus. Mapleson performed a meta-analysis of MAC and age and showed a consistent decline in the concentration of inhalational agent required for one MAC as age increased. A plot of the logarithm of agent concentration shows a linear decline with age (Fig. 9-1). A more helpful way to think about MAC and age might be Nichalls' idea of iso-MAC charts. His diagram for sevoflurane and desflurane is illustrated in Fig. 9-2.[15] For example, in order to maintain a total MAC of 1.2 in an 80-year-old patient, the required end-expired concentration of desflurane is 2% and 6.25% when using nitrous oxide 67% and 0% in oxygen, respectively. In contrast, to maintain a total MAC of 1.2 in a 40-year-old patient, the required end-expired concentration of desflurane is approximately 3.8% and 8% when using nitrous oxide 67% and 0% in oxygen, respectively. Note that from Fig. 9-2, the end-expired concentration needed to obtain a desired MAC decreases with age, regardless of whether nitrous oxide is included in the inhalational mixture.

It is generally assumed that the cardiovascular effects of inhalational anesthetics are magnified in the elderly population. However, no good studies exist which clearly quantify what the differences are, if any, in cardiovascular responses between elderly and younger patients.

CARDIAC PROTECTION IN AGING: INHALATIONAL AGENTS MAY NOT HELP

Inhalational agents have complex effects on the heart with changes that range from the organ level, including myocardial blood flow, to changes at the cellular level, including biochemical pathways. Some of the changes at the organ level are easily deduced. For example, total myocardial blood flow might be reduced if hypotension occurred from the vasodilation that can accompany inhaled agents. Yet this hypotension would be recognized and treated. Less predictable changes in myocardial blood flow can occur, in particular,

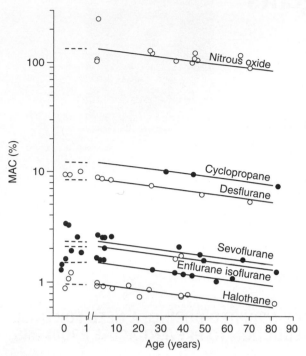

FIGURE 9-1 Effect of age on MAC: comparison of fitted lines with published values. Continuous lines = fitted values, from 1 to 80 years, for each an anesthetic as a whole, based on data for age > year; broken lines = extrapolation to age zero. A 10-times expanded time scale has been used for ages less than 1 year to separate the many published values in that age group. The open and closed circles are used for alternate anesthetics. *(Reproduced with permission from Ref. 16.)*

the change in regional myocardial perfusion known as *steal*. Myocardial steal occurs when an ischemic area of myocardium is dependent on collateral flow from a normal area[17] (Fig. 9-3). Steal has been a particular concern with isoflurane.

While steal has been demonstrated in animals, the clinical implications are unclear.[18] Classic studies like Slogoff and Keats, with about 1000 patients, find no difference in incidence of ischemia when comparing patients receiving halothane, enflurane, isoflurane,

or sufentanil.[19] But, on further inspection, hemodynamic changes might have masked any effect of steal.

Off-pump surgery may provide a better chance of finding differences in anesthetic technique than conventional surgery using cardiopulmonary bypass because lower levels of troponin T occur with this procedure. Kendal used troponin T as a measure of myocardial damage during off-pump coronary artery bypass surgery.[20] No differences among the groups receiving propofol, isoflurane, or isoflurane with thoracic epidural anesthesia were found, although only 30 patients were in the study. These and similar studies have led Agnew to state that "It is evident that the isoflurane coronary steal controversy has been resolved and that isoflurane can be used in high-risk patients with coronary heart disease as long as blood pressure and heart rate are maintained."[17]

On the other hand, a general concern in human studies of steal has been the failure to maintain hemodynamic stability. Isoflurane can induce hypotension and it is the hypotension, not the steal, that results in ischemia. This had led some authors to wonder if hemodynamic changes might have masked any effect of steal. Diana et al. in a study where blood pressure and heart rate were tightly controlled to within 20% of baseline, noted that the incidence of ischemic events, determined by electrocardiogram (ECG), echocardiography, and coronary sinus lactate measurement, was higher in patients receiving isoflurane (50%) compared with those receiving enflurane (20%).[21] Consistent with the idea of steal during hemodynamic stability, Teo presents a case report of a patient with steal-prone anatomy who had dramatic ischemic ECG changes shortly after the addition of isoflurane despite maintenance of arterial pressure. These changes resolved after discontinuing isoflurane and administration of nitroglycerin.[22] A more recent study by Murugesan compared 10 patients with angiographically demonstrated steal-prone anatomy with 40 controls undergoing coronary artery bypass graft (CABG) with 1.2% isoflurane.[23] Half of the *steal-prone* patients had ischemia while none of the control patients did. These results suggest that in a certain patient population, steal may be a clinically important problem.

Inhalational agents may protect vital organs, like the heart, the brain, and the kidney, from damage occurring during ischemia and reperfusion by inducing biochemical and gene expression changes.

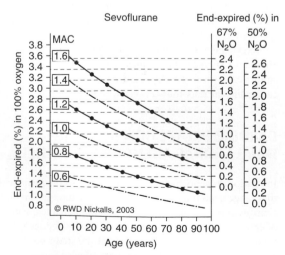

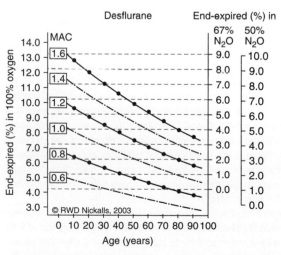

FIGURE 9-2 Iso-MAC charts for sevoflurane (left) and desflurane (right). In the sevoflurane iso-MAC chart, the vertical shifts for the nitrous oxide 50% and 67% scales are 0.86 and 1.16, respectively. In the desflurane iso-MAC chart, the vertical shifts for the nitrous oxide 50% and 67% scales are 3.15 and 4.22, respectively. *(Reproduced with permission from Ref. 15.)*

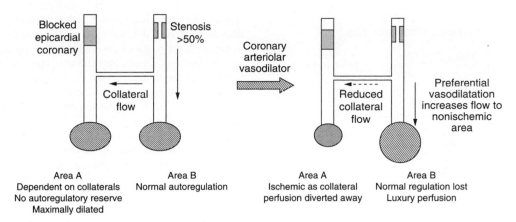

FIGURE 9-3 Schematic diagram illustrating coronary steal. Arrows represent coronary blood flow. *(Reproduced with permission from Ref. 17.)*

In particular, cardiac protection and preconditioning has been the subject of intense investigation over last 20 years. Briefly, when inhalational agents are given before or during myocardial ischemia, there seems to be less subsequent myocardial damage. For example, Kersten discovered that dogs given a 30-min exposure to isoflurane, followed by discontinuation of isoflurane for 30 min prior to coronary occlusion, had smaller infarctions than control dogs.[24] These results suggest some prolonged action of isoflurane. While the possible mechanisms to explain this observation are beyond the scope of this discussion, Zaugg provides a concise explanation of the molecular mechanism of anesthetic-induced preconditioning (Fig. 9-4).[25] For a more detailed discussion on the topic, the reader is referred to any one of several reviews on the subject.[25–28] Anesthetic-induced preconditioning appears to occur through multiple signaling pathways related to nitric oxide, protein kinase C (PKC), free radicals, activation of adenosine receptors, and adenosine triphosphate (ATP)-sensitive potassium (K_{ATP}) channels. However, of primary importance, is the activation of K_{ATP} channels by volatile anesthetics in the sarcolemma and mitochondria. Activation of the sarcolemmal K_{ATP} channels decreases intracellular Ca^{++} influx by decreasing the resting membrane potential and shortening the cell's action potential. Activation of the mitochondrial K_{ATP} channels enhances the restoration of mitochondrial energy production following ischemia and reperfusion through a variety of mechanisms.

While preconditioning is complex phenomena, whether it makes a difference clinically is still not clear. In cardiac surgery, there are conflicting data concerning the role of anesthetic-induced preconditioning in myocardial protection. For example, Zaugg reviews studies of cardioprotection with anesthetic-induced preconditioning in coronary artery bypass surgery and finds no consistent association between mechanical measures such as cardiac index and ejection fraction or biochemical measures such as creatinine phosphokinase MB (CPK-MB) (Table 9-1).[27] Of the studies presented in Table 9-1, Belhomme's study is notable as it used not only traditional measures of ischemia like troponin and CPK, but took tissue samples from the right atria to look for evidence of changes in signaling pathways known to be affected by preconditioning.[29] Belhomme compared 10 patients receiving a 5-min exposure to isoflurane before cross-clamping for CABG to 10 matched control patients. Right atrial biopsy samples were examined for ecto-5'-nucleotidase activity, as a measure of PKC activation. While ecto-5'-nucleotidase was significantly increased after isoflurane preconditioning, there was no significant difference between the groups for troponin I or CPK-MB

though there was a trend toward lower values in the isoflurane group.

Aside from these signaling pathways, an anti-inflammatory effect of volatile agents may be clinically important in myocardial protection during cardiopulmonary bypass. For example, Garcia compared 37 patients exposed to sevoflurane with 35 controls.[30] The sevoflurane group had statistically better event-free survival during the 1-year follow-up. Interestingly, transcription levels for a platelet-endothelial cell adhesion molecule were reduced in the sevoflurane group. Garcia speculates that reduction in inflammation, particularly in patients undergoing cardiopulmonary bypass, where blood is in contact with synthetic surfaces, may be a mechanism for improved survival with volatile agents. But reduction of inflammation by volatile agents may not be clinically significant in noncardiac surgery.

These results underscore how difficult it is to extrapolate experimental data to clinical care. While there is some evidence that volatile anesthetics offer protective effects against myocardial ischemia in patients undergoing coronary artery bypass surgery, there currently are no data concerning protective effects of volatile anesthetics in noncardiac surgery.[29,31] The incidence of surgical procedures in elderly patients increases, concomitant with a high prevalence of coronary heart disease.[32] In these patients with high risk for perioperative cardiac events, myocardial infarction occurs in 6.6% even after noncardiac surgery, and it is likely that volatile anesthetics offer beneficial effects in clinical ischemia-reperfusion situations.[33]

Preconditioning protection may be lost in aged myocardium. Even worse, increased deleterious effects of ischemia were reported in preconditioned aged rat hearts.[34] This effect appears to be due to the insufficient translocation of PKC isoforms in response to the preconditioning stimulus.[35] These experimental findings are supported by two clinical studies in which the antiarrhythmic and infarct-limiting effects of prodromal angina were lost in elderly patients with myocardial infarction.[36,37] In contrast, JimeÂnez-Navarro and colleagues found that the occurrence of angina 1 week before myocardial infarction still conferred protection against in-hospital adverse outcomes in patients aged >70 years.[38] However, a more recent clinical study in patients undergoing percutaneous transluminal coronary angioplasty (PTCA), comparing ischemic preconditioning in younger (45 ± 5 years [M ± SD]) and elderly patients (71 ± 3 years), also suggests that ischemic preconditioning is attenuated in the aged human myocardium, most probably as a result of age-related inhibitory effects upstream of the mitochondrial K_{ATP} channels.[39]

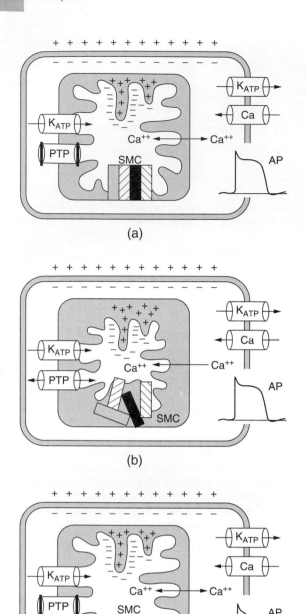

(a)

(b)

(c)

FIGURE 9-4 Cytoprotective mechanisms of cardiac preconditioning. The sarcolemmal and mitochondrial K_{ATP} channels, the sarcolemmal voltage-dependent CA++ channel, and the mitochondrial permeability transition pore (PTP) are shown. The differently marked bars in the mitochondrial intermembrane space represent the supramolecular complex (SMC). SMC contains the proton pump, ATP synthase, the adenine nucleotide transporter, and mitochondrial creatine kinase. Boldness and direction of arrows represent relative intensity and direction of ion flux. (A) Normal conditions: The cytosolic Ca++ concentration is governed mainly by duration of the action potential (AP) and the resting membrane potential. The CA++ uniporter is dependent on the mitochondrial inner membrane potential. (B) Ischemia-reperfusion: The increased cytosolic Ca++ concentration induces disruption of the SMC. The opens and induces dissipation of the inner membrane potential leading to cell death. (C) Anesthetic-induced preconditioning: Cardioprotection occurs via two mechanisms. First, by activation of the sarcolemmal K_{ATP} channel, which reduces the intracellular Ca++ by stabilizing the resting membrane potential below −80 mV and shortening of the AP. Second, by activation of the mitochondrial K_{ATP} channel, which leads to reassembly of the SMC, closure or maintenance of the closed state of the PTP, and restored mitochondrial energy production. *(Reproduced with permission from Ref. 25.)*

While the mechanisms of ischemic and inhalational agent preconditioning may have differences, they share many of the same fundamental steps.[25] Because of the limited data in the elderly and changes in the extent of volatile agent preconditioning, we will consider ischemic preconditioning in the elderly as an analogous situation.

Riess and Juhaszova provide some discussion of aging in their reviews of cardiac preconditioning.[40,41] Specifically, Riess points out the work of Loubani showing that human atrial myocardium tolerance for ischemia does not decline with age.[42] But Riess also cites Schulman, Sniecinski, and Abete who show a declining or no preconditioning effect with increasing age.[36,43,44] In particular, Schulman shows middle-aged rats have a blunted response and aged rats have no response to ischemic preconditioning. Similarly Sniecinski showed aged rats do not have a response to inhaled anesthetic preconditioning. Later, in his own work, Riess finds a reduced effect of inhaled anesthetics in aged guinea pig hearts.[41,45]

The extent of the effect of age on preconditioning appears to be strongly dependent on the exact experimental situation. For instance, Abete's work shows "Food restriction and exercise training alone are able, at least in part, to restore IP (ischemic preconditioning) in hearts from senescent rats. More importantly, the action of food restriction and exercise training on IP in the aging heart is additive, and therefore early IP is completely restored."[46–50]

Human data, from observational studies, show decreasing effects of preconditioning with increasing age with a few exceptions. For example, Abete considered that preinfarction angina is a kind of naturally occurring ischemic preconditioning. Previous work had shown that the presence of preinfarction angina did reduce infarct size and improve in-hospital outcomes, yet the elderly have a greater mortality rate for coronary artery disease. Could the greater mortality be the result of loss of preconditioning in the elderly? In a retrospective analysis of 503 patients admitted to the coronary care unit, those under age 65 showed better outcomes if they had angina in the preceding 48 h of their infarction: lower rates of congestive heart failure, shock, and the combined end point of in-hospital death. Yet those at or over age 65 had no improvement with preinfarction angina, suggesting a loss of preconditioning with age.[51]

Subsequent work from Abete showed that preconditioning was retained in those elderly patients who had similar attributes to the animal studies discussed earlier. For example, thin elderly, those in a study's lowest body mass index (BMI) quartile, retained preconditioning and had lower rates of in-hospital death and cardiogenic shock with preinfarction angina.[52] Similar findings were true for the active elderly: those with high ratings on the Physical Activity Scale for the Elderly (PASE) showed a similar protective effect of preinfarction angina.[47]

The Juhaszova diagram (Fig. 9-5) provides a summary of the relationship between age and myocardial preconditioning.[41] There is evidence that increasing age both lowers the threshold needed for injury, while also increasing the threshold required for protection. In addition, various factors may act to modify these thresholds.

NEUROPROTECTION

A full discussion of neuroprotection, the ability to prevent sequellae of an ischemic insult of the brain, is beyond the scope of this article. Given the potential devastating effect of neurologic injury during surgery, it is not surprising that neuroprotection has been examined for decades and has a large and complex literature.[53] Of additional concern here is that the elderly brain is more sensitive to ischemic insult.[54,55]

Table 9-1

Clinical Studies Evaluating Volatile Anesthetic-Induced Preconditioning

Clinical Study (Study Design)	No. of Patients	Preconditioning: Drug/Doses/ Duration	Basal Anesthesia	No. of Diseased Vessel/Grafts (mean)	Cross-Clamp Time/ Treated/Untreated (min)	Cardioplegia/Core Temperature	Outcome Measures	Result
Tomai et al. (randomized, unblinded)	40	Isoflurane 1.5% (ventilator), 15 min, 10 min washout before CPB	Diazepam, fentanyl, pancuronium	2–3/3.4–3 7	49/53	Antegrade, cold, with blood, intermittent, 32–33°C	Cardiac index LVEF before/ after CPB cTnI/CK-MB preop-96 hostop	No change No change ↓only patients with LVEF<50′
Belhomme et al. (randomized, unblinded)	20	Isoflurane 2.7% (2.5 MAC) (membrane oxygenator), 5 min, 10 min washout before ACC	Flunitrazepam, fentanyl, pancuronium	?/2.5–2.7	48/52	Retrograde, cold, with blood, intermittent, 33–34°C	cTnI/CK-MB preop-72 Ch postop Ecto-5′-NT before/after preconditioning	Tendency to postop ↑after preconditioning
Haroun-Bizri et al. (randomized blinded?)	49	Isoflurance, 0.5–2%* (ventilator), whole pre-CPB time, discontinued before CPB (washout until ACC)	Thiopental, midazolam, sufentanil, cisatracurium	?/2.7–2.8	32/35	Antegrade, cold, no blood, intermittent, 28°C	Cardiac index before/after CPB ST changes before/after CPB Reperfusion arrhythmias after release of ACC	↑after CPB ↓after CPB No change
Penta de peppo et al. randomized, unblinded		Enflurane 1.3 (0.5–2)%† (ventilator), 5 min, before CPB, 1.5–1.8 min washout before ACC	Diazepam, fentanyl, pancuronium	2–3/3.7–4.2	111/125	Antegrade, cold, with blood, intermittent, 26°C	Cardiac output preop/postop LV contractility (pressure-area relation) before/after CPB cTnI/CK-MB preop-96 h postop	No change ↑after CPB No change

ACC = aortic across-clamping; CK-MB = phosphocreatine kinase MB isoenzyme; CPB = cardiopulmonary bypass; cTnI = cardiac troponin I; ecto-5′-NT = ecto-5′-n-nucleotidase; LVEF = left ventricular ejection fraction.
*0.5–2% isoflurane to maintain systolic arterial blood pressure within 20–25% ACC.
†To reduce systolic blood pressure by 20–25% ACC.
Source: Reproduced with permission from Ref. 27.

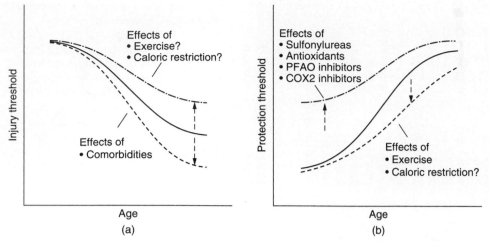

FIGURE 9-5 Changes in the injury and protection threshold in aging heart. (A) Aging diminishes the heart's threshold to sustain injury (e.g., from ischemia reperfusion injury). Lifestyle modifications including exercise and possibly caloric restriction may partially diminish the aging effect. Comorbidities (such as diabetes) have negative influence. (B) Aging increases the heart's threshold to activate protection-signaling mechanisms. Various pharmacological agents (e.g., sulfonylureas, antioxidants, partial fatty acid oxidation inhibitors (PFAO), and COX2 inhibitors) that can interfere with cardioprotective signaling-pathways can exacerbate this trend and further increase the protection threshold. Exercise and caloric restriction might attenuate the age-dependent trends. *(Reproduced with permission from Ref. 41.)*

Most volatile agents, isoflurane in particular, have multiple actions that might favor neuroprotection: reduction in cerebral metabolic rate of oxygen, $CMRO_2$; redistribution of cerebral blood flow; inhibition of N-methyl-D-aspartate (NMDA) action; and potentiation of γ-aminobutyric acid (GABA) action. Sadly, much of the literature, even when including nonanesthetic drugs, is wanting for useful, positive results. Volatile agents have been assumed to have neuroprotective properties, but the initial studies were flawed. Neurologic damage occurs by both an early pathway, characterized by excitotoxicity, and a late pathway, characterized by apoptosis (programmed cell death).[56] Since cerebral ischemia can cause cell death long after the initial event, an experiment must be of long enough duration to include late pathways of cell death: this may be days or weeks. For example, Kawaguchi et al. showed that isoflurane appeared to be neuroprotective 2 days after focal ischemia, but the effect is lost at 2 weeks after ischemia. Thus, the end result is no protection. Warner summarizes the literature on neuroprotection with anesthetic agents this way: "We currently have no evidence that anesthetics alone can provide meaningful long-term neuroprotection against cerebral ischemia. Although the use of anesthetics for neuroprotection poses little additional hazard, beyond that which is already encountered by their requisite use to provide anesthesia, reliance upon anesthetics to increase permanent tolerance of human brain to an ischemic insult is unjustified on the basis of existing scientific evidence."[53]

POSSIBLE CHRONIC EFFECTS OF INHALATIONAL AGENTS

Are inhalational agents long-acting toxins? Certainly anesthetics can be dangerous, and in some situations such as the Moscow theater raid of 2002, even fentanyl and halothane might be considered chemical weapons.[57–61] But are inhalational agents, when used clinically, associated with unexpected toxic problems? In a controversial study, Monk looked at factors associated with 1-year mortality in 1064 patients and found comorbidity, systolic hypotension, and *cumulative deep hypnotic time* (total time that a patient's bispectral index [BIS] value was less

than 45) were statistically significant in a proportional hazards model.[7] Monk speculates that long-term effects of anesthetics may be due to inflammation, perhaps mediated by tumor necrosis factor-α (TNF-α) or interleukin-6 (IL-6). While controversial and with many unresolved issues, the idea that inhaled anesthetics have effects far beyond their pharmacologic clearance and elimination is concerning. In Monk's study, 90.9% of patients received inhalational anesthesia for maintenance, and the median case length was 3.1 h. However, no data are presented concerning the actual anesthetic dose administered. Perhaps considering an Occupational Safety and Health Administration (OSHA) exposure measure, like the integral of a time versus concentration curve or a weighted average concentration would help to determine the relationship between anesthetic exposure and mortality.[62–65,66]

Reversibility is the classic hallmark of anesthesia. The idea of inhaling a vapor, having it distribute through the body, reaching the brain and spinal cord, rendering the patient unconscious, and by simply turning off the vapor, having the patient return to consciousness is fundamental to the modern practice of anesthesiology. Until work in the last decade, little was known about the mechanism of action of inhaled anesthetics. But almost all ideas about mechanism of action have centered around reversible biochemical processes.[4,5] In fact, we often consider the half-life of most current anesthetic agents to be short, and their elimination to be rapid. Yet at the same time when these reversible mechanisms were being considered, others were concerned about chronic changes after anesthesia. For example, Bedford in 1955 found anesthesia was associated with 18 case histories of extreme dementia, and many more cases of lesser severity.[2] Even then, several anesthesia providers objected to the idea that such chronic changes were secondary to anesthesia.

Several studies have looked at Alzheimer's disease from an epidemiologic perspective and surprisingly included exposure to general anesthesia. Bohnen found an association between receiving anesthesia before the age of 50 and earlier onset of Alzheimer's disease, particularly for halogenated agents and barbiturates as quantified by total minutes of anesthesia (Table 9-2).[67] Yet other studies have not found this association, perhaps because they did not quantify exposure.[68,69]

How might inhaled anesthetics cause chronic problems? Eckenhoff considered that if the "presumed mechanism of neurodegenerative

Table 9-2

Correlation Analysis between Cumulative Early and Midlife Exposure to Different Types of General and Major Regional Anesthetic Agents and the Age of Onset of Dementia in Incident Cases of Alzheimer's Disease (N = 252)

	Early and Midlife Exposure 50 Years and Below	Exposure After 50 Years of Age	Total Exposure
General Anesthesia			
Ether	−0.09 ns	0.14*	0.02 ns
Narcotic	−0.00 ns	0.06 ns	0.06
Barbiturates	−0.23‡	0.20†	0.01 ns
Halogenated agents	−0.21‡	−0.11 ns	−0.14 ns
Total general	−0.26‡	0.04 ns	−0.05
Major Regional Anesthesia			
Spinal	−0.13*	0.14*	0.04 ns
Epidural/sacral	0.09 ns	0.04 ns	0.06 ns
Extremity block	−0.01 ns	0.04 ns	−0.05 ns
Total regional	−0.08	0.09 ns	0.03 ns
Cumulative Anesthesia			
(General plus major regional)	−0.26‡	0.03 ns	−0.07 ns

*$p < 0.05$.
†$p < 0.01$.
‡$p < 0.001$.
Source: Reproduced with permission from Ref. 67

disorders is uncontrolled oligomerization of normal proteins," then inhaled anesthetics might also cause oligomerization of amyloid β-proteins. Indeed, halothane and isoflurane did enhance oligomerization and cytotoxicity of Alzheimer's disease–associated proteins, including some action at clinical concentrations.[70]

Postoperative cognitive dysfunction is discussed elsewhere (see Chap. 22). While some large studies show no difference between general and regional anesthetics and the incidence of postoperative cognitive dysfunction, some concern about inhaled anesthetics being associated with long-term effects is worth considering.[71–73] Pratico suggests that changes in central cholinergic activity may be a mechanism for the cognitive dysfunction after general anesthesia. However, the interaction of inhaled anesthetics with each subtype of muscarinic receptor shows no clear pattern.[74]

PROBLEMS WITH THE LITERATURE

Unfortunately, much of the literature that might be helpful in looking at long-term effects of inhaled anesthetics is of poor quality. If we are going to consider inhaled anesthetics as toxic, then we need

exposure data such as the product of time and concentration (really the integral of the concentration-time curve). Studies seldom collect this information. Marcantonio in 1998 noted no difference in delirium between general (apparently largely with isoflurane) and regional anesthesia, but there are no details.[75] For example, Canet's work "There were no restrictions on the type of general anesthetics" and only the presence or absence of volatile agents was noted, so an intriguing but statistically insignificant difference remains (cognitive dysfunction 8.7% vs. 5.6%, p = 0.27).[72]

There are some intriguing data from animal studies. Jevtovic-Todorovic's work began showing that infant rats receiving an anesthetic with midazolam, nitrous oxide, and isoflurane resulted in "apoptotic neurodegeneration in the developing brain, deficits in hippocampal synaptic function, and persistent memory/learning impairments."[76] Later she found that nitrous oxide and ketamine, both NMDA receptor agents, cause more severe damage in aged rats.[77]

There is additional evidence for long-term changes in brain function after anesthesia. Culley notes that in both young and aged rats, 2-h exposure to 1.2% isoflurane with 70% nitrous oxide produces lasting impairment in the ability to acquire and perform a spatial memory task. Interestingly, this is not an age-specific phenomena, and is not explained by pharmacokinetics.[78] Rather, Culley's data suggest that there is a persistent anesthesia-induced change in memory function.

Finally, inhaled anesthetics appear to alter gene expression. Sakamoto observed a limited number of changes in gene expression in the blood, spleen, kidneys, liver, lungs, heart, and brain of rats anesthetized for 0, 2, and 6 h with sevoflurane.[79] As might be expected, in the liver, changes in gene expression were related to drug-metabolizing enzymes. But in the lung, endothelin-1 gene expression was upregulated. This gene is associated with response to toxins, and may be upregulated in response to the high concentration of sevoflurane in the lungs. In the brain, three genes were upregulated and six downregulated. These genes encode transcription factors and genes related to circadian rhythm. The genes affected by inhalational anesthesia in the brain have previously been reported to increase with amphetamine, cocaine, and morphine withdrawal, but decrease with intravenous agents. These results suggest that the longer-term action of inhalational anesthetics may be caused by a cascade of gene expression.

UNRESOLVED ISSUES

The major problem with the anesthesia literature is not simply the complexity of the biochemistry and physiology, but the difficulty in defining who the elderly are. The fundamental issue is the definition of the term "elderly." While the geriatric literature uses specific terms, much of the anesthesiology literature does not. For example, in the geriatric literature, Suzman in 1985 used the term "oldest-old" for those over age 85. In 2001, Kinsella suggested that "There is a growing awareness that the term "elderly" is an inadequate generalization that conceals the diversity of a broad age group." Indeed, one can be American Association of Retired Persons (AARP) eligible at age 50, a member of the older population at 55 years, young-old at 65–74 years, and oldest-old over age 80 or 85.[80–82] Current anesthesia literature has not consistently used these now-traditional categories.

Another problem is that[63,64,83] even in the same age groups, say the oldest-old, some patients are fit but others, such as the frail elderly, "have outlived their social and financial supports" and have significant medical problems.[80,84] Yet the anesthesia literature draws no difference between these populations. For instance, there is a large difference in functional ability between the community-dwelling elderly and the nursing home elderly. These are not comparable populations. In fact, searches for the names of volatile anesthetics found 23,244 references with Institute for Scientific Information (ISI) and 28,048 references with PubMed, but only two of these papers made mention of any of the common geriatric terms "oldest-old," "young-old," "community dwelling," "frail elderly," "frailty," or "frail."[85,86] The inhalational agent names used in the search were: isoflurane, Forane, enflurane, Ethrane, halothane, Fluothane, sevoflurane, Ultane, desflurane, and Suprane.

While further research will reveal a greater understanding of the interaction of age and inhalational agents, a consistent set of categories for clinical trials in the elderly is still needed to allow comparison of outcomes.

KEY POINTS

▸ For all inhalational agents, elderly patients need less agent to produce a given depth of anesthesia.

▸ Anesthetic-induced coronary steal, myocardial preconditioning, and neuroprotection have complex mechanisms, and in the elderly, the clinical relevance of these phenomena is unclear.

▸ Volatile agents may have unexpected chronic consequences that are unrelated to their pharmacokinetics, especially in the brain. This may be a possible explanation for cognitive dysfunction.

▸ A major issue with the anesthesia literature is the failure to adequately define and characterize the elderly population studied. This includes both age and functional state categories.

KEY ARTICLES

▸ Zaugg M, Lucchinetti E, Uecker M, et al. Anaesthetics and cardiac preconditioning. Part I. Signaling and cytoprotective mechanisms. *Br J Anaesth*. 2003;91(4):551–565.

▸ Zaugg M, Lucchinetti E, Garcia C, et al. Anaesthetics and cardiac preconditioning. Part II. Clinical implications. *Br J Anaesth*. 2003; 91(4):566–576.

▸ Sakamoto A, Imai J, Nishikawa A, et al. Influence of inhalation anesthesia assessed by comprehensive gene expression profiling. *Gene*. 2005;356:39–48.

▸ Monk TG, Saini V, Weldon BC, Sigl JC. Anesthetic management and one-year mortality after noncardiac surgery. *Anesth Analg*. 2005;100(1):4–10.

REFERENCES

1. Snow J. On the inhalation of chloroform and ether with description of an apparatus. *Lancet*. 1848:177–80.
2. Bedford PD. Adverse cerebral effects Of anaesthesia on old people. *Lancet*. 1955;269(6884):259–263.
3. Eger EI. Characteristics of anesthetic agents used for induction and maintenance of general anesthesia. *Am J Health-Syst Pharm*. 2004;61:S3–S10.
4. Pauling L. Hydrate microcrystal theory of general anesthesia. *Anesth Analg*. 1964;43(1):1–10.
5. Pauling L. Molecular theory of general anesthesia—anesthesia is attributed to formation in brain of minute hydrate crystals of clathrate type. *Science*. 1961;134(347):15–21.
6. Gomez RS, Guatimosim C, Gomez MV. Mechanism of action of volatile anesthetics: role of protein kinase C. *Cell Mol Neurobiol*. 2003;23(6):877–885.
7. Monk TG, Saini V, Weldon BC, Sigl JC. Anesthetic management and one-year mortality after noncardiac surgery. *Anesth Analg*. 2005;100(1):4–10.
8. Monk TG. Postoperative cognitive dysfunction is more common in the elderly following major surgery. *Anesthesiology*. 2000;93(3A):U126.
9. Stemp LI. Anesthetic depth and long-term mortality. *Anesth Analg*. 2005; 101(5):1559.
10. Berry AJ. Observational studies identify associations, not causality. *Anesth Analg*. 2005;101(4):1238.
11. Stevens WC, Dolan WM, Gibbons RT, et al. Minimum alveolar concentrations (MAC) of isoflurane with and without nitrous-oxide in patients of various ages. *Anesthesiology*. 1975;42(2):197–200.
12. Eger EI. Age, minimum alveolar anesthetic concentration, and minimum alveolar anesthetic concentration-awake. *Anesth Analg*. 2001;93(4):947–953.
13. Fragen RJ, Dunn KL. The minimum alveolar concentration (MAC) of sevoflurane with and without nitrous oxide in elderly versus young adults. *J Clin Anesth*. 1996;8(5):352–356.
14. Lerou JGC. Nomogram to estimate age-related MAC. *Br J Anaesth*. 2004; 93(2):288–291.
15. Nickalls RWD, Mapleson WW. Age-related iso-MAC charts for isoflurane, sevoflurane, and desflurane in man. *Br J Anaesth*. 2003;91(2):170–174.
16. Mapleson WW. Effect of age on MAC in humans: a meta-analysis. *Br J Anaesth*. 1996;76(2):179–185.
17. Agnew NM, Pennefather SH, Russell GN. Isoflurane and coronary heart disease. *Anaesthesia*. 2002;57(4):338–347.
18. Buffington CW, Romson JL, Levine A, et al. Isoflurane induces coronary steal in a canine model of chronic coronary-occlusion. *Anesthesiology*. 1987;66(3):280–292.
19. Slogoff S, Keats AS, Dear WE, et al. Steal-prone coronary anatomy and myocardial-ischemia associated with 4 primary anesthetic agents in humans. *Anesth Analg*. 1991;72(1):22–27.
20. Kendall JB, Russell GN, Scawn NDA, et al. A prospective, randomized, single-blind pilot study to determine the effect of anaesthetic technique on troponin T release after off-pump coronary artery surgery. *Anaesthesia*. 2004;59(6):545–549.
21. Diana P, Tullock WC, Gorcsan J, et al. Myocardial-ischemia—a comparison between isoflurane and enflurane in coronary-artery bypass patients. *Anesth Analg*. 1993;77(2):221–226.
22. Teo A, Koh KF. Isoflurane and coronary steal. *Anaesthesia*. 2003;58(1):95–96.
23. Murugesan C, Murthy K, Garg R, et al. Influence of isoflurane on ischaemic heart disease in patients with coronary steal prone anatomy. *Ann Card Anaesth*. 2004;7:51–54.
24. Kersten JR, Schmeling TJ, Pagel PS, Warltier DC. Isoflurane mimics myocardial ischemic preconditioning via activation of K-ATP channels. *Anesthesiology*. 1997;87(3):A579.
25. Zaugg M, Lucchinetti E, Uecker M, et al. Anaesthetics and cardiac preconditioning. Part I. Signaling and cytoprotective mechanisms. *Br J Anaesth*. 2003;91(4):551–565.
26. Warltier DC, Kersten JR, Pagel PS, Gross GJ. Anesthetic preconditioning: serendipity and science. *Anesthesiology*. 2002;97(1):1–3.
27. Zaugg M, Lucchinetti E, Garcia C, et al. Anaesthetics and cardiac preconditioning. Part II. Clinical implications. *Br J Anaesth*. 2003;91(4):566–576.
28. Bienengraeber MW, Weihrauch D, Kersten JR, et al. Cardioprotection by volatile anesthetics. *Vasc Pharmacol*. 2005;42(5-6):243–252.
29. Belhomme D, Peynet J, Louzy M, et al. Evidence for preconditioning by isoflurane in coronary artery bypass graft surgery. *Circulation*. 1999; 100(19 suppl):II 340–344.
30. Garcia C, Julier K, Bestmann L, et al. Preconditioning with sevoflurane decreases PECAM-1 expression and improves one-year cardiovascular outcome in coronary artery bypass graft surgery. *Br J Anaesth*. 2005; 94(2):159–165.
31. Haroun-Bizri S, Khoury SS, Chehab IR, et al. Does isoflurane optimize myocardial protection during cardiopulmonary bypass? *J Cardiothorac Vasc Anesth*. 2001;15(4):418–421.
32. Mangano DT. Perioperative cardiac morbidity. *Anesthesiology*. 1990; 72(1):153–184.
33. Badner NH, Knill RL, Brown JE, et al. Myocardial infarction after noncardiac surgery. *Anesthesiology*. 1998;88(3):572–578.
34. Tani M, Suganuma Y, Hasegawa H, et al. Changes in ischemic tolerance and effects of ischemic preconditioning in middle-aged rat hearts. *Circulation*. 1997;95(11):2559–2566.
35. Przyklenk K, Li GH, Simkovich BZ, Kloner RA. Mechanisms of myocardial ischemic preconditioning are age related: PKC-epsilon does not play a requisite role in old rabbits. *J Appl Physiol*. 2003;95(6):2563–2569.

36. Abete P, Cacciatore F, Ferrara N, et al. Angina offers protections against myocardial infarctions in adult but not in elderly: a loss of preconditioning mechanism in the aging heart? *Circulation.* 1997;96[suppl I]:I-140-I-144.

37. Ishihara M, Sato H, Tateishi H, et al. Beneficial effect of prodromal angina pectoris is lost in elderly patients with acute myocardial infarction. *Am Heart J.* 2000;139(5):881–888.

38. Jimenez-Navarro M, Gomez-Doblas JJ, Alonso-Briales J, et al. Does angina the week before protect against first myocardial infarction in elderly patients? *Am J Cardiol.* 2001;87(1):11–15.

39. Lee TM, Su SF, Chou TF, et al. Loss of preconditioning by attenuated activation of myocardial ATP-sensitive potassium channels in elderly patients undergoing coronary angioplasty. *Circulation.* 2002;105(3):334–340.

40. Riess ML, Stowe DF, Warltier DC. Cardiac pharmacological preconditioning with volatile anesthetics: from bench to bedside? *Am J Physiol Heart Circ Physiol.* 2004;286(5):H1603–H1607.

41. Juhaszova M, Rabuel C, Zorov DB, et al. Protection in the aged heart: preventing the heart-break of old age? *Cardiovasc Res.* 2005;66(2):233–244.

42. Loubani M, Ghosh S, Galinanes M. The aging human myocardium: tolerance to ischemia and responsiveness to ischemic preconditioning. *J Thorac Cardiovasc Surg.* 2003;126(1):143–147.

43. Schulman D, Latchman DS, Yellon DM. Effect of aging on the ability of preconditioning to protect rat hearts from ischemia-reperfusion injury. *Am J Physiol Heart Circ Physiol.* 2001;281(4):H1630–H1636.

44. Sniecinski R, Liu H. Reduced efficacy of volatile anesthetic preconditioning with advanced age in isolated rat myocardium. *Anesthesiology.* 2004;100(3):589–97.

45. Riess ML, Camara AKS, Rhodes SS, et al. Increasing heart size and age attenuate anesthetic preconditioning in guinea pig isolated hearts. *Anesth Analg.* 2005;101(6):1572–1576.

46. Abete P, Calabrese C, Ferrara N, et al. Exercise training restores ischemic preconditioning in the aging heart. *J Am Coll Cardiol.* 2000;36(2): 643–650.

47. Abete P, Ferrara N, Cacciatore F, et al. High level of physical activity preserves the cardioprotective effect of preinfarction angina in elderly patients. *J Am Coll Cardiol.* 2001;38(5):1357–1365.

48. Abete P, Testa G, Ferrara N, et al. Cardioprotective effect of ischemic preconditioning is preserved in food-restricted senescent rats. *Am J Physiol Heart Circ Physiol.* 2002;282(6):H1978–H1987.

49. Abete P, Testa G, Galizia G, et al. Tandem action of exercise training and food restriction completely preserves ischemic preconditioning in the aging heart. *Exp Gerontol.* 2005;40(1-2):43–50.

50. Wan RQ, Camandola S, Mattson MP. Intermittent food deprivation improves cardiovascular and neuroendocrine responses to stress in rats. *J Nutr.* 2003;133(6):1921–1929.

51. Abete P, Ferrara N, Cacciatore F, et al. Angina-induced protection against myocardial infarction in adult and elderly patients: a loss of preconditioning mechanism in the aging heart? *J Am Coll Cardiol.* 1997;30(4): 947–954.

52. Abete P, Cacciatore F, Ferrara N, et al. Body mass index and preinfarction angina in elderly patients with acute myocardial infarction. *Am J Clin Nutr.* 2003;78(4):796–801.

53. Warner DS. Perioperative neuroprotection: are we asking the right questions? *Anesth Analg.* 2004;98(3):563–565.

54. Davis M, Mendelow AD, Perry RH, et al. Experimental stroke and neuroprotection in the aging rat-brain. *Stroke.* 1995;26(6):1072–1078.

55. Jin KL, Minami M, Xie L, et al. Ischemia-induced neurogenesis is preserved but reduced in the aged rodent brain. *Aging Cell.* 2004;3(6):373–377.

56. Kawaguchi M, Furuya H, Patel PM. Neuroprotective effects of anesthetic agents. *J Anesth.* 2005;19(2):150–156.

57. Langford RE. *Introduction to Weapons of Mass Destruction: Radiological, Chemical, and Biological.* Hoboken, New Jersey: John Wiley & Sons, Inc; 2004.

58. GlobalSecurity.org. Weapons of Mass Destruction (WMD): Choking Agents. In; 2005.

59. Global Security Newswire by National Journal Group. Russia I: Officials Deny Fentanyl Usage Violates Treaty. In; 2005.

60. Global Security Newswire by National Journal Group. Russia I: Theater Gas Was Probably Powerful Narcotic, Experts Say. In; 2005.

61. Myers SL. 2005. New York Times March 9, 2005.

62. Monk TG, Weldon BC, Saini V, Sigl JC. The evidence that deep anesthesia impacts long-term mortality is not compelling—response. *Anesth Analg.* 2005;101(6):1880–1881.

63. Cohen NH. Anesthetic depth and long-term mortality—in response. *Anesth Analg.* 2005;101(5):1559–1560.

64. Levy WJ. Is anesthetic-related mortality a statistical illness? *Anesth Analg.* 2005;101(4):1238.

65. Monk TG, Weldon BC, Saini V, Sigl JC. Editorial board reproached for publication of BIS-mortality correlation—response. *Anesth Analg.* 2005;101(4):1239–1240.

66. OSHA. Available at http://www.osha.gov/dts/osta/anestheticgases/index.html

67. Bohnen N, Warner MA, Kokmen E, Kurland LT. Early and midlife exposure to anesthesia and age-of-onset of Alzheimer's disease. *Int J Neurosci.* 1994;77(3-4):181–185.

68. Gasparini M, Vanacore N, Schiaffini C, et al. A case-control study on Alzheimer's disease and exposure to anesthesia. *Neurol Sci.* 2002;23(1): 11–14.

69. Tyas SL, Manfreda J, Strain LA, Montgomery PR. Risk factors for Alzheimer's disease: a population-based, longitudinal study in Manitoba, Canada. *Int J Epidemiol.* 2001;30(3):590–597.

70. Eckenhoff RG, Johansson JS, Wei HF, et al. Inhaled anesthetic enhancement of amyloid-beta oligomerization and cytotoxicity. *Anesthesiology.* 2004;101(3):703–709.

71. Williams-Russo P, Sharrock NE, Mattis S, et al. Cognitive effects after epidural vs. general anesthesia in older adults: a randomized trial. *J Am Med Assoc.* 1995;274(1):44.

72. Canet J, Raeder J, Rasmussen LS, et al. Cognitive dysfunction after minor surgery in the elderly. *Acta Anaesthesiol Scand.* 2003;47(10):1204–1210.

73. Crul BJP, Hulstijn W, Burger IC. Influence of the type of anesthesia on postoperative subjective physical well-being and mental function in elderly patients. *Acta Anaesthesiol Scand.* 1992;36(7):615–620.

74. Pratico C, Quattrone D, Lucanto T, et al. Drugs of anesthesia acting on central cholinergic system may cause postoperative cognitive dysfunction and delirium. *Med Hypotheses.* 2005;65(5):972–982.

75. Marcantonio ER, Orav EJ, Cook EF, et al. The association of intraoperative factors with the development of postoperative delirium. *Am J Med.* 1998;105(5):380.

76. Jevtovic-Todorovic V, Hartman RE, Izumi Y, et al. Early exposure to common anesthetic agents causes widespread neurodegeneration in the developing rat brain and persistent learning deficits. *J Neurosci.* 2003;23(3):876–882.

77. Jevtovic-Todorovic V, Carter LB. The anesthetics nitrous oxide and ketamine are more neurotoxic to old than to young rat brain. *Neurobiol Aging.* 2005;26(6):947.

78. Culley DJ, Baxter MG, Yukhananov R, Crosby G. Long-term impairment of acquisition of a spatial memory task following isoflurane-nitrous oxide anesthesia in rats. *Anesthesiology.* 2004;100(2):309–314.

79. Sakamoto A, Imai J, Nishikawa A, et al. Influence of inhalation anesthesia assessed by comprehensive gene expression profiling. *Gene.* 2005;356: 39–48.

80. Suzman R, Riley MW. Introducing the oldest old. *Milbank Mem Fund Q Health Soc.* 1985;63(2):177–186.

81. Kinsella K, Velkoff VA. *An Aging World: 2001,* U.S. Census Bureau, Series P95/01-1. In: Bureau USC, ed. Washington, DC: U.S. Government Printing Office; 2001.

82. AARP. AARP Membership. In: AARP; 2005.

83. Cohen NH. Anesthetic depth is not (yet) a predictor of mortality! *Anesth Analg.* 2005;100(1):1–3.

84. Rockwood K. What would make a definition of frailty successful? *Age Ageing.* 2005;34(5):432–434.

85. Thomson Scientific. ISI Web of Knowledge. In: Thomson Scientific; 2005.

86. National Library of Medicine. Entrez PubMed. In: National Library of Medicine; 2005.

Local Anesthetics and the Elderly

Asha Padmanabhan

The aging population presents the anesthesiologist with a challenge. The normal physiologic and pathophysiologic processes of the aging body can present an array of problems in perioperative management. One of the decisions the anesthesiologist has to make is the selection of the type of anesthetic. Ultimately, the choice of the anesthetic technique will depend on many factors such as the nature of the surgery, the comorbid conditions, the length of the procedure, the expertise of the surgeon, the comfort level of the anesthesiologist with the technique, and the patient's wishes. This chapter focuses on the anatomical, physiological, and pharmacological alterations with aging pertinent to regional anesthesia, and the modifications in technique necessary to make the administration of regional anesthesia in this population as safe as possible.

ANATOMIC AND PHYSIOLOGIC CHANGES

Changes in the vertebral spine with aging

The human spine is a complicated structure composed of the vertebrae and intervertebral discs. Alterations to the form and composition of the individual components of the spine occur as a part of the process of aging. The intervertebral discs become drier with age. They become more fibrous and less resilient due to the increase in collagen and loss of elastin. These changes make the discs stiffer and more resistant to deformation. The intervertebral disc height is diminished, leading to decreased space between the posterior spinous processes, which may lead to difficulty in needle insertion. There is an overall decrease in bone density in the vertebral bodies. The vertebral end plates deform by microfracture and gradually bow into the vertebral body, imparting a concave shape to the superior and inferior surfaces of the vertebral body. There is increased calcification of the ligamentum flavum leading to difficulty in introducing the needle through the tissue. As the intervertebral disc height diminishes, the ligamentum flavum may buckle and constrict the vertebral canal.[1]

Due to the biochemical and structural changes in the joints of the spine, there is a reduction in mobility, and associated decrease in flexion leading to a greater difficulty in positioning.

Extradural space

The process of aging causes anatomic changes in the structure of the extradural space. The connective tissue around the intervertebral foramina becomes dense and firm with age, partially reducing the size of the intervertebral foramina. The extradural compliance increases and the extradural resistance decreases with age as the fatty tissue in the extradural space degenerates (Fig. 10-1).[2]

Hogan studied the influence of age, vertebral level and disease on the epidural anatomy by examining the spine of 26 patients by cryomicrotome section (Figs. 10-2 and 10-3). He found that distortion and compression of the epidural space occurs with aging. The distortion occurs because of the buckling of the ligamentum flavum, changes in the disc and the facet joints. All these changes constrict the vertebral canal and may make it difficult to thread an epidural catheter.[1] All of these changes may also cause maldistribution in the spread of local anesthetic. There may also be a greater longitudinal spread of local anesthetic with more extensive neural block in the elderly due to progressive occlusion of the intervertebral foramina.

Saitoh et al. investigated the relationship between the leakage of iohexol through the intervertebral foramina and age, and between the degree of leakage and the extent of longitudinal spread (Figs. 10-4 and 10-5). They found a correlation between age and longitudinal spread, but there was no correlation between leakage through the intervertebral foramina and age, or between leakage and longitudinal spread. They postulated that the longitudinal extradural spread of local anesthetics in the elderly may not be attributed to decreased leakage through the intervertebral foramina.[3]

Igarashi et al. examined the extradural space with an extraduroscope at the L2–3 level. They found that the amount of fatty tissue in the extradural space was reduced and the space became widely patent with increasing age (Fig. 10-6).[4]

This may affect the longitudinal spread of local anesthetics in the elderly. The dura also appears to become more permeable to local anesthetic because of an increase in the size of the arachnoid villi.[4] This increase in permeability might increase the transdural diffusion of local anesthetic in the elderly and lead to a subdural site of action of the local anesthetic as opposed to the mainly paravertebral site in the young.

Subarachnoid space

There may be a reduction in the volume of the cerebrospinal fluid (CSF) with aging as well as an increase in its specific gravity. The dural sleeve covering the roots of the spinal cord may also decrease in thickness with aging. As mentioned above, the dura is also more permeable to local anesthetic.

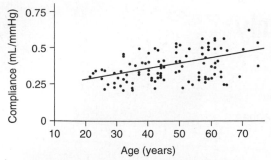

(a)   Correlation between age and extradural compliance
($r = 0.40$; $y = 0.00406x + 0.20145$; $P < 0.01$).

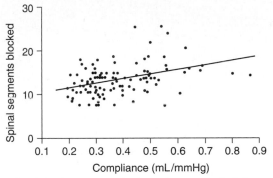

(b)   Correlation between extradural compliance and extent of
analgesia ($r = 0.40$; $y = 11.44x + 9.09$; $P < 0.01$).

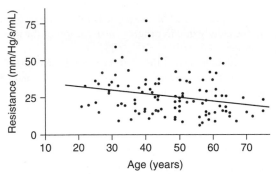

(c)   Correlation between age and extradural resistance
($r = -0.22$; $y = -0.24x + 38.10$; $P < 0.05$).

FIGURE 10-1 (A) Correlation between age and extradural compliance (top graph).
(B) Correlation between extradural compliance and extent of analgesia (middle graph).
(C) Correlation between age and extradural resistance (bottom graph). *(Adapted from Ref. 2.)*

Anatomical considerations pertinent to peripheral nerve blocks

Generally, the changes in the anatomy with aging do not provide an impediment for the performance of peripheral nerve blocks in the elderly. However, arthritic changes in the body with aging may make the positioning of the patient more difficult for the performance of peripheral nerve blocks. Bony landmarks might become more prominent, thus aiding in the identification of the appropriate site.

Changes in the neural tissue

There are various physiological changes in the central nervous system (CNS) that occur with aging. These are

- A decrease in the diameter and the number of myelinated fibers in the dorsal and ventral nerve roots. One-third of the myelinated nerve fibers in the body have disappeared by 90 years of age.
- The distance between the Schwann cells in the myelinated fibers decreases with aging, leading to an increase in the number of cationic acceptor sites available to be blocked by the local anesthetic.
- The mucopolysaccharides in the connective tissue sheaths of the nerves deteriorate with aging allowing more local anesthetic to penetrate the nerve sheath.
- There is a decline in the neuronal population with aging, and there is a progressive slowing of the conduction velocities of peripheral motor and sensory nerves and an increase in the onset latencies of F waves and sensory-evoked potentials with advancing age.
- There is a significant increase in the size of the arachnoid villi, which in turn leads to the dura becoming more permeable to the local anesthetic.
- The regeneration capability of the nerves decreases with aging.[5-7]

All of these changes may contribute to an increased sensitivity to local anesthetics in the elderly.

LOCAL ANESTHETIC AGENTS

Pharmacokinetics

The study of the pharmacokinetics of a local anesthetic drug enables us to determine the safest and the most efficacious dose of that drug. Pharmacokinetics includes the study of absorption, distribution, metabolism, and clearance.

Absorption

Once injected at a site, the local anesthetic is quickly absorbed into the blood stream and taken up by the highly perfused tissues such as the brain, lung, kidney, and liver. This redistribution is responsible for the rapid disappearance of the drug from the blood stream.

Unlike other drugs, the primary effects of local anesthetic agents occur at the site of injection. Once injected at a depot site, the drug undergoes local and systemic disposition. The local disposition, that is, the uptake of the drug into the neuronal tissue, is responsible for the nerve blockade, whereas the systemic disposition contributes to potential side effects. The processes of bulk movement, binding, diffusion, and metabolism influence the local disposition of the drug. Thus, any factor that increases the uptake of the local anesthetic into the blood stream and away from the neural tissue will decrease the amount of drug available for blocking the nerve. This in turn will affect the onset, intensity, and the duration of the nerve block. The uptake of local anesthetic from the site of injection depends on:

- Dose: This is the most important factor in determining the speed of onset, the intensity, and the duration of the nerve block. Studies have not shown a significant difference in the onset or quality of a block when a large dilute volume of local anesthetic is injected versus a small concentrated volume. Thus, it is likely that it is the total dose which is important.
- pK_a, and pH Adjustment: The closer the pK_a of a given anesthetic is to the pH of the injected tissue, the greater the proportion of it that exists in base form. The base form has the greatest penetration of the neural membranes. Adding sodium bicarbonate can increase the pH of local anesthetic solutions. This can speed the onset of the block.

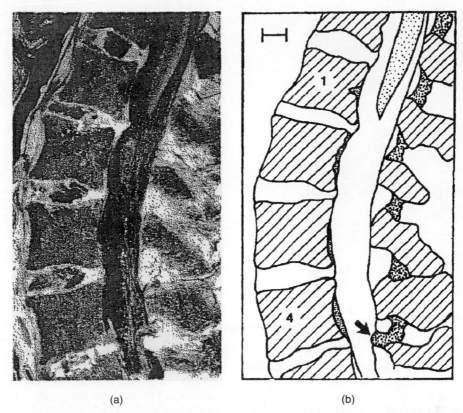

(a)   (b)

FIGURE 10-2 Midline sagittal cryomicrotome section (A) and index drawing (B) of lumbar vertebral column of a 76-year-old female showing degenerative disc disease. The L1 and L4 vertebral bodies are indicated by "1" and "4." Radial tears through the annulus fibrosus of the intervertebral discs are seen at L1–L2 and L3–L4 levels with end-stage disc disease at L4–L5. Loss of disc height has produced distortion of the ligamenta flava, with buckling of the redundant L4–L5 ligamentum flavum into the vertebral canal (arrow). Spinous processes of L3 through L5 are touching. *(Adapted from Ref. 1.)*

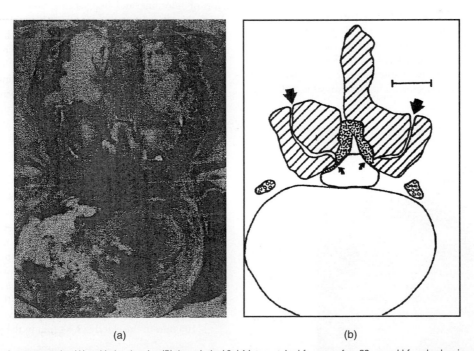

(a)   (b)

FIGURE 10-3 Axial cryomicrotome section (A) and index drawing (B) through the L3–L4 intervertebral foramen of an 86-year-old female showing advanced degenerative joint and disc disease. The intervertebral disc is partially calcified. The facet joint (heavy arrow) show loss of cartilage, subarticular erosions, and osteophyte development. Sclerotic bone occupies the expanded articular processes. The ligamenta flava are degenerated and thickened. These features reduce the volume of the posterior epidural compartment, compress the dural sac (small arrows), and compromise the intervetebral foramina. *(Adapted from Ref. 1.)*

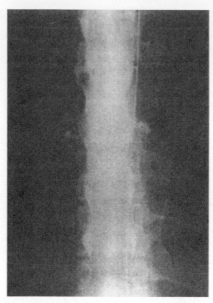

FIGURE 10-4 Extradural radiograph in a 42-year-old woman. Leakage is seen from one intervertebral foramen. *(Adapted from Ref. 3.)*

▶ Site of Injection: The rate of absorption of a local anesthetic also depends on the site of injection. The order of absorption decreases from intercostal > caudal > epidural > brachial plexus > sciatic and femoral nerve blocks > subarachnoid space. The absorption rate is fastest from the intercostal space because of the relative lack of fat in the space and the large number of blood vessels draining it. This is independent of the local anesthetic agent used. Though the epidural space is vascular, most of the venous plexuses traverse it rather than drain it. The epidural space also has a large quantity of fat, which sequesters the local anesthetic.

At a standard dose and at a particular site, absorption also depends on: partition coefficient of the local anesthetic; factors affecting local diffusion, that is, presence of fat and scar tissue capable of binding and later releasing the local anesthetic; pH of the local environment; vascularity of the tissue; total area of absorption; regional blood flow, which is the most rate-limiting factor; addition of vasoconstrictors like

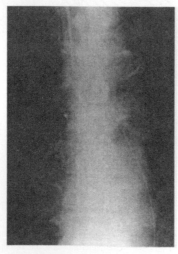

FIGURE 10-5 Extradural radiograph in a 76-year-old man. Leakage is seen from several intervertebral foramina. *(Adapted from Ref. 3.)*

epinephrine and phenylephrine; and vasodilating property of the individual local anesthetic and its lipid solubility.

Absorption from the Epidural Space There is little or no metabolism of the local anesthetic occurring in the epidural space. Therefore, almost the entire injected dose is absorbed eventually. Local anesthetics undergo *flip-flop kinetics* in the epidural space, that is, their absorption rate constant is smaller than the elimination rate constant.[8,9] Hence, Burm et al. developed a stable isotope method, using deuterium-labeled isotopes of bupivacaine, to study simultaneously the absorption and disposition of lidocaine and bupivacaine following subarachnoid and epidural injection. They found that the absorption and distribution of both the drugs were consistent with a two-compartment model and two parallel first-order absorption processes. They concluded that the systemic absorption of these drugs was biphasic. There is a rapid initial absorption phase followed by a slower phase. The rapid initial absorption phase from the site of injection is due to the uptake of the drug by the blood vessels. The slower, or late absorption phase, is due to the uptake of the drug sequestered in the epidural fat.[10] The rapid initial absorption rates were similar for all the agents, but slow absorption phase was slower for bupivacaine and etidocaine than for lidocaine.

Veering et al. used the stable isotope method to investigate the effect of age on the pharmacokinetics of bupivacaine.[10] According to this study, age did not influence the systemic absorption or disposition of bupivacaine. The half-lives of the fast and slow absorption processes and the absorbed fraction did not change with age. Thus, the maximum plasma concentration (C_{max}) and the corresponding time to C_{max} (T_{max}) were unaffected by aging (Table 10-1).

Absorption from the Subarachnoid Space Similar to the epidural space, local anesthetics are not metabolized in the subarachnoid space and almost the entire injected dose is absorbed. Burm et al. used the stable isotope method described above to study the absorption of lidocaine and bupivacaine from the subarachnoid space. From this study it appears that the initial absorption after subarachnoid injection for both agents is slower than that with epidural injection. This difference could be due to the differences in vascularity of the two spaces. Lidocaine did not show the rapid absorption phase. Its absorption was more characteristic of a single-order absorption process. Bupivacaine, on the other hand, demonstrated a biexponential process indicating two parallel absorption processes similar to that in the epidural space. This process was slower than in the epidural space. These differences might be due to higher lipid solubility and protein binding of bupivacaine that makes it bind to tissues near the site of injection.[11]

The systemic absorption of hyperbaric bupivacaine from the subarachnoid space studied by Veering et al. using the stable isotope method demonstrates a decrease in the slow absorption rate with aging but a faster late absorption rate. The net result is a decrease in the mean absorption rate. The C_{max} did not change with age, whereas the T_{max} increased with age (107 min in the elderly vs. 65 min in the young adults). A previous study by Veering indicates that baricity affects the pharmacokinetics of bupivacaine in the elderly (Table 10-2). With glucose-free bupivacaine, the C_{max} increased with age (96 min in the elderly vs. 75 min in the young adults) as did the T_{max} (105 min in the elderly vs. 84 min in the young adults).[12,13]

Distribution and protein binding

After the local anesthetic agent is absorbed from the site of injection, it is distributed by the blood to various tissues. It is initially taken up

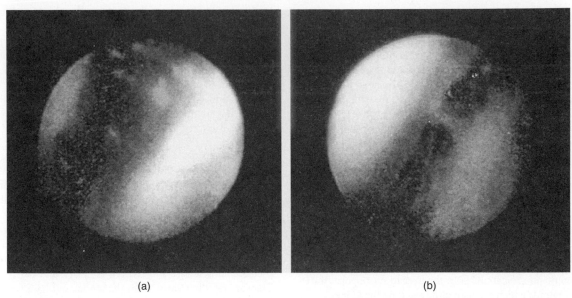

(a)   (b)

FIGURE 10-6 Photographs obtained via an extradurascope in a 77-year-old man. (A) The extradural space is seen as a widely patent canal. (B) Fibrous connective tissues extend across the patent canal. *(Adapted from Ref. 4.)*

by the highly perfused, rapidly equilibrating tissues such as the lung, brain, kidney, and liver. This is the α-phase of distribution and it is responsible for initial redistribution of local anesthetic from the blood.

The lung is one of the first organs to be exposed to the drug because it is well perfused. It also presents a large tissue mass to the drug in the systemic circulation. The extravascular pH of the lung is low relative to the plasma pH and it traps the local anesthetic ions. It sequesters the local anesthetic temporarily and thus acts as a buffer. This is particularly important when a large quantity of the drug might access the systemic circulation, as with intravenous regional anesthesia and intercostal blocks, and affords some protection against the development of toxic concentrations.

After distributing in and out of the rapid equilibrating tissues, the local anesthetic is taken up by the slow equilibrating tissues, which receive a lesser proportion of the cardiac output. These include the skeletal muscle and fat which act as storage buffers. This is the β-phase of distribution.

The third phase of distribution or the γ-phase is the phase of clearance, which includes metabolism and excretion. This phase is independent of the route of administration.[14,15]

Local anesthetics are bound to plasma proteins. The degree of binding is one of the factors which determine the rate at which the drug will distribute to various tissues. The unbound or free fraction

of the drug is responsible for the pharmacological effects and the toxic effects. α-1-acid glycoprotein (AAG) is the major plasma protein complex that binds local anesthetics. They bind to its high affinity, low capacity receptor sites. To a lesser extent, they also bind to the low affinity, high capacity sites on albumin. AAG concentrations are increased in various disease and physiological states such as the postoperative period, cancer, trauma, myocardial infarction, uremia, and inflammatory disease, and decreased during pregnancy or when taking oral contraceptives. Accordingly, the proportion of the free drug in circulation will decrease or increase. The binding of local anesthetics to AAG is sensitive to changes in plasma pH.

As the body ages, there is a reduction in the muscle mass, an increase in the body fat, and a reduction in the total body water. This will affect the distribution of lipophilic local anesthetics, which will have a larger volume of distribution (Vd) which may in turn lead to a longer clearance time.

A study by Davis et al. showed a slight increase in the plasma binding of lidocaine with age.[16] Several other studies have shown that AAG concentrations did not change with age, provided there were no coexisting diseases.[16–18] Veering et al. further showed that serum binding of bupivacaine is independent of age uncomplicated by disease.[19] However, since many elderly patients have coexisting diseases which may elevate AAG levels, there might be a decrease in the free fraction of the local anesthetic in plasma. The significance of this is unclear.

Table 10-1

Changes in Pharmacokinetics of Local Anesthetics after Epidural Administration with Age

Drug	C_{max}	T_{max}	Terminal 1/2	CL
Bupivacaine[26,112]	↔	↔	↑	↓
Lidocaine[113]	↔	↔	↑	↓
Levobupivacaine[32]	↔	↓	↔	↔

Note: C_{max}: maximum plasma concentration; T_{max}: time to maximum plasma concentration; Terminal 1/2: terminal half-life; CL: clearance ↔: no change; ↑: increased; ↓: decreased.

Table 10-2

Effect of Age on the Absorption of Bupivacaine from the Subarachnoid Space

Drug	C_{max}	T_{max}	Terminal 1/2	CL
Hyperbaric[12]	↔	↑	↑	↓
Glucose-free[13]	↑	↑	↓	↓

Note: C_{max}: maximum plasma concentration; T_{max}: time to maximum plasma concentration; Terminal 1/2: terminal half-life; CL: clearance ↔: no change; ↑: increased; ↓: decreased.

Plasma albumin levels do decrease with aging.[17] However, since only a relatively small proportion of local anesthetic is bound to albumin, it would not affect the disposition significantly.

The role of plasma protein binding in prevention of local anesthetic toxicity is unclear. Theoretically, it may limit toxic levels of local anesthetic reaching the brain in case of inadvertent intravenous injection. However, at the concentrations reaching the brain and heart after intravenous injection, plasma binding is likely to be saturated. Tucker et al. showed that only 20% of lidocaine and 50% of bupivacaine would be protein bound after a 400-mg dose of lidocaine and 150-mg dose of bupivacaine intravenous.

Also, in rat studies, the binding of lidocaine to AAG is rapidly reversible and drug uptake by the brain is not rate-limited.[20] Plasma binding alone may not control CNS penetration by lidocaine as evidenced by lumbar CSF concentrations exceeding the unbound plasma lidocaine concentration.[21]

Metabolism

Local anesthetics are metabolized in the liver to more polar, water-soluble compounds which are then eliminated by the kidney.

Amide Metabolism The amide local anesthetics are biotransformed in the endoplasmic reticulum of the hepatocytes. There are three main processes involved: aromatic hydroxylation, *N*-dealkylation, and amide hydrolysis. The rate of metabolism among the different local anesthetics is roughly the following: prilocaine > etidocaine > lidocaine > mepivacaine > bupivacaine. A large number of metabolites are formed during the biotransformation of local anesthetics. Metabolites may have similar or different actions as compared to the parent drug. They may also have toxic effects similar to the parent drug.

Eighty percent of an administered dose of lidocaine is converted to metabolites. There are three main metabolic byproducts: monoethylglycinexylidide (MEGX), glycine-xylidide (GX), and xylidine. MEGX accounts for 70% of unbound lidocaine found in plasma. It has a short half-life, slightly longer than that of lidocaine, and is eliminated by further metabolism. In animals, MEGX has been shown to have antiarrhythmic and anticonvulsant activities comparable to lidocaine. Its toxicity may be additive to that of lidocaine. GX concentrations in plasma are much lower than lidocaine, though it has a longer half-life of about 10 h. Fifty percent of GX in plasma is excreted unchanged; therefore, it may accumulate during continuous infusions of lidocaine, especially in the renally impaired patient. GX is much less antiarrhythmic than lidocaine and does not have convulsant activity.[21]

Bupivacaine metabolites have been much less studied than those of lidocaine. One of its metabolites is 2,6-pipecolylxylidide (PPX) and it has a longer half-life than bupivacaine. PPX concentrations in plasma after epidural injection are only one-tenth that of bupivacaine.

Prilocaine is hydrolyzed to *o*-toluidine and *N*-propylalanine. *O*-toluidine is then oxidized to two toluene derivatives, 2-amino-3-hydroxytoluene and 2-amino-5-hydroxytoluene, which oxidize hemoglobin to methemoglobin. Prilocaine doses more than 600 mg may result in methemoglobinemia.

The major route of metabolism for mepivacaine appears to be benzene ring hydroxylation. The metabolites of mepivacaine include PPX, a 3-hydroxy compound, a 4-hydroxy compound, and neutral lactams. PPX and the 4-hydroxy compound may have 68% and 36%, respectively, the toxicity of mepivacaine.

Etidocaine is highly lipid soluble; therefore, only minute amounts are excreted unchanged in the urine. About 20 metabolites of etidocaine have been found in the urine, but the clinical and toxic significance of these metabolites is unknown.

Ropivacaine is metabolized by cytochrome P4501A in the liver. Its major metabolites are PPX and 3-hydroxyropivacaine. Unbound PPX and 3-hydroxyropivacaine have less pharmacological activity than ropivacaine in animal models.

The pharmacokinetics of levobupivacaine are similar to that of bupivacaine. It is extensively metabolized and the metabolites are excreted in the urine. 3-Hydroxylevobupivacaine is its major metabolite.

Ester Metabolism Cocaine is metabolized by plasma and liver cholinesterases. Ester hydrolysis and *N*-demethylation are the major routes of breakdown. Ester hydrolysis yields benzoylecgonine, which is further broken down to ecgonine methyl ester and ecgonine. *N*-demethylation yields Norcocaine which is the only metabolite believed to have significant pharmacologic activity, but it is not a major by-product.

The procaine derivatives are metabolized partly in the blood by pseudocholinesterase and red cell esterases, and partly in the liver. They are rapidly cleared from the blood, and have very short half-lives. The hydrolysis products of procaine and 2-chloroprocaine are said to be pharmacologically inactive.

Effects of Aging on Metabolism of Local Anesthetics Studies show lower MEGX concentrations in the elderly population with higher free lidocaine concentrations, leading to a lower MEGX/lidocaine concentration ratio. The activity of cytochrome P450 3A4, which is responsible for the metabolism of lidocaine to MEGX, has been reported to decrease with age. This can correlate with the findings that total plasma clearance of epidural lidocaine decreased and terminal half-life increased with age, as demonstrated in several studies.[22–24] The metabolites of the other local anesthetics have not been extensively studied in the elderly population.

Clearance

Clearance is independent of the route of administration. Clearance of a drug from the body depends on blood flow, protein binding, biotransformation, and elimination. Local anesthetics are eliminated from the body mostly by metabolism. Only 1–6% of the administered dose is excreted unchanged by the kidneys, with the amide local anesthetics being cleared predominantly by the liver. Hepatic clearance depends on the hepatic extraction ratio (HER). This ratio, in turn, depends on the degree of protein binding. Moderately protein-bound agents like lidocaine (65% protein bound) and mepivacaine (77%) have a higher HER than bupivacaine (95%) and etidocaine (94%). For drugs with a high HER, the clearance is limited by, and varies with, hepatic blood flow. On the other hand, the clearance of drugs with a low HER such as bupivacaine (HER less than 50%) is rate-limited by the concentration of the unbound drug. The order of clearance for amides is bupivacaine < mepivacaine < lidocaine < etidocaine < prilocaine. The terminal elimination half-lives of all agents after intravenous injection are between 2 and 3 h.

Some studies have shown that the elimination half-life of lidocaine increases, and its plasma clearance decreases, with age. One study showed a decrease in clearance of lidocaine with aging only in the male population, while some other studies did not show any change in clearance with aging.[25] Aging might cause a reduction in hepatic blood flow, a decrease in liver volume, and a decrease in intrinsic metabolic activity which might decrease the clearance of lidocaine, though this has not been supported by studies. Studies on bupivacaine have also shown an increase in its terminal half-life and a decrease in plasma clearance with aging after epidural and subarachnoid administration (Fig. 10-7).[12,26] This decline in clearance with age might be related more to a decrease in the capacity of the liver to metabolize bupivacaine rather than the decrease in hepatic blood flow. The clearance of levobupivacaine has also been shown to decrease with age after epidural administration.[12,26] These changes in clearance may not be clinically significant with a single epidural or subarachnoid dose of local anesthetic, but continuous infusion or multiple doses might lead to an accumulation of the drug in the plasma, leading to toxic levels. Therefore, care must be taken when continuous infusions or repeated intermittent doses are administered in the elderly.

▶ Pharmacodynamics

The elderly are more sensitive to the effects of local anesthetic drugs. The basis for this sensitivity is not clear though the changes in pharmacokinetics mentioned above may play a role. It is likely that a combination of the physiological changes which occur with aging, as well as changes in pharmacokinetics and pharmacodynamics are all responsible for this increased sensitivity. The various anatomical and physiological changes in the CNS which occur with aging have been enumerated previously. It appears likely that the alterations in clinical effects of local anesthetics with aging are a result of changes in neuronal sensitivity.

Epidural dose requirements

The segmental dose requirement (SDR) is defined as the volume of local anesthetic needed to block one spinal dermatome for epidural anesthesia. Bromage demonstrated a linear decrease in the SDR with age between 18 and 80 years (Fig. 10-8). He found he could reasonably predict the dose for a single-shot epidural between the ages of 18 and 80 years. Beyond 80 years though, the individual variation was too large to accurately predict the dose based on his formula.[27] Sharrock tested this relationship with 0.75% bupivacaine. He found a significant linear relationship between the dose and the number of spinal segments blocked in patients between 20 and 40 years; but over 50 years of age, no positive correlation was found between the dose and the segments anesthetized. Over 60 years of age, T3–T4

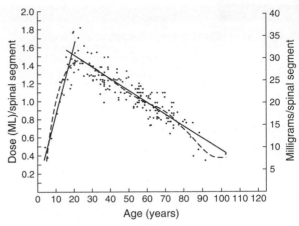

FIGURE 10-8 Segmental dose requirements related to age between 4 and 102 years. Computer fitted linear (——) and curvilinear (---------) regression lines have been drawn thorough the data points. (Adapted from Ref. 27.)

levels of anesthesia were obtained, irrespective of the dose used.[28] A study by Park using lidocaine with epinephrine also showed a minimal effect of age on the level of epidural anesthesia achieved with a standard dose.[29] Another study by Anderson et al. also showed an insignificant correlation between age and segmental dose requirement using mepivacaine with adrenaline.[30] Levobupivacaine appears to have similar clinical actions as bupivacaine, though it is said to be less toxic than an equivalent dose of bupivacaine. It also appears to have a longer duration of action in the epidural space when compared to bupivacaine.[31] The pharmacokinetics of levobupivacaine in the elderly appear to be similar to bupivacaine with a higher level of analgesia but relatively little change in the onset and duration of sensory and motor blocks.[32] Epidural ropivacaine has 0.6 times the potency of bupivacaine.[33] With advancing age, the clinical profile of ropivacaine changes. The upper level of analgesia and the intensity of motor block increase.[34] Thus, the epidural doses of ropivacaine need to be adjusted accordingly in the elderly. Though a standardized formula cannot be used to predict the required dose of any local anesthetic, it is clear that the dose requirements for epidural anesthesia in the elderly are decreased (Table 10-3). However, because of the increased sensitivity to local anesthetics in the elderly, the quality of the block may not be affected by the reduced dose.

Spinal dose requirements

There is an increased spread of local anesthetic in the subarachnoid space depending on the baricity of the solution (Table 10-4). Veering et al. demonstrated an increase in the maximum height of analgesia obtained and an increase in the duration of analgesia with hyperbaric bupivacaine in the elderly. Hyperbaric bupivacaine was also associated with a faster onset of motor block.[12,35] Studies on isobaric or glucose-free bupivacaine in spinal anesthesia in the elderly showed a faster onset to complete motor block. However, the correlation of maximal spread of analgesia with age was not clinically significant.[13,36] Isobaric mepivacaine has also been shown to have a faster onset and a higher block when used in the elderly.[37]

Intrathecal levobupivacaine in the elderly has been found to have a similar onset, duration, and degree of motor and sensory block as bupivacaine.[38] Intrathecal ropivacaine appears to be less potent than bupivacaine. It has been suggested to be 0.5 times as potent as bupivacaine for spinal anesthesia.[39] McNamee et al. found that a dose of 17.5 mg of ropivacaine provided surgical anesthesia of

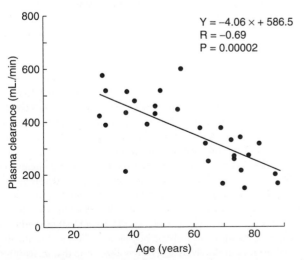

FIGURE 10-7 Relationship between total plasma clearance to bupivacaine and age with epidural anesthesia. (Adapted from Ref. 26.)

Table 10-3

Changes in Epidural Block Characteristics with Age

Drug	Max Height of Analgesia	Time to Max Caudal Spread	Time to Motor Block	Time to Recovery	Duration of Block	Intensity of Motor Block
Bupivacaine[26,112]	↑	↓	↓	↑	↔,↓	↑
Ropivacaine[34]	↑	↔	↔			↑
Levobupivacaine[32]	↑	↔		↔	↔	↔

Note: ↔: no change; ↑: increased; ↓: decreased.

similar quality, but shorter duration than the same dose of bupivacaine when used for spinal anesthesia in the elderly population (mean age 66 years) for hip surgery. There was no significant difference in time to onset of the block. However, the sensory block lasted for 3 h (range 1.5–4.6) in the ropivacaine group as opposed to 3.5 h (range 2.7–5.2) in the bupivacaine group.[40] Ropivacaine has been compared to levobupivacaine as well and seems to have the same clinical profile.[41] Sell et al. recently published a study wherein the minimum local anesthetic dose (MLAD) of levobupivacaine and ropivacaine was determined for hip replacement surgery in the elderly using a continuous spinal anesthesia technique. The MLAD is the local anesthetic dose that is effective in 50% of the patients. They found the MLAD of levobupivacaine to be 11.7 mg and that of ropivacaine to be 12.8 mg. One of six patients in whom anesthesia was initially adequate in this study however required additional local anesthetic to complete the surgery.[42]

Peripheral nerve block dose requirements

The elderly may need a lesser dose of local anesthetic. This is because of the reduction in the diameter and number of myelinated nerve fibers, slowing of nerve conduction, availability of more cationic receptor sites, and the increased sensitivity of peripheral nerves to local anesthetic agents due to decline in neuronal population which occur with aging. Paqueron et al. compared the onset and duration of brachial plexus block with ropivacaine in elderly and young patients. They found the elderly group to have a longer duration of both sensory blocks (390 min in elderly vs. 150 min in the young) as well as longer duration of motor block (357 min in the elderly vs. 150 min in the young).[43] Thus, smaller doses of local anesthetic may be necessary for peripheral nerve blockade in the elderly. There have not been many other clinical studies to substantiate the need for smaller doses. Caution must be exercised when using infusions or repeated doses of local

anesthetic. There may be a cumulative toxicity due to reduced clearance of the local anesthetic.

▶ Additives to local anesthetics

Epinephrine and phenylephrine

Vasoconstrictors like epinephrine and phenylephrine have been added to local anesthetic drug mixtures to prolong the duration of the block as well as to improve its quality. Since there is no metabolism of the local anesthetic at the site of injection, its absorption is dependent on the local blood flow. Epinephrine or phenylephrine will cause vasoconstriction at the site of injection and slow down the absorption of the local anesthetic. The prolongation of local anesthetic effect by epinephrine depends on extent of local perfusion (infiltration > epidural > intercostals), absorptive surface area, and the specific local anesthetic. Epinephrine increases the duration of block with procaine, chloroprocaine, mepivacaine, and lidocaine. Its effect with bupivacaine and etidocaine depends on the concentration of solution used. With dilute concentrations, the duration will be increased. With stronger concentrations (0.5 and 0.75%), the greater lipid solubility and protein binding of the drug by itself has a longer duration of action and epinephrine is superfluous. Epinephrine has also been shown to have a direct dose-dependent action on the spinal cord antinociceptors. This action of epinephrine adds to its analgesic effect.

The dose of epinephrine used is 0.2–0.5 mg. Phenylephrine is used in doses varying from 0.5 to 5 mg.

Epinephrine can augment the increase in the heart rate and fall in blood pressure seen with epidural anesthesia. However, a study by Tomoda et al. showed that the reduction in systolic blood pressure caused by epinephrine in the epidural solution was less pronounced with age, whereas the increase in heart rate and fall in diastolic blood pressure was not influenced by age.[44]

Epinephrine is also used in epidural test doses to rule out intravascular placement. Aging has been shown to reduce the reliability of epinephrine in the test dose. Studies have shown a decrease in responsiveness of the β-receptors with increasing age. Guinard et al. demonstrated a reduction in the magnitude of heart rate increase after a dose of intravenous epinephrine in the elderly.[45] Hence, a negative test dose must be considered with caution.

There have been conflicting reports on the effect of epinephrine in prolonging the duration of spinal anesthesia. Apparently, epinephrine does prolong the duration of anesthesia when used as an adjuvant with tetracaine, but not significantly with lidocaine or bupivacaine.[46] However, a subsequent study by Racle et al. found that the addition of 0.3 mg of epinephrine to isobaric bupivacaine did increase the duration of the block in elderly patients. They also found that increasing the dose of epinephrine beyond 0.4 mg did not result in a corresponding increase in duration of anesthesia. Thus, a ceiling effect may exist.

Table 10-4

Changes in Subarachnoid Block Characteristics with Age

Drug	Onset of Block	Duration of Block	Maximum Block Height
Hyperbaric bupivacaine[12,35]	↑	↑	↑
Isobaric bupivacaine[13,36]	↑		↔
Mepivacaine[37]	↑		↑

Note: ↔: no change; ↑: increased; ↓: decreased.

Racle also studied the effect of addition of epinephrine to lidocaine and found a clinically significant prolongation of anesthesia.[47,48]

Clonidine

Clonidine is an α-adrenoreceptor agonist. It has been shown to potentiate the sensory and motor block effect of local anesthetics by 30–50%. Its mechanism of action has not been confirmed though it may act by inhibiting the afferent cell firing at the level of the dorsal horn. Side effects of clonidine are hypotension, bradycardia, and sedation. These side effects are dose-dependent and easily treated.

Clonidine has been used as an adjunct with lidocaine, bupivacaine, levobupivacaine, and ropivacaine for epidural surgical anesthesia and postoperative analgesia in various studies. It has been combined with local anesthetic alone and with a combination of local anesthetic and opioids. Clonidine prolongs the duration of the motor and sensory epidural block and intensifies the quality of the block. Postoperatively, clonidine has been shown to produce analgesia beyond the duration of the local anesthetic block, prolonging the time before the first request of additional analgesia. Clonidine acts synergistically with fentanyl, sufentanil, butorphanol, and morphine and has been shown to reduce the dose requirements of epidural opioids.[49–52] A meta-analysis to determine the most efficacious dose of epidural clonidine required to provide good analgesia with minimal side effects failed to provide the answer because of the tremendous variability in study design. Epidural clonidine doses have ranged from boluses of 75 µg to 800 µg or 1 µg/kg to 8 µg/kg. Clonidine in epidural infusions has ranged from 0.3 µg/kg/h to 2 µg/kg/h.[53]

When used alone for intrathecal anesthesia, clonidine does not provide adequate surgical anesthesia. Hence, it has been used in conjunction with local anesthetic agents. Clonidine has been used in combination with bupivacaine, tetracaine, and ropivacaine for spinal anesthesia in elderly patients for joint replacement surgeries. It has been shown to prolong the motor and sensory block and also intensify the quality of the block.[49] A combination of bupivacaine and clonidine significantly increases the duration of the motor block as compared to plain bupivacaine or bupivacaine with epinephrine in the elderly.[54] Clonidine has also been shown to have a synergistic and additive effect with intrathecal opioids.[49,55] Strebel et al. studied the dose-response relationship of small doses of intrathecal clonidine with bupivacaine in spinal anesthesia. A dose of 150 µg of clonidine is the preferred dose when added to isobaric bupivacaine to adequately prolong both the block time and the time interval to first request of supplemental analgesia.[56] De Kock et al. found that a small dose of clonidine (15 µg) combined with ropivacaine provided adequate anesthesia for ambulatory surgery.[49]

Clonidine has been used as an adjunct to local anesthetic for brachial plexus, intercostal, peribulbar, cervical plexus, femoral, and combined femoral-sciatic and psoas compartment blocks. It appears to have an analgesic effect when used in peripheral nerve blocks, though the evidence is conflicting. A systematic review of clonidine in brachial plexus blocks by Murphy et al. found five studies where clonidine had an analgesic effect and one that was negative. They concluded that clonidine is useful as an adjunct to prolong analgesia in doses up to 150 µg.[57] Subsequent studies on brachial plexus blocks are still ambiguous as are previous studies involving other types of peripheral nerve blocks. Tschernko et al. added clonidine to bupivacaine for intercostal nerve blocks and found a significant short-term improvement in postthoracotomy pain and arterial oxygenation as compared to patients who received plain bupivacaine or patients who received plain bupivacaine and

intramuscular clonidine.[58] Gentili et al. used 150 µg of clonidine with lidocaine for intravenous regional anesthesia and found this combination to improve the tolerance for a tourniquet in lower arm procedures.[59] Casati et al. in a randomized, double-blinded study using 30 patients demonstrated a 3-h delay in the first analgesic effect postoperatively after foot surgery where 1 µg/kg of clonidine was added to 0.75% ropivacaine in a sciatic-femoral nerve block.[60] They had a similar finding when the same dose of clonidine was added to ropivacaine for axillary nerve block.[61] However, several studies do not show a consistent prolongation of peripheral nerve block with the addition of clonidine. Duma et al. added clonidine to levobupivacaine and bupivacaine in axillary brachial plexus blocks in 80 patients. They found a wide variability on the duration of the block without consistent prolongation of the block effect in the groups that received clonidine as compared to the groups who received plain local anesthetic.[62] Similar findings have been reported in other studies.[63,64] Ilfeld et al. found no clinically significant benefit in analgesia or in reducing oral analgesic requirements when 1 µg/mL of clonidine was added to 0.2% ropivacaine infusion for postoperative analgesia via an infraclavicular peridural catheter.[65] Similar results were found by the same investigators with a larger dose of clonidine (2 µg/mL) used as an adjunct to ropivacaine in continuous interscalene perineural infusions.[66]

In conclusion, the role of clonidine as an adjunct to local anesthetics in improving the anesthesia and postoperative analgesia during peripheral nerve blocks and in reducing the need for supplemental analgesia remains unclear.

Ketamine

Ketamine is a noncompetitive N-methyl-D-aspartate (NMDA) receptor antagonist, which has been used as an adjunct to local anesthetics in epidural and intrathecal anesthesia. When combined with bupivacaine, it has been shown to reduce the onset time of epidural anesthesia and increase the height of the sensory block.[67] However, a study by Weir et al. compared three doses of ketamine (0.3 mg/kg, 0.5 mg/kg, and 0.67 mg/kg) in combination with bupivacaine for epidural block in 60 elderly patients undergoing total knee replacements. They did not find any improvement in the rate of onset or maximum height of the sensory block, or any increase in the duration of analgesia from the ketamine-bupivacaine mixtures as compared to the plain bupivacaine group.[68] Analogous to the epidural results, studies on intrathecal ketamine are conflicting. It has been used as the sole anesthetic for lower limb surgery, but has shown a tendency for high incidence of CNS disturbances. Hence, even though there are no cardiovascular depressive effects, which might be advantageous in the elderly, its use has been limited.[69,70]

S (+) ketamine is one of the two enantiomers of ketamine with threefold analgesic potency of R (−) ketamine. Use of the S (+) ketamine enantiomer as an adjunct has given more encouraging results. Togal et al. studied the effects of adding 0.1 mg/kg of preservative-free S (+) ketamine to bupivacaine for intrathecal block in 40 elderly patients undergoing transurethral resection of the prostate (TURP). They found that this addition to low-dose bupivacaine shortened the onset time of motor and sensory block, shortened the duration of the block, and provided less motor blockade in elderly males.[71] Himmelseher et al. found that the combination of 0.25 mg/kg of S (+) ketamine with ropivacaine given as a single dose epidurally before total knee arthroplasty had better quality postoperative analgesia and less consumption of ropivacaine infusion than patients who received plain ropivacaine.[72] More studies in the general population and in the elderly population are needed to confirm these findings.

Opioids

Opioids have been used in the intrathecal and epidural route for over 30 years. Wang et al. were the first to conduct a study on intrathecal morphine in cancer patients. They reported significant analgesia with 0.5–1 mg intrathecal morphine.[73] Since that time, the use of intrathecal and extradural opioids has been extensive.

Intrathecal opioids act on the μ-opioid receptors in the spinal cord. They appear to selectively modulate C and A fibers with little effect on the dorsal root axons or somatosensory-evoked potentials.[74]

Both hydrophilic opioids such as morphine and lipophilic opioids like fentanyl and sufentanil have been used in the intrathecal and extradural spaces. Hydrophilic opioids have a slow onset of analgesia due to low lipid solubility, but this analgesia has a longer duration with the risk of delayed respiratory depression due to slow cephalad spread in the CSF. Lipophilic opioids have a fast onset of analgesia, which is relatively short-lived. The risk of delayed respiratory depression with these is relatively low. Opioids, when administered as adjuncts to local anesthetics in the epidural or spinal space, have a synergistic effect. Thus, smaller, subtherapeutic doses of local anesthetics are frequently adequate to provide good surgical anesthesia.[75,76]

Side Effects   The primary side effects of spinal opioids include ventilatory depression, urinary retention, pruritus, and nausea and vomiting. The risk factors which predispose to respiratory depression include older age group, thoracic administration, large doses, hydrophilic opioids like morphine, reduced ventilatory capacity, preexisting respiratory disease, and concomitant administration of opioids or other CNS-depressant drugs by other routes.[77,78] Gustafsson et al., after a nationwide study of spinal opioid use in Sweden, reported figures of late ventilatory depression in 4–7% patients after intrathecal morphine and in 0.25–0.40% after extradural morphine. The time of onset of respiratory depression seems to be variable. It was usually seen within 6–10 h after the opioid dose, but has been seen up to 12 h later because of slow rostral spread of morphine in the CSF. After extradural administration of morphine, respiratory depression has been seen from 5 h up to even 24 h later.[77,79]

Urinary retention is seen in 20–40% of patients after 2–6 mg of extradural morphine.[78] The incidence of urinary retention does not appear to be dose-related as evidenced by a study by Martin et al. who found the same incidence with extradural morphine doses from 0.5 to 8 mg.[80] The urinary retention caused by opioids also appears to respond to naloxone.

Pruritus may be localized or generalized. Gustafsson et al. reported an incidence of 2–5% and greater in their survey after extradural morphine.[81] In other studies, the incidence has varied widely, with a 100% incidence seen after 10 mg extradural morphine to 28% after the same dose in another study. One percent of the patients experienced pruritus after 2 mg and 5 mg of extradural morphine.[77]

Morphine Intrathecal   In the elderly, morphine has been used extensively as an additive in spinal anesthesia to decrease the dose of local anesthetic and incidence of hypotension. Slappendel et al. tested four doses of morphine (0.025, 0.05, 0.1, and 0.2 mg) combined with 20 mg bupivacaine for total hip arthroplasty under spinal anesthesia in 143 elderly patients (mean age 63 years) in a prospective, randomized, double-blinded, dose-finding study. This study found that the optimal dose was 0.1 mg which provided excellent postoperative analgesia with minimal side effects.[82] Mendieta Sanchez et al. had a similar finding.[83] Murphy et al. conducted a study similar to the one by Slappendel using a lower dose of bupivacaine (15 mg) with 50–200 μg of morphine in 60 patients older than 65 years. They concluded 100 μg provided the best analgesia with least side effects in older patients undergoing total hip arthroplasty.[84] Sakai et al. tested minidose morphine (0.05 mg

vs. 0.1 mg) with tetracaine 10 mg in 42 elderly patients (mean age 72 years) undergoing TURP under spinal anesthesia. They found the dose of 0.05 mg morphine to be sufficient to provide analgesia without the side effects of respiratory depression and hypoxemia and significantly less pruritus in this population.[85] This minidose might be adequate for relatively less painful procedures such as TURP, but might not be adequate for more invasive and painful procedures (Table 10-5).

Epidural   As with intrathecal administration, epidural morphine has a synergistic effect with local anesthetics. Ready et al. found a correlation between age and effective epidural morphine dose. In a retrospective study of 66 patients after abdominal hysterectomy, they found an inverse relationship between 24-h epidural morphine dose and age. Thus, elderly patients seem to have greater analgesia from the same dose of epidural morphine than do younger patients.[86] This also correlates to the finding that the analgesic response to parenteral opioids increases with increasing age.[87] Moore et al. found a significant difference in epidural morphine requirements between the elderly and young patients after abdominal surgery. Using a single epidural dose of 0.07 mg/kg or 5 mg/70 kg of morphine injected epidurally, they found that elderly patients had significantly better postoperative analgesia than younger patients. Most elderly patients needed supplemental analgesia only toward the end of the first postoperative day (21 h).[88] The reason for this sensitivity to morphine is not yet clear. The elderly may have a decreased perception to pain.[89] The clearance of morphine may also be decreased in the elderly, which may lead to a longer duration of action. Reduction of morphine clearance of up to 50% in the elderly has been reported.[90] On the other hand, these findings may be related to brain drug levels. Gustafsson et al. found that in patients over 40 years of age, the concentration of morphine in the CSF was higher after epidural administration as compared to younger patients.[81]

Ventilatory depression after epidural morphine is still of concern, especially in the elderly. Gustaffson et al. reported an incidence of 0.25–0.40% of ventilatory depression in their survey population (6000–9150 patients). These patients received between 2 and 4 mg of extradural morphine, with smaller doses being used for thoracic epidurals. Twenty-two patients developed respiratory depression within 1 h of the last dose of extradural morphine. Of these, nine had also received systemic opioids. Seven patients developed respiratory depression more than 6 h after the last doses of extradural morphine. Of these, five had received systemic opioids. Thus, the concomitant

Table 10-5

Optimal Doses for Intrathecal Morphine in Elderly Patients

Author	Morphine Doses	Local Anesthetic	Surgery	Optimal Dose
Slappendel et al.	0.025, 0.05, 0.1, 0.2 mg	Bupivacaine 20 mg	Total hip arthroplasty	0.1 mg
Mendieta Sanchez	0, 0.1 mg	Bupivacaine	Total hip arthroplasty	0.1 mg
Murphy et al.	0, 50, 100, 200 μg	Bupivacaine 15 mg	Total hip arthroplasty	100 μg
Sahai	0.05, 0.1 mg	Tetracaine 10 mg	TURP	0.05 mg
Kirson et al.	0, 0.1, 0.2 mg	Lidocaine 75 mg	TURP	0.1 mg

Source: Adapted from Refs. 82–85,114.

administration of systemic opioids seems to be a risk factor for the development of ventilatory depression. The other risk factors identified in this study include age of 70 years or more, previously impaired respiratory function, and thoracic administration.[78]

In the above-mentioned survey, the incidence of pruritus after extradural morphine was found to be between 2% and greater than 5%. About 10% of patients had postoperative urinary retention requiring bladder catheterization.

Fentanyl Fentanyl is a lipophilic opioid which has a fast onset of action when injected intrathecally. Its duration of action is short as it is rapidly cleared from the CSF. Fentanyl, when combined with local anesthetics for spinal anesthesia, has a synergistic effect. It enhances the sensory block produced by local anesthetics without increasing the motor block. Fentanyl has been used in doses ranging from 10 to 50 μg intrathecally. From studies in the general population, fentanyl, when added to local anesthetics for surgical spinal anesthesia, appears to facilitate faster onset of the block, improve the quality of the block intraoperatively, and prolong the postoperative analgesia without prolonging the time to discharge.[91]

Because of its lipophilicity, the side-effect profile of intrathecal fentanyl is somewhat different from morphine. Respiratory depression is not common with the current doses being used. In the elderly, fentanyl doses of 25 μg or less does not affect the CO_2 ventilatory response curves.[92] The risk of respiratory depression may be increased with concomitant systemic administration of opioids. Sedation, like respiratory depression, has also not been reported with the small doses of intrathecal fentanyl currently in use. Urinary retention does not seem as common with fentanyl as it is with morphine. There was no significant increase in time to urination when fentanyl was added to hyperbaric lidocaine or bupivacaine.[93,94] Mild pruritus after intrathecal fentanyl is common.[93]

Intrathecal As with morphine, many studies have been conducted in the elderly to find the lowest possible optimal dose of fentanyl to be used as an adjunct to local anesthetic in spinal anesthesia. The addition of fentanyl has allowed the use of lower doses of the local anesthetic, hence decreasing the side effects (Table 10-6). For shorter, less invasive surgery-like urological procedures, small doses of local anesthetic (4–5 mg bupivacaine) when combined with small doses of fentanyl (10–25 μg) seem to provide adequate surgical anesthesia with minimal hypotension.[95,96] Walsh et al. found no difference in hypotension in their study comparing 10 mg hyperbaric bupivacaine with and without fentanyl.[97] However, they used a larger dose of bupivacaine when compared with the previous studies[95,96] for similar procedures in the same patient population. This may explain why they did not find any hemodynamic difference in their two groups. A subsequent study by Kararmaz et al.[98] had findings similar to the previous studies.[95,96] For hip fracture surgery in the elderly, Ben-David et al.[99] and Chico et al.[100] found minidoses of bupivacaine (4 and 5 mg) adequate for surgical anesthesia when combined with 15 and 20 μg of fentanyl, respectively, with significantly less hypotension. Martyr et al.[101] did not find any difference in their two groups using 7.5 mg bupivacaine with 20 μg of fentanyl and 12.5 mg bupivacaine without fentanyl. However, the previous studies had used isobaric bupivacaine as opposed to the hyperbaric used by Martyr, which might have migrated cephalad and caused sympathetic blockade sufficient to cause hypotension.

Epidural Extradural fentanyl may primarily act at supraspinal sites after being almost completely absorbed from the spinal sites and redistributed to the brain. If this is the case, the question has been asked whether there is any advantage to using extradural fentanyl when the same effect would be obtained with intravenous or intramuscular injection. Many studies have come up with conflicting reports. Ginosar et al. compared previously reported studies and hypothesized that fentanyl, when administered in the epidural space as a bolus injection, works by a spinal mechanism, whereas if it is administered as a continuous infusion, it works by a supraspinal mechanism. They confirmed these findings in a study on 10 healthy volunteers.[102]

Sufentanil When administered intrathecally sufentanil is rapidly cleared from the CSF, and hence does not provide adequate postoperative analgesia.[103] Olofsson et al. studied low-dose bupivacaine spinal anesthesia with sufentanil for hip repair in elderly patients. They found that a dose of 7.5-mg hyperbaric bupivacaine with 5 μg of sufentanil provided reliable spinal anesthesia for this surgery with significantly less hypotension.[104] It has also been used in continuous intrathecal infusions after orthopedic surgery and seems to provide good analgesia,[105] but with a high incidence of nausea and vomiting.[106] Sufentanil intrathecally has also been known to cause respiratory depression, which may develop within 30 min of injection, and requires close monitoring.[107] Epidural sufentanil has efficacy in providing postoperative pain relief. Kampe et al. used a continuous epidural infusion of 0.1% ropivacaine with 0.5 μg/mL of sufentanil for postoperative analgesia in 32 patients (mean age 65 years) undergoing total hip replacement with good results. The addition of sufentanil led to a six-fold reduction in total postoperative opioid requirement with negligible motor block. 0.2% ropivacaine with 1.5 μg/mL of sufentanil also provided good analgesia after total knee replacement.[108–110]

DRUG INTERACTIONS AND LOCAL ANESTHETICS

The older patient often takes a variety of medications. Some of these medications may interact with the local anesthetic agents. Studies of these interactions specifically in the elderly population are lacking. However, some of these interactions are well-known in the general population and can be extrapolated to the elderly. These drug interactions may be potentially significant in the elderly population and certainly need to be considered when the use of local anesthetics in this population is anticipated.

In therapeutic doses, propranolol is known to directly inhibit mixed-function oxidase activity in the hepatocyte. It also decreases liver blood flow by reducing the cardiac output and by intrahepatic β2-receptor blockade. As a result, propranolol reduces the clearance of lidocaine by about 40%. It may also reduce the clearance of bupivacaine. Other β-blockers may have less marked effects on the hepatic blood flow, and may not affect the metabolism of local anesthetics significantly.

Cimetidine, an H2-receptor antagonist, directly inhibits the microsomal enzymes, thus decreasing the metabolism of lidocaine. It reduces the clearance of lidocaine after either intravenous or epidural administration by 20–30% in humans. Animal studies indicate cimetidine may also inhibit the metabolism of bupivacaine. Ranitidine, another H2-receptor antagonist, has no effect on local anesthetic metabolism.

Phenytoin, an anticonvulsant, is known to induce the activity of hepatic microsomal enzymes. Unbound lidocaine clearance increases by 25% in patients receiving phenytoin. Phenytoin also induces α-1-acid glycoprotein synthesis, which may lower the unbound lidocaine fraction.

Ecothiophate inhibits plasma pseudocholinesterase and will inhibit the breakdown of ester-type local anesthetics.

Drugs that displace local anesthetics from their protein binding sites may cause an increase in their unbound plasma fraction. Quinidine, disopyramide, and bupivacaine are known to increase free lidocaine concentration.[14,111]

Table 10-6

Studies in the Elderly To Define Optimum Dose of Fentanyl and Local Anesthetic in Intrathecal Anesthesia

Authors	Year	Local Anesthetic	Dose of Fentanyl	Surgery	# pts	Study Type	Findings
Varrassi et al.	1992	Bupivacaine (hyperbaric) 15 mg	50, 25, 2.5 µg, saline	Urological	28	Randomized, double-blind, controlled	50 µg caused early respiratory depression
Fernandez-Galinski et al.	1996	Bupivacaine 12.5 mg	25 µg	Knee and hip repl acement	40	Prospective, randomized, double-blind	Sensory/motor block onset/duration not altered, postoperative pain decreased
Kuusniemi et al.	2000	Bupivacaine 10, 7.5, 5 mg	25 µg	Urological	80	Prospective, randomized, double-blind	25 µg fentanyl added to 5 mg bupivacaine resulted in short-lasting motor block with same sensory level as larger doses of bupivacaine
Chen T-Y et al.	2000	Tetracaine 8, 4 mg	10 µg	TURP	45	Prospective, randomized, double-blind	10 µg fentanyl with 4 mg tetracaine provided adequate anesthesia with fewer side effects
Ben-David et al.	2000	Isobaric bupivacaine 4 mg	20 µg	Hip fracture repair	20	Prospective, randomized	Minidose bupivacaine with fentanyl 20 µg provided adequate anesthesia with significantly less hypotension
Martyr et al.	2001	Hyperbaric bupivacaine 7.5 mg with fentanyl and 12.5 mg without	20 µg	Hip fracture	42		No difference in hypotension between the two groups with similar levels of sensory block
Alonso Chico et al.	2003	Bupivacaine 5 mg with fentanyl, 7.5 mg without fentanyl	15 µg	Hip fracture	60		Significantly less hypotension in the fentanyl group
Walsh et al.	2003	Hyperbaric bupivacaine 10 mg with fentanyl, 15 mg without fentanyl	25 µg	TURP	30		No difference in hemodynamic stability or pulmonary function in the two groups
Kararmaz et al.	2003	Plain bupivacaine 4 mg with fentanyl, 7.5 mg without	25 µg	TURP	40		4 mg bupivacaine with fentanyl provided adequate anesthesia with minimal side effects

Source: Adapted from Refs. 92,95–101,115.

CONCLUSION

The process of aging leads to alterations in the pharmacokinetics and pharmacodynamics of local anesthetics. Use of local anesthetic agents is a good alternative to general anesthesia in this patient population. However, the techniques as well as the doses of the drugs used need to be modified in the elderly.

KEY POINTS

▶ The process of aging causes anatomic changes in the structure of the extradural space, which constrict the vertebral canal and may make it difficult to thread an epidural catheter and may also cause maldistribution in the spread of local anesthetic. There may also be a greater longitudinal spread of local anesthetic with more extensive neural block in the elderly due to progressive occlusion of the intervertebral foramina.

- Age does not influence the systemic absorption or disposition of bupivacaine from the epidural space. With aging, the systemic absorption of hyperbaric bupivacaine from the subarachnoid space shows a decrease in the slow absorption rate but a faster late absorption rate.

- Changes in clearance of local anesthetics with aging may not be clinically significant with a single epidural or subarachnoid dose, but continuous infusion or multiple doses might lead to an accumulation of the drug in the plasma, leading to toxic levels. Therefore, care must be taken when continuous infusions or repeated intermittent doses are administered in the elderly.

- Though a standardized formula cannot be used to predict the required dose of any local anesthetic, it is clear that the dose requirements for epidural anesthesia in the elderly are decreased. However, because of the increased sensitivity to local anesthetics in the elderly, the quality of the block may not be affected by the reduced dose.

- There is an increase in the maximum height of analgesia obtained, and an increase in the duration of analgesia with hyperbaric bupivacaine in the elderly. However, there is no correlation between maximal spread of analgesia and age with isobaric or glucose-free bupivacaine spinal anesthesia.

- The elderly may need a lesser dose of local anesthetic for peripheral nerve blocks because of the reduction in the diameter and number of myelinated nerve fibers, slowing of nerve conduction, availability of more cationic receptor sites, and the increased sensitivity of peripheral nerves to local anesthetic agents with aging. Aging has been shown to reduce the reliability of epinephrine in the epidural test dose.

- In the elderly, morphine has been used extensively as an additive in spinal anesthesia to decrease the dose of local anesthetic and incidence of hypotension. As with intrathecal administration, epidural morphine has a synergistic effect with local anesthetics. Ventilatory depression after epidural morphine is still of concern, especially in the elderly.

- Fentanyl has a fast onset of action when injected intrathecally. Its duration of action is short as it is rapidly cleared from the CSF. Fentanyl, when combined with local anesthetics for spinal anesthesia, enhances the sensory block produced by local anesthetics without increasing the motor block. The side-effect profile of intrathecal fentanyl is somewhat different from morphine, and respiratory depression is not common with the current doses being used.

- When administered intrathecally sufentanil is rapidly cleared from the CSF, and hence does not provide adequate postoperative analgesia. Intrathecal sufentanil has also been known to cause respiratory depression and requires close monitoring.

- The older patient is often taking a variety of medications. Drug interactions need to be considered when the use of local anesthetics in this population is anticipated.

KEY ARTICLES

- Fukuda T, Kakiuchi Y, Miyabe M, et al. Free lidocaine concentrations during continuous epidural anesthesia in geriatric patients. *Reg Anesth Pain Med.* 2003;28:215–220.

- Veering BT. Pharmacological aspects of local anesthetics in the elderly. *Acta Anaesthesiol Belg.* 1998;49:117–122.

- Paqueron X, Boccara G, Bendahou M, et al. Brachial plexus nerve block exhibits prolonged duration in the elderly. *Anesthesiology.* 2002;97:1245–1249.

- Murphy PM, Stack D, Kinirons B, Laffey JG. Optimizing the dose of intrathecal morphine in older patients undergoing hip arthroplasty. *Anesth Analg.* 2003;97:1709–1715.

REFERENCES

1. Hogan QH. Epidural anatomy examined by cryomicrotome section. Influence of age, vertebral level, and disease. *Reg Anesth.* 1996;21:395–406.
2. Hirabayashi Y, Shimizu R, Matsuda I, Inoue S. Effect of extradural compliance and resistance on spread of extradural analgesia. *Br J Anaesth.* 1990;65:508–513.
3. Saitoh K, Hirabayashi Y, Shimizu R, et al. Extensive extradural spread in the elderly may not relate to decreased leakage through intervertebral foramina. *Br J Anaesth.* 1995;75:688–691.
4. Igarashi T, Hirabayashi Y, Shimizu R, et al. The lumbar extradural structure changes with increasing age. *Br J Anaesth.* 1997;78:149–152.
5. Bromage PR. *Epidural Analgesia.* Philadelphia: W.B. Saunders; 1978.
6. La Fratta, Canestrani RE. A comparison of sensory and motor nerve conduction in man. *Phys Med Rehabil.* 1966;47:286–290.
7. Dorfman LJ, Bosley TM. Age-related changes in peripheral and central nerve conduction in man. *Neurology.* 1979;29:38–44.
8. Tucker GT, Mather LE. Pharmacology of local anaesthetic agents. pharmacokinetics of local anaesthetic agents. *Br J Anaesth.* 1975;47(Suppl.): 213–224.
9. Tucker GT, Mather LE. Clinical pharmacokinetics of local anaesthetics. *Clin Pharmacokinet.* 1979;4:241–278.
10. Burm AG, Vermeulen NP, Van Kleef JW, et al. Pharmacokinetics of lignocaine and bupivacaine in surgical patients following epidural administration. Simultaneous investigation of absorption and disposition kinetics using stable isotopes. *Clin Pharmacokinet.* 1987;13:191–203.
11. Burm AG, Van Kleef JW, Vermeulen NP, et al. Pharmacokinetics of lidocaine and bupivacaine following subarachnoid administration in surgical patients: simultaneous investigation of absorption and disposition kinetics using stable isotopes. *Anesthesiology.* 1988;69:584–592.
12. Veering BT, Burm AG, Spierdijk J. Spinal anaesthesia with hyperbaric bupivacaine. Effects of age on neural blockade and pharmacokinetics. *Br J Anaesth.* 1988;60:187–194.
13. Veering BT, Burm AG, Van Kleef JW, et al. Spinal anesthesia with glucose-free bupivacaine: effects of age on neural blockade and pharmacokinetics. *Anesth Analg.* 1987;66:965–970.
14. Tucker GT, Mather LE. Properties, absorption, and disposition of local anesthetic agents. In: Cousins MJ, Bridenbaugh PO, eds. *Neural Blockade in Clinical Anesthesia and Management of Pain.* 2nd ed. Philadelphia: Lippincott; 1998:55–98.
15. Ferrante FM. Pharmacology of local anesthetics. In: Longnecker DE, Tinker JH, Morgan GE, eds. *Principles and Practice of Anesthesiology.* 2nd ed. Mosby, St Louis 1998.
16. Davis D, Grossman SH, Kitchell BB, et al. The effects of age and smoking on the plasma protein binding of lignocaine and diazepam. *Br J Clin Pharmacol.* 1985;19:261–265.
17. Veering BT. The effect of age on serum concentrations of albumin and (alpha)1-acid glycoprotein. *Br J Clin Pharmacol.* 1990;29:201.
18. Verbeeck RK, Cardinal JA, Wallace SM. Effect of age and sex on the plasma binding of acidic and basic drugs. *Eur J Clin Pharmacol.* 1984;27: 91–97.
19. Veering BT, Burm AG, Gladines MP, Spierdijk J. Age does not influence the serum protein binding of bupivacaine. *Br J Clin Pharmacol.* 1991; 32:501–503.
20. Pardridge WM, Sakiyama R, Fierer G. Transport of propranolol and lidocaine through the rat blood-brain barrier. Primary role of globulin-bound drug. *J Clin Invest.* 1983;71:900–908.
21. Laurikainen E, Marttila R, Lindberg R, Kanto J. Penetration of lidocaine and its active desethylated metabolite into cerebrospinal fluid in man. *Eur J Clin Pharmacol.* 1983;25:639–641.

22. Fukuda T, Kakiuchi Y, Miyabe M, et al. Free lidocaine concentrations during continuous epidural anesthesia in geriatric patients. *Reg Anesth Pain Med.* 2003;28:215–220.

23. Fukuda T, Kakiuchi Y, Miyabe M, et al. Plasma lidocaine, monoethyl-glycinexylidide, and glycinexylidide concentrations after epidural administration in geriatric patients. *Reg Anesth Pain Med.* 2000;25:268–273.

24. Sotaniemi EA, Lumme P, Arvela P, Rautio A. Age and CYP3A4 and CYP2A6 activities marked by the metabolism of lignocaine and coumarin in man. *Therapie.* 1996;51:363–366.

25. Veering BT. The role of ageing in local anaesthesia. *Pain Rev.* 1999; 6:167.

26. Veering BT, Burm AG, Vletter AA, et al. The effect of age on the systemic absorption, disposition, and pharmacodynamics of bupivacaine after epidural administration. *Clin Pharmacokinet.* 1992;22:75–84.

27. Bromage PR. Ageing and epidural dose requirements: segmental spread and predictability of epidural analgesia in youth and extreme age. *Br J Anaesth.* 1969;41:1016–1022.

28. Sharrock NE. Epidural anesthetic dose responses in patients 20 to 80 years old. *Anesthesiology.* 1978;49:425–428.

29. Park WY, Hagins FM, Rivat EL, Macnamara TE. Age and epidural dose response in adult men. *Anesthesiology.* 1982;56:318–320.

30. Andersen S, Cold GE. Dose response studies in elderly patients subjected to epidural analgesia. *Acta Anaesthesiol Scand.* 1981;25:279–281.

31. Kopacz DJ, Allen HW, Thompson GE. A comparison of epidural levobupivacaine 0.75% with racemic bupivacaine for lower abdominal surgery. *Anesth Analg.* 2000;90:642–648.

32. Simon MJ, Veering BT, Stienstra R, et al. Effect of age on the clinical profile and systemic absorption and disposition of levobupivacaine after epidural administration. *Br J Anaesth.* 2004;93:512–520.

33. Polley LS, Columb MO, Naughton NN, et al. Relative analgesic potencies of ropivacaine and bupivacaine for epidural analgesia in labor: implications for therapeutic indexes. *Anesthesiology.* 1999;90:944–950.

34. Simon MJ, Veering BT, Stienstra R, et al. The effects of age on neural blockade and hemodynamic changes after epidural anesthesia with ropivacaine. *Anesth Analg.* 2002;94:1325–1330, table of contents.

35. Racle JP, Benkhadra A, Poy JY, Gleizal B. Spinal analgesia with hyperbaric bupivacaine: influence of age. *Br J Anaesth.* 1988;60:508–514.

36. Pitkanen M, Haapaniemi L, Tuominen M, Rosenberg PH. Influence of age on spinal anaesthesia with isobaric 0.5% bupivacaine. *Br J Anaesth.* 1984;56:279–284.

37. Boss EG, Schuh FT. The effect of age on the spread of spinal anesthesia using isobaric 2% mepivacaine. *Anaesthesist.* 1993;42:162–168.

38. Glaser C, Marhofer P, Zimpfer G, et al. Levobupivacaine versus racemic bupivacaine for spinal anesthesia. *Anesth Analg.* 2002;94:194–198, table of contents.

39. McDonald SB, Liu SS, Kopacz DJ, Stephenson CA. Hyperbaric spinal ropivacaine: a comparison to bupivacaine in volunteers. *Anesthesiology.* 1999;90:971–977.

40. McNamee DA, McClelland AM, Scott S, et al. Spinal anaesthesia: comparison of plain ropivacaine 5 mg ml(−1) with bupivacaine 5 mg ml(−1) for major orthopaedic surgery. *Br J Anaesth.* 2002;89:702–706.

41. Milligan KR. Recent advances in local anaesthetics for spinal anaesthesia. *Eur J Anaesthesiol.* 2004;21:837–847.

42. Sell A, Olkkola KT, Jalonen J, Aantaa R. Minimum effective local anaesthetic dose of isobaric levobupivacaine and ropivacaine administered via a spinal catheter for hip replacement surgery. *Br J Anaesth.* 2005;94:239–242.

43. Paqueron X, Boccara G, Bendahou M, et al. Brachial plexus nerve block exhibits prolonged duration in the elderly. *Anesthesiology.* 2002;97:1245–1249.

44. Tomoda MK, Ueda W, Hirakawa M. Hemodynamic effect of epidurally administered epinephrine in middle-aged and elderly patients. *Acta Anaesthesiol Scand.* 1989;33:647–651.

45. Guinard JP, Mulroy MF, Carpenter RL. Aging reduces the reliability of epidural epinephrine test doses. *Reg Anesth.* 1995;20:193–198.

46. Greene NM. Uptake and elimination of local anesthetics during spinal anesthesia. *Anesth Analg.* 1983;62:1013–1024.

47. Racle JP, Benkhadra A, Poy JY. Subarachnoid anaesthesia produced by hyperbaric lignocaine in elderly patients. Prolongation of effect with adrenaline. *Br J Anaesth.* 1988;60:831–835.

48. Racle JP, Benkhadra A, Poy JY, Gleizal B. Effect of increasing amounts of epinephrine during isobaric bupivacaine spinal anesthesia in elderly patients. *Anesth Analg.* 1987;66:882–886.

49. Eisenach JC, De Kock M, Klimscha W. Alpha(2)-adrenergic agonists for regional anesthesia. A clinical review of clonidine (1984–1995). *Anesthesiology.* 1996;85:655–674.

50. Carabine UA, Milligan KR, Moore J. Extradural clonidine and bupivacaine for postoperative analgesia. *Br J Anaesth.* 1992;68:132–135.

51. Dobrydnjov I, Axelsson K, Gupta A, et al. Improved analgesia with clonidine when added to local anesthetic during combined spinal-epidural anesthesia for hip arthroplasty: a double-blind, randomized, and placebo-controlled study. *Acta Anaesthesiol Scand.* 2005;49:538–545.

52. Milligan KR, Convery PN, Weir P, et al. The efficacy and safety of epidural infusions of levobupivacaine with and without clonidine for postoperative pain relief in patients undergoing total hip replacement. *Anesth Analg.* 2000;91:393–397.

53. Armand S, Langlade A, Boutros A, et al. Meta-analysis of the efficacy of extradural clonidine to relieve postoperative pain: an impossible task. *Br J Anaesth.* 1998;81:126–134.

54. Racle JP, Poy JY, Benkhadra A, et al. Prolongation of spinal anesthesia with hyperbaric bupivacaine by adrenaline and clonidine in the elderly. *Ann Fr Anesth Reanim.* 1988;7:139–144.

55. Harada Y, Nishioka K, Kitahata LM, et al. Visceral antinociceptive effects of spinal clonidine combined with morphine, [D-Pen2, D-Pen5] enkephalin, or U50,488H. *Anesthesiology.* 1995;83:344–352.

56. Strebel S, Gurzeler JA, Schneider MC, et al. Small-dose intrathecal clonidine and isobaric bupivacaine for orthopedic surgery: a dose-response study. *Anesth Analg.* 2004;99:1231–1238, table of contents.

57. Murphy DB, McCartney CJ, Chan VW. Novel analgesic adjuncts for brachial plexus block: a systematic review. *Anesth Analg.* 2000;90:1122–1128.

58. Tschernko EM, Klepetko H, Gruber E, et al. Clonidine added to the anesthetic solution enhances analgesia and improves oxygenation after intercostal nerve block for thoracotomy. *Anesth Analg.* 1998;87:107–111.

59. Gentili M, Bernard JM, Bonnet F. Adding clonidine to lidocaine for intravenous regional anesthesia prevents tourniquet pain. *Anesth Analg.* 1999;88:1327–1330.

60. Casati A, Magistris L, Fanelli G, et al. Small-dose clonidine prolongs postoperative analgesia after sciatic-femoral nerve block with 0.75% ropivacaine for foot surgery. *Anesth Analg.* 2000;91:388–392.

61. Casati A, Magistris L, Beccaria P, et al. Improving postoperative analgesia after axillary brachial plexus anesthesia with 0.75% ropivacaine. A double-blind evaluation of adding clonidine. *Minerva Anestesiol.* 2001;67:407–412.

62. Duma A, Urbanek B, Sitzwohl C, et al. Clonidine as an adjuvant to local anaesthetic axillary brachial plexus block: a randomized, controlled study. *Br J Anaesth.* 2005;94:112–116.

63. Erlacher W, Schuschnig C, Orlicek F, et al. The effects of clonidine on ropivacaine 0.75% in axillary perivascular brachial plexus block. *Acta Anaesthesiol Scand.* 2000;44:53–57.

64. Culebras X, Van Gessel E, Hoffmeyer P, Gamulin Z. Clonidine combined with a long acting local anesthetic does not prolong postoperative analgesia after brachial plexus block but does induce hemodynamic changes. *Anesth Analg.* 2001;92:199–204.

65. Ilfeld BM, Morey TE, Enneking FK. Continuous infraclavicular perineural infusion with clonidine and ropivacaine compared with ropivacaine alone: a randomized, double-blinded, controlled study. *Anesth Analg.* 2003;97:706–712.

66. Ilfeld BM, Morey TE, Thannikary LJ, et al. Clonidine added to a continuous interscalene ropivacaine perineural infusion to improve postoperative analgesia: a randomized, double-blind, controlled study. *Anesth Analg.* 2005;100:1172–1178.

67. Yanli Y, Eren A. The effect of extradural ketamine on onset time and sensory block in extradural anaesthesia with bupivacaine. *Anaesthesia.* 1996;51:84–86.

68. Weir PS, Fee JP. Double-blind comparison of extradural block with three bupivacaine-ketamine mixtures in knee arthroplasty. *Br J Anaesth.* 1998;80:299–301.

69. Bion JF. Intrathecal ketamine for war surgery. A preliminary study under field conditions. *Anaesthesia.* 1984;39:1023–1028.

70. Hawksworth C, Serpell M. Intrathecal anesthesia with ketamine. *Reg Anesth Pain Med.* 1998;23:283–288.
71. Togal T, Demirbilek S, Koroglu A, et al. Effects of S(+) ketamine added to bupivacaine for spinal anaesthesia for prostate surgery in elderly patients. *Eur J Anaesthesiol.* 2004;21:193–197.
72. Himmelseher S, Ziegler-Pithamitsis D, Argiriadou H, et al. Small-dose S(+)-ketamine reduces postoperative pain when applied with ropivacaine in epidural anesthesia for total knee arthroplasty. *Anesth Analg.* 2001;92:1290–1295.
73. Wang JK, Nauss LA, Thomas JE. Pain relief by intrathecally applied morphine in man. *Anesthesiology.* 1979;50:149–151.
74. Hamber EA, Viscomi CM. Intrathecal lipophilic opioids as adjuncts to surgical spinal anesthesia. *Reg Anesth Pain Med.* 1999;24:255–263.
75. Tejwani GA, Rattan AK, McDonald JS. Role of spinal opioid receptors in the antinociceptive interactions between intrathecal morphine and bupivacaine. *Anesth Analg.* 1992;74:726–734.
76. Maves TJ, Gebhart GF. Antinociceptive synergy between intrathecal morphine and lidocaine during visceral and somatic nociception in the rat. *Anesthesiology.* 1992;76:91–99.
77. Cousins MJ, Mather LE. Intrathecal and epidural administration of opioids. *Anesthesiology.* 1984;61:276–310.
78. Gustafsson LL, Schildt B, Jacobsen K. Adverse effects of extradural and intrathecal opiates: report of a nationwide survey in Sweden. *Br J Anaesth.* 1982;54:479–486.
79. Rawal N, Wattwil M. Respiratory depression after epidural morphine—an experimental and clinical study. *Anesth Analg.* 1984;63:8–14.
80. Martin R, Salbaing J, Blaise G, et al. Epidural morphine for postoperative pain relief: a dose-response curve. *Anesthesiology.* 1982;56:423–426.
81. Gustafsson LL, Grell AM, Garle M, et al. Kinetics of morphine in cerebrospinal fluid after epidural administration. *Acta Anaesthesiol Scand.* 1984;28:535–539.
82. Slappendel R, Weber EW, Dirksen R, et al. Optimization of the dose of intrathecal morphine in total hip surgery: a dose-finding study. *Anesth Analg.* 1999;88:822–826.
83. Mendieta Sanchez JM, Fernandez-Liesa JI, Marco G, et al. Efficacy of 0.1 mg of subarachnoid morphine combined with bupivacaine on postoperative analgesia in total hip arthroplasty. *Rev Esp Anestesiol Reanim.* 1999;46:433–437.
84. Murphy PM, Stack D, Kinirons B, Laffey JG. Optimizing the dose of intrathecal morphine in older patients undergoing hip arthroplasty. *Anesth Analg.* 2003;97:1709–1715.
85. Sakai T, Use T, Shimamoto H, et al. Minidose (0.05 mg) intrathecal morphine provides effective analgesia after transurethral resection of the prostate. *Can J Anaesth.* 2003;50:1027–1030.
86. Ready LB, Chadwick HS, Ross B. Age predicts effective epidural morphine dose after abdominal hysterectomy. *Anesth Analg.* 1987;66:1215–1218.
87. Bellville JW, Forrest WH, Jr, Miller E, Brown BW, Jr. Influence of age on pain relief from analgesics. A study of postoperative patients. *JAMA.* 1971;217:1835–1841.
88. Moore AK, Vilderman S, Lubenskyi W, et al. Differences in epidural morphine requirements between elderly and young patients after abdominal surgery. *Anesth Analg.* 1990;70:316–320.
89. Sherman ED, Robillard E. Sensitivity to pain in the aged. *Can Med Assoc J.* 1960;83:944–947.
90. Kaiko RF, Wallenstein SL, Rogers AG, et al. Narcotics in the elderly. *Med Clin N Am.* 1982;66:1079–1089.
91. Hamber EA, Viscomi CM. Intrathecal lipophilic opioids as adjuncts to surgical spinal anesthesia. *Reg Anesth Pain Med.* 1999;24:255–263.
92. Varrassi G, Celleno D, Capogna G, et al. Ventilatory effects of subarachnoid fentanyl in the elderly. *Anaesthesia.* 1992;47:558–562.
93. Liu S, Chiu AA, Carpenter RL, et al. Fentanyl prolongs lidocaine spinal anesthesia without prolonging recovery. *Anesth Analg.* 1995;80:730–734.
94. Ben-David B, Solomon E, Levin H, et al. Intrathecal fentanyl with small-dose dilute bupivacaine: better anesthesia without prolonging recovery. *Anesth Analg.* 1997;85:560–565.
95. Kuusniemi KS, Pihlajamaki KK, Pitkanen MT, et al. The use of bupivacaine and fentanyl for spinal anesthesia for urologic surgery. *Anesth Analg.* 2000;91:1452–1456.
96. Chen TY, Tseng CC, Wang LK, et al. The clinical use of small-dose tetracaine spinal anesthesia for transurethral prostatectomy. *Anesth Analg.* 2001;92:1020–1023.
97. Walsh KH, Murphy C, Iohom G, et al. Comparison of the effects of two intrathecal anaesthetic techniques for transurethral prostatectomy on haemodynamic and pulmonary function. *Eur J Anaesthesiol.* 2003;20:560–564.
98. Kararmaz A, Kaya S, Turhanoglu S, Ozyilmaz MA. Low-dose bupivacaine-fentanyl spinal anaesthesia for transurethral prostatectomy. *Anaesthesia.* 2003;58:526–530.
99. Ben-David B, Frankel R, Arzumonov T, et al. Minidose bupivacaine-fentanyl spinal anesthesia for surgical repair of hip fracture in the aged. *Anesthesiology.* 2000;92:6–10.
100. Alonso Chico A, Cruz Pardos P, Alvarez Grau J, et al. Comparison of the hemodynamic response in subarachnoid anesthesia with bupivacaine versus bupivacaine with fentanyl in traumatology surgery in elderly patients. *Rev Esp Anestesiol Reanim.* 2003;50:17–22.
101. Martyr JW, Clark MX. Hypotension in elderly patients undergoing spinal anaesthesia for repair of fractured neck of femur. A comparison of two different spinal solutions. *Anaesth Intensive Care.* 2001;29:501–505.
102. Ginosar Y, Riley ET, Angst MS. The site of action of epidural fentanyl in humans: the difference between infusion and bolus administration. *Anesth Analg.* 2003;97:1428–1438.
103. Hansdottir V, Hedner T, Woestenborghs R, Nordberg G. The CSF and plasma pharmacokinetics of sufentanil after intrathecal administration. *Anesthesiology.* 1991;74:264–269.
104. Olofsson C, Nygards EB, Bjersten AB, Hessling A. Low-dose bupivacaine with sufentanil prevents hypotension after spinal anesthesia for hip repair in elderly patients. *Acta Anaesthesiol Scand.* 2004;48:1240–1244.
105. Standl TG, Horn E, Luckmann M, et al. Subarachnoid sufentanil for early postoperative pain management in orthopedic patients: a placebo-controlled, double-blind study using spinal microcatheters. *Anesthesiology.* 2001;94:230–238.
106. Vercauteren MP, Geernaert K, Hoffmann VL, et al. Postoperative intrathecal patient-controlled analgesia with bupivacaine, sufentanil, or a mixture of both. *Anaesthesia.* 1998;53:1022–1027.
107. Ferouz F, Norris MC, Leighton BL. Risk of respiratory arrest after intrathecal sufentanil. *Anesth Analg.* 1997;85:1088–1090.
108. Kampe S, Kiencke P, Delis A, et al. The continuous epidural infusion of ropivacaine 0.1% with 0.5 microg × mL(−1) sufentanil provides effective postoperative analgesia after total hip replacement: a pilot study. *Can J Anaesth.* 2003;50:580–585.
109. Kampe S, Veltkamp A, Kiencke P, et al. Continuous epidural infusion of ropivacaine with sufentanil 1.5 microg × mL(−1) for postoperative analgesia after total knee replacement. *Can J Anaesth.* 2003;50:617–618.
110. Kampe S, Weigand C, Kaufmann J, et al. Postoperative analgesia with no motor block by continuous epidural infusion of ropivacaine 0.1% and sufentanil after total hip replacement. *Anesth Analg.* 1999;89:395–398.
111. Bowdle TA, Freund PR. Effects of age on local anesthetic agents. In: *Geriatric Anesthesiology.* Ed. McClesky CH. Baltimore: Williams & Wilkings; 1997:367–380.
112. Nydahl PA, Philipson L, Axelsson K, Johansson JE. Epidural anesthesia with 0.5% bupivacaine: influence of age on sensory and motor blockade. *Anesth Analg.* 1991;73:780–786.
113. Veering BT. Pharmacological aspects of local anesthetics in the elderly. *Acta Anaesthesiol Belg.* 1998;49:117–122.
114. Kirson LE, Goldman JM, Slover RB. Low-dose intrathecal morphine for postoperative pain control in patients undergoing transurethral resection of the prostate. *Anesthesiology.* 1989;71:192–195.
115. Fernandez-Galinski D, Rue M, Moral V, et al. Spinal anesthesia with bupivacaine and fentanyl in geriatric patients. *Anesth Analg.* 1996;83:537–541.

SECTION 4

PREOPERATIVE ASSESSMENT

Age and Anesthetic Risk

CHAPTER

11

Renee Blanding

THE HISTORICAL PERSPECTIVE OF ADVANCED AGE AND ITS INFLUENCE ON SURGICAL OUTCOME

The risk of surgery and anesthesia has changed dramatically over the last 150 years, and the influence of advanced age has weighed heavily on the medical decisions of the past and present. In the mid-nineteenth century, advanced age alone was a strong contraindication for operative treatment for several reasons. The average life expectancy in 1850 for whites was approximately 40 years; the operative and medical experience with patients 65 years and older was limited based on numbers alone. In 1850, out of a total U.S. population of 23.2 million, only 600,000 were elderly (Table 11-1),[1] with many persons succumbing to infectious diseases of the lung, cholera, and yellow fever. Operative procedures were met with a prohibitively high mortality because of unsanitary hospital conditions, where hand washing between patients was not well understood as a deterrent to infectious diseases. Many patients died from the postoperative complications and not from the primary disease of admission.[2,3] The postoperative or convalescence period was protracted, often 3 weeks in the hospital and 3 weeks at home, a time susceptible to infection and embolic phenomenon; the risks of surgery and recuperation greatly overshadowed the benefits of the procedure.

During the 1920s and 1930s, the U.S. population 65 years and older reached over 6 million with a life expectancy of close to 59 and 47 years for whites and blacks, respectively, yet the decision to perform elective surgery on patients of advanced age was still met with reluctance [4–6]; elective procedures such as inguinal hernia repairs were often declined in 50 year olds because of a high operative mortality, which often approached 50%.[2,3] Despite the discouraging statistics, a confluence of events over time was instrumental in changing the mind-set concerning surgery on the elderly. Tremendous public health strides with regard to water and sanitation had effects on the general population with eventual decreases in infant mortality and midlife-related mortality. Advances in pharmaceutical use such as digitalis and penicillin, introduced in the mid-nineteenth and twentieth centuries, had beneficial effects on the general health and longevity of the elderly and the population at large. Developments in the field of anesthesiology, with the use of ether and chloroform in the mid-nineteenth century, allowed greater tolerance and success of surgical procedures. The use of these earlier agents was not benign; ether

was known to be irritating and flammable, and chloroform was noted to have toxicity on the liver. Mid-nineteenth century discoveries by Lister who applied the antiseptic carbolic acid to the wound prior to incision, and Pasteur who pioneered sterilization techniques as well as Halsted who later introduced the use of gloves during surgery, all contributed to decreasing the risk of morbidity and mortality in surgical candidates (Fig. 11-1).

In addition to medical, anesthetic, and surgical advances, textbooks were written specifically for the diagnosis and treatment of illnesses in older patients. In 1849, Dr. George Day published *Diseases of Advanced Life*, and in 1881, Dr. JM Charcot outlined the differences in pathology between older and younger adults in *Clinical Lectures on the Diseases of Old Age*.[7] In 1909, when the population of elderly U.S. citizens exceeded 3 million, Ignatz Nascher, known as the father of modern geriatrics, recognized the need for a specialty devoted to the elderly and coined the expression geriatrics. He published an article in *The Medical Record of New York* titled *Geriatrics*, and in 1914 wrote *Geriatrics: The Diseases of Old Age and Their Treatment*.[8,9] In 1915, Nascher founded the New York Geriatrics Society. The works by Day, Charcot, and Nascher established a discipline that allowed the medical and surgical treatment of the elderly. By 1937, surgical literature which focused on the elderly was being published. *Surgery in Patients of Advanced Age* was published in 1937 with favorable mortality results in patients 70 years and older.[6] This sentinel article helped change attitudes regarding surgical risk for the elderly population. This article was followed by an impressive report in *JAMA* in 1939 that described a successful prostatectomy in a patient at age 110.[10] The patient survived without major postoperative sequelae, and was noted to be alive and well 1 year after surgery. In 1945, a surgeon, Dr. Louis Carp wrote the *Basic Principles of Geriatric Surgery*.[1] Carp noted that the problem of the care of the aged was becoming increasingly important as the life span increased. The surgeon stated that old age did not preclude surgical procedures and provided indications for surgery in the elderly which included: when the disease was an immediate threat to life, and when the disease produced continued discomfort, pain, disability, economic loss, and interference with normal routine. Carp reported an overall mortality rate of 22.6% from his hospital in New York on the *bad-risk* elderly patients, with increasing mortality rate with increasing age. Mortality rate nearly doubled when comparing the 61–70-years group to the 81–90 year olds (Table 11-2). The contributing causes of operative death were heart failure, bronchopneumonia, and pulmonary edema. Additionally, the author listed anesthesia

Table 11-1

Historical Data on Age Composition of the Population (All Numbers in Millions)

Year	Total Population	<20 years	20–49 years	50–64 years	65 and Older
1850	23.2	12.1	8.9	1.4	0.6
1900	76.0	33.7	32.0	7.1	3.1
1930	122.8	47.6	54.0	14.4	6.6
1950*	138.3	40.1	63.2	22.4	12.5
1970*	151.4	40.6	59.8	28.6	22.4

*Values recalculated, not observed.
Source: Data reproduced from Ref. 6.

Table 11-2

Historical Operative Mortality Statistics from Goldwater Memorial Hospital

Age	Average Mortality Rates	Overall Mortality Rate
61–70	18.89%	
71–80	25.89%	22.66%
81–90	34.86%	

Note: Data reported from 450 major operative procedures in *bad-risk* patients, of which 13% were emergent.
Source: Adapted from Ref. 1.

as a major factor in the success of geriatric surgery and described the delivery of anesthetics as scientific and accurate. Cyclopropane was the preferred anesthetic because of its lesser toxicity and smooth postoperative recovery. Carp was not the only surgeon reporting his findings on the elderly; his bibliography contained at least 25 references on the surgical treatment of the elderly. By 1950, two major textbooks had been penned on geriatric medicine.[11,12]

The population of the elderly has increased sixfold since the early enumerations of the U.S. population began. Currently, 12% of the population in the United States is 65 years or older; by 2050, this number is expected to increase to 23%,[13] with an average life expectancy of 77 and 71 years for whites and blacks, respectively. The elderly undergo one-third of all surgical procedures annually, and one-third of all health expenditures in this country are spent on this age group.[14] Within the span of 20 years, the number of elderly patients requiring surgery has nearly doubled from 19% to 36%. Fifty percent of patients in general surgical practices are in this age group.[5] Despite decreasing mortality and morbidity rates for some procedures, the risk of an adverse outcome is greater in this age group. Because the medical care of these individuals is becoming more frequent, it is imperative to know which factors influence poor outcomes with respect to mortality and morbidity. This chapter explores the influence of advanced age as a risk parameter in operative outcome, methods of risk assessment, the impact of comorbidity as well as anesthetic management and surgical intervention in the elderly population.

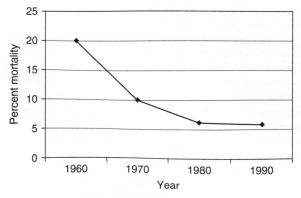

FIGURE 11-1 Overall mortality rates in the elderly over time. *(Adapted from Ref. 24.)*

DEFINITIONS OF PERIOPERATIVE OUTCOME AND FACTORS THAT INFLUENCE OUTCOME

▶ Definitions

Perioperative outcome is generally described as mortality, that is death occurring within 30 days of the surgical procedure, and/or morbidity, which involves anesthetic or surgical complications that occur also within the 30-day period. Morbidity may also include events that occur intraoperatively.[15] Within recent years, more data and studies are reporting on outcomes at 1 year. The vast majority of adverse outcomes involve the cardiovascular, pulmonary, and neurological systems.

▶ Factors that influence outcome

Emergency surgery is one of the most important factors influencing surgical outcome in the elderly. Older patients often have a more advanced stage of disease at presentation and a higher incidence of emergency surgery. In fact, the percentage of operations done on an emergent basis in patients over 85 is twice that of patients over 65,[4,5] and patients over 65 are twice as likely to present for emergent surgery when compared to younger patients.[16] Rosenthal reports that operative mortality and morbidity increase at least threefold when the surgery is performed under emergent conditions, and earlier studies from the 1980s show mortality rates ranging from 21% to 45% for emergency surgery in the elderly.[17] Additionally, there is a two- to fivefold increased risk of cardiac complications and a fivefold increased need for postoperative ventilation following emergency surgery in the elderly.[15,18] Another factor influencing outcome is the development of multiple complications during the hospital course. While studying patients aged 80 and older undergoing noncardiac surgery, Hamel et al. showed that patients who experience complications have a higher 30-day mortality than those who did not (26% vs. 4%), and for nearly half of the complications, mortality approached 33%.[19] In a study involving patients with hip complaints, Lawrence et al. reported that mortality was 15% versus 0.5% in subjects with and without complications respectively, and that patients with multiple complications and renal failure had the highest mortality rates, 29–38%.[20] Fleischmann et al. examined the outcomes and effects on length of stay in patients with a mean age of greater than 65 years undergoing noncardiac surgery and determined that cardiac and noncardiac complications occurred 2% and 13% of the time, respectively, while both types of complications occurred in 1% of the patients. Among the types of cardiac complications, patients with pulmonary edema were at the highest risk of developing noncardiac complications. Length of stay for patients experiencing cardiac and noncardiac complications was nearly three times (11 days) that of a patient without complications (4 days), while patients with both cardiac and noncardiac complications had an average length of stay of 15 days.[21]

Outcome in the elderly is influenced by the often atypical clinical presentation at the time of surgical intervention. Presentations such as atypical angina or silent ischemia may not be a prominent feature of the preoperative evaluation and may manifest postoperatively as a myocardial infarction (MI) with associated mortality of 50%.[22]

The presence of heart disease strongly affects the elderly. Coronary artery disease (CAD) may exist in up to 80% of patients over the age of 80; the incidence of heart failure may be as high as 10% in the elderly.[23,24] In a hallmark study examining outcomes in the elderly, Pedersen noted that the highest incidence of cardiovascular morbidity occurred in patients with a history of heart disease such as congestive heart failure (CHF) and ischemic heart disease, and that octogenarians had a nearly eightfold increase in cardiovascular complications when compared to patients under the age of 50 years, that is, 16.7% versus 2.6%.[25]

The aging process increases the probability that a person will require an operative procedure, and the type of surgery is another factor that influences morbidity and mortality. In a study examining the impact of age on perioperative complications, Polanczyk et al. showed that poor outcomes were associated with abdominal, intrathoracic, and abdominal aneurysm repair, and elderly patients who undergo these procedures are 2.6, 1.4, and 3.3 times as likely to have a major complication. Advanced age was significantly associated with a higher risk for cardiogenic pulmonary edema, MI, ventricular arrhythmias, bacterial pneumonia, and respiratory failure, and in-hospital mortality after these types of procedures.[26]

METHODS OF RISK ASSESSMENT

Risk assessment and stratification, particularly in the elderly, is essential to formulate proper management strategies. Approaches vary in assessing operative risk from overall medical status schemes to those which incorporate both physiology and type of operation. In addition, risk indices can be organ-specific, for example, cardiac, pulmonary, or neurological. This section highlights some of the currently used risk assessment tools and how age influences risk assessment.

► ASA

The American Society of Anesthesiologists (ASA) classification was introduced in 1941 by Saklad[27] and modified in the 1960s. It is a preoperative assessment of overall comorbidity and physical status (Table 11-3). The original purpose was to focus primarily on the physical status and discourage the use of *operative risk* because of the excessive number of variables to be considered, the tremendous degree of

variation in hospitals and physicians, and the complete lack of agreement on definition of terms. Although the ASA classification was not designed to be a specific measure of perioperative risk, it is one of the most reliable and accurate predictors of surgical mortality.[5,14,28–30] Wolters et al. compared ASA class and other perioperative variables such as renal insufficiency, anemia, and class of operation as predictors of outcome. Risk odds ratios (ORs) were determined for each variable; the highest ORs for developing a postoperative complication were associated with increased ASA class.[31] The study determined that an ASA IV implied an OR of 4.26 (95% confidence interval [CI] 2.96–6.13), ASA III class an OR of 2.24 (1.71–2.96), and ASA II a ratio of 1.5 (1.21–2.03) for postoperative complications. In a study by Hamel involving 80 year olds, 10 patient characteristics were studied as predictors of mortality; ASA class was the strongest predictor; each ASA level was associated with an adjusted OR of 1.9.[19] Although the original paper by Saklad does not specifically mention the influence of age on physical status, there is a strong tendency for increasing age to be associated with a higher ASA score.[32] There is also a strong association between the incidence of adverse events after surgery with age and ASA score[22] (Fig. 11-2). These findings have been substantiated through multiple studies.[28,33,34] During his study of 90 year olds, Hosking et al. report that ASA status was highly predictive of short-term outcomes, with ASA class II patients experiencing a 3.2% rate of 48-h complications as opposed to 18.3% for ASA class IV patients.[15] The ASA classification has been criticized for its subjective nature, but studies such as the National VA Surgical Quality Improvement Program (NSQIP) rank ASA classification as either the first or second most important predictive factor for mortality and among the top three factors for morbidity for combined analysis of all types of surgical procedures.[5] Despite its universal application, the ASA is limited in that it does not explore the intraoperative aspects with regard to surgical procedure that invariably add to risk.

► Charlson comorbidity index

The ASA classification assigns a grade or class for the physical state based on comorbidity, but was not meant to be a predictor of risk. On the other hand, the Charlson comorbidity index (CCI) quantifies the burden of medical conditions and their influence on mortality and complications. Relative risks were assigned for many of the common comorbid states, and based on the relative risk a weighted index was developed that considers the number and severity of diseases and impact on mortality (Table 11-4). In the CCI only two variables, age and comorbid state, are significant in predicting death.[35,36] A Charlson comorbidity score of 3 or more confers a 16-fold increased

Table 11-3

The American Society of Anesthesiologists Classification

I	Normal healthy patient
II	Mild systemic disease
III	Severe systemic disease but not incapacitating
IV	Incapacitating systemic disease that is a threat to life
V	Moribund, not expected to survive 24 h with or without operation

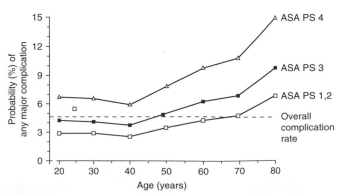

FIGURE 11-2 Relationship between the incidence of adverse events after surgery with age and ASA score. *(Reprinted with permission from Ref. 22.)*

Table 11-4

Weighted Charlson Comorbidity Index

Relative Risk	Assigned Weight	Medical Condition
1.2≥RR≤1.5	1	Myocardial infarction
		CHF, COPD, diabetes, Dementia, PVD
1.5≥RR≤2.5	2	Hemiplegia, moderate or severe renal
		Diabetes with end-organ damage
		Any tumor, leukemia, lymphoma
2.5≥RR≤3.5	3	Moderate liver disease
RR≥6	6	Metastatic solid tumor, AIDS

Source: Adapted from Ref. 35.

risk of 1-year mortality following anesthesia.[37] The study by Polanczyk et al., which examined age and perioperative complications, showed that the number of comorbid conditions and average CCI score increase with age.

▶ Goldman/Detsky/Lee cardiac risk index

Organ-specific risk indices are widely used for the cardiovascular system. The Goldman cardiac risk index was introduced in 1977 in an effort to identify patients at high risk for developing adverse postoperative cardiac outcomes.[38] The index identifies nine risk factors that are correlated with poor cardiac outcomes (Table 11-5); point values are assigned for the presence of each risk factor and four subsequent

Table 11-5

Goldman's Original Multifactorial Index

	Points
History	
Myocardial infarction with 6 months	10
Age over 70	5
Physical examination	
S-3 or jugular venous distention	11
Important aortic stenosis	3
Electrocardiogram	
Rhythm other than sinus or sinus plus APBs on last preoperative electrocardiogram	7
More than five premature ventricular bpm at any time preoperatively	7
Poor general medical status*	3
Intraperitoneal, intrathoracic, or aortic surgery	3
Emergency operation	4
Total	53

*PO_2 <60 mm Hg, PCO_2 >50 mm Hg, K <3.0 meq/1, HCO_3 <20 meq/1, BUN >50 mg/dL (18 mmol/1), creatinine >3 mg/dL (260 mmol/1), abnormal SGOT, signs of chronic liver disease, bedridden from noncardiac causes.
Source: Adapted from Ref. 38.

risk categories are derived. Class I represents the lowest risk category and class IV has the greatest number of risk factors and the greatest number of cardiac complications and death. The maximum score for Goldman's index is 53. Age is factored into this risk index as age greater than 70 years is assigned a baseline point value of 5. In 1986, Detsky et al. modified Goldman's index to include variables such as angina and pulmonary edema.[38–40] Patients are grouped into three risk categories based on the total points (Table 11-6). Several criticisms for both indices exist. Both were validated more than 10 years ago and the specific numerical risk attached to a high score may not be as applicable to today's practice. Pretest probabilities for severe cardiac complications reported by Detsky in 1986 are now overestimated in several of the surgeries such as carotid endarterectomy (CEA).[41,42] Additionally, neither of the indices have shown discrimination between low and intermediate groups; this is important considering that most events occur in the intermediate group which the index will miss.[43] For this reason, both Palda and Detsky feel that the indices may be used as a first assessment and supplemented with a more sensitive index such as the American Heart Association/ American College of Cardiology (ACC/AHA) guidelines, which recommend a strategy of stratification based on the presence or absence of clinical indicators.[44,45] Ali et al. examined the ACC/AHA guidelines as a predictor of postoperative cardiac outcome and found that the classification scheme performed extremely well with a sensitivity of 87% in predicting adverse cardiac events.[46] The Lee index was introduced to the literature in 1999 in an attempt to simplify the preoperative cardiac risk assessment.[47] A point is assigned to each clinical variable, a score is computed, and a complication rate ranging from

Table 11-6

Detsky's Modified Multifactorial Index

	Point
Coronary artery disease	
Myocardial infarction within 6 months	10
Myocardial infarction more than 6 months	5
Canadian Cardiovascular Society angina	
Class III	10
Class IV	20
Unstable angina within 6 months	10
Alveolar pulmonary edema	
Within 1 week	10
Ever	5
Valvular disease	
Suspected critical aortic stenosis	20
Arrhythmias	
Rhythm other than sinus or sinus plus APBs* on last preoperative electrocardiogram	5
More than five premature ventricular contractions at any time prior to surgery	5
Poor general medical status†	5
Age over 70	5
Emergency operation	10

*APB = atrial premature beat.
†As described in Goldman's original multifactorial index.
Source: Adapted from Ref. 40.

0.4% for 0 points to 11% for a score >3 is determined (Table 11-7). Boersma et al. examined the Lee index and found it to be predictive of cardiovascular mortality, but felt its classification of surgical procedures to be suboptimal.[48]

Postoperative pneumonia index

Because the elderly are particularly vulnerable to postoperative pulmonary complications, particularly pneumonia, recent risk assessment strategies have focused on developing validated models that accurately predict postoperative complications. Postoperative pulmonary complications are at least as common as are postoperative cardiac sequelae,[21,49,50] and 20–40% of affected patients with postoperative pneumonia die within 30 days of surgery.[51] Lawrence et al. studied patients undergoing abdominal surgery who had either one cardiac or pulmonary complication and found that 59% of the patients had pulmonary complications as opposed to the 15% for the cardiac complications. Postoperative deaths were more often due to pulmonary morbidity and contributed to twice the length of stay when compared to cardiac complications. As discussed in Chap. 5, the postoperative pneumonia risk index (PPRI) identifies preoperative risk factors and their impact on postoperative pulmonary outcome.[49,52,53] Of importance to the current discussion, considerable weight is given to age in this risk index. McAlister et al. investigated the incidence and risk for pulmonary complications and reported several complications that increased the odds of developing an adverse pulmonary outcome. Among variables examined, age greater than 65 (OR = 5.73) was significant in predicting a pulmonary complication.[54]

Delirium risk predictors

Risk indices to predict postoperative neurological dysfunction have also been developed.[55,56] Methods to predict postoperative cognitive dysfunction in the elderly were developed because an acute confusional state or delirium is noted to be one of the most common postoperative complications in the elderly occurring 15–25% after elective procedures and 25–65% following emergency procedures.[57–59] This phenomenon is associated with mortality rates ranging from 10% to 65% greater complication rates, poor functional recovery, and longer hospital stay.[24] Not only does delirium represent a postoperative complication but its presence may also lead to complications involving the cardiopulmonary systems. A delirium prediction rule was developed by Marcantonio et al. in an effort to determine which factors influenced the incidence of postoperative delirium.[60] Age greater than 70 years is an important risk variable in predicting postoperative delirium. A detailed discussion of delirium is presented in Chap. 22.

POSSUM

Another approach to risk stratification is to combine physiologic and operative variables. The Physiological and Operative Severity Score for the enUmeration of Mortality and Morbidity or POSSUM explores physiologic as well as operative variables to calculate the risk of mortality and morbidity of surgical patients.[32,61,62] Among the physiologic portions of the index, age is included and the score increases with increased age; the operative score contains six variables including operative magnitude, blood loss, and timing of operation whether elective or emergent (Table 11-8). POSSUM is a comprehensive tool that examines preoperative and intraoperative variables, but may overestimate the mortality rate in lower risk patients. Despite its criticism, the POSSUM criteria have been cited as the most appropriate scoring system available for assessing risk in noncardiac surgical patients.[32]

SAS

In an effort to categorize the degree of cardiovascular disability and functional status, Goldman et al. developed the Specific Activity Scale (SAS) shortly after the development of the cardiac risk index.[63] The approximate metabolic costs of a variety of personal care, housework, and recreational activities were determined and functional class is determined. As the functional status decreases, the SAS classification increases (Table 11-9). SAS is significantly worse in older patients, and the SAS is a correlate of the combined outcome of postoperative complications or in-house mortality.[26,45]

Table 11-7

Lee Index

One point for each of the following:
High risk surgery
History of ischemic heart disease
Congestive heart failure
Cerebrovascular disease
Insulin-dependent diabetes mellitus
Serum creatinine >2.0 mg/dL

Total Points	Complication*
0	0.4%
1	1%
2	7%
>3	11%

*Myocardial infarction, pulmonary edema, ventricular fibrillation or primary cardiac arrest, complete heart block.
Source: Adapted from Ref. 47.

Table 11-8

Variables and Point Values Assigned in the General Surgery POSSUM Scoring System

Operative Severity				
Score	1	2	4	8
Operative magnitude	Minor	Intermediate	Major	Major+
No. of operations within 30 days	1		2	>2
Blood loss per operation, mL	<100	101–500	501–999	>1000
Peritoneal contamination	No	Serious	Local pus	Free bowel content, pus or blood
Presence of malignancy	No	Primary cancer only	Node metastases	Distant metastases
Timing of operation	Elective		Emergency resuscitation possible, operation <24 h	Emergency immediate, operation <2 h

(Continued)

Table 11-8

Variables and Point Values Assigned in the General Surgery POSSUM Scoring System (*Continued*)

Physiological

Score	1	2	4	8
Age, y	≤60	61–70	≥71	
Cardiac signs	Normal	Cardiac drugs or Steroids	Edema: warfarin	JVP
CXR	Normal		Borderline cardiomegaly	Cardiomegaly
Respiratory signs	Normal	SOB exertion	SOB stairs	SOB rest
CXR	Normal	Mild COPD	Mod COPD	Any other change
Systolic BP, mmHg	110–130	131–17 100–109	≥171 90–99	≤89
Pulse, beats/min	50–80	81–100 40–49	101–120	≤121 ≤39
Coma score	15	12–14	9–11	≤8
Urea nitrogen, mmol/L	<7.5	7.6–10	10.1–15	≥15.1
Na, mEq/L	>136	131–135	126–130	≤125
K, mEq/L	3.5–5	3.2–3.4 5.1–5.3	2.9–3.1 5.4–5.9	≤2.8 ≥6
Hb, g/dL	13–16	11.5–12.9 16.1–17	10–11.4 17.1–18	≤9.9 ≥18.1
WCC X10^{12}/L	4–10	10.1–20 3.1–3.9	>20.1 ≤3	
ECG	Normal		AF (60–90)	Any other change

Table 11-9

Summary of Specific Activity Scale

Classification	Description	Activity*
Class I	Completion of any activity requiring ≥7 metabolic equivalents (ME)	Run/walk 5 mi/h (9) Up 8 steps with 24 lb (10) Carry 80 lb (8) Shovel snow (7)
Class II	Completion of ≥5≤7 ME	Walk level ground 4 m/h (5–6) Walk up 8 steps without pause (5)
Class III	Completion of ≥2≤5 ME	Down a flight of stairs (4.5) Housework (4) Walk 2.5 m/h (3–3.5) Shower without stopping (3.5)
Class IV	Inability to complete activity ≥2 ME	Dress without stopping (2–2.3)

*Approximate metabolic equivalents in ( ). ME = metabolic equivalents.
Source: Adapted from Ref. 63.

From the above discussion, the risk stratification schemes provide objective organ-specific, physiologic, or intraoperative criteria when considering perioperative risk and outcome. All with the exception of the ASA classification incorporate advanced age as an important risk parameter because advanced age is an independent predictor of increased postoperative morbidity and mortality.

ADVANCED AGE AND COMORBIDITY

Comorbidity and advanced age are independent predictors of post-operative morbidity and mortality.[18] This section examines some of the important chronic illnesses prevalent among the elderly and their impact on perioperative mortality and morbidity.

▶ Heart failure

Approximately 500,000 new cases of heart failure are diagnosed each year, and the number of existing cases is over 5 million. Over 75% of these cases exist in patients 65 years and older. One-year mortality rates among patients hospitalized for heart failure in population-based studies are reported to be 35–40%.[64] There are 10 million noncardiac surgeries performed each year, and a large majority of these procedures are performed on patients 65 years and older. Because much of the focus has been put on perioperative risk and CAD, few studies have evaluated perioperative risk in heart failure patients. One such study examined the mortality of patients with heart failure and compared the results with patients with CAD and the controls.[65] The results showed that the heart failure group had a higher Charlson index score, were more likely to be discharged to a nursing facility, and had a higher rate of emergency procedures than the CAD group or the control group. Additionally, the patients with heart failure had higher 30-day mortality rates when compared to the CAD and control group (11.7% versus 6.6% and 6.2%, respectively) (Fig. 11-3). Mortality during surgery admission and readmission rates within 30 days was higher in the CHF group. Hernandez et al. showed that the outcome statistics for patients with CAD and the controls were similar, and the presence of heart failure substantially increases the risk of mortality when compared to the other groups. Leung et al. determined that CHF was an important preoperative predictor of postoperative neurological and cardiac outcomes in the elderly.[66] Both studies suggest that more investigation and risk-based strategies with a focus on heart failure are needed. Lee et al. whose goal was to identify predictors of mortality and to design a model for risk assessment[64] developed one such model for heart failure. In this model, advanced age has an important interaction with the presence of heart failure in predicting mortality at both 30 days and 1 year. Several comorbidities were associated with increased mortality in the patient with heart failure such as dementia, cirrhosis, cerebrovascular disease, COPD, and cancer. This promising system provides insight for exploration of the variables, which place the heart failure patient at risk, and its impact on mortality. Ideally, the information can be adapted to outcomes in the perioperative setting.

▶ Atrial fibrillation

Perioperative atrial arrhythmias are estimated to affect 1 million elderly Americans per year and are associated with increased hospital stay. The prevalence of AF is approximately 0.4% in the general

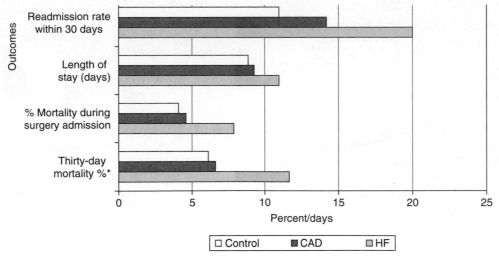

FIGURE 11-3 Comparison of outcomes in elderly patients with congestive heart failure (HF) and coronary artery disease (CAD). *(Adapted from Ref. 65.)*

population. It occurs in fewer than 1% of patients 60 years and younger. However, after the age of 80, the prevalence increases to 6%.[67] Because of possible hemodynamic instability in the elderly, perioperative rapid atrial arrhythmias can be life threatening in this population.[68,69] Postoperative atrial arrhythmias, primarily atrial fibrillation and flutter, are seen in 6.1% of elderly patients undergoing major abdominal or peripheral surgery. The incidence is noted to be 30% in coronary artery bypass graft (CABG) surgery and 65% in valvular surgery. Risk factors related to the development of perioperative AF are hypertension and CHF. However, the only independent risk factor most strongly associated with the onset of postoperative atrial fibrillation is advanced age. In a study to determine a risk stratification system for patients likely to develop postoperative AF, Amar and Zhang found age >60, preoperative heart rate >74 bpm, and those who develop postoperative pneumonia to be at greater risk of postoperative AF. Passman et al. developed a clinical prediction rule for postoperative AF; heart rate and male gender increased the OR 1.8 and 1.9 times, respectively, age 55–74 had an OR of 4.8, while patients older than 75 years were nine times more likely to develop AF.[70]

▶ COPD

COPD affects 10.2 million adults in the United States, and in patients 65–75 years and >75 years was a primary or contributing cause of hospitalization in 19.9% and 18.2% of patients, respectively.[71] Elderly patients with COPD are three to four times more likely to develop pulmonary complications; in 10 studies ranging over 30 years in elderly patients 65 years and older, the rate of postoperative pulmonary complications averaged 25% with a mortality of 7%.[49]

▶ Diabetes

Diabetes mellitus (DM) affects between 17 and 35 million people in the United States. Nearly one-fifth of the U.S. population >60 years of age have diabetes, and it is predicted that older individuals will comprise two-thirds of the diabetic population in developed countries by 2025.[72] DM is a major risk factor for cardiovascular disease, and 80% of deaths in patients with DM are from cardiovascular disease. Patients with diabetes have the same risk for MI as nondiabetics who have an MI.[73] A direct relationship between fasting blood glucose and the risk of sustaining an MI has been shown in several studies.[74,75] There may also be a direct relationship between blood

glucose and the severity and the extent of infarction.[75] Carson et al. compared the outcomes of diabetics versus nondiabetics following CABG and reported a higher morbidity and rate of infection among the diabetic group.[76] Additionally, the insulin-dependent diabetics had a higher rate of mortality than patients on oral medications. Dubey et al. conducted a study examining the effects of diabetes on outcome after hip fracture, the study derived from the Geriatric Hip Fracture Group, determined that diabetic hip fracture patients were at increased risk from dying during hospitalization compared to patients who have no history of diabetes.[77]

PREOPERATIVE LABORATORY TESTING AS A PREDICTOR OF OUTCOME IN THE ELDERLY

Between $3 and $11 billion are spent annually on preoperative testing in the United States; approximately one-third of this sum is spent on geriatric surgical patients.[78] Preoperative laboratory testing in healthy patients 60 years and older routinely includes testing for hemoglobin and hematocrit, glucose, blood urea nitrogen (BUN), and creatinine and 12-lead electrocardiogram (ECG). However, the usefulness of such routine testing has come under scrutiny for several reasons: few studies have been able to demonstrate that abnormal preoperative tests were associated with adverse postoperative outcomes and approximately $290 million can be potentially saved if this strategy of testing were eliminated.

▶ Laboratory tests

Several of the risk indices previously discussed assign point scores to abnormal laboratory values. However, recent studies suggest that laboratory values are not significant predictors of perioperative complications. Dzankic et al. performed a study to determine the prognostic significance of abnormal preoperative laboratory tests in elderly patients undergoing noncardiac surgery.[78] Fifty-five percent of the tests were performed in patients ASA > II. The study concluded that only ASA class > II and surgical risk were significant predictors of risk, despite abnormal results for creatinine, hemoglobin, and glucose. The authors recommended that testing in geriatric patients be performed based on clinical indications, not routine. However, this does not hold for all routine laboratory tests. Gibbs

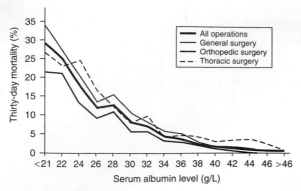

FIGURE 11-4 Thirty-day mortality rate by preoperative serum albumin level for all operations and three subspecialties. *(Reprinted with permission from Ref. 79.)*

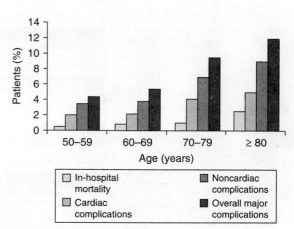

FIGURE 11-5 Major postoperative complications and in-hospital mortality in patients undergoing noncardiac surgery. *(Reprinted with permission from Ref. 26.)*

et al. studied the association of preoperative serum albumin concentration and surgical outcome in 54,215 cases from the National VA Surgical Risk Study and found that this measurement was a strong predictor of surgical outcome in most surgeries.[79] A decrease in serum albumin from concentration greater than 46 g/L to less than 21 g/L was associated with an exponential increase in mortality from less than 1% to 29% (Fig. 11-4). From such decreases in albumin, morbidity increased from 10% to 65%. Marrelli et al. substantiated the presence of hypoalbuminemia as a predictor of poor outcome in a study. The study examined outcome in patients 80 years and older following surgery for gastrointestinal carcinoma and found that albuminemia <32 g/L increased the risk of postoperative complications 2.9 times.[80]

► ECG

Because the number of ECG abnormalities increase with age, the prevalence of ECG abnormalities may be higher in patients >85 years than in those 65 years of age.[81] Liu et al. performed a study on geriatric patients undergoing noncardiac surgery to determine whether the presence of abnormal preoperative ECG findings predicted postoperative adverse cardiac outcomes. Despite the fact that 75% of the ECGs had abnormalities of which 69% were considered major, none of the abnormalities were predictive of an adverse cardiovascular event. In this study, ASA class III or greater and a history of CHF were strongly associated with cardiac complications.[82] In the elderly population, standard ECG has low sensitivity.

► Echocardiography

Echocardiography is commonly done prior to surgery to assess wall motion abnormalities, ejection fraction, and left ventricular hypertrophy in an attempt to identify patients who are at high risk for perioperative cardiac morbidity and mortality. Halm et al. examined the usefulness of this instrument as a prognostic tool for cardiac risk.[83] The study revealed that no echocardiography measurement significantly predicted ischemic outcomes. The study concluded that ejection fraction alone as a prognostic tool is limited. However, preoperative echocardiography may provide independent information about the risk of postoperative cardiac complications in selected patients.[84]

RISK STRATIFICATION BY SPECIFIC AGE

The term elderly is used liberally in the geriatric literature. It is assumed that this generic term is used for individuals 65 years or greater. In addition, definitions such as aged and the very old are used

for groups 75–84 years and 85 years and above, respectively.[14] The lack of standardization in the geriatric literature can be confusing because census data groups the elderly starting at the age of 65, the traditional start of old age, while much of the scientific data report physiologic changes by the chronological decade. Recently, however, the literature is beginning to refer to these individuals by the chronological decade of age, that is, sexagenarians (60–69), septagenerians (70–79), octogenarians (80–89), nonagenarians (90–99), and centenarians (100 and older). For the purposes of this chapter, both nomenclatures are used.

Up through the age of 60 years, both basal organ function and physiologic reserve (defined as the difference between basal and maximal organ function) are well maintained.[14] After 60 years, physiologic reserve declines, and it is likely that a patient over the age of 74 has on average three disabilities or diseases.[16] In a study examining the effect of age on perioperative complications, Polancyzk showed in the 50–59 years age group a 5.6% rate of major or fatal perioperative complications with in-hospital mortality less than 2%.[26] Earlier studies by Pedersen demonstrated a similar overall mortality of 2.2%.[25] Cardiac and noncardiac complications were approximately 3% and 3.8%, respectively, in Polanczyk's study. This study clearly showed that fatal and major complications increase with age; the younger reference group of 50–59 year olds had a lower mortality and complications while the age groups 70–79 years and greater than 80 years had higher overall mortality of 9.6% and 12.5%, respectively (Fig. 11-5). Additionally, this work showed that Charlson comorbidity and ASA scores increased with age.

● THE EFFECT OF ANESTHETIC TECHNIQUE AND INTRAOPERATIVE EVENTS ON OUTCOME IN THE ELDERLY

There is a considerable debate on the impact of anesthetic technique on mortality and morbidity in the elderly patient. This controversy is covered in Chap. 21. Suffice it to say that comparable outcome statistics exist between general and regional anesthetic techniques. Factors such as the type of surgery and comorbid state of the patient not only influence the ultimate outcome of the procedure but also the choice of anesthetic technique. In addition, intraoperative hemodynamic events and choice of anesthetic agents as a result of choice of anesthetic technique may influence outcome in the elderly. In a study examining predictive factors for adverse postoperative events in patients 80 years and older, Liu et al. found that vasopressor use during surgery increased the odds of death eight times (CI 1.4–50.8, P value 0.02) and the incidence of a postoperative pulmonary event 12 times (CI 2.5–63, P value 0.002).[23] Further studies suggest that factors such as the duration of the anesthetic and intraoperative tachycardia are predictive of adverse postoperative outcomes.[60,64,85] When examining the effects of general and regional anesthesia on outcome, it must be kept in mind that because of anatomic and physiologic changes associated with aging, the response by the elderly patient to the applied anesthetic can influence outcome. The function of both the sympathetic and parasympathetic nervous systems decrease with age. This impairment may become evident as pronounced hypotension in response to the vasodilator effects of the inhalation agent or the regional technique.[86] Carpenter et al. determined that patients over 40 years of age were 2.5 times more likely to develop hypotension during spinal anesthesia.[87] Although the study was not performed exclusively in the elderly population, it is likely that because of the aging process the effects will be augmented in this population. Another effect of the changes in autonomic function in the elderly is impaired thermoregulation. Concomitant illnesses, such as hypothyroidism and diabetes, augment the response to decreased thermoregulation. Patients who experience mild reductions in core body temperature are three times as likely to have a perioperative cardiac event.[88,89] The geriatric population is noted to have decreased ability to vasoconstrict to inhalation agents, thereby allowing increased cooling during anesthesia.[90] Conversely, ability to rewarm is impaired in the elderly. Decreased requirements for intravenous and inhalation agents in the elderly must be kept in mind during anesthetic management.

AGE AND SURGICAL PROCEDURES

Overall operative mortality increases with advanced age, but outcome varies widely based on the type, location, and magnitude of the surgical procedure. Several risk classification systems consider the type of surgical procedure as a major determinant of risk and outcome. Copeland, the developer of the POSSUM risk assessment model, stratified type of surgery into minor, intermediate, and major magnitude.[61,62] The ACC/AHA guidelines incorporate the surgical procedure in its risk stratification.[46,44] In addition to considering age greater than 70 years as a risk parameter, the Goldman risk index (Table 11-5) ascribes a greater scoring to surgeries in the abdomen and thorax.[38] Arozullah et al. established that the procedures associated with the greatest likelihood of postoperative pulmonary complications were abdominal aneurysm repair, thoracic, and upper abdominal surgeries, all of which are regarded as high risk or major procedures.[52] Because a large majority of the diseases requiring surgical intervention present in the later years, many of the highly invasive procedures, such as cancer resections and major cardiovascular procedures, are performed primarily on the elderly. Fortunately, the mortality and morbidity has improved for some surgical procedures such as CABG and CEA. However, for certain cancer surgeries, no significant changes have occurred in the mortality and morbidity.[91] Just as the risk of the surgery is based on the magnitude and severity, the outcome varies according to the procedure as well. This section explores the mortality and morbidity in the elderly with respect to common surgeries performed in this population.

▶ Ambulatory surgery

The most common ambulatory surgeries performed on patients aged 65 and older are extraction of the lens (1,977,000), insertion of prosthetic lens (1,501,000), endoscopy of the large intestine (8,22,000), and endoscopy of the small intestine (6,14,000) (Advance Data 300). Severe or life-threatening adverse outcomes such as MI or cardiac arrest are rare in the ambulatory surgery setting and are not ideal choices for assessing the quality of ambulatory surgery. A more appropriate outcome measure in the ambulatory surgery setting is the length of postoperative stay. Increasing age, type, and duration of surgery were noted to be significant predictors of increased postoperative stay.[92] In a study examining the adverse events in ambulatory surgery, the most common intraoperative adverse events contributing to increased length of stay are hypertension and dysrhythmia, while postoperative nausea and vomiting (PONV) were the most common postoperative events causing increased length of stay. The frequency of intraoperative events increased linearly with age, while the frequency of postoperative events showed a decreasing tendency with increasing age. Additionally, two medical conditions, CHF and smoking status were associated with length of stay. Patients with CHF had the highest incidence of intraoperative events. The study compared outcomes between elderly and younger patients, and their findings suggest that the elderly have a higher incidence of any intraoperative event and intraoperative cardiac events when compared to younger subjects. The elderly subjects were noted to have a lower incidence of PONV and dizziness.

Cataract surgery is the most commonly performed operation in elderly people in developed countries. Nearly 2 million cataract extractions were performed in 2003 almost entirely on an outpatient setting. Morbidity and mortality associated with cataract surgery is extremely low, approximately 0.10%. However, patients who present for cataract procedures tend to have multiple comorbidities. Anesthesia management strategies for cataract surgery are associated with adverse intraoperative medical events. Katz et al. examined the outcome in patients who received local anesthesia topically or by injection with or without intravenous sedative—hypnotics, opioids, or Benedryl.[93] Overall, there was no difference observed in the prevalence of intraoperative events between topical and injection local anesthesia without sedatives. There was a significant increase in adverse events such as hypertension, hypotension, angina, and bradycardia with the use of intravenous sedatives when used in conjunction with topical or injection local anesthesia. The greatest increase occurred with the combination of opiates and sedatives.[93] Despite the increase in medical events, the incidence of medical problems remained low, 1.95% and 1.23% for intraoperative and postoperative complications, respectively.

▶ Hip and knee replacements

The total number of hip and knee replacements performed in 2003 was 220,000 and 418,000, respectively. Of these, the number of patients 65 years and older undergoing hip and knee arthroplasty was 129,000 or 59% and 255,000 or 61%, respectively (Advance Data 359). Information from the National Discharge Survey, the principal source for data from nonfederal, short stay hospitals, estimates that $9.9 billion were spent on hip and knee replacement surgery in 2000. Thirty-day mortality and morbidity, length of stay, and rate of revision measure outcome parameters for these procedures. Outcome statistics for hip fractures are studied as far as 2 years past the injury and subsequent repair because many of the surviving hip patients experience reduced mobility and lose their ability to function. As many as 45% of those in community settings at the time of their fracture are discharged to institutions after hip fracture repair, and 15–25% remain institutionalized for a year postfracture.[94]

In a study examining preoperative risks and outcome of patients undergoing hip and knee repair in VA patients, Weaver et al. concluded that age and coexistent disease were associated with serious complications including pulmonary embolism, MI, and stroke.[95] The mortality rate for 6876 patients undergoing total hip replacement was approximately 1%, and the most frequent complications were urinary tract infection, pneumonia, and deep venous thrombosis. Thirty-eight percent of the readmission complications were caused by mechanical complications of the internal device and graft, while 12% of the readmissions were due to infection of the internal joint prosthesis. Weaver's study also examined the mortality rate in 11,591 total knee patients and reported an extremely low mortality rate of <0.5%. Approximately 1% of the patients were readmitted in the year following surgery and the majority of readmissions were due to infections (43%) and mechanical complications (18%).[95] Similar mortality and morbidity rates were found in a study by Millar who reported mortality rates for hip and knee replacements of 1.5% and 0.5%, respectively.[96] Millar's study found that the length of stay increased with increasing age. The average length of stay for 65–69 year olds undergoing hip replacement was 9.2 days, while for patients 85 and older, the stay nearly doubled to 17.2 days. For knee replacements, 65–69 year olds stayed on average 8.2 days, while patients aged 85 and older had a length of stay 11.6 days.[96] Parvizi et al. conducted a review of 22,540 total knee arthroplasties between 1969 and 1997 to identify patients who died within 30 days.[97] The overall mortality rate in this comprehensive study was 0.21%, that is, 47 of 22,540 patients. All deaths occurred in patients who received cemented implants, and no deaths occurred in patients who received an uncemented implant. Thirty-nine of the forty-seven patients were older than 70; the 30-day mortality rate for this age group was 0.54%. More than 90% of the patients who died had a history of cardiopulmonary disease. Three of the deaths occurred intraoperatively during cementing of the tibial component and following deflation of the tourniquet. The study also examined the outcome statistics from revision knee surgery and discovered that the mortality rate was significantly lower than primary knee replacement. Despite the fact that revision knee procedures are longer and may involve greater blood loss, only 4 of the 47 patients died within 30 days for a mortality rate of 0.09% in this study. Parvizi postulates that the risk is higher in primary knee arthroplasty due to the effects of embolization of fat and marrow contents from a previously inviolate medullary canal.[97]

Although the outcome from unilateral knee replacement has a mortality of <0.5%, increased perioperative morbidity and mortality occur during simultaneous bilateral knee replacement, particularly early postoperative death. Bilateral knee replacement ideally has the advantage of only one operative visit, shorter duration of hospitalization, which may result in decreased overall health costs. However, the costs may be offset by need for intensive care admission, increased need for homologous blood transfusion, and subsequent transfer to a rehabilitation center.[98] Several studies have examined outcome following bilateral knee replacement and report that the risk of early postoperative death is increased nearly threefold.[98] When compared with unilateral knee replacement, there is an increased risk of postoperative cardiac events (3.3-fold), gastrointestinal bleeding (1.6-fold), thromboembolic events (1.4-fold), and cerebrovascular accident (CVA) or confusion (1.3-fold) for patients undergoing simultaneous bilateral knee replacement. The study performed by Parvizi which studied outcome for unilateral, revision, and bilateral knee procedures determined that the mortality rate for bilateral knee procedures was significantly higher than unilateral procedures, 0.49% versus 0.19%.[97] Oakes and Hanssen report

that the relative risk of bilateral simultaneous replacement as compared to unilateral knee replacement increases with advanced age.[98] According to their study, there have been few studies to specifically define an absolute age or set of medical comorbidities that suggest that a patient may be at higher risk of perioperative morbidity with bilateral knee replacement. Several studies suggest an age of 70–75 years to minimize risk of adverse events. Pavone et al. conducted a study on simultaneous or one-stage bilateral knee replacements on patients with an average age of 66 years.[99] With respect to comorbidites, 86% had one or more preoperative comorbidities: 30% had one comorbid state, 30% had two comorbid states, 18% with three, 7% with four, and 1% with five. All patients were done with an epidural anesthetic to reduce the risk of thrombosis. The complications were divided into major and minor based on severity and impact on the overall hospital stay; the most frequent major complication was deep venous thrombosis, which occurred in 13% of the patients. Cardiac complications and atrial fibrillation was present in 5.6% and 4.6% of the patients, respectively; 80.4% of the patients were discharged to a rehabilitation facility. No perioperative deaths or MIs were recorded in this study. There were no statistically significant associations between the rate of major complications and variables such as age and number of comorbid states. Patients that were ASA class I had a tendency to have less complications in comparison to patients that were class II or III. Patients younger than 60 years had fewer complications than patients aged 75 years and older. Lynch et al. performed a study specifically looking at complications after concomitant cemented bilateral knee replacements in patients aged 80 and older, and compared their findings to age-matched subjects who underwent cemented unilateral knee replacements.[100] Their paired analysis showed that CHF and delirium occurred more frequently in the bilateral group. The study also compared the overall complication rate with younger patients undergoing the same procedure and determined that the overall complication rate was higher when compared to younger patients.[100]

Several recommendations have been made to improve outcome. The replacements should be done sequentially during the same anesthetic, rather than with simultaneous surgical teams. Inflations of both tourniquets at the same time may increase afterload for the left ventricle, and expose the patient to an increase in procoagulants following tourniquet deflation.[99] Oakes and Hanssen advocated the use of intraoperative pulmonary artery catheter to monitor pulmonary vascular resistance (PVR), which may correlate with the presence of fatty emboli.[98] Additionally, the use of an epidural anesthetic may decrease the risk of postoperative deep venous thrombosis (Table 11-10).

Mortality in elderly patients following hip fracture repair is much higher compared with elective hip replacement. Lawrence et al. studied the medical outcomes and complications after hip fracture repair and discovered that the 30-day mortality for patients without

Table 11-10

Factors Associated with Increased Mortality after Knee Arthroplasty

Age greater than 70 years

Primary arthroplasty

Use of cement

Preexisting cardiopulmonary disease

Simultaneous bilateral total knee arthroplasty

Source: Adapted from Ref. 97.

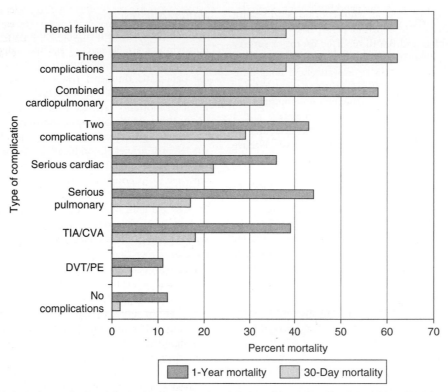

FIGURE 11-6 The relationship between complications following hip fracture repair and 30-day and 1-year mortality. *(Adapted from Ref. 2.)*

complications was 1.7%.[20] Cardiac and pulmonary complications occurred in 8% and 4% of the patients, respectively. The overall inpatient mortality was 3.3%. The 30-day and 1-year mortality increased based on the type and number of complications. Patients with two complications had 30-day mortality rates of 29% and 1-year mortality of 43%. Patients with renal failure or three or more complications had the highest mortality, 38% and 62% at 30 days and 1 year, respectively.[20] (Fig. 11-6).

▶ Laparascopic cholecystectomy

Gallstone disease increases with advancing age. Because the elderly often present with atypical symptoms making diagnosis more difficult and delayed, elderly patients are more likely than younger patients to present with complicated cholelithiasis. Since its beginning in 1988, laparascopic cholecystecomy (LC) has become one of the most common abdominal surgeries performed in the elderly. A total of 154,000 procedures were performed in this age group in 2003. The complication rate and length of stay from LC are significantly lower than with open cholecystectomy where mortality rates range from 0.5% to 10%. Several studies examining the outcome following LC in the elderly have been performed.[101–105] Most studies report a higher conversion rate in the elderly to open cholecystectomy due to acute cholecystitis, or the presence of chronic inflammation and adhesions. Brunt et al. reported an overall conversion rate to open procedures in elderly patients as 5.7%, as compared to a 2% conversion rate in patients younger than 65.[103] In patients 80 and older, there was a conversion rate of 16%. Despite a longer hospital stay and higher conversion rate to open cholecystectomy in the elderly, the reduction in morbidity and mortality in LC as compared to open is encouraging. The average complication rate for LC is 15% versus an average of 26% for open.[103] The overall mortality rate for LC is 1.8%, while the open procedure averages an overall mortality

rate of 4.4%.[102] A review of several studies reveals that the complication rate often exceeds 20% in cases where the presentation is acute cholecystitis or cholelithiasis.[102,104,105] Complications are usually graded with increasing severity from 1 to 4; the most common being grade 1 presentations, are urinary retention, umbilical wound infection, and delirium, while grade 2 complications involved hemorrhage, postsite hernias and retained common bile stones, and bile leak. Both grade 1 and 2 complications were more common in the elderly, particularly in the patients 80 years and older.[103,105]

▶ Major abdominal surgery

Survival following major abdominal surgery in the elderly depends on age, health status, and characteristics of the surgery, including the location and whether the procedure is elective or emergent. Overall 30-day mortality rates with emergency abdominal procedures can be as high as 29%, and one-third of the patients experience complications, whereas elective abdominal operations in the elderly have mortality rates around 7.5% (Table 11-11).[106] Similar

Table 11-11
Factors That Influence Surgical Mortality of the Acute Abdomen in the Elderly
Age greater than 80 years
Associated disease
ASA class
Colorectal surgery
Malignant disease
Severity of surgical condition

findings were reported by Zerbib et al. who reported perioperative mortality in octogenarians of 26.6% with a perioperative complication rate of 29.5%.[107] Abbas and Booth reported on major surgery in patients 80 and older; their findings show a higher mortality for ASA IV and V patients, 46% and 33%, respectively.[106] Long-term survival was significantly affected by the presence of comorbidities. Median survival for the ASA II and III patients was 48 months and 23 months; ASA IV and V patients had survived only 7 and 3 months following emergency surgery. Despite the discouraging mortality rates for elderly patients on an emergent basis, elective abdominal surgeries can have favorable outcomes in this age group.

Hepatic resection

The operative mortality for patients undergoing hepatic resection increases incrementally with age.[108] The overall mortality for subsegmental resection is 1.4%. The mortality increases to 4.4% for major resection. When the outcome is examined by age, the operative mortality rate increased to more than 10% for patients 65 years and older as compared to 3.6% in patients aged 55–64 and 0.7% in patients 55 years and younger. If an extended right hepatic lobectomy is performed, the operative mortality can increase to more than 30% in patients aged 65 and older. Most of the deaths are noted to occur from hepatic insufficiency.[108]

Gastrectomy

Several features with regard to gastric cancer surgery deserve mention; incidence and mortality rates rise incrementally with age and the overall mortality rate (8.6%) has changed little over time.[42,91] Similarly, Marrelli et al. report an in-house mortality rate of 8.4% and an overall mortality rate of 11.6% in Italians.[80] The overall morbidity rate was 30.4% with the most common complications due to cardiac, bleeding, or prolonged ileus. Otani et al. who studied gastric carcinoma in octogenarians list delirium, respiratory dysfunction, and cardiac dysfunction as the three most common postoperative complications.[109]

Colorectal surgery

Age is recognized as the most significant risk factor for the development of colorectal cancer. Sixty percent of the patients requiring surgical intervention for colon cancer are 70 years and older. One of the most comprehensive studies examining outcomes in elderly patients undergoing colorectal surgery used data from 28 independent studies, which included 34,194 patients from Great Britain, Ireland, and the United States. The study shows that there was a significant trend toward increasing rates of emergent versus elective surgery with advancing age, and older patients tend to present with more advanced disease. The review also demonstrated that as age increased, the incidence of respiratory, cardiovascular, cerebrovascular, and thromboembolic complications increased. Just as in the study by Finlayson and Birkmeyer, the mortality rate for colorectal surgery increased with advanced age with similar mortality rates reported for both studies.[42]

Mortality rates vary according to the location of the colon surgery. In a study done by Tekkis et al., which examined the operative mortality in colorectal cancer, the highest 30-day mortality rates were reported for palliative bypass, palliative stoma, and Hartmann's pouch with observed mortality rates of 26.7%, 22.9%, and 15.7%, respectively.[110] Considerably lower 30-day mortality rates ranging from 4.8% to 8.5% were reported for the curative procedures involving hemicolectomy, anterior, and anterior posterior resection.[110]

Pancreatic resection

Approximately three-quarters of the patients with pancreatic adenocarcinoma are 60 years of age and older, and as the population increases, an increasing number of elderly patients are presenting for pancreatic duodenal resection. The outcome statistics have improved dramatically from the 1960s and 1970s when most centers reported mortality rates for pancreaticoduodenctomy in the range of 20–40%, with postoperative morbidity as high as 60%. Currently, the mortality for patients aged 70 and older ranges from 4% to 9%.[42,111] DiCarlo et al. conducted a study on pancreatic resection in the elderly and noted that the resection rate of the cancer decreased with age.[111] Although not statistically significant, patients 80 years and older had a lower resection rate 11% as compared to 32% in younger patients. In this particular study, elderly patients also had a higher rate of hemorrhagic events and reoperation. Sohn et al. presented findings from a retrospective study over a 10-year period on pancreatic resection in patients above 80 years and compared their results with patients younger than 80 years.[112] There was a statistically significant difference in the incidence of benign disease in the younger subset (20%) when compared to the older group (7%). Although the mortality rate for the older group was higher (4.3%) as compared to the younger group (1.6%), these differences were not significant. However, the incidence of perioperative complications for the two groups, 57% in older group versus 41% in younger group, was different. The older patients had a higher incidence of delayed gastric emptying, pancreatic fistula formation, and wound infection. Additionally, the older group had significantly longer length of hospital stay. Multiple studies have shown that the elderly patient can successfully undergo pancreatic cancer resection.

Long-term survival in this operation has also been examined. Over 70% of the patients 80 years and greater survive 1 year following surgery, but only 20% survive 5 years postsurgery. Patients younger than 80 years have better survival rates of 81% and 45% at the same time intervals.

▶ Cardiac surgery

The data presented in the National Hospital Discharge Survey (NHDS) for 2003 estimates that 467,000 CABGs were performed in that year. Of that number, 257,000 or 55% were performed on patients 65 years and older. An almost equal percentage of coronary stents and ballon angioplasty procedures were done in this age group (Table 11-12).

Improvements in bypass techniques and perioperative care have resulted in reductions in mortality and morbidity. Studies of CABG procedures indicate that operative mortality fell at least 20% between 1980 and the mid-1990s.[91] Goodney et al. studied operative mortality in 14 high-risk cardiovascular procedures in Medicare

Table 11-12			
2003 National Hospital Discharge Survey, Advance Data 359			
Procedure	Total Number Performed	Number Performed in 65 and Older	%
CABG	467,000	257,000	55
Coronary stents	574,000	296,000	52
Angioplasty	664,000	346,000	52

Table 11-13

Thirty-Day Operative Mortality by Age Group for Selected Cardiovascular Procedures (Results Reported in Percent)

Age	CABG + SVGel	CABG + SVGem	CABG + LIMAel	CABG + LIMAem	AVR	MVR	AVR + MVR	CABG + AVR	CABG + MVR	CABG + AVR + MVR
60–69	2.5	8.3	2.1	5.4	2.5	7	14.9	7.3	19.2	25
70–79	5.2	17.5	3.4	13	7.3	11.2	19.4	11.4	23.3	0
>80	8.2	24.1	2.3	0	5.7	16.7	0	9.7	33.3	0

Note: el = elective, em = emergency.
Source: Adapted from Ref. 117.

patients 65 and older for a 5-year period from 1994 to 1999.[91] The study showed declines in mortality for all six cardiovascular procedures. Significant declines were shown in three of the procedures, namely CABG, carotid endarterectomy (CEA), and mitral valve replacement (MVR). Because of those declines, patients of advanced age, even nonagenarians and centenarians are presenting for cardiac surgery. Survival analysis extends beyond the initial operative experience. Studies are now focusing on functional outcome and long-term survival, particularly 1, 5, and 20 years postsurgery.[113,114]

Even in light of the favorable statistics, Weintraub et al. found that age was the most powerful contributor to decreased survival, and that mortality rates rose with increasing age.[115] The study determined that for each decade of life, the hazard ratio increased by 1.46 as a correlate of mortality. In addition to age, Fruitman et al. determined that renal failure and emergent procedure were significant risk factors for early death.[116]

The earlier studies describing CABG date back to 1968. The initial procedures described saphenous vein autograft (SVG) and since that time, the use of the left internal mammary artery (LIMA) has been introduced with improvements in overall outcome. Octogenarians who had CABG with LIMA had significantly lower operative mortality than similar age groups having elective CABG with vein graft. Two- and five-year survival rates were also more favorable for the CABG with LIMA group.[117] Age influences outcome for off-bypass or beating heart procedures and valve replacements.[117,118] Stamou et al. compared the in-house mortality for off-bypass in octogenarians and patients who were younger.[118] The mortality rate increased with age. The mortality rate for sexagenarians was 0.3%, septuagenarians 3%, and octogenarians 6%.

Outcome in valve replacement is influenced by age and the type of cardiac procedure performed. Craver examined the outcome in the elderly for CABG, isolated valve, and CABG plus valve (Table 11-13).[117] Although the findings were not all significant, they illustrate an age-related increase in mortality based on the severity of the cardiac procedure, particularly the procedures involving the mitral valve or double valve procedures. Causes of death include heart failure, multisystem organ failure, stroke, MI, and pneumonia. Atrial fibrillation and delirium are common postoperative complications, both of which have been shown to be age-dependent.

▶ Thoracotomy for esophagectomy and lung resection

Goodney et al. determined that esophagectomy and thoracotomy for malignant tumor were two cancer surgeries that did not experience a decrease in mortality over recent years.[91] The study also concluded that both surgeries continue to have some of the highest mortality rates (Table 11-14). Adam et al. studied a small group of octogenarians who had undergone esophagectomy for cancer.[119] The in-house mortality was 16%, and the mortality rate for elective surgery was 10.7%. These findings are similar to the rates reported by Finlayson et al. who reported an overall mortality rate for ages 65–99 of 13.6%.[42]

The incidence of postoperative complications following esophagectomy is increased in the elderly.[119] The risk of anastomotic leak is approximately five times greater in patients 70 years and older, and those who experience this complication have an increased risk of in-house mortality.[119] Bonavina et al. studied 900 geriatric patients who had undergone esophagectomy and determined outcome for patients less than 65 and patients older than 65.[120] Although the study showed no difference in mortality between the two age groups, there was not a higher incidence of cardiovascular complications in the older subset. In addition, esophagectomy patients showed a mortality rate of 1.8% and an overall morbidity rate of 26%.[120] Although the complication rate is somewhat age-dependent, 5-year survival rates, which range from 17% to 35%, are no different in the younger versus older patients.[119,120] Laparoscopic-assisted surgical approaches to esophageal carcinoma are now being performed by primarily two techniques: right thoracotomy and left cervicotomy with transmediastinal endosection. Although the data are limited due to small sample size, the results are encouraging; no hospital deaths occurred. The reported morbidity rate is 20% and 30% for thoracotomy and cervicotomy patients, respectively.[120] This surgical approach demonstrates the potential for reducing mortality in the geriatric patient.

In 2003, a large percentage of the deaths from lung cancer occurred in the geriatric population; 20% alone occurred in patients 80 years and older. As the elderly population increases, more candidates of advanced age will present for lung resection. Because earlier

Table 11-14

Cancer Surgeries with the Highest Overall Mortality

Surgery	Overall Mortality
Gastrectomy	8.6%
Pancreatic resection	9.35%
Esophagectomy	13.6%
Thoracotomy	13.7%

mortality and morbidity rates approached 20% and 50%, respectively, there has been considerable reluctance to offer lung resection surgery to elderly candidates. Older patients are only one-third as likely to undergo resection as younger patients.[121]

Outcomes of lung resection are age dependent. Earlier studies (1983) by Ginsberg et al. show an 8.1% mortality rate for octogenarians as compared to 1.6% for patients less than 65 years.[122] A later study by Finlayson examining outcomes in 1.2 million patients in the Medicare system supports this finding.[42] Finlayson's study results are from patients having had pneumonectomy, not lobectomy or wedge resection. Additionally, the data from the 85–99-year-old group had a small sample size. Data from this age group is limited because in the past, age greater than 80 years was a relative contraindication to surgery. Outcome analysis is noted to be more favorable if lobectomy is performed.[123] Brock et al. reported their findings from a retrospective study spanning 22 years, which examined the surgical outcome in patients 80 years and older.[123] Lobectomies were performed 69% of the time followed by wedge resections 16% and segmentectomy 7.5%. All surgeries were elective. The 30-day mortality rate was 8.8%, and 44% of the patients experienced one or more complications primarily cardiopulmonary in nature. Nearly three-quarters of the patients were discharged to home without need for rehabilitation services. Based on previous studies, lobectomy has nearly half the mortality for subjects of similar age.

Just as endoscopic surgery for esophageal cancer is noted to decrease mortality, the same holds true for video-assisted thoracic surgery (VATS), which has been shown to produce less pain and interruption of pulmonary function. Koren et al. conducted a study of thoracic surgery in octogenarians and reported a mortality rate of 2% and a morbidity rate of 5.5% for major complications such as bleeding and air leaks.[124] A minor complication rate of 12% involving arrhythmias and minor air leaks occurred. The average length of stay was noted to be 2.6 days, whereas patients undergoing thoracotomy generally stay 8–14 days.

▶ Major vascular procedures

Carotid endarterectomy

Stroke is the second leading cause of death worldwide, and the risk of stroke appears to increase with age. CEA was introduced in the 1950s for the prophylaxis of stroke.[125,126] Although CEA had been shown to be of clear benefit in selected patients, elderly patients with occlusive carotid artery disease were often excluded out of fear of increased rates of complications and decreased long-term benefit. Schneider et al. compared the outcomes of octogenarians and younger patients undergoing CEA and reported that the older group was more likely to have anatomically critical disease, that is, 80–99% stenosis.[125] Additionally, the older group was more likely to have CHF. The study revealed that the number of octogenarians undergoing CEA is increasing over time, and the perioperative length of stay is decreasing in this age group. The study also revealed that the perioperative morbidity and mortality rates after CEA were indistinguishable between the octogenarians and younger group, less than 2%, despite the fact that three-fourths of the older patients had symptomatic disease and had a higher degree of stenosis. Kazmers et al. conducted a similar but more comprehensive study in 9152 patients.[127] The study examined the outcome following carotid surgery in octogenarians and younger patients. Illness severity, MI, and surgical complications of the central nervous system (CNS) were associated with a greater likelihood of mortality following the procedure.

The in-hospital mortality rate for patients less than 80 years was 1.0%, while in patients 80 years and older it was 3.0%. Stroke mortality rate after CEA in this study was 3.68% in octogenarians and 1.68% for younger patients. The most common complication in this study was MI not stroke. A higher percentage of patients with a postoperative MI died (17.6%, p <0.0001) versus patients with a postoperative stroke (10.3%, p <0.0001). Finlayson et al. reported mortality rates of 1.0–2.2% in the elderly population ranging from 65 to 99 years.[42] Survival after CEA in the elderly population is encouraging, reported at 90% at 1 year, 76% at 2 years, and 62% after 3 years.[127]

Abdominal aortic aneurysms

NHDS estimated that over 150,000 aneurysm cases were diagnosed in U.S. hospitals in 1994 and over 50,000 were treated surgically. Of all the aneurysm surgeries, 75% were performed on either ruptured or nonruptured abdominal aneurysms.[128] Because of age-related alterations in the vessel wall involving a reduction in the synthesis of elastin, abdominal aortic aneurysm (AAA) is primarily a disease of old age.[129–131] Surgical mortality rates vary from 1.2% for lower extremity aneurysm repair to 68–80% for ruptured AAA. The overall mortality rate for nonruptured AAA is approximately 8.4%.[128,129,132,133] In-house mortality for ruptured thoracic aneurysms is over 50%; nonruptured thoracic aneurysm repair has an overall mortality of 23%. Length of stay and mortality increase as age increases.[42,133,134]

Endovascular stent graft repair (ESG) or endovascular aneurysm repair (EVAR) has been performed in the United States since 1992 and is a less invasive alternative to open repair. The success of the procedure is defined as freedom from endoleaks, which is blood flow outside the lumen of the graft primarily caused by inadequate proximal or distal fixation (type I), retrograde flow from the aneurysm sac (type II), or tears within the graft (type III). The absence of graft infection or thrombosis, aneurysm rupture, conversion to open procedure, or lack of graft migration is also a measure of success.[135] Marin et al. examined the results of an ESG study spanning over 10 years involving repair of aortic and thoracic aneurysms and reported a 2.3% perioperative mortality rate.[135] Major adverse events such as cardiac complications following ESG repair were less than 4%. Type I or III endoleaks occurred in 6.9% and 15% of aortic and thoracic graft repairs, respectively; type II endoleaks, which may be less clinically significant, occurred in 21% and 10% of abdominal and thoracic procedures, respectively. Minor et al. who studied EVAR in octogenarians[136] reported similar findings. Thirty-day mortality was 3.3% and endoleaks were common. The study also concluded that this technique is associated with lower intraoperative blood loss and shorter length of hospital stay. Published results on a small number of endovascular procedures performed on hemodynamically stable, infrarenal ruptured aneurysms showed that there was no statistical difference between early mortality and morbidity, but hospital stay, intensive care unit (ICU) stay, estimated blood loss, and operative time were shorter in the EVAR group.[137]

▶ Neurosurgical procedures

Pathology requiring cranial surgery poses significant risks and potential long-term disability for all age groups. However, older age is an independent predictor of poor outcome after neurosurgery with respect to mortality, morbidity, and cognitive impairment.[138] According to a study done by Buczko on cranial surgery among Medicare beneficiaries, the most common diagnoses for elderly neurosurgery patients are subdural hemorrhage (15.3%), intracerebral

Table 11-15

Risk Factors for Death Following Subarachnoid Hemorrhage

Increased age

Position of the aneurysm

Clinical grade on admission

Arterial hypertension

Thickness of clot on CT scan

Associated diseases

Source: Criteria derived from Kassel NF, Torner JC, Haley EC. The International Cooperative Study on the Timing of Aneurysm Surgery, Part I: Overall management results. *J Neurosurg.* 1990;73:18–36.

hemorrhage (7.6%), benign neoplasm of the brain (7.5%), secondary neoplasm of the brain and spinal cord (6.8%), and subarachnoid hemorrhage (SAH) (5.8%).[139] The two largest groups of cranial surgery patients are 70–74 years and 75–79 years comprising 22.3% and 20.5% of the surgeries, respectively.[139] More than 40% of the admissions were emergent, 22.6% urgent, and 37% elective. A nearly equal number of patients are discharged to postacute care facilities (44.6%) and home (42.3%), while the remainder require inpatient facilities or home health care. The mortality rate for all elderly age groups is 10.9%.

Vogel et al. reviewed intracerebral aneurysms in the geriatric group.[138] According to the study, the incidence of SAH secondary to intracranial aneurysm rupture increases up to 50–70 years, followed by a decline thereafter. The study explored outcomes in ruptured aneurysms and reported a 25–50% mortality rate, while as many as 20% remain severely disabled. Table 11-15 lists the risk factors for death after SAH. For both ruptured and unruptured aneurysms, surgical clipping or endovascular coiling are the treatment modalities. Timing of selective embolization of ruptured aneurysm depends on the Hunt and Hess (HH) grade on admission. According to a study by Lubicz et al., which examined endovascular treatment of ruptured aneurysms in the elderly, patients with a HH grade of I–III may be considered for endovascular occlusion at an early stage; HH grade of IV or V should be delayed.[140] The study reported a mortality rate of 20.5% and a good outcome in 59% of the patients.[140] Sedat et al. compared the outcomes of patients greater than 65 years versus younger subjects for outcome following endovascular treatment for aneurysm; elderly patients had a higher mortality of 23% versus 14% for the younger group.[141] Overall, 84% of the elderly patients with a higher clinical grade on admission had unfavorable outcomes with a 42% mortality rate as opposed to 60% and 33% for the younger group, respectively. A higher incidence of thromboembolic events occurred in the older group, and fewer patients had a return to normal life in the elderly group. The study concluded that although endovascular treatment appears to be effective in preventing recurrent aneurysmal bleeding, patients older than 65 years presented more risks than the younger population.

SURGEON AND HOSPITAL VOLUME

Although there is no evidence to suggest that age affects the relationship between surgical volume and outcome, the elderly undergo many of the high-risk cardiovascular and cancer surgeries, and mortality decreases as the surgical volume increases.[142] Birkmeyer et al. cite number of cases and technical skill of the surgeon as well as the use of specific intraoperative processes as important determinants of outcome.[142] Hospital volume is dependent on surgical volume but is also influenced by hospital-based services such as ICU, respiratory and nursing care. Surgeon and hospital volume vary according to the procedure, and volume is a predictor of outcome for some but not all surgical procedures. Katz et al. examined the association between hospital and surgeon procedure volume and outcome for total knee replacement (TKR).[143] The study reported that the mortality risk for patients who had TKR in hospitals in which 25 or more procedures had been performed was 30% lower than for patients who had the procedure in hospitals in which between 1 and 25 procedures were done. Additionally, the risk of pneumonia and deep infection declined steadily with hospital volume. Higher case volumes and lower mortality rates are also observed in craniotomy for aneurysm clipping, CABG, pancreatic resection, and esophagectomy.[142–145] High-risk procedures such as pneumonectomy and esophagectomy, requiring longer hospital stay and specialized services, are influenced by both surgeon and hospital volume.

CONCLUSION

The influence of advanced age on risk and outcome is unquestionably multifactorial with several variables weighing more significantly than others (Table 11-16). Advanced age, particularly over 70 years, has been shown to be an independent predictor of poor outcome, namely because as age increases, the number of comorbid states is likely to increase. The nature and magnitude of the surgery, whether it is emergent or high risk, is a determinant of outcome and based on the age of the patient and surgery, mortality and morbidity have been shown to increase (Fig. 11-7).

Table 11-16

Summary of Risk Factors That Influence Outcome in the Elderly

Parameter	Predictors of Poor Outcome
ASA	III, IV
Age	>70 years
Cardiac	S3 gallop, recent MI, >5 PVCs before surgery, rhythm other than sinus, critical aortic stenosis, unstable angina
Pulmonary	Intraoperative NG tube, COPD, FEV <1 L, pulmonary edema within 1 week of surgery
Neurological	Impaired preoperative cognitive state, high risk surgery
Specific Activity Scale	Class III, IV
Comorbid states	COPD, CAD, diabetes, AF
Laboratory findings	Hypoalbuminemia
Surgery	Emergency, abdominal, intrathoracic, magnitude, and duration

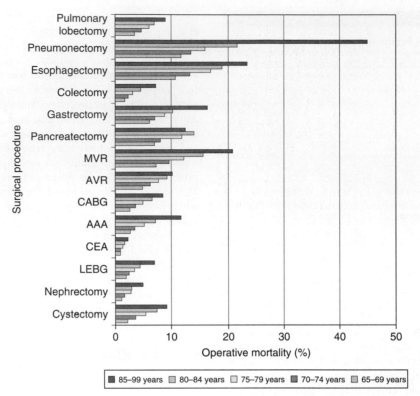

FIGURE 11-7 Age-specific 30-day mortality for various surgical procedures. MVR = mitral valve replacement; AVR = aortic valve replacement; CABG = coronary artery bypass graft; AAA = abdominal aortic aneurysm; CEA = carotid endarterectomy; LEBG = lower extremity bypass graft. *(Adapted from Ref. 42.)*

KEY POINTS

▶ Nearly all of the risk assessment models consider advanced age as an independent risk factor for adverse perioperative outcome.

▶ The ASA classification and Goldman cardiac risk index and subsequent modifications are widely used measures for risk assessment.

▶ The Charlson comorbidity index is used widely in the development of risk models and clinical outcome studies and demonstrates that the number and severity of comorbidities as well as advanced age contribute to mortality.

▶ Complications and mortality rates increase with ASA III and IV, SAS III, and higher Charlson comorbidity scores.

▶ The POSSUM is not used widely in the United States but provides helpful clinical parameters for consideration in risk assessment.

▶ Knowledge and familiarization with the parameters used for each of the risk models will allow practical risk stratification in the clinical setting, which should improve outcome.

▶ Outcome studies indicate that heart failure patients have a higher morbidity and mortality when compared to patients with CAD.

▶ Advanced age is the one of the strongest preoperative predictors for the development of atrial fibrillation.

▶ The morbidity and mortality for elderly patients with COPD is approximately 25% and 7%, respectively.

▶ Although many risk indices consider abnormal laboratory values as a part of their scoring design, routine laboratory testing and preoperative ECGs and echocardiogram have limited value in predicting postoperative outcomes in the elderly.

▶ The preoperative serum albumin level is a strong predictor of mortality and morbidity because it reflects the general health and nutrition of the patient.

▶ Comparable outcome statistics exist between general and regional anesthetic techniques.

▶ The effects of the anesthetic agents and intraoperative conditions such as hypothermia can influence outcome in the elderly patient.

▶ Morbidity and mortality in the elderly is dependent on the type of surgery. Outcome statistics have improved over time with the exception of high-risk cancer surgery; however, newer endoscopic and endovascular surgical techniques decrease operative time, length of hospital stay, and complication rates.

KEY REFERENCES

▶ Richardson JD, Cocanour CS, Kern JA, et al. Perioperative risk assessment in elderly and high-risk patients. *J Am Coll Surg.* 2004;199:133–146.

▶ Hamel MB, Henderson WG, Khuri SF, Daley J. Surgical outcomes for patients aged 80 and older: morbidity and mortality from major noncardiac surgery. *J Am Geriatr Soc.* 2005;53:424–429.

▶ Polanczyk CA, Marcantonio E, Goldman L, et al. Impact of age on perioperative complications and length of stay in patients undergoing noncardiac surgery. *Ann Intern Med.* 2001;134:637–643.

▶ Finlayson EV, Goodney PP, Birkmeyer JD. Hospital volume and operative mortality in cancer surgery: a national study. *Arch Surg.* 2003;138:721–725; discussion 726.

► Goodney PP, Siewers AE, Stukel TA, et al. Is surgery getting safer? National trends in operative mortality. *J Am Coll Surg.* 2002;195: 219–227.

REFERENCES

1. Carp L. Basic principles in geriatric surgery. *Ann Surg.* 1946;123:1101.
2. Ellman R. *Surgical Care. A Practical Physiologic Guide.* New York: Appleton Century Crofts; 1951.
3. Ochsner A. Is risk of indicated operation too great in the elderly? *Geriatrics.* 1967;22:121–130.
4. Rosenthal RA, Kavic SM. Assessment and management of the geriatric patient. *Crit Care Med.* 2004;32:S92–S105.
5. Rosenthal RA. Surgical approaches to the surgical patient. In: Cassell C, Leipzig R, Cohen H, Larson E, Meier D, eds. *Geriatric Medicine: an Evidence-Based Approach.* 4th ed. New York: Springer-Verlag; 2003:239–257.
6. Brooks B. Surgery in patients of advanced age. *Ann Surg.* 1937;105:481.
7. Chase P, Mitchell K, Morley JE. In the steps of giants: the early geriatrics texts. *J Am Geriatr Soc.* 2000;48:89–94.
8. Nascher I. Geriatrics. *N Y Med J.* 1909;90:358.
9. Achenbaum WA. Commentary: Morley's "A brief history of geriatrics". *J Gerontol A Biol Sci Med Sci.* 2004;59:1153; discussion 1132–1152.
10. Clark JB. Prostatectomy at age of 110. *JAMA.* 1939;123:1101.
11. Thewlis MW. *The Care of the Aged (Geriatrics).* St. Louis: CV Mosby; 1946.
12. Stieglitz EJ. *Geriatric Medicine.* Philadelphia: WB Saunders; 1948.
13. Weber DM. Laparoscopic surgery: an excellent approach in elderly patients. *Arch Surg.* 2003;138:1083–1088.
14. Muravchick S. Preoperative assessment of the elderly patient. *Anesthesiol Clin N Am.* 2000;18:71–89, vi.
15 . Hosking MP, Warner MA, Lobdell CM, et al. Outcomes of surgery in patients 90 years of age and older. *JAMA.* 1989;261:1909–1915.
16. Beliveau MM, Multach M. Perioperative care for the elderly patient. *Med Clin N Am.* 2003;87:273–289.
17. Rigberg D, Cole M, Hiyama D, McFadden D. Surgery in the nineties. *Am Surg.* 2000;66:813–816.
18. Richardson JD, Cocanour CS, Kern JA, et al. Perioperative risk assessment in elderly and high-risk patients. *J Am Coll Surg.* 2004;199:133–146.
19. Hamel MB, Henderson WG, Khuri SF, Daley J. Surgical outcomes for patients aged 80 and older: morbidity and mortality from major non-cardiac surgery. *J Am Geriatr Soc.* 2005;53:424–429.
20. Lawrence VA, Hilsenbeck SG, Noveck H, et al. Medical complications and outcomes after hip fracture repair. *Arch Intern Med.* 2002;162: 2053–2057.
21. Fleischmann KE, Goldman L, Young B, Lee TH. Association between cardiac and noncardiac complications in patients undergoing noncardiac surgery: outcomes and effects on length of stay. *Am J Med.* 2003; 115:515–520.
22. John AD, Sieber FE. Age associated issues: geriatrics. *Anesthesiol Clin N Am.* 2004;22:45–58.
23. Liu LL, Leung JM. Predicting adverse postoperative outcomes in patients aged 80 years or older. *J Am Geriatr Soc.* 2000;48:405–412.
24. Liu LL, Wiener-Kronish JP. Perioperative anesthesia issues in the elderly. *Crit Care Clin.* 2003;19:641–656.
25. Pedersen T, Eliasen K, Henriksen E. A prospective study of mortality associated with anaesthesia and surgery: risk indicators of mortality in hospital. *Acta Anaesthesiol Scand.* 1990;34:176–182.
26. Polanczyk CA, Marcantonio E, Goldman L, et al. Impact of age on peri-operative complications and length of stay in patients undergoing non-cardiac surgery. *Ann Intern Med.* 2001;134:637–643.
27. Saklad M. Grading of patients for surgical procedures. *Anesthesiology.* 1941;2:281–284.
28. Menke H, Klein A, John KD, Junginger T. Predictive value of ASA classification for the assessment of the perioperative risk. *Int Surg.* 1993;78: 266–270.
29. Prause G, Offner A, Ratzenhofer-Komenda B, et al. Comparison of two preoperative indices to predict perioperative mortality in non-cardiac thoracic surgery. *Eur J Cardiothorac Surg.* 1997;11:670–675.
30. Prause G, Ratzenhofer-Comenda B, Pierer G, et al. Can ASA grade or Goldman's cardiac risk index predict peri-operative mortality? A study of 16,227 patients. *Anaesthesia.* 1997;52:203–206.
31. Wolters U, Wolf T, Stutzer H, Schroder T. ASA classification and perioperative variables as predictors of postoperative outcome. *Br J Anaesth.* 1996;77:217–222.
32. Jones HJ, de Cossart L. Risk scoring in surgical patients. *Br J Surg.* 1999; 86:149–157.
33. Hall JC, Hall JL. ASA status and age predict adverse events after abdominal surgery. *J Qual Clin Pract.* 1996;16:103–108.
34. Bufalari A, Ferri M, Cao P, et al. Surgical care in octogenarians. *Br J Surg.* 1996;83:1783–1787.
35. Charlson ME, Pompei P, Ales KL, MacKenzie CR. A new method of classifying prognostic comorbidity in longitudinal studies: development and validation. *J Chronic Dis.* 1987;40:373–383.
36. Charlson ME, Sax FL, MacKenzie CR, et al. Morbidity during hospitalization: can we predict it? *J Chronic Dis.* 1987;40:705–712.
37. Monk TG, Saini V, Weldon BC, Sigl JC. Anesthetic management and one-year mortality after noncardiac surgery. *Anesth Analg.* 2005;100:4–10.
38. Goldman L, Caldera DL, Nussbaum SR, et al. Multifactorial index of cardiac risk in noncardiac surgical procedures. *N Engl J Med.* 1977;297: 845–850.
39. Detsky AS, Abrams HB, McLaughlin JR, et al. Predicting cardiac complications in patients undergoing non-cardiac surgery. *J Gen Intern Med.* 1986;1:211–219.
40. Detsky AS, Abrams HB, Forbath N, et al. Cardiac assessment for patients undergoing noncardiac surgery. A multifactorial clinical risk index. *Arch Intern Med.* 1986;146:2131–2134.
41. Kumar R, McKinney WP, Raj G, et al. Adverse cardiac events after surgery: assessing risk in a veteran population. *J Gen Intern Med.* 2001;16:507–518.
42. Finlayson EV, Goodney PP, Birkmeyer JD. Hospital volume and operative mortality in cancer surgery: a national study. *Arch Surg.* 2003;138: 721–725; discussion 726.
43. Palda VA, Detsky AS. Perioperative assessment and management of risk from coronary artery disease. *Ann Intern Med.* 1997;127:313–328.
44. Eagle KA, Berger PB, Calkins H, et al. ACC/AHA guideline update for perioperative cardiovascular evaluation for noncardiac surgery—executive summary. A report of the American College of Cardiology/American Heart Association Task Force on practice guidelines (committee to update the 1996 guidelines on perioperative cardiovascular evaluation for noncardiac surgery). *Anesth Analg.* 2002;94:1052–1064.
45. Wiklund RA, Stein HD, Rosenbaum SH. Activities of daily living and cardiovascular complications following elective, noncardiac surgery. *Yale J Biol Med.* 2001;74:75–87.
46. Ali MJ, Davison P, Pickett W, Ali NS. ACC/AHA guidelines as predictors of postoperative cardiac outcomes. *Can J Anaesth.* 2000;47:10–19.
47. Lee TH, Marcantonio ER, Mangione CM, et al. Derivation and prospective validation of a simple index for prediction of cardiac risk of major noncardiac surgery. *Circulation.* 1999;100:1043–1049.
48. Boersma E, Kertai MD, Schouten O, et al. Perioperative cardiovascular mortality in noncardiac surgery: validation of the Lee cardiac risk index. *Am J Med.* 2005;118:1134–1141.
49. Smetana GW. Preoperative pulmonary assessment of the older adult. *Clin Geriatr Med.* 2003;19:35–55.
50. Smetana GW. Preoperative pulmonary evaluation. *N Engl J Med.* 1999;340:937–944.
51. Lawrence VA, Hilsenbeck SG, Mulrow CD, et al. Incidence and hospital stay for cardiac and pulmonary complications after abdominal surgery. *J Gen Intern Med.* 1995;10:671–678.
52. Arozullah AM, Daley J, Henderson WG, Khuri SF. Multifactorial risk index for predicting postoperative respiratory failure in men after major noncardiac surgery. The national veterans administration surgical quality improvement program. *Ann Surg.* 2000;232: 242–253.
53. Arozullah AM, Khuri SF, Henderson WG, Daley J. Participants in the National Veterans Affairs Surgical Quality Improvement Program. Development and validation of a multifactorial risk index for predicting postoperative pneumonia after major noncardiac surgery. *Ann Intern Med.* 2001;135:847–857.
54. McAlister FA, Bertsch K, Man J, et al. Incidence of and risk factors for pulmonary complications after nonthoracic surgery. *Am J Respir Crit Care Med.* 2005;171:514–517.
55. Bohner H, Hummel TC, Habel U, et al. Predicting delirium after vascular surgery: a model based on pre- and intraoperative data. *Ann Surg.* 2003;238:149–156.

56. Olin K, Eriksdotter-Jonhagen M, Jansson A, et al. Postoperative delirium in elderly patients after major abdominal surgery. *Br J Surg.* 2005; 92:1559–1564.

57. Marcantonio ER, Flacker JM, Michaels M, Resnick NM. Delirium is independently associated with poor functional recovery after hip fracture. *J Am Geriatr Soc.* 2000;48:618–624.

58. Marcantonio ER, Flacker JM, Wright RJ, Resnick NM. Reducing delirium after hip fracture: a randomized trial. *J Am Geriatr Soc.* 2001;49: 516–522.

59. Zakriya K, Sieber FE, Christmas C, et al. Brief postoperative delirium in hip fracture patients affects functional outcome at three months. *Anesth Analg.* 2004;98:1798–1802.

60. Marcantonio ER, Goldman L, Mangione CM, et al. A clinical prediction rule for delirium after elective noncardiac surgery. *JAMA.* 1994;271: 134–139.

61. Copeland GP. The POSSUM system of surgical audit. *Arch Surg.* 2002; 137:15–19.

62. Copeland GP, Jones D, Walters M. POSSUM: a scoring system for surgical audit. *Br J Surg.* 1991;78:355–360.

63. Goldman L, Hashimoto B, Cook EF, Loscalzo A. Comparative reproducibility and validity of systems for assessing cardiovascular functional class: advantages of a new specific activity scale. *Circulation.* 1981; 64:1227–1234.

64. Lee DS, Austin PC, Rouleau JL, et al. Predicting mortality among patients hospitalized for heart failure: derivation and validation of a clinical model. *JAMA.* 2003;290:2581–2587.

65. Hernandez AF, Whellan DJ, Stroud S, et al. Outcomes in heart failure patients after major noncardiac surgery. *J Am Coll Cardiol.* 2004;44: 1446–1453.

66. Leung JM, Dzankic S. Relative importance of preoperative health status versus intraoperative factors in predicting postoperative adverse outcomes in geriatric surgical patients. *J Am Geriatr Soc.* 2001;49:1080–1085.

67. Furberg CD, Psaty BM, Manolio TA, et al. Prevalence of atrial fibrillation in elderly subjects (the cardiovascular health study). *Am J Cardiol.* 1994;74:236–241.

68. Amar D. Perioperative atrial tachyarrhythmias. *Anesthesiology.* 2002;97: 1618–1623.

69. Amar D, Zhang H, Leung DH, et al. Older age is the strongest predictor of postoperative atrial fibrillation. *Anesthesiology.* 2002;96:352–356.

70. Passman RS, Gingold DS, Amar D, et al. Prediction rule for atrial fibrillation after major noncardiac thoracic surgery. *Ann Thorac Surg.* 2005; 79:1698–1703.

71. Mannino DM. COPD: epidemiology, prevalence, morbidity and mortality, and disease heterogeneity. *Chest.* 2002;121:121S–126S.

72. Gregg EW, Beckles GL, Williamson DF, et al. Diabetes and physical disability among older U.S. adults. *Diabetes Care.* 2000;23:1272–1277.

73. Woods SE, Smith JM, Sohail S, et al. The influence of type 2 diabetes mellitus in patients undergoing coronary artery bypass graft surgery: an 8-year prospective cohort study. *Chest.* 2004;126:1789–1795.

74. Subramaniam B, Pomposelli F, Talmor D, Park KW. Perioperative and long-term morbidity and mortality after above-knee and below-knee amputations in diabetics and nondiabetics. *Anesth Analg.* 2005;100: 1241–1247.

75. Gu W, Pagel PS, Warltier DC, Kersten JR. Modifying cardiovascular risk in diabetes mellitus. *Anesthesiology.* 2003;98:774–779.

76. Carson JL, Scholz PM, Chen AY, et al. Diabetes mellitus increases short-term mortality and morbidity in patients undergoing coronary artery bypass graft surgery. *J Am Coll Cardiol.* 2002;40:418–423.

77. Dubey A, Aharonoff GB, Zuckerman JD, Koval KJ. The effects of diabetes on outcome after hip fracture. *Bull Hosp Jt Dis.* 2000;59:94–98.

78. Dzankic S, Pastor D, Gonzalez C, Leung JM. The prevalence and predictive value of abnormal preoperative laboratory tests in elderly surgical patients. *Anesth Analg.* 2001;93:301–308.

79. Gibbs J, Cull W, Henderson W, et al. Preoperative serum albumin level as a predictor of operative mortality and morbidity: results from the national VA surgical risk study. *Arch Surg.* 1999;134:36–42.

80. Marrelli D, Roviello F, De Stefano A, et al. Surgical treatment of gastrointestinal carcinomas in octogenarians: risk factors for complications and long-term outcome. *Eur J Surg Oncol.* 2000;26:371–376.

81. Fleischmann KE. Noninvasive cardiac testing in the geriatric patient. *Am J Geriatr Cardiol.* 2003;12:28–32.

82. Liu LL, Dzankic S, Leung JM. Preoperative electrocardiogram abnormalities do not predict postoperative cardiac complications in geriatric surgical patients. *J Am Geriatr Soc.* 2002;50:1186–1191.

83. Halm EA, Browner WS, Tubau JF, et al. Echocardiography for assessing cardiac risk in patients having noncardiac surgery. Study of perioperative ischemia research group. *Ann Intern Med.* 1996;125: 433–441.

84. Rohde LE, Polanczyk CA, Goldman L, et al. Usefulness of transthoracic echocardiography as a tool for risk stratification of patients undergoing major noncardiac surgery. *Am J Cardiol.* 2001;87:505–509.

85. Moller JT, Cluitmans P, Rasmussen LS, et al. Long-term postoperative cognitive dysfunction in the elderly ISPOCD1 study. ISPOCD investigators. International study of post-operative cognitive dysfunction. *Lancet.* 1998;351:857–861.

86. Priebe HJ. The aged cardiovascular risk patient. *Br J Anaesth.* 2000;85: 763–778.

87. Carpenter RL, Caplan RA, Brown DL, et al. Incidence and risk factors for side effects of spinal anesthesia. *Anesthesiology.* 1992;76:906–916.

88. Doufas AG. Consequences of inadvertent perioperative hypothermia. *Best Pract Res Clin Anaesthesiol.* 2003;17:535–549.

89. Frank SM, Fleisher LA, Breslow MJ, et al. Perioperative maintenance of normothermia reduces the incidence of morbid cardiac events. A randomized clinical trial. *JAMA.* 1997;277:1127–1134.

90. Prough DS. Anesthetic pitfalls in the elderly patient. *J Am Coll Surg.* 2005;200:784–794.

91. Goodney PP, Siewers AE, Stukel TA, et al. Is surgery getting safer? National trends in operative mortality. *J Am Coll Surg.* 2002;195:219–227.

92. Chung F, Mezei G, Tong D. Adverse events in ambulatory surgery. A comparison between elderly and younger patients. *Can J Anaesth.* 1999; 46:309–321.

93. Katz J, Feldman MA, Bass EB. Adverse intraoperative medical events and their association with anesthesia management in cataract surgery. *Ophthalmology.* 2001;108:1721–1726.

94. Magaziner J, Hawkes W, Hebel JR, et al. Recovery from hip fracture in eight areas of function. *J Gerontol A Biol Sci Med Sci.* 2000;55: M498–M507.

95. Weaver F, Hynes D, Hopkinson W. Preoperative risks and outcomes of hip and knee arthroplasty in the veterans health administration. *J Arthroplasty.* 2003;18:693–708.

96. Millar WJ. Hip and knee replacement. *Health Rep.* 2002;14:37–50.

97. Parvizi J, Sullivan TA, Trousdale RT, Lewallen DG. Thirty-day mortality after total knee arthroplasty. *J Bone Joint Surg Am.* 2001;83-A:1157–1161.

98. Oakes DA, Hanssen AD. Bilateral total knee replacement using the same anesthetic is not justified by assessment of the risks. *Clin Orthop Relat Res.* 2004;428:87–91.

99. Pavone V, Johnson T, Saulog PS, Bottner F. Perioperative morbidity in bilateral one-stage total knee replacements. *Clin Orthop Relat Res.* 2004;421:155–161.

100. Lynch NM, Trousdale RT, Ilstrup DM. Complications after concomitant bilateral total knee arthroplasty in elderly patients. *Mayo Clin Proc.* 1997;72:799–805.

101. Hazzan D, Geron N, Golijanin D, et al. Laparoscopic cholecystectomy in octogenarians. *Surg Endosc.* 2003;17:773–776.

102. Maxwell JG, Tyler BA, Rutledge R, et al. Cholecystectomy in patients aged 80 and older. *Am J Surg.* 1998;176:627–631.

103. Brunt LM, Quasebarth MA, Dunnegan DL, Soper NJ. Outcomes analysis of laparoscopic cholecystectomy in the extremely elderly. *Surg Endosc.* 2001;15:700–705.

104. Magnuson TH, Ratner LE, Zenilman ME, Bender JS. Laparoscopic cholecystectomy: applicability in the geriatric population. *Am Surg.* 1997;63:91–96.

105. Mayol J, Martinez-Sarmiento J, Tamayo FJ, Fernandez-Represa JA. Complications of laparoscopic cholecystectomy in the ageing patient. *Age Ageing.* 1997;26:77–81.

106. Abbas S, Booth M. Major abdominal surgery in octogenarians. *N Z Med J.* 2003;116:U402.

107. Zerbib P, Kulick JF, Lebuffe G, et al. Emergency major abdominal surgery in patients over 85 years of age. *World J Surg.* 2005;29: 820–825.

108. Fortner JG, Lincer RM. Hepatic resection in the elderly. *Ann Surg.* 1990;211:141–145.

109. Otani Y, Kubota T, Kumai K, et al. Surgery for gastric carcinoma in patients more than 85 years of age. *J Gastroenterol Hepatol.* 2000;15:507–511.
110. Tekkis PP, Poloniecki JD, Thompson MR, Stamatakis JD. Operative mortality in colorectal cancer: prospective national study. *Br Med J.* 2003;327:1196–1201.
111. DiCarlo V, Balzano G, Zerbi A, Villa E. Pancreatic cancer resection in elderly patients. *Br J Surg.* 1998;85:607–610.
112. Sohn TA, Yeo CJ, Cameron JL, et al. Should pancreaticoduodenectomy be performed in octogenarians? *J Gastrointest Surg.* 1998;2:207–216.
113. Falcoz PE, Chocron S, Stoica L, et al. Open heart surgery: one-year self-assessment of quality of life and functional outcome. *Ann Thorac Surg.* 2003;76:1598–604; discussion 1604.
114. Avery GJ, II, Ley SJ, Hill JD, et al. Cardiac surgery in the octogenarian: evaluation of risk, cost, and outcome. *Ann Thorac Surg.* 2001;71:591–596.
115. Weintraub WS, Clements SD, Jr, Crisco LV, et al. Twenty-year survival after coronary artery surgery: an institutional perspective from Emory university. *Circulation.* 2003;107:1271–1277.
116. Fruitman DS, MacDougall CE, Ross DB. Cardiac surgery in octogenarians: can elderly patients benefit? Quality of life after cardiac surgery. *Ann Thorac Surg.* 1999;68:2129–2135.
117. Craver JM, Puskas JD, Weintraub WW, et al. 601 octogenarians undergoing cardiac surgery: outcome and comparison with younger age groups. *Ann Thorac Surg.* 1999;67:1104–1110.
118. Stamou SC, Hill PC, Dangas G, et al. Stroke after coronary artery bypass: incidence, predictors, and clinical outcome. *Stroke.* 2001;32:1508–1513.
119. Adam DJ, Craig SR, Sang CT, et al. Esophagectomy for carcinoma in the octogenarian. *Ann Thorac Surg.* 1996;61:190–194.
120. Bonavina L, Incarbone R, Saino G, et al. Clinical outcome and survival after esophagectomy for carcinoma in elderly patients. *Dis Esophagus.* 2003;16:90–93.
121. Port JL, Kent M, Korst RJ, et al. Surgical resection for lung cancer in the octogenarian. *Chest.* 2004;126:733–738.
122. Ginsberg RJ, Hill LD, Eagan RT, et al. Modern thirty-day operative mortality for surgical resections in lung cancer. *J Thorac Cardiovasc Surg.* 1983;86:654–658.
123. Brock MV, Kim MP, Hooker CM, et al. Pulmonary resection in octogenarians with stage I nonsmall cell lung cancer: a 22-year experience. *Ann Thorac Surg.* 2004;77:271–277.
124. Koren JP, Bocage JP, Geis WP, Caccavale RJ. Major thoracic surgery in octogenarians: the video-assisted thoracic surgery (VATS) approach. *Surg Endosc.* 2003;17:632–635.
125. Schneider JR, Droste JS, Schindler N, Golan JF. Carotid endarterectomy in octogenarians: comparison with patient characteristics and outcomes in younger patients. *J Vasc Surg.* 2000;31:927–935.
126. Cina CS, Clase CM, Haynes BR. Refining the indications for carotid endarterectomy in patients with symptomatic carotid stenosis: a systematic review. *J Vasc Surg.* 1999;30:606–617.
127. Kazmers A, Perkins AJ, Huber TS, Jacobs LA. Carotid surgery in octogenarians in veterans affairs medical centers. *J Surg Res.* 1999;81:87–90.
128. Lawrence PF, Gazak C, Bhirangi L, et al. The epidemiology of surgically repaired aneurysms in the United States. *J Vasc Surg.* 1999;30:632–640.
129. van der Vliet JA, Boll AP. Abdominal aortic aneurysm. *Lancet.* 1997;349:863–866.
130. Berry AJ, Smith RB, III, Weintraub WS, et al. Age versus comorbidities as risk factors for complications after elective abdominal aortic reconstructive surgery. *J Vasc Surg.* 2001;33:345–352.
131. Cota AM, Omer AA, Jaipersad AS, Wilson NV. Elective versus ruptured abdominal aortic aneurysm repair: a 1-year cost-effectiveness analysis. *Ann Vasc Surg.* 2005;19:858–861.
132. Dueck AD, Kucey DS, Johnston KW, et al. Survival after ruptured abdominal aortic aneurysm: effect of patient, surgeon, and hospital factors. *J Vasc Surg.* 2004;39:1253–1260.
133. Kazmers A, Jacobs L, Perkins A. The impact of complications after vascular surgery in veterans affairs medical centers. *J Surg Res.* 1997;67:62–66.
134. Tambyraja AL, Murie JA, Chalmers RT. Outcome and survival of patients aged 65 years and younger after abdominal aortic aneurysm rupture. *World J Surg.* 2005;29:1245–1247.
135. Marin ML, Hollier LH, Ellozy SH, et al. Endovascular stent graft repair of abdominal and thoracic aortic aneurysms: a ten-year experience with 817 patients. *Ann Surg.* 2003;238:586–593; discussion 593–595.
136. Minor ME, Ellozy S, Carroccio A, et al. Endovascular aortic aneurysm repair in the octogenarian: is it worthwhile? *Arch Surg.* 2004;139: 308–314.
137. Vaddineni SK, Russo GC, Patterson MA, et al. Ruptured abdominal aortic aneurysm: a retrospective assessment of open versus endovascular repair. *Ann Vasc Surg.* 2005;19:782–786.
138. Vogel T, Verreault R, Turcotte JF, et al. Intracerebral aneurysms: a review with special attention to geriatric aspects. *J Gerontol A Biol Sci Med Sci.* 2003;58:520–524.
139. Buczko W. Cranial surgery among medicare beneficiaries. *J Trauma.* 2005;58:40–46.
140. Lubicz B, Leclerc X, Gauvrit JY, et al. Endovascular treatment of ruptured intracranial aneurysms in elderly people. *Am J Neuroradiol.* 2004;25:592–595.
141. Sedat J, Dib M, Lonjon M, et al. Endovascular treatment of ruptured intracranial aneurysms in patients aged 65 years and older: follow-up of 52 patients after 1 year. *Stroke.* 2002;33:2620–2625.
142. Birkmeyer JD, Siewers AE, Finlayson EV, et al. Hospital volume and surgical mortality in the united states. *N Engl J Med.* 2002;346:1128–1137.
143. Katz JN, Barrett J, Mahomed NN, et al. Association between hospital and surgeon procedure volume and the outcomes of total knee replacement. *J Bone Joint Surg.* 2004;86-A:1909–1916.
144. Taylor CL, Yuan Z, Selman WR, et al. Mortality rates, hospital length of stay, and the cost of treating subarachnoid hemorrhage in older patients: institutional and geographical differences. *J Neurosurg.* 1997;86:583–588.
145. Cross DT, III, Tirschwell DL, Clark MA, et al. Mortality rates after subarachnoid hemorrhage: variations according to hospital case volume in 18 states. *J Neurosurg.* 2003;99:810–817.

Issues of Specific Importance to the Elderly in Preoperative Assessment

Frederick E. Sieber

INTRODUCTION

The objective of the preoperative assessment is to optimize patient care in preparation for surgery. Preoperative history and physical examination including laboratory findings comprise the basic information used to make decisions regarding surgical risk in the elderly. However, there are other, not so well appreciated, components of the preoperative examination which are of greater importance to the elderly that are often overlooked. The most important issue to the geriatric patient is not necessarily the underlying surgical risk. Rather, the elderly patients are more concerned with maintaining their independence and current level of functional ability following surgery. This chapter discusses the elements of preoperative assessment which are useful in predicting long-term functional outcome, living situation, and overall quality of life in the elderly surgical patient. It is the opinion of this author that as data continue to be gathered on quality of life issues in the elderly surgical patient, surgical decisions will incorporate this information to an ever greater extent.

STUDIES EXAMINING QUALITY OF LIFE FOLLOWING SURGERY

Quality of life is an important outcome measure in many series examining surgery in the elderly population. This new focus differs from the traditional morbidity and mortality reports and is being driven in part by economic factors. Quality of life issues are an important determinant of health-care expenditures following surgery. Some typical examples of studies examining quality of life for the elderly and the compelling results are described below.

In the field of vascular surgery, Williamson et al.[1] examined long-term functional outcome in 140 nonemergent open repairs of infrarenal abdominal aortic aneurysms. All patients were asymptomatic and fully ambulatory preoperatively. The study used telephone interviews to assess patient functional status. The mean length of time for follow-up was 33.9 months. There were 7 operative deaths and 46 deaths for a 38% overall mortality rate during the time of follow-up. Thirteen percent of patients required hospital discharge to a skilled nursing facility for a mean length of time of 3.66 ± 2.9 months. Of the original 140 patient cohort, only 87 patients of the original cohort were able to be contacted. Twenty-one percent of patients never fully recovered from surgery. Although all patients were fully ambulatory preoperatively, only 41% of patients interviewed could walk without assistance on follow-up. But, most

important, only 37% of patients would undergo the surgery again. The results as shown in Table 12-1 are particularly worthy of note as asymptomatic elderly patients, nearing the end of life, were studied. These individuals fear loss of independence more than loss of life. The economic implications are compelling when one begins to address costs of nursing home care as well as the social costs, given the large number of patients never fully recovering from surgery.

In the field of orthopedic surgery, Holtzman et al.[2] used postoperative telephone interviews in 1120 Medicare patients to assess activity levels, walking ability, and activities of daily living (ADLs) at 1 year following total hip arthroplasty. Table 12-2 demonstrates that patients with an abnormal preoperative functional status are more likely to have less than optimal postoperative outcomes. Thus, a worse preoperative functional status is predictive of a worse outcome in terms of both function and pain after total hip arthroplasty. The expectations concerning functional outcome in patients undergoing total hip arthroplasty who are already substantially disabled must be dampened. This study has compelling economic implications as it suggests that it may be better for a patient to choose total hip arthroplasty before they begin to require the assistance of others. The results of surgery are not as good once the patient has crossed the threshold of requiring assistance with activities of daily living, even if functional status and pain improve postoperatively.

Lawrence et al.[3] prospectively studied the time course of recovery to preoperative levels of functional independence in 372 elderly patients following major elective abdominal operations. The investigators examined both performance-based measures (handgrip strength, timed up and go, functional reach) and self-reported measures (ADLs and instrumental activities of daily living [IADLs]) up to 6 months postoperatively. This study had several interesting findings. For one, there was a unique time line of recovery for each measure evaluated. For instance, cognitive status recovered in 3 weeks whereas IADLs took 3–6 months to recover. Second, substantial numbers of patients (10–50% depending on the measure being evaluated) had a protracted postoperative recovery and had not returned to their preoperative status by 6 months. This late disability was more likely to be observed with performance-based measures in comparison to self-reported measures. Lawrence et al.[3] found several independent predictors of ADLs and IADLs recovery. The strongest predictor of both recovery and time to recovery of ADLs and IADLs was postoperative complications. Other predictors included preoperative physical conditioning, presence of dementia or depression, elevated creatinine level, and depressed serum albumin. Of note, postoperative complications,

Table 12-1

Long-Term (33.9 months) Functional Outcome with Open Repair of Infrarenal Abdominal Aortic Aneurysms

	N
Total number in series (all were asymptomatic and functioned independently preoperatively)	140
Operative deaths	7 (5)
Deaths during follow-up	46 (33)
Patients discharged to nursing home	17 (12)
Patients able to walk without assistance at follow-up	58 (41)
Patients who never fully recover from surgery	29 (21)
Patients who would choose to have surgery again	52 (37)

Note: ( ) denotes percent of total.
Source: Data from Ref. 1.

preoperative physical conditioning, and depression are potentially modifiable. Lawrence's study has clear implications for the growing number of elderly patients undergoing major abdominal operations. The results suggest that these patients fully recover their abilities to care for themselves and their affairs by 3 months, but they will not return to preoperative strength and physical conditioning levels until at least 6 months postoperatively. In addition, more attention should be paid to identifying and modifying known predictors of increased time to recovery in the elderly following major abdominal surgery.

Falcoz et al.[4] used preoperative and postoperative questionnaires to look at quality of life issues 1 year following open heart surgery in 264 elderly patients. Surprisingly, quality of life was improved after operation in only 50% of patients. Thirty-six percent of patients continued to experience limiting symptoms of angina or dyspnea at 1 year. Most important, the preoperative quality of life measures including self-assessed level of physical functioning and pain had greater predictive value of 1-year cardiac functional status than clinical variables. Falcoz's study suggests that formal preoperative quality of life assessment

Table 12-2

The Relationship of Pain and Functional Outcome 1 Year Following Total Hip Arthroplasty to Preoperative Functional Status

	Was Outcome Variable Abnormal Preoperatively?	
Outcome variable	No	Yes
Any pain walking	8%	21%
Participate in moderate activity less than daily	11%	16%
Needs assistance with walking	16%	35%
Need assistance with housework	18%	38%
Needs assistance with grocery shopping	14%	35%

Source: Data from Ref. 2.

should be considered to help determine risk stratification with regard to long-term cardiac functional status following open heart surgery. The results of Falcoz et al.[4] have been corroborated by other authors who have demonstrated that patients greater than 75 years of age derive less benefit from coronary artery bypass graft (CABG) in terms of quality of life at 1 year postoperatively compared with their younger counterparts.[5]

Morbidity and mortality are only the tip of the iceberg when scrutinizing surgical outcomes. The above studies demonstrate that in the elderly surgical population, the decision to offer surgery needs to be evaluated in terms of improvement in quality of life. As observed with open heart procedures, the benefits of surgery on functional outcomes appear to dwindle with age. Large vascular procedures should be evaluated in terms of their impact on both family and living situation. On the other hand, the data suggest that total joint replacement should be considered sooner, rather than later to optimize outcome. In addition, the time course of recovery following major abdominal procedures is lengthier than previously appreciated. Given the above studies, how does one predict postoperative quality of life during the preoperative assessment? What is the relationship between preoperative and postoperative functional level and quality of life? The studies discussed below have tried to answer this question.

MODELS PREDICTING FUNCTIONAL IMPAIRMENT AND QUALITY OF LIFE

To examine quality of life issues it is necessary to determine predictors of functional outcome and independence in the elderly. The best models currently available have been developed in medical populations and incorporate both pre- and posthospitalization functional criteria. The principles derived from these medical models are applicable to surgical patients. These studies emphasize that level of function is an important predictor of long-term outcome.

Initial studies focused on the relationship between functional level and the primary outcome variable of mortality. Inouye et al. validated the contribution of functional measurements in predicting 90-day and 2-year mortality in hospitalized patients aged 70 or greater.[6] In this prospective study, the authors looked at the combined effect of several functional components. The functional components studied included any impairment of IADLs, cognitive impairment (Mini-Mental State Examination [MMSE] <20), and depression (Geriatric Depression Scale ≥ 7). The authors showed that these three measures of functional capacity were strong predictors of mortality in elderly hospitalized patients, even without severity of illness indices. Walter et al.[7] developed an all-inclusive index for predicting 1-year mortality following hospital discharge in medical patients aged greater than 70 years. This far-reaching study showed that the cause of death in the elderly following hospitalization is multifactorial and may be secondary to demographic, medical, functional, or laboratory variables. The independent risk factors for 1-year mortality included male sex, number of dependent ADLs at discharge, congestive heart failure, cancer, creatinine level higher than 3.0 mg/dL, and low albumin level. Of pertinence to this discussion is the finding that inability to perform ADLs has as much impact in predicting death as all other variables except the presence of metastatic cancer or severe malnutrition.

The data suggest that there is a strong relationship between baseline functional level (as determined by ADLs, IADLs, and presence of dementia) and mortality. What about the relationship between baseline functional level and ability to maintain independence? Many outcome studies have documented the importance of preexisting level of function in determining speed of recovery after injury or rate of functional decline in the elderly. One approach that has been used is to look at important mediators of recovery from disability. Hardy and Gill[8] identified independent predictors of time to and duration of recovery of independent ADLs function among newly disabled community-dwelling persons aged 70 years or greater. There were 420 newly disabled subjects who were studied over an average follow-up period of 53 months. In terms of time to recovery, 81.4% of subjects had full recovery of their ADLs after 4.9 ± 0.5 months. Shorter time to recovery was predicted by habitual physical activity, mild disability, and hospitalization at time of disability. In terms of duration of recovery, 73.4% of subjects suffered recurrent disability by 7.3 ± 8.5 months. Longer duration of recovery was predicted by younger age, habitual physical activity, higher baseline functional level, and shorter duration of disability. The take-home message from Hardy and Gill[8] is that habitual physical activity is the most important independent predictor of time to recovery and duration of recovery of independence among newly disabled older persons. There is further evidence that physical activity is an important determinant of functional outcome. Gill et al.[9] evaluated the association between the occurrence of restricted activity and functional decline over an 18-month period. They looked at 680 patients aged 70 years or older and found that restricted activity is an important predictor of functional decline in older persons who are not otherwise at high risk for ADLs disability. Data from Israel provide additional support for the importance of physical activity in the elderly. Stessman et al.[10] measured the effect of regular exercise on the ability to maintain independent function. This study examined 287 patients at 70 years of age and then looked at the effect of exercise on ease of performance of ADLs and IADLs as these individuals aged to 77 years. All subjects remained active and independent at age 77. However, ease of performance of functions of daily living changed with aging. It was found that regular exercise, 4 days/week, was associated with greater ease in independent performance of ADLs in both men and women as they age. In surgical patients, other studies have looked at the relationship between preoperative functional level and postoperative complications in the elderly. Leung et al.[11] prospectively examined the prevalence and predictors of adverse postoperative outcomes in surgical patients aged 70 years or greater undergoing noncardiac surgery. Preoperative functional status was associated with postoperative neurological events. For instance, of the frequent neurological events that occur in elderly surgical patients, that is, stroke and delirium, the most important preoperative predictors are whether a patient is a nursing home resident and whether a patient has decreased preoperative functional status.

Baseline functional status is an important determinant of long-term independence and level of function. Baseline functional status is composed of many components. Independence in ADLs and IADLs are one indicator of level of function. Another important component is cognitive function. Both educational level and cognitive impairment affect level of function over time in the elderly. In a study of 862 elderly patients admitted to a medical service, an educational level less than high school was an independent risk factor for poor functional recovery 6 months following hospitalization.[12] Even mild dementia is an important determinant of functional recovery following hospitalization for medical illness. Seventy-three adults aged 65 years and older who were independent

in ADLs before hospitalization and dependent at discharge were studied to determine risk factors for lack of recovery of independent functioning after hospitalization for acute medical illness. Cognition, prehospital mobility, and discharge physical performance were the best predictors of patients who are less likely to recover functional independence after hospitalization. In particular, patients with lower cognition as evidenced by a MMSE score <24 have an 87% likelihood of not recovering independent ADLs function 1 month after hospital discharge.[13] These studies point out the relationship between cognitive ability and long-term functional outcomes.

Table 12-3 summarizes the predictors of functional outcome in the elderly as discussed in the above mentioned studies. Notice that baseline level of physical activity, independent function, and cognition are associated with many types of long-term functional outcomes. It is these elements of preoperative assessment which are most useful in predicting long-term functional outcome, living situation, and overall quality of life in the elderly surgical patient. The following sections discuss tools for assessment of functional level and cognition.

Table 12-3

Functional Outcome Predictors in the Elderly

Predictors	Outcome	Reference
IADLs/ADLs impairment Dementia Depression Sex Congestive heart failure Cancer Creatinine Albumin	Mortality	Inouye[6] Walter[7]
Age Habitual physical activity Baseline functional level Severity and duration of disability Hospitalization at time of disability	Functional recovery from a new disability	Hardy and Gill[8]
Restricted activity Regular exercise	Functional decline over time	Gill[9] Stessman[10]
Education level Dementia Prehospitalization mobility Physical performance on hospital discharge	Functional recovery following hospitalization	Chaudhry[12] Hansen[13]
Preoperative functional status Living situation	Postoperative stroke and delirium	Leung[11]

ASSESSMENT OF FUNCTIONAL AND ACTIVITY LEVEL IN THE PREOPERATIVE EXAM

The best screening tool for determining independence and functional level for the preoperative assessment is to question the patient concerning ADLs and IADLs. ADLs represent activities involved in physical day-to-day self-care whereas the IADLs represent more complex tasks. Tables 12-4 and 12-5 outline the types of questions to ask. When using the questions outlined, scoring and interpretation is done in the following manner. For ADLs, the total score ranges from 0 to 6, and for IADLs, from 0 to 8. As shown in Tables 12-4 and 12-5, in some categories, only the highest level of function receives a 1; in others, two or more levels have scores of 1 because each describes competence that represents some minimal level of function. These screens are useful for indicating specifically how a person is performing at the present time. When they are also used over time, they serve as documentation of a person's functional improvement or deterioration. IADLs and ADLs assessment are important for their predictive ability. For instance, any ADLs impairment is associated with a relative risk of 1.9 (1.2–2.9; 95% confidence interval) for 90-day mortality in medical patients. Any IADLs impairment is associated with a relative risk of 2.4 (1.4–4.2; 95% confidence interval) for 90-day mortality in medical patients.[6] Furthermore, any impairment of 1–2 ADLs is associated with a 1.47 (1.08–2.01; 95% confidence interval) hazard ratio of recovering independent function from a disability.[8]

For some anesthesiologists, a complete functional assessment can be an onerous task. Some data suggest that the entire battery of ADLs and IADLs questions is not necessary to obtain, and a more focused approach can be taken in the preoperative examination. For instance, self-reported walking ability may be the best predictor of overall mobility in community-dwelling older adults, even if they have existing difficulties with ADLs and mobility.[14] Overall mobility includes walking, ability to maintain stance, and rising from a chair. In particular, it is important to inquire about the ability to walk upstairs and to walk half a mile. Self-reported walking ability is important to assess because data suggest that walking-related items are predictive of both mortality and nursing home admission.[15] This simple assessment may be more helpful for the anesthesiologist who is "pressed for time."

ASSESSMENT OF COGNITIVE FUNCTION IN THE PREOPERATIVE EXAM

The level of cognitive functioning is easily assessed using simple tests such as the MMSE and/or the Mini-Cog. The MMSE[16] is an eleven-question instrument that tests five areas of cognitive function: orientation, registration, attention and calculation, recall, and language. The maximum score is 30. A score of 23 or lower may indicate cognitive dysfunction. The MMSE is shown in Table 12-6. It takes 3–5 min to perform. Prior educational level influences the MMSE score in that normal scores are often seen in patients with higher educational achievement. In comparison, elderly patients with lower levels of educational achievement can have low MMSE scores without a decline in cognitive function. The educational and age norms for the MMSE are provided in Table 12-7.

The Mini-Cog Assessment Instrument for Dementia takes approximately 3 min to perform and is relatively uninfluenced by level of education or variation in language. The Mini-Cog test combines an uncued three-item recall test with a clock drawing test and is demonstrated in Table 12-8.[17] Unlike the MMSE, the Mini-Cog test only determines the presence or absence of dementia and does not appraise its severity. In comparison to the MMSE, the Mini-Cog test is an easier and quicker screen for dementia.

▶ Interventions on the part of the anesthesiologist

The studies outlined above demonstrate that preoperative functional level and dementia are important determinants of postoperative quality of life. What difference does this information make to the anesthesiologist given that these variables are not immediately treatable? These variables help to paint the global outcome picture, and as such, help in defining surgical risk for the elderly. This information will allow geriatric patients and their families a more realistic view of their expected quality of life, something which assumes greater importance as one nears death.

OTHER IMPORTANT PREOPERATIVE ASSESSMENTS IN THE ELDERLY

▶ Nutritional assessment in the elderly

As seen in Table 12-3, malnutrition, as assessed by albumin level, is an important predictor of mortality. Even though poor nutritional status can be quickly and appropriately managed, nutritional status of the elderly is an often neglected component of the preoperative assessment. The incidence of malnutrition in the hospitalized elderly is quite high and has been reported to be greater than 40%.[18] The definition of malnutrition in the elderly is not uniform. Most definitions of malnutrition involve both laboratory indices and components of the history and physical. Of importance to the anesthesiologist, in hospitalized patients, a history of decreased caloric intake and the presence of hypoalbuminemia and hypocholesterolemia are primary determinants of malnutrition.

No single laboratory test is adequately sensitive or specific to diagnose malnutrition. The biochemical markers used to assess malnutrition (Table 12-9) may decrease as a result of other pathology such as trauma, sepsis, or infection. Diagnosis of malnutrition must take into account the patient's overall medical picture.

There are numerous accepted instruments to determine malnutrition, and nutritional status, as diagnosed by these instruments, has been associated with hospital outcomes in the elderly. For instance, poor nutritional status, as detected by the Mini-Nutritional Assessment Instrument, is predictive of increased in-hospital mortality, a higher rate of discharge to nursing homes, and increased length of stay in elderly in-hospital patient populations.[19] The Mini-Nutritional Assessment is composed of several components, including anthropomorphic measurements (weight, height, weight loss), global assessment (lifestyle, medication, and mobility), diet assessment, and self-perception of health and nutrition. Each component of the test is assessed a specific number of points. The maximum score which can be obtained is 30 points. According to the score obtained, a patient is placed into one of three categories: well nourished (≥ 24 points); at risk for malnutrition (17–23.5 points); malnourished (<17 points). The complete instrument and an explanation of its administration are provided on the website http://www.mna-elderly.com. The test takes approximately 10 min to administer. The Mini-Nutritional Assessment was designed to determine nutritional status in frail elderly patients in whom nutritional intervention is contemplated. So, for the anesthesiologist performing preoperative assessments, the Mini-Nutritional Assessment is probably not a satisfactory "routine" instrument to use. Rather, it should probably be reserved for use in detecting malnutrition under the type of circumstances for which it was originally designed.

Table 12-4

Activities of Daily Living (ADLs)

In each category, circle the item that most closely describes the person's highest level of functioning and record the score assigned to that level (either 1 or 0) in the blank at the beginning of the category.

A. Toilet

1. Care for self at toilet completely; no incontinence	1
2. Needs to be reminded, or needs help in cleaning self, or has rare (weekly at most) accidents	0
3. Soiling or wetting while asleep more than once a week	0
4. Soiling or wetting while awake more than once a week	0
5. No control of bowels or bladder	0

B. Feeding

1. Eats without assistance	1
2. Eats with minor assistance at meal times and/or with special preparation of food, or help in cleaning up after meals	0
3. Feed self with moderate assistance and is untidy	0
4. Requires extensive assistance for all meals	0
5. Does not feed self at all and resists efforts of others to feed him or her	0

C. Dressing

1. Dresses, undresses, and selects clothes from own wardrobe	1
2. Dresses and undresses self, with minor assistance	0
3. Needs moderate assistance in dressing and selection of clothes	0
4. Needs major assistance in dressing, but cooperates with efforts of others to help	0
5. Completely unable to dress self and resists efforts of others to help	0

D. Grooming (Neatness, Hair, Nails, Hands, Face, Clothing)

1. Always neatly dressed, well-groomed, without assistance	1
2. Grooms self-adequately with occasional minor assistance, e.g., with shaving	0
3. Needs moderate and regular assistance or supervision with grooming	0
4. Needs total grooming care, but can remain well-groomed after help from others	0
5. Actively negates all efforts of others to maintain grooming	0

E. Physical Ambulation

1. Goes about grounds or city	1
2. Ambulates within residence on or about one block distant	0
3. Ambulates with assistance of (check one)	0
a. ( ) another person, b. ( ) railing, c. ( ) cane, d. ( ) walker, e. ( ) wheelchair	
1.___Gets in and out without help. 2.___ Needs help getting in and out.	
4. Sits unsupported in chair or wheelchair, but cannot propel self without help	0
5. Bedridden more than half the time	0

F. Bathing

1. Bathes self (tub, shower, sponge bath) without help	1
2. Bathes self with help getting in and out of tub	0
3. Washes face and hands only, but cannot bathe rest of body	0
4. Does not wash self, but is cooperative with those who bathe him or her	0
5. Does not try to wash self and resists efforts to keep him or her clean	0

Note: For scoring interpretation see text.

Table 12-5

Instrumental Activities of Daily Living (IADLs)

In each category, circle the item that most closely describes the person's highest level of functioning and record the score assigned to that level (either 1 or 0) in the blank at the beginning of the category.

A. Ability To Use Telephone
1. Operates telephone on own initiative; looks up and dials numbers — 1
2. Dials a few well-known numbers — 1
3. Answers telephone, but does not dial — 1
4. Does not use telephone at all — 0

B. Shopping
1. Takes care of all shopping needs independently — 1
2. Shops independently for small purchases — 0
3. Needs to be accompanied on any shopping trip — 0
4. Completely unable to shop — 0

C. Food Preparation
1. Plans, prepares, and serves adequate meals independently — 1
2. Prepares adequate meals if supplied with ingredients — 0
3. Heats and serves prepared meals or prepares meals, but does not maintain adequate diet — 0
4. Needs to have meals prepared and served — 0

D. Housekeeping
1. Maintains house alone or with occasional assistance (e.g., heavy work domestic help) — 1
2. Performs light daily tasks such as dishwashing, bedmaking — 1
3. Performs light daily tasks, but cannot maintain acceptable level of cleanliness — 1
4. Needs help with all home maintenance tasks — 1
5. Does not participate in any housekeeping tasks — 0

E. Laundry
1. Does personal laundry completely — 1
2. Launders small items; rinses socks, stockings, etc. — 1
3. All laundry must be done by others — 0

F. Mode of Transportation
1. Travels independently on public transportation or drives own car — 1
2. Arranges own travel via taxi, but does not otherwise use public transportation — 1
3. Travels on public transportation when assisted or accompanied by another — 1
4. Travel limited to taxi or automobile with assistance of another — 0
5. Does not travel at all — 0

G. Responsibility for Own Medication
1. Is responsible for taking medication in correct dosages at correct time — 1
2. Takes responsibility if medication is prepared in advance in separate dosages — 0
3. Is not capable of dispensing own medication — 0

H. Ability to Handle Finances
1. Manages financial matters independently (budgets, writes checks, pays rent and bills, goes to bank); collects and keeps track of income — 1
2. Manages day-to-day purchases, but needs help with banking, major purchases, etc. — 1
3. Incapable of handling money — 0

Note: For scoring and interpretation see text.

Table 12-6

Mini-Mental State Exam

Questions (Total of 30 Points)

A. Orientation (10 points, 1 point for each correct answer)
   1. Year, season, date, day of week, and month
   2. State, county, town, or city
   3. Hospital or clinic, floor

B. Registration (3 points)
   1. Name three objects: apple, table, penny
   2. Each one spoken distinctly and with brief pause
   3. Patient repeats all three (one point for each)
   4. Repeat process until all three objects learned
   5. Record number of trials needed to learn all three objects

C. Attention and Calculation (5 points)
   1. Spell WORLD backwards: DLROW
   2. Points given up to first misplaced letter
   3. Example: DLORW scored as 2 points only

D. Recall (3 points, 1 point for each object recalled)
   1. Recite the three objects memorized in Registration above

E. Language (9 points)
   1. Patient names two objects when they are displayed
      a. Example: pencil and watch (1 point each)
   2. Repeat a sentence: "No ifs, ands, or buts" (1 point)
   3. Follow three stage commands (3 points)
      a. Take a paper in your right hand
      b. Fold it in half
      c. Put it on the floor
   4. Read and obey the following:
      a. Close your eyes (1 point)
      b. Write a sentence (1 point)
      c. Copy the design (picture of two overlapped pentagons) (1 point)

Table 12-7

Educational and Age Norms for the Mini-Mental State Exam

Educational and Age Norms

1. Fourth Grade Education
   a. Ages 18–69: Median MMSE Score 22–25
   b. Ages 70–79: Median MMSE Score 21–22
   c. Age over 79: Median MMSE Score 19–20
2. Eighth Grade Education
   a. Ages 18–69: Median MMSE Score 26–27
   b. Ages 70–79: Median MMSE Score 25
   c. Age over 79: Median MMSE Score 23–25
3. High School Education
   a. Ages 18–69: Median MMSE Score 28–29
   b. Ages 70–79: Median MMSE Score 27
   c. Age over 79: Median MMSE Score 25–26
4. College Education
   a. Ages 18–69: Median MMSE Score 29
   b. Ages 70–79: Median MMSE Score 28
   c. Age over 79: Median MMSE Score 27

Source: Data from Ref. 16.

or pitting edema is also important. With the subjective global assessment of nutrition, there is no numerical weighting scheme for combining the history and physical examination results into one of the Subjective Global Assessment categories. Rather, they are combined subjectively into an overall global assessment. The simplicity and ease of the Subjective Global Nutritional Assessment may make it the best instrument for preoperative anesthetic assessment when used in combination with some simple laboratory values such as albumin level and complete blood counts.

Assessment of frailty

The concept of frailty and its assessment is still in evolution. Frailty refers to a loss of physiologic reserve which makes a person more vulnerable to disability during and following stress. In general, frailty may encompass signs and symptoms such as exercise intolerance, immobility, weakness, weight loss, muscle wasting, or frequent falls. Patients who are frail are more likely to be hospitalized, fall, develop disability, and die than their peers. Currently, there is no consensus as to the definition of frailty. To better define this syndrome, an international working group consisting of geriatricians and epidemiologists was formed and called the Interventions on Frailty Working Group. This working group believes that any operational definition of frailty must include the impairments in physiological domains most frequently cited in the frailty literature.[21] These domains comprise the reported components of the frailty syndrome and include mobility such as lower extremity performance and gait disturbance; muscle weakness; poor exercise tolerance; unstable balance; and factors related to body composition such as weight loss, malnutrition, and muscle wasting.[21] Physical frailty is not necessarily associated with cognitive dysfunction.[21] Table 12-11

The subjective global assessment of nutritional status is another validated instrument which has been used to assess malnutrition and its relationship to mortality and poor functional status in the elderly.[18] The subjective global assessment of nutritional status uses relevant features of the typical history and physical examination to divide patients into three classes: class A—well nourished; class B—moderately (or suspected of being) malnourished; class C—severely malnourished.[20] Notice that the classifications of the subjective global assessment are analogous to those of the Mini-Nutritional Assessment.

The components of the Subjective Global Nutritional Assessment are shown in Table 12-10. The first four components deal with patient history including functional capacity (component four, Table 12-10). Patients who are unable to eat will often complain of fatigue, weakness, and decreased functional capacity. The physical examination component focuses on specific findings of malnourishment. The best areas to look for loss of subcutaneous fat are the triceps region of the arms and the midaxillary line at the costal margin. In terms of muscle wasting, the best muscles to examine for loss of bulk and tone are the quadriceps femoris and the deltoids. Examination for the presence of ascites

Table 12-8

Mini-Cog Scoring Algorithm

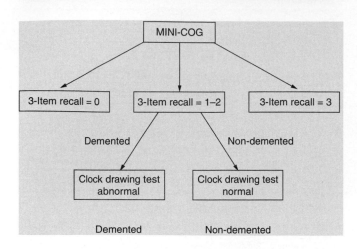

Administration

The test is administrated as follows:

1. Instruct the patient to listen carefully to three unrelated words and then to repeat the words.

2. Instruct the patient to draw the face of a clock, either on a blank sheet of paper or on a sheet with the clock circle already drawn on the page.

   After the patient puts the numbers on the clock face, ask him or her to draw the hands of the clock to read a specific time, such as 11:20. These instructions can be repeated but no additional instructions should be given. Give the patient as much time as needed to complete the task. The CDT serves as the recall distractor.

3. Ask the patient to repeat the three previously presented words.

Scoring

Give 1 point for each recalled word after the CDT distractor. Score 1–3.

The CDT is considered normal if all numbers are present in the correct sequence and position, and the hands readably display the requested time.

---

outlines some suggested criteria used to define frailty in the elderly. Using this operationalized definition of frailty it is estimated that the incidence of frailty in the community-dwelling population greater than 65 years is 6.9%.[22] When followed over a period of 3 years, frailty is predictive of disability, hospitalization, and death.[22] There are scant data concerning the effect of frailty on surgical outcomes. However, note that many of the domains included in the frailty definition such as poor mobility, exercise tolerance, malnutrition, and

Table 12-9

Laboratory Markers For Malnutrition

Complete blood count	(nutritionally related anemia)
Albumin	(prognostic value)
Transferrin	
Prealbumin	(monitoring nutritional recovery)
Cholesterol	(prognostic value)

Table 12-10

Features of Subjective Global Assessment

History

1. Weight change

   Overall loss in past 6 months: amount = ____ kg; ____%

   Change in past 2 weeks: ____ Increase

   ____ No change

   ____ Decrease

2. Dietary intake change (relative to normal)

   ____ No change

   ____ Change ____ Duration ____ Weeks

   ____ Type ____ Suboptimal solid diet ____ Full liquid diet

   ____ Hypocaloric liquids ____ Starvation

3. Gastrointestinal symptoms (that persisted for >2 weeks)

   ____ None ____ Nausea ____ Vomiting ____ Diarrhea ____ Anorexia

4. Functional capacity

   ____ No dysfunction (e.g., full capacity)

   ____ Dysfunction ____ Duration = ____ Weeks

   ____ Type ____ Working suboptimally

   ____ Ambulatory

   ____ Bedridden

Physical (for each trait specify: 0 = normal, 1 + = mild, 2 + = moderate, 3 + = severe)

   ____ Loss of subcutaneous fat (triceps, chest)

   ____ Muscle wasting (quadriceps, deltoids)

   ____ Ankle edema

   ____ Sacral edema

   ____ Ascites

Subjective Global Assessment rating (select one)*

   ____ A = well nourished

   ____ B = moderately (or suspected of being) malnourished

   ____ C = severely malnourished

*Class A indicates those with less than 5% weight loss or more than 5% total weight loss, but recent gain and improvement in appetite; class B, those with 5–10% weight loss without recent stabilization or gain, poor dietary intake, and mild (1+) loss of subcutaneous tissue; and class C, ongoing weight loss of more than 10% with severe subcutaneous tissue loss and muscle wasting often with edema.
Source: Derived from Ref. 20.

---

muscle weakness have been discussed earlier in this chapter. In the author's opinion, the concept of frailty will assume greater importance in assessment of surgical outcomes as more research on this topic becomes available.

KEY POINTS

▶ The decision to offer surgery to the elderly patient needs to be evaluated in terms of improvement in quality of life.

▶ Baseline level of physical activity, independent function, and cognition are associated with many types of long-term functional outcomes. It is these elements of preoperative assessment which

Table 12-11

Criteria Used to Define Frailty

Weight loss criterion: The patient is asked the question, "In the last year, have you lost more than 10 lb unintentionally (i.e., not due to dieting or exercise)?" If yes, then frail for weight loss criterion.

Exhaustion criterion: The patient is asked to read the following two statements: (1) I felt that everything I did was an effort; (2) I could not get going. The question is asked, "How often in the last week did you feel this way?" 0 = rarely or none of the time (<1 day). 1 = some or little of the time (1–2 days). 2 = a moderate amount of the time (3–4 days), or 3 = most of the time. Subjects answering "2" or "3" to either of these questions are categorized as frail by the exhaustion criterion.

Physical activity criterion: The patients are asked about their weekly physical activity. Those with low physical activity are considered frail by physical activity criterion.

Walk time criterion: The patient is asked to walk a short distance and timed. Slower walkers are considered frail by walk time criterion.

Grip strength criterion: The patient's grip strength is measured. Subjects with decreased grip strength are considered frail by grip strength criterion.

Note: Frailty is defined as a clinical syndrome in which three or more of the above frailty criteria are met.
Source: Adapted from Ref. 22.

---

are most useful in predicting long-term functional outcome, living situation, and overall quality of life in the elderly surgical patient.

▸ The best screening tool for determining independence and functional level for the preoperative assessment is to question the patient concerning ADLs and IADLs.

▸ Self-reported walking ability may be the best predictor of overall mobility in community-dwelling older adults.

▸ The level of cognitive function is easily assessed using simple tests such as the MMSE or Mini-Cog test.

▸ Poor nutritional status is predictive of increased in-hospital mortality, a higher rate of discharge to nursing homes, and increased length of stay in elderly in-hospital patient populations.

▸ No single laboratory test is adequately sensitive or specific to diagnose malnutrition. Diagnosis of malnutrition must take into account the patient's overall medical picture. The Mini-Nutritional Assessment and the Subjective Global Assessment are accepted instruments to determine malnutrition in the elderly.

KEY ARTICLES

▸ Walter LC, Brand RJ, Counsell SR, et al. Development and validation of a prognostic index for 1-year mortality in older adults after hospitalization. *JAMA.* 2001;285:2987–2994.

▸ Alexander NB, Guire KE, Thelen DG, et al. Self-reported walking ability predicts functional mobility performance in frail older adults. *J Am Geriatr Soc.* 2000;48:1408–1413.

▸ Borson S, Scanlan J, Brush M, et al. The mini-cog: a cognitive "vital signs" measure for dementia screening in multilingual elderly. *Int J Geriatr Psychiatry.* 2000;15:1021–1027.

▸ Van Nes MC, Herrmann FR, Gold G, et al. Does the mini nutritional assessment predict hospitalization outcomes in older people? *Age Ageing.* 2001;30:221–226.

REFERENCES

1. Williamson WK, Nicoloff AD, Taylor LM, Jr, et al. Functional outcome after open repair of abdominal aortic aneurysm. *J Vasc Surg.* 2001;33: 913–920.
2. Holtzman J, Saleh K, Kane R. Effect of baseline functional status and pain on outcomes of total hip arthroplasty. *J Bone Joint Surg Am.* 2002;84-A: 1942–1948.
3. Lawrence VA, Hazuda HP, Cornell JE, et al. Functional independence after major abdominal surgery in the elderly. *J Am Coll Surg.* 2004;199: 762–772.
4. Falcoz PE, Chocron S, Stoica L, et al. Open heart surgery: one-year self-assessment of quality of life and functional outcome. *Ann Thorac Surg.* 2003;76:1598–1604; discussion 1604.
5. Jarvinen O, Saarinen T, Julkunen J, et al. Changes in health-related quality of life and functional capacity following coronary artery bypass graft surgery. *Eur J Cardiothorac Surg.* 2003;24:750–756.
6. Inouye SK, Peduzzi PN, Robison JT, et al. Importance of functional measures in predicting mortality among older hospitalized patients. *JAMA.* 1998;279:1187–1193.
7. Walter LC, Brand RJ, Counsell SR, et al. Development and validation of a prognostic index for 1-year mortality in older adults after hospitalization. *JAMA.* 2001;285:2987–2994.
8. Hardy SE, Gill TM. Factors associated with recovery of independence among newly disabled older persons. *Arch Intern Med.* 2005;165: 106–112.
9. Gill TM, Allore H, Guo Z. Restricted activity and functional decline among community-living older persons. *Arch Intern Med.* 2003;163:1317–1322.
10. Stessman J, Hammerman Rozenberg R, Maaravi Y, Cohen A. Effect of exercise on ease in performing activities of daily living and instrumental activities of daily living from age 70 to 77: the Jerusalem longitudinal study. *J Am Geriatr Soc.* 2002;50:1934–1938.
11. Leung JM, Dzankic S. Relative importance of preoperative health status versus intraoperative factors in predicting postoperative adverse outcomes in geriatric surgical patients. *J Am Geriatr Soc.* 2001;49:1080–1085.
12. Chaudhry SI, Friedkin RJ, Horwitz RI, Inouye SK. Educational disadvantage impairs functional recovery after hospitalization in older persons. *Am J Med.* 2004;117:650–656.
13. Hansen K, Mahoney J, Palta M. Risk factors for lack of recovery of ADL independence after hospital discharge. *J Am Geriatr Soc.* 1999;47: 360–365.
14. Alexander NB, Guire KE, Thelen DG, et al. Self-reported walking ability predicts functional mobility performance in frail older adults. *J Am Geriatr Soc.* 2000;48:1408–1413.
15. Guralnik JM, Simonsick EM, Ferrucci L, et al. A short physical performance battery assessing lower extremity function: association with self-reported disability and prediction of mortality and nursing home admission. *J Gerontol.* 1994;49:M85–M94.
16. Folstein MF, Folstein SE, McHugh PR. ìMini-mental state." A practical method for grading the cognitive state of patients for the clinician. *J Psychiatr Res.* 1975;12:189–198.
17. Borson S, Scanlan J, Brush M, et al. The mini-cog: a cognitive "vital signs" measure for dementia screening in multilingual elderly. *Int J Geriatr Psychiatry.* 2000;15:1021–1027.
18. Covinsky KE, Martin GE, Beyth RJ, et al. The relationship between clinical assessments of nutritional status and adverse outcomes in older hospitalized medical patients. *J Am Geriatr Soc.* 1999;47:532–538.
19. Van Nes MC, Herrmann FR, Gold G, et al. Does the mini nutritional assessment predict hospitalization outcomes in older people? *Age Ageing.* 2001;30:221–226.
20. Detsky AS, Smalley PS, Chang J. The rational clinical examination. Is this patient malnourished? *JAMA.* 1994;271:54–58.
21. Ferrucci L, Guralnik JM, Studenski S, et al. Designing randomized, controlled trials aimed at preventing or delaying functional decline and disability in frail, older persons: a consensus report. *J Am Geriatr Soc.* 2004;52:625–634.
22. Fried LP, Tangen CM, Walston J, et al. Frailty in older adults: evidence for a phenotype. *J Gerontol A Biol Sci Med Sci.* 2001;56:M146–M156.

Polypharmacy

James E. Heavner

INTRODUCTION

Polypharmacy refers to multiple drug use. This includes self-prescription and/or use of more than one drug by individuals for health or recreational purposes, or the prescription and/or administration of two or more drugs by health-care professionals. Anesthesiologists are trained in the science and art of administering multiple drugs while patients are in their care. They continuously monitor patients to assure that desired responses are achieved and undesired effects are avoided or minimized. With few exceptions, drugs administered to achieve intraoperative anesthesia goals have rapid onset and short duration of action. Because of the continuous monitoring during anesthesia and favorable pharmacokinetic properties of the drugs used for anesthesia care, undesirable drug interactions usually are quickly detected and responses to adjustments to reduce or stop the interactions are rapid.

POLYPHARMACY

Patients presenting for anesthesia care may already be taking multiple drugs for one or more chronic conditions. The probability that this is so increases as the age of patients increases. Studies show that people 65 years of age or older frequently have multiple chronic illness for which they are taking multiple drugs. One report states that the average patient 65 years of age or older takes about eight different drugs daily.[1] In addition to multiple medications and increased risk for adverse drug events, comorbidity is associated with poor quality of life, physical disability, and increased risk for mortality.[2–4]

Anderson and Howath[5] reported that in 1999, 48% of Medicare beneficiaries aged 65 years or older had at least three chronic medical conditions and 21% had five or more. Eleven of the most common diseases are listed in Table 13-1. Treatment of a single disease may require polypharmacy such as administration of a second drug to deal with side effects of another, for example, a laxative to treat constipation due to opioid use for chronic pain therapy (Table 13-2).

Anesthesiologists must have a broad knowledge about how one drug influences the action of another, how comorbidities influence drug responses, and how age-related changes in organ and system function alter drug responses. The scope of the knowledge must extend beyond the drugs used in anesthesia care. The knowledge is essential for making decisions about drugs and doses to use—what drug(s) a patient is taking must be stopped before anesthesia and the consequences of discontinuing the drug with respect to anesthetic management and ongoing medical care. Thus, this discussion of polypharmacy includes the use of drugs for chronic disease states.

DRUG INTERACTIONS

Polypharmacy and drug interactions go hand in hand. Drug interactions may produce desired responses or unwanted side effects (adverse drug reactions [ADRs]) by increasing or decreasing the effects of one or all drugs the patient is receiving. Multidrug therapy may be required to treat comorbidities and may be used to increase therapeutic effects or reduce toxicity.

Boyd et al.[6] recently presented data illustrating how multiple comorbid diseases in older patients present challenges to using an appropriate spectrum of drugs for the care of the patients. They examined how clinical practice guidelines (CPGs) address comorbidity in older patients and explored what happens when multiple single-disease CPGs are applied to a hypothetical 79-year-old woman with five common diseases—hypertension, type 2 diabetes mellitus, osteoporosis, osteoarthritis, and chronic obstructive pulmonary disease (COPD). The patient would take 12 separate medications. Table 13-3 shows interactions that could result. The interactions include between a medication and a disease other than the target disease, between medications for different diseases, and between food and medications.

Of nine CPGs reviewed by Boyd et al.,[6] seven discussed older adults or comorbid disease. CPGs for two diseases of interest from an anesthetic perspective, depression and dementia, were not reviewed. Only four CPGs (diabetes, osteoarthritis, atrial fibrillation, and angina) addressed older individuals with multiple comorbidities (Tables 13-4 and 13-5). The investigators observed that CPGs rarely address treatment of patients with three or more chronic diseases, that is, half of the population older than 65 years.

The foregoing indicates how difficulties with polypharmacy escalate with the number of diseases a patient has and the number of drugs the patient takes. Estimates of how the difficulties in predicting drug interaction increase vary from exponential (n^2; n is the number of drugs) to approaching nearly unpredictable beyond more than two drugs.

Table 13-1

Common Chronic Diseases in Medicare Beneficiaries 65 Years of Age or Older

Hypertension

Chronic heart failure

Stable angina

Atrial fibrillation

Hypercholesterolemia

Diabetes mellitus

Osteoarthritis

Chronic obstructive pulmonary disease

Osteoporosis

Depression

Dementia

Source: Data from Ref. 6.

Table 13-2

Drugs Given to Treat the Side Effects of Other Medications

α-Adrenergic antagonists (such as terazosin or tamsulosin) to treat urinary retention related to anticholinergic agents

Antiemetics to treat nausea associated with digoxin

Antitussives to treat cough induced by ACE inhibitors (such as captopril)

Chronic use of antacids, H2-receptor antagonists (such as ranitidine), or proton pump inhibitors (such as omeprazole) to treat dyspepsia related to use of aspirin or NSAIDs (such as ibuprofen)

Laxatives to treat verapamil-induced constipation

Sedative agents to manage the activating effects of some antidepressants (such as fluoxetine)

Source: Reproduced with permission from Ref. 20.

Table 13-3

Potential Treatment Interactions for a Hypothetical 79-Year-Old Woman with Five Chronic Diseases

Type of Disease	Medications with Potential Interactions	Type of Interaction		
		Medication and Other Disease	Medications for Different Diseases	Medication and Food
Hypertension	Hydrochlorothiazide, lisinopril	Diabetes: diuretics increase serum glucose and lipids*	Diabetes medications: hydrochlorothiazide may decrease effectiveness of glyburide	NA
Diabetes	Glyburide, Metformin, aspirin, and atorvastatin	NA	Osteoarthritis medications: NSAIDs plus aspirin increase risk of bleeding Diabetes medications: glyburide plus aspirin may increase the risk of hypoglycemia; aspirin may decrease effectiveness of lisinopril	Aspirin plus alcohol: increased risk of gastrointestinal tract bleeding Atorvastatin plus grapefruit juice: muscle pain, weakness Glyburide plus alcohol: low blood sugar, flushing, rapid breathing, tachycardia Metformin plus alcohol: extreme weakness and heavy breathing Metformin plus any type of food: medication absorption decreased
Osteoarthritis	NSAIDs	Hypertension: NSAIDs raise blood pressure†; NSAIDs plus hypertension increase risk of renal failure	Diabetes medications: NSAIDs in combination with aspirin increase risk of bleeding Hypertension medications: NSAIDs decrease efficacy of diuretics	NA
Osteoporosis	Calcium, alendronate	NA	Diabetes medications: calcium may decrease efficacy of aspirin; aspirin plus alendronate can cause upset stomach Osteoporosis medications: calcium may lower serum alendronate level	Alendronate plus calcium: take on empty stomach (>2 h from last meal) Alendronate: avoid orange juice Calcium plus oxalic acid (spinach and rhubarb) or phytic (bran and whole cereals): eating these foods may decrease amount of calcium absorbed (>2 h from last meal)
Chronic obstructive pulmonary disease	Short-acting β-agonists	NA	NA	NA

Abbreviations: NA = no interaction is known; NSAIDs = nonsteroidal anti-inflammatory drugs.

*Thiazide-type diuretics may worsen hyperglycemia, but effect thought to be small and not associated with increased incidence of cardiovascular events.

†This interaction is noted to be particularly relevant for individuals with diabetes; no recommendation for treatment is given.

Source: Reproduced with permission from Ref. 6.

Table 13-4

Relevance of Clinical Practice Guidelines for the Treatment of Older Patients with Diabetes Mellitus, Hypertension, Osteoarthritis, Osteoporosis, and Chronic Obstructive Pulmonary Disease (COPD)

	Chronic Disease Addressed by Guideline				
	Diabetes Mellitus	Hypertension	Osteoarthritis	Osteoporosis	COPD
Guideline addressed treatment for type of patient?	Older: yes Multiple comorbidities: yes Both: yes	Older: yes Multiple comorbidities: no Both: no	Older: yes Multiple comorbidities: yes Both: yes	Older: no Multiple comorbidities: no Both: no	Older: no Multiple comorbidities: no Both: no
Quality of evidence discussed for type of patient?	Older: yes Multiple comorbidities: yes Quality of evidence poor, requires extrapolation for nutrition recommendations	Older: yes Multiple comorbidities: no Quality of evidence good for treating hypertension in older patients	Older: no Multiple comorbidities: no	Older: no Multiple comorbidities: no	Older: no Multiple comorbidities: no
Specific recommendations for patients with one comorbid condition?	Yes Diseases: hypercholesterolemia, hypertension, congestive heart failure, chronic kidney disease, cardiovascular disease, peripheral vascular disease, benign prostatic hypertrophy	Yes Diseases: coronary artery disease, diabetes mellitus, metabolic syndrome, sleep apnea, chronic kidney disease, gout, left ventricular hypertrophy, erectile dysfunction, peripheral vascular disease, congestive heart failure, stroke, dementia,* renal transplantation, renal artery stenosis, urinary outflow obstruction	Yes Diseases/drugs: anticoagulants, glucocorticoids, peptic ulcer disease, chronic kidney disease, hypertension, congestive heart failure	No	No
Specific recommendations for patients with several comorbid conditions?	Yes	No	No	No	No
Time needed to treat to benefit from treatment in the context of life expectancy discussed?	Yes	No	No	No	No

*Limited to the possible effects of antihypertensive treatment on preventing cognitive decline, not management of hypertensive patients with mild cognitive impairment or dementia.
†Limited to patients at highest risk of gastrointestinal tract bleeding with certain therapies.
Source: Reproduced with permission from Ref. 6.

CLINICALLY SIGNIFICANT ADVERSE DRUG INTERACTIONS AND POLYPHARMACY: GENERAL

Drugs may either indirectly (precipitant drugs) cause adverse responses to another drug (object drug) or be the direct cause of the adverse response.[7] The cause of the indirect effect may be modification of the absorption, distribution, metabolism excretion (pharmacokinetic), or actual clinical effect (pharmacodynamic). Nonsteroidal anti-inflammatory drugs and antibiotics (especially rifampin) are common precipitant

drugs. Likely object drugs for serious drug interactions are drugs with a narrow therapeutic range or a low therapeutic index (Table 13-6). Warfarin, fluoroquinolones, antiepileptic drugs, oral contraceptives, cisapride, and statins are common object drugs. Table 13-7 contains a list of selected serious drug interactions.

The prevalence of ADRs in outpatients 65 years of age or older is between 5% and 35%.[8] An expert panel identified 21 ADR risk factors in this patient population including 12 medication-related factors and 9 patient characteristics (Table 13-8). Polypharmacy, multiple chronic

Table 13-5

Relevance of Clinical Practice Guidelines for the Treatment of Older Patients with Atrial Fibrillation, Chronic Heart Failure, Angina, and Hypercholesterolemia

	Chronic Disease Addressed by Guidelines			
	Atrial Fibrillation	Chronic Heart Failure	Angina	Hypercholesterolemia
Guideline addressed treatment for type of patient?	Older: yes Multiple comorbidities: yes Both: yes	Older: yes Multiple comorbidities: yes Both: no	Older: yes Multiple comorbidities: yes* Both: yes*	Older: yes Multiple comorbidities: yes† Both: no
Quality of evidence discussed for type of patient?	Older: yes Multiple comorbidities: yes Average age of patients in clinical trials younger than population average, trials excluded those athigh risk for bleeding	Older: yes Multiple comorbidities: no Absence of older persons in large clinical trials	Older: yes Multiple comorbidities: no Few older patients were included in clinical trials for one possible intervention	Older: yes‡ Multiple comorbidities: no
Specific recommendations for patients with one comorbid condition?	Yes Diseases: congestive heart failure, hypertension, diabetes mellitus, angina, left ventricular hypertrophy, Wolff-Parkinson-White syndrome, hypertrophic cardiomyopathy, hyperthyroidism, pregnancy, chronic obstructive pulmonary disease	Yes Diseases: hypertension, diabetes mellitus, hypercholesterolemia, angina, atrial fibrillation, chronic obstructive pulmonary disease	Yes Diseases: hypertension, diabetes mellitus, hypercholesterolemia, congestive heart failure, aortic valve stenosis, valvular heart disease, asthma, heart block, hypertrophic cardiomyopathy, atrial fibrillation, peripheral vascular disease,hyperthyroidism, chronic kidney disease, depression, migraines	Yes Diseases: hypertension, diabetes mellitus, cardiovascular disease
Specific recommendations for patients with several comorbid conditions?	No	Yes: only for combination of cardiovascular diseases	Yes*	Yes: only for combination of diabetes mellitus and cardiovascular disease†
Time needed to treat to benefit from treatment in the context of life expectancy discussed?	No	No	No	No

*Limited to weighting severe comorbidity likely to limit life expectancy when considering treatment procedures that would lead to revascularization; asking patients in follow-up about presence of new comorbid illnesses; and the effect of severity of or treatment for comorbidities on angina. Older patients with severe angina and several comorbid illnesses may be satisfied with a reduction in symptoms that enables an improvement in physical disability.
†Limited to multiple comorbid conditions that increase cardiovascular risk (no discussion of comorbidities other than combination of diabetes mellitus and cardiovascular disease.
‡Secondary prevention trials included older persons. Guideline reports that PROSPER authors state that statin use can be extended to older persons. Conflicting data on cancer risk with statins; statins have no effect on cognition or progression of disability.
Source: Reproduced with permission from Ref. 6.

medical problems, prior ADRs, and dementia were the most prevalent patient characteristics.

Many drugs are biotransformed by cytochrome P-450 enzymes (Table 13-9), and therefore the enzymes are a site where drug interactions occur. In addition to genetic variability in these enzymes, their activity may be increased (induced) by some drugs and inhibited by others (Table 13-10). Cadieux[9] reviewed potential interactions between antidepressants and other drugs resulting from effects on cytochrome P-450 enzymes. Antidepressants are commonly administered to the elderly as up to 20% of persons 65 years of age or older are affected by clinical depression.[10] Modifications of drug action due to

Table 13-6

Examples of Classes of Drugs with Narrow Therapeutic Indexes

Tricyclic antidepressants

Anticoagulants

Antiarrhythmic agents

Note: Even small elevations in free plasma concentrations can cause potentially serious adverse reactions.
Source: Data from Ref. 21.

Table 13-7

Overview of Selected Serious Drug Interactions

Interaction	Potential Effect	Time to Effect	Recommendations and Comments
Warfarin (Coumadin) plus ciprofloxacin (Cipro), clarithromycin (Biaxin), erythromycin, metronidazole (Flagyl), or trimethoprim-sulfamethoxazole (Bactrim, Septra)	Increased effect of warfarin	Generally within 1 week	Select alternative antibiotic.
Warfarin plus acetaminophen	Increased bleeding, increased INR	Any time	Use lowest possible acetaminophen dosage and monitor INR.
Warfarin plus acetylsalicylic acid (aspirin)	Increased bleeding, increased INR	Any time	Limit aspirin dosage to 100 mg/day and monitor INR.
Warfarin plus NSAID	Increased bleeding, increased INR	Any time	Avoid concomitant use if possible; if coadministration is necessary, use a cyclooxygenase-2 inhibitor and monitor INR.
Fluoroquinolone plus divalent/trivalent cations or sucralfate (Carafate)	Decreased absorption of fluoroquinolone	Any time	Space administration by 2–4 h.
Carbamazepine (Tegretol) plus cimetidine (Tagamet), erythromycin, clarithromycin, or fluconazole (Diflucan)	Increased carbamazepine levels	Generally within 1 week	Monitor carbamazepine levels.
Phenytoin (Dilantin) plus cimetidine, erythromycin, clarithromycin, or fluconazole	Increased phenytoin levels	Generally within 1 week	Monitor phenytoin levels.
Phenobarbital plus cimetidine, erythromycin, clarithromycin, or fluconazole	Increased phenobarbital levels	Generally within 1 week	Clinical significance has not been established. Monitor phenobarbital levels.
Phenytoin plus rifampin (Rifadin)	Decreased phenytoin levels	Generally within 1 week	Clinical significance has not been established. Monitor phenytoin levels.
Phenobarbital plus rifampin	Decreased phenobarbital levels	Generally within 1 week	Monitor phenobarbital levels.
Carbamazepine plus rifampin	Decreased carbamazepine levels	Generally within 1 week	Clinical significance has not been established. Monitor carbamazepine levels.
Lithium plus NSAID or diuretic	Increased lithium levels	Any time	Decrease lithium dosage by 50% and monitor lithium levels.
Oral contraceptive pills plus rifampin	Decreased effectiveness of oral contraception	Any time	Avoid if possible. If combination therapy is necessary, have the patient take an oral contraceptive pill with a higher estrogen content (>35 µg of ethinyl estradiol) or recommend alternative method of contraception.
Oral contraceptive pills plus antibiotics	Decreased effectiveness of oral contraception	Any time	Avoid if possible. If combination therapy is necessary, recommend use of alternative contraceptive method during cycle.
Oral contraceptive pills plus troglitazone (Rezulin)	Decreased effectiveness of oral contraception	Any time	Have the patient take an oral contraceptive pill with a higher estrogen content or recommend alternative method of contraception.
Cisapride (Propulsid) plus erythromycin, clarithromycin, fluconazole, itraconazole (Sporanox), ketoconazole (Nizoral), nefazodone (Serzone), indinavir (Crixivan), or ritonavir (Norvir)	Prolongation of QT interval along with arrhythmias secondary to inhibited cisapride metabolism	Generally within 1 week	Avoid. Consider whether metoclopramide (Reglan) therapy is appropriate for the patient.
Cisapride plus class IA or class III antiarrhythmic agents, tricyclic antidepressants, or phenothiazine	Prolongation of QT interval along with arrhythmias	Any time	Avoid. Consider whether metoclopramide therapy is appropriate for the patient.

Table 13-7

Overview of Selected Serious Drug Interactions (*Continued*)

Interaction	Potential Effect	Time to Effect	Recommendations and Comments
Sildenafil (Viagra) plus nitrates	Dramatic hypotension	Soon after taking sildenafil	Absolute contraindication.
Sildenafil plus cimetidine, erythromycin, itraconazole, or ketoconazole	Increased sildenafil levels	Any time	Initiate sildenafil at a 25-mg dose.
HMG-CoA reductase inhibitor plus niacin, gemfibrozil (Lopid), erythromycin, or itraconazole	Possible rhabdomyolysis	Any time	Avoid if possible. If combination therapy is necessary, monitor the patient for toxicity.
Lovastatin (Mevacor) plus warfarin	Increased effect of warfarin	Any time	Monitor INR.
SSRI plus tricyclic antidepressant	Increased tricyclic antidepressant level	Any time	Monitor for anticholinergic excess and consider lower dosage of tricyclic antidepressant.
SSRI plus selegiline (Eldepryl) or nonselective monoamine oxidase inhibitor	Hypertensive crisis	Soon after initiation	Avoid.
SSRI plus tramadol (Ultram)	Increased potential for seizures; serotonin syndrome	Any time	Monitor the patient for signs and symptoms of serotonin syndrome.
SSRI plus St. John's wort	Serotonin syndrome	Any time	Avoid.
SSRI plus naratriptan (Amerge), rizatriptan (Maxalt), sumatriptan (Imitrex), or zolmitriptan (Zomig)	Serotonin syndrome	Possibly after initial dose	Avoid if possible. If combination therapy is necessary, monitor the patient for signs and symptoms of serotonin syndrome.

Note: INR = International Normalized Ratio; NSAID = nonsteroidal anti-inflammatory drug; HMG-CoA = 3-hydroxy-3-methylglutaryl coenzyme A reductase inhibitor; SSRI = selective serotonin reuptake inhibition.
Source: Reproduced with permission from Ref. 7.

cytochrome P-450 genetic variability may mimic drug interactions.[11] Differences in cytochrome P-450 enzymes produce 20–50-fold variations in serum levels of some drugs among different patients.[12]

CLINICALLY SIGNIFICANT ADVERSE DRUG INTERACTIONS AND POLYPHARMACY: ANESTHESIA

According to Muravchick,[13] individuals 65 years of age and older undergo almost one-third of the 25 million surgical procedures performed annually. Statistics indicate that anesthesia- and surgery-related mortality (death within 30 days of operation) increases in patients when grouped by age, for example, 60–69, 70–79 years, etc. Major surgery and emergency surgery are associated with increased mortality in the elderly. The overall mortality rate associated with anesthesia is 1 in 250,000, which decreased from 1 in 10,000 in a decade.[14] This represents significant reduction at a time when the number of older patients presenting for anesthesia care was increasing.

The decreased mortality due to anesthesia is attributed to multiple factors, including improved monitoring technology, introduction of drugs with short half-lives and more drugs that do not depend on biotransformation by liver enzymes to terminate their action, better selection and use of drugs for specific objectives (e.g., muscle relaxation, analgesia, anxiolysis, sedation) rather than depending on a few less selective drugs, improved training, expanded knowledge about drug interactions, increased information about factors that influence individual responses to drugs administered by anesthesiologists (e.g., genetic, lifestyle, age-related

change in system function, and comorbidity), and improved techniques for perioperative and intraoperative pain control.

One hallmark of patients 65 years of age and older is variability in changes associated with advancing age, both among individuals and among different organ systems in an individual.[15] Some elderly patients are totally independent, have maintained significant levels of physical activity, have preserved lean muscle mass and cardiopulmonary function, and have physiologic responses similar to those of younger individuals. Gender-related differences in younger patients may disappear in older ones, for example, sex-related differences in postoperative pain and morphine requirements.[16] It is impossible to memorize all of the nuances of anesthetic management of the elderly and interaction between anesthetic drugs and other drugs. Various reference sources are available, for example, *Manual of Drug Interactions for Anesthesiology.*[17] Generalities about pre-, intra-, and postoperative care help individualize anesthesia management in the elderly (Table 13-11). First and foremost, it is important to acknowledge that chronological age is not the primary determinant of response to anesthesia. Secondly, drugs with narrow therapeutic range and low therapeutic index are likely to object drugs for serious drug interactions.

Decrease in perioperative risk in the elderly requires rigorous preoperative assessment of organ function and reserve, good intraoperative control of concomitant disorders such as coronary artery disease, ischemic heart disease, hypertension, COPD and/or diabetes mellitus, and vigilant postoperative monitoring and pain management.[18] Elderly patients have reduced ability to maintain homeostasis, are at increased risk for complications, and complications are not well-tolerated. Thus, perioperative care must focus on minimizing the stresses of surgery and avoiding stresses of complications.[15]

Table 13-8

Adverse Drug Reaction (ADR) Risk Factors in Rank Order on a 5-Point Likert Scale* from the Delphi Survey

Risk Factor	MeanScale Score	95% CI
Medication-related factors		
Class of medication		
Anticholinergics	4.9	4.7–5.0
Benzodiazepines	4.9	4.7–5.0
Antipsychotics	4.7	4.4–5.0
Sedative/hypnotics	4.7	4.4–5.0
Non-ASA, non-COX-2 NSAIDs	4.5	4.2–4.8
TCAs	4.5	4.2–4.8
Opioid analgesics	4.5	4.2–4.8
Corticosteroids	4.4	4.1–4.7
Specific medications		
Chlorpropamide	4.7	4.4–5.0
Theophylline salts	4.6	4.3–4.9
Warfarin salts	4.6	4.2–5.0
Lithium salts	4.4	4.0–4.8
Patient characteristics		
Polypharmacy	5.0	5.0–5.0
Dementia	4.7	4.4–5.0
Multiple chronic medical problems	4.7	4.4–5.0
Renal insufficiency (CrCl <50 mL/min)	4.7	4.3–5.0
Recent hospitalization	4.5	4.2–4.8
Advanced age (>85 years)	4.5	4.2–4.8
Multiple prescribers	4.5	4.2–4.8
Regular use of alcohol (>1 fl oz/day)	4.4	4.1–4.7
Prior ADR	4.4	4.0–4.8

Note: Non-ASA, non-COX-2 NSAIDs = nonacetylsalicylic acid, noncyclooxygenase-2 nonsteroidal anti-inflammatory drugs; TCAs = tricyclic antidepressants; CrCl = creatinine clearance.
*Scale: 1 = definitely not a risk, 2 = doubtful as a risk, 3 = equivocal—may or may not be a risk, 4 = probably a risk, and 5 = definitely a risk.
Source: Reproduced with permission from Ref. 8.

As a result of responses to multiple drug treatment, multiple comorbidities, and natural history of certain diseases, symptoms observed on preoperative assessment may be diminished in intensity, nonspecific, indirect, or atypical, and therefore ignored or attributed to advanced age. Medical history may be difficult to obtain if the patient is cognitively impaired or suffers from hearing loss.[15] Compliance with drug instructions and use of nonprescription drugs and natural remedies may be difficult to determine. Presentation for emergency surgery obviously limits the extent of history that can be obtained and preanesthetic preparation such as discontinuation of medication that normally would be discontinued.

Among important polypharmacy considerations for an anesthetic management plan for an elderly patient are complications that can develop in patients taking warfarin or antidepressants (monoamine oxidase inhibitors [MAOI] and serotonin selective reuptake inhibitors [SSRI]) and residual effects of drugs administered for anesthesia care in the postoperative period.

Warfarin, a drug taken by many elderly patients for blood clotting prophylaxis, has a narrow therapeutic range. Overmedication with warfarin can interfere with hemostasis, and undermedication can increase the risk of deep venous thrombosis (DVT). Many factors can exaggerate the effects of warfarin therapy. Some examples are displacement of warfarin from plasma protein by other drugs that bind to the proteins (including many drugs administered for anesthesia care), antibiotic inhibition of vitamin K production by intestinal flora, synergistic action between warfarin and aspirin, and reduction in plasma protein by hemodilution or malnutrition.

The potential for SSRI and MAOI antidepressants to exaggerate the action of many drugs acting on the central nervous and cardiovascular systems is well known. Of particular potential importance in the elderly are interactions between these drugs and the phenylpiperidine series of opioids (meperidine, tramadol, methadone, dextromethorphan, and propoxyphene). Interaction between these analgesics and antidepressants has been implicated in serotonin toxicity reactions, including some fatalities.[19] For example, fentanyl administration to a patient taking an MAOI before surgery reputedly was responsible for the death of the patient. Serotonin toxicity is characterized by clonus, hyperreflexia, hyperthermia, and agitation.

Residual effects of neuromuscular blocking drugs and anesthetics plus postoperative opioid administration can depress respiration and have been implicated as one of many causes of delirium in the postoperative period.

A conflict regarding aspirin is evident in the literature.[18] One recommendation is to stop aspirin use 7 days before surgery to prevent complications due to bleeding. On the other hand, it is suggested that prophylactic use of low-dose aspirin (or low-dose, low-molecular-weight heparin) be used to reduce the risk of DVT in certain elderly patients. Noteworthy is that postoperative pain control and residual anesthetic effects are responsible for MIs being silent, a common cardiac complication in elderly patients.[18]

CONCLUSION

One approach to anesthetic management in the patients with so many issues related to polypharmacy is to start with low doses of drugs and administer the drugs slowly, that is, "start low and go slow."

KEY POINTS

► There is high probability that patients 65 years of age or older presenting for anesthesia care will have multiple chronic comorbidities for which they take multiple medications.

► Anesthesia care requires a broad knowledge of how comorbidities and age-related changes in system and organ function influence drug responses.

► Polypharmacy and drug interactions go hand in hand.

► CPGs rarely deal with chronic comorbidities in the elderly.

► Difficulties with polypharmacy escalate with the number of diseases a patient has and the number of drugs the patient takes.

► Likely object drugs for serious drug interactions are drugs with a narrow therapeutic range or a low therapeutic index.

► An expert panel identified 21 ADR risk factors in outpatients 65 years of age or older including 12 medication-related factors and 9 patient characteristics.

Table 13-9

Drugs that Are Substrates for Cytochrome Isoenzymes

Enzyme	Substrates	
CYP1A2	Antidepressants	Amitriptyline HCl,* clomipramine HCl,* desipramine HCl,* imipramine HCl*
	Antipsychotics	Clozapine,* haloperidol*
	Benzodiazepines	Chlordiazepoxide, diazepam
	Other	Caffeine, propranolol, tacrine HCl, theophylline,* R-warfarin*
CYP2C9	Antidepressants	Amitriptyline,* clomipramine,* imipramine*
	Other	Diazepam, losartan potassium, omeprazole, phenytoin,* S-warfarin*
CYP2C19	Antidepressants	Amitriptyline,* citalopram HBr, clomipramine,* imipramine*
	Other	Omeprazole, propranolol, S-mephenytoin
CYP2D6	Analgesics	Codeine, dextromethorphan, fentanyl, hydrocodone, meperidine HCl, methadone HCl, morphine sulfate, oxycodone HCl
	Antiarrhythmics	Flecainide acetate,* mexiletine, propafenone HCl*
	Antidepressants	Fluoxetine HCl, fluvoxamine maleate, hydroxybupropion,* paroxetine HCl, trazodone HCl, venlafaxine, tricyclic antidepressants*
	Antipsychotics	Chlorpromazine HCl,* haloperidol,* perphenazine,* risperidone,* thioridazine HCl*
	β-Blockers	Bisoprolol fumarate, labetalol HCl, metoprolol, pindolol, propranolol, timolol maleate
CYP3A4	Analgesics	Acetaminophen, alfentanil HCl, codeine, dextromethorphan
	Antiarrhythmics	Disopyramide, lidocaine HCl, quinidine
	Anticonvulsants	Carbamazepine,* ethosuximide*
	Antidepressants	Citalopram, desipramine,* nefazodone HCl, sertraline HCl, trazodone
	Antifungal drugs	Itraconazole, ketoconazole
	Antihistamines	Loratadine
	Benzodiazepines	Alprazolam, clonazepam, midazolam HCl, triazolam
	Calcium channel blockers	Amlodipine, felodipine, isradipine, mibefradil, verapamil HCl
	Chemotherapeutics	Busulfan,* doxorubicin HCl,* etoposide,* paclitaxel, tamoxifen citrate, vinblastine sulfate,* vincristine sulfate*
	Cholesterol-lowering drugs	Atorvastatin calcium,* fluvastatin sodium,* lovastatin,* pravastatin sodium,* simvastatin*
	Immunosuppressants	Cyclosporine, tacrolimus
	Macrolide antibiotics	Clarithromycin, erythromycin, troleandomycin
	Steroids	Estradiol, cortisol, methylprednisolone, prednisone, testosterone
	Other	Cisapride,* rifampin, R-warfarin*

Note: However, specific drug combinations that should be closely monitored or avoided have been identified. Most notably, coadministration of monoamine oxidase inhibitors (MAOIs) and other antidepressants is absolutely contraindicated because of the risk of severe, potentially deadly pharmacodynamic interactions (e.g., hyperpyretic crisis, severe convulsions). A minimum washout period of 14 days should precede a switch from an MAOI to any of these agents; for drugs with a longer half-life, a washout period of at least 5 weeks should precede a switch to MAOI therapy.

*Has low therapeutic-to-toxic ratio; thus, combination with antidepressants that might significantly inhibit its metabolism should be undertaken with extreme caution or avoided if possible.

Source: Reproduced with permission from Ref. 9.

► Many drugs are biotransformed by cytochrome P-450 enzymes, and therefore the enzymes are a site where drug interactions occur.

► Modifications of drug action due to cytochrome P-450 genetic variability may mimic drug interactions.

► One hallmark of patients 65 years of age and older is variability in changes associated with advancing age, both among individuals and among different organ systems in an individual.

► Chronological age is not the primary determinant of response to anesthesia.

► Gender-related differences in younger patients may disappear in older ones.

► Among important polypharmacy considerations for an anesthetic management plan for an elderly patient are complications that can develop in patients taking warfarin or antidepressants and residual effects of drugs administered for anesthesia care in the postoperative period.

► Elderly patients have reduced ability to maintain homeostasis, are at increased risk for complications, and complications are not well-tolerated.

Table 13-10

Inhibitors of Cytochrome Isoenzymes

Enzyme	Inhibitors	
CYP1A2	Antibiotics	Ciprofloxacin, clarithromycin, erythromycin, levofloxacin, norfloxacin
	Antidepressants	Citalopram,* fluoxetine HCl,* fluvoxamine maleate, mirtazapine,* paroxetine HCl,* sertraline HCl*
	Other	Cimetidine, grapefruit juice, ketoconazole
CYP2C9	Antidepressants	Fluoxetine,* fluvoxamine, paroxetine,* sertraline*
	Other	Amiodarone HCl, chloramphenicol, fluconazole, omeprazole
CYP2C19	Antidepressants	Fluoxetine, fluvoxamine, paroxetine,* sertraline*
	Other	Fluconazole, omeprazole
CYP2D6	Antiarrhythmics	Amiodarone, propafenone HCl, quinidine
	Antidepressants	Clomipramine HCl, desipramine HCl, desmethylcitalopram,* fluoxetine, S-norfluoxetine, fluvoxamine,* mirtazapine,* paroxetine, sertraline, venlafaxine*
	Antipsychotics	Fluphenazine, haloperidol
	Other	Cimetidine
CYP3A4	Antiarrhythmics	Amiodarone
	Antibiotics/ antibacterials	Clarithromycin, erythromycin, metronidazole, norfloxacin, troleandomycin
	Antidepressants	Fluoxetine,* fluvoxamine, mirtazapine,* nefazodone HCl, paroxetine,* sertraline*
	Antifungal drugs	Fluconazole, ketoconazole, itraconazole
	Other	Grapefruit juice, quinine

*Weak inhibitor.
Source: Reproduced with permission from Ref. 9.

Table 13-11

Factors Critical for Obtaining Best Outcomes from Anesthetic Care of Elderly Patients

1. Preoperative preparation of the patient to optimize medical and physiological status

2. Minimize perioperative starvation and the stresses of hypothermia, hypoxemia, and pain

3. Meticulous perioperative care to avoid complications from perturbations of fluid and electrolyte imbalance, impaired cardiovascular and respiratory function, and inappropriate pharmacotherapy

4. Careful anesthetic judgment and technique to achieve desired goals and avoid technical complications

5. Optimize physical and cognitive function

Source: Data from Ref. 15.

KEY REFERENCES

▶ Boyd et al.[6] This article discusses how multiple comorbid diseases in older patients present challenges to using an appropriate spectrum of drugs for the care of the patients.

▶ Hajjar et al.[8] This article discusses adverse drug reaction risk factors in older outpatients.

▶ Watters et al.[15] This article presents a concise overview of perioperative considerations for the elderly surgical patient.

▶ Jin and Chung.[18] This article presents a broad overview of how to minimize perioperative adverse events in the elderly.

REFERENCES

1. Salzman C. Medication compliance in the elderly. *J Clin Psychiatry.* 1995; 56(Suppl. 1):18–22.
2. Gijsen R, Hoeymans N, Schellevis FG, et al. Causes and consequences of comorbidity: a review. *J Clin Epidemiol.* 2001;54:661–674.
3. Hoffman C, Rice D, Sung HY. Persons with chronic conditions: their prevalence and costs. *JAMA.* 1996;276:1473–1479.
4. Field TS, Gurwitz JH, Harrold LR, et al. Risk factors for adverse drug events among older adults in the ambulatory setting. *J Am Geriatr Soc.* 2004;52:1349–1354.
5. Anderson G, Horvath J. Chronic conditions: making the case for ongoing care. *Robert Wood Johnson Foundation's Partnership for Solutions.* Princeton, NJ; 2002. http://www.rwjf.org/research.
6. Boyd CM, Darer J, Boult C, et al. Clinical practice guidelines and quality of care for older patients with multiple comorbid diseases: implications for pay for performance. *JAMA.* 2005;294:716–724.
7. Ament PW, Bertolino JG, Liszewski JI. Clinically significant drug interactions. *Am Fam Physician.* 2000;61:1745–1754.
8. Hajjar ER, Hanlon JT, Artz MB, et al. Adverse drug reaction risk factors in older outpatients. *Am J Geriatric Pharmacotherap.* 2003;1: 82–89.
9. Cadieux RJ. Antidepressant drug interactions in the elderly. *Postgrad Med.* 1999;106:231–249.
10. Butler RN, Lewis MI. Late-life depression: when and how to intervene. *Geriatrics.* 1995;50:44–55.
11. Samer CF, Piguet V, Dayer P, et al. Polymorphisme genetique et interactions medicamenteuses: luer importance dans le traitement de la douleur: [Genetic polymorphism and drug interactions: their importance in the treatment of pain]. *Can J Anaesth.* 2005;52:806–821.
12. Ingelman-Sundberg M. Pharmacogenetics of cytochrome P-450 and its applications in drug therapy: the past, present, and future. *Trends Pharmacol Sci.* 2004;25:193–200.
13. Muracchick S. Gerontology. Syllabus on Geriatric Anesthesiology. http://www.apicella.com/felice/Syllabus4-071301.htm, Version 7/13/01.
14. Luchsinger J, Pexton C. HRO is key concept in health care. *APSF Newsletter.* September 2004:25–27.
15. Watters JM, McClaran JC, Man-Son-Hing M. The elderly surgical patient. In: American College of Surgeons. *ACS Surgery: Principles and Practice.* Available at www.medscape.com/viewarticle/508534.
16. Aubrun F, Salvi N, Coriat P, et al. Sex- and age-related differences in morphine requirements for postoperative pain relief. *Anesthesiology.* 2005; 103:156–160.
17. Mueller RA, Lundberg DBA. *Manual of Drug Interactions for Anesthesiology.* New York: Churchill Livingstone; 1992.
18. Jin F, Chung F. Minimizing perioperative adverse events in the elderly. *Br J Anaesth.* 2001;87:608–624.
19. Gillman PK. Monoamine oxidase inhibitors, opioid analgesics, and serotonin toxicity. *Br J Anaesth.* 2005;95:434–441.
20. Buchardt RL, Jones KW. Nine key questions to address polypharmacy in the elderly. *JAAPA.* 2005;5:32–37.
21. Numeroff CB, DeVane CL, Pollock BG. Newer antidepressants and the cytochrome P-450 system. *Am J Psychiatry.* 1995;153:311–320.

Preoperative Screening for Outpatient Surgery in Geriatric Patients

L. Reuven Pasternak

INTRODUCTION

Outpatient surgery has increased dramatically in the United States over the past two decades, from 16% in 1980 and 50% in 1990 to an estimated 63% in 2000.[1] Associated with this phenomenon is an increased complexity of the surgical procedures and the medical conditions associated with patients undergoing procedures. Among the conditions of great interest and concern is the presence of patients of advanced age with the usual medical conditions associated with the aging patient. Even where prospective studies have demonstrated the technical feasibility of the surgical procedure, there has been little in the way of analysis of the extent to which age alone poses a risk factor associated with morbidity and mortality. In a retrospective analysis of over 750,000 patients undergoing outpatient surgery by Fleisher et al., postoperative distress as measured by emergency room visit and/or admission was associated with type of surgery and type and duration of anesthesia, but not for age >65.[2]

These same considerations exist for the same-day admission patient who, presumably, is undergoing even more stressful surgical procedures. Given the lack of definitive information on the relative risk of surgery in the ambulatory population, the performance of complex procedures in the older population is carried out in a wide array of hospitals.[3] This is in stark contrast with the well-demonstrated improved outcomes associated with pediatric surgery and anesthesia performed in designated "children's centers" with surgical, anesthesia, and other specialists who specialize in this age group.

Thus, the preoperative assessment of the surgical patient for ambulatory surgery poses a formidable challenge for anesthesiologists and health systems. The purpose of this assessment is to proactively identify risks associated with the perioperative period and, where possible, actively intervene to address those concerns. The list of issues associated with improved outcomes when "tightly" managed is growing and will be covered in other chapters in this book. Suffice it to say that foremost among these are hypertension, glycemic control (diabetes mellitus), and reactive airway disease (asthma). The ability to address these concerns during the preoperative and perioperative period is of increasing importance.

As the administration of anesthesia may involve a risk for the patient that equals or even excels that of the surgery itself, the pre-anesthesia evaluation is a crucial first step that may affect the clinical safety and organizational integrity of the entire surgical system. At a time when increasing pressure is being placed on system productivity and safety, declining reimbursement and increasingly scarce anesthesia resources are putting a strain on the ability to meet this demand.

Thus, while attention is provided to ensure that only appropriately prepared patients are allowed to undergo anesthesia, organizational morbidity has been the price of preventing clinical morbidity as cancellations, delays, and unnecessary "preemptive" testing have become increasingly common. Added to this strain has been the professional and personal pressure placed on anesthesiologists to resolve these issues on the day of surgery.

Several issues have combined to cause this previously simple process to become more complex:

► While the surgeon has retained the opportunity to examine and assess the patient before the scheduling of surgery, the anesthesiologist often does not have the same access to the patient that had previously existed with routine preoperative admissions.

► The selection of procedures by third-party payers to be done on an outpatient and same-day admission basis is generally determined on the presumed complexity of the procedure and not the patient's other underlying medical problems or potential issues associated with anesthesia. Consequently, the anesthesiologist is often asked to manage patients with complex medical conditions undergoing less complex surgery with little prior information.

► Organized health plans often seek to retain as much of the control of the process as possible, including determining when and where tests and consultations are to be done.

► Many hospitals and surgical units have yet to organize and develop preoperative evaluation units due to the expense of staff and space at a time when financial constraints are increasingly severe.

► There has been no consistent system for risk assessment to determine appropriate preoperative management.

► Multiple professional societies have developed specific and often contradictory guidelines on preoperative evaluation for their members.

To further compound the issues there are multiple strategies and guidelines for assessment of the patient undergoing surgery, often from organizations outside of the anesthesia community and, at times, with little input from anesthesiologists or consideration of anesthesia-related issues.

PHILOSOPHY

The purpose of the preoperative evaluation is to identify and reduce the risks associated with anesthesia and surgery. The preanesthesia evaluation is that portion of the general process of preoperative evaluation that is designed to address issues related to the perioperative management of the surgical patient by anesthesiologists. All preanesthesia activities, including evaluation prior to the day of surgery, testing, and consultation, should be undertaken only on the reasonable expectation that they will enhance the safety, comfort, and efficiency of the process for the patient, clinical staff, and overall system. Decisions concerning preanesthesia management should be associated with a consideration of how any aspect of the evaluation will affect the management and outcome of the perioperative process. Evaluations and interventions that do not have a demonstrated beneficial effect do not have value to the patient, clinician, or manager and should not be undertaken on the basis of custom or convenience.

The preanesthesia evaluation is therefore a focused assessment to address issues relevant to the safe administration of anesthesia and performance of surgery. The use of this interaction to perform unrelated general medical screening and intervention should be undertaken only in association with appropriate primary and specialty care support. Only anesthesia staff may determine a patient's fitness for administration of anesthesia and appropriate anesthesia technique. The performance of a history and physical examination by other health-care providers does not constitute a clearance for administration of anesthesia but provides information to the anesthesia staff to make that determination.

When evaluating patients for ambulatory surgery, it should be remembered that, while important, the anesthesiologist has only a temporary relationship with the patient. Their continuing care, including assessment of new or acute exacerbations of chronic conditions, should be done by their primary care provider and associated consultants with whom they will have a long-term relationship. Patients should be apprised of the fact that the preoperative evaluation is not a substitute for their regular primary physician. Requests by patients for performance of tests not deemed necessary for the performance of surgery or administration of surgery should also be referred to their primary health care source.

RISK CLASSIFICATION

While the purpose of the preanesthesia evaluation is to reduce risk, current risk classification systems are ill-equipped to provide assistance with patient classification. The first attempt to quantify risks associated with surgery was undertaken by Meyer Saklad[4] in 1941 at the request of the American Society of Anesthesiology (ASA). This effort was the first by any medical specialty to stratify risk for its patients. Saklad's system did so on the basis of mortality secondary to anesthesia based on associated preoperative medical condition. Type of anesthesia and nature of surgery were not considerations in this system and the divisions were based on empirical experience rather than on specific sets of data and reflect the techniques and standards of practice as of 50 years ago. Four preanesthesia risk categories were established ranging from category 1 (least likely to die) to category 4 (highest expectation of mortality).

The current ASA classification system is a modification of this work, adding an additional fifth category for moribund patients undergoing surgery in a desperate attempt to preserve life. Numerous studies have demonstrated an association of mortality with ASA class independent of anesthetic technique.[5–17] However, this data has limited application as it relates to mortality as its sole outcome and is based on anesthetic techniques as practiced more than 20 years ago. Apfelbaum[18] and Meridy,[19] for example, have noted a lack of correlation between ASA status and cancellations, unplanned admissions, and other perioperative complications in outpatient surgery.

Thus, while useful as a broad assessment of preoperative medical status, the current ASA classification is limited in its ability to truly establish risk or serve as a basis for formulating clinical guidelines without an associated risk index for the surgical procedure. In addition, while concerning itself with the identification of risk, there is a remarkable lack of data delineating outcomes in ambulatory surgery and anesthesia. When the ASA Task Force on Preanesthesia Evaluation recently issued its recommendations for all preoperative assessment, it initially tried to do so using an evidence-based approach linking specific tests and interventions with designated outcomes. The literature in this area for all of anesthesia was such that of over 1200 articles identified in this area fewer than 30 fit the criteria for use. Lack of information of sufficient scientific validity mandated that the guideline development had to yield to an advisory that was based on consensus opinion subject to further scientific investigation and validation using evidence-based studies at a future date. For purposes of risk stratification, the ASA adopted a modification of the risk index system for patient medical severity and surgical severity as used by the other most commonly used algorithm for patient preoperative assessment, the AHA/ACC guidelines for preoperative assessment of the cardiac patient for noncardiac surgery.[20]

PATIENT AND PROCEDURE SELECTION

The nature of patient and procedure selection is a function of medical status, surgical procedure, and, in the case of outpatient surgery, availability of appropriate postoperative assistance. While ambulatory surgical procedures are by definition not emergencies, many are nonetheless relatively urgent in nature. The delay of some procedures, such as biopsies for staging of oncology treatments, may unnecessarily delay and inappropriately compromise the care of the patient. Surgeons and anesthesiologists must make a judgment as to whether delay will truly reduce the risk for the patient or merely postpone the inevitable task of dealing with a potentially difficult challenge in the operating room. Finally, while mandates for early discharge by regulatory and managed care groups are based almost wholly on postoperative physiologic status, patient comfort and availability of appropriate assistance at home should be major considerations in this process.

▶ Time of the evaluation

It has been a common assumption that a preoperative visit prior to the day of surgery confers some added measure of safety and comfort for patients. On the basis of this assumption, patients have often been asked to take the time and expense required to comply with such requirements while hospitals and anesthesiologists have had to staff centers able to handle this demand.

The literature on the utility of preoperative evaluation prior to the day of surgery is scant and at best inconclusive. Fisher's study[21] demonstrated for outpatients and inpatients that prior preanesthesia evaluation by anesthesia staff reduced cancellations, tests, and consultations. This study was thus useful in demonstrating the need for a screening mechanism that allowed for patient assessment prior to the day of surgery. However, in asserting that this needs to be done by anesthesia staff, it should be remembered that studies comparing this system to others with more selective criteria for requiring an actual visit prior to the day of surgery have not been done. Similarly, studies asserting that no preanesthesia evaluation was necessary involve small numbers of healthy patients undergoing minor procedures.[22,23] Some of the most comprehensive work in this area has been by Twersky et al.,[24] which indicates that patient evaluations on the day of surgery may be performed in a manner that is safe and effective. Even in these studies, patients were not stratified by medical status or surgical procedure and were not relevant for the larger patient population managed by most anesthesiologists.

Consequently, recommendations that all patients required preoperative evaluations by anesthesia staff prior to surgery cannot be considered justified on the basis of this data alone. The requirement for a preoperative evaluation prior to the day of surgery should be based on the need to obtain appropriate information and provide instructions in a manner that cannot be done without this direct personal contact.

In discussions with major academic and private practice medical center directors, it has been observed by this author that the percentage of patients required having an on-site visit prior averages about 25–33%. The preoperative assessment must be a balance between patient convenience and the need to have information available in a timely fashion to allow for planning appropriate preoperative and perioperative management. While the ideal system may include a preoperative evaluation prior to the day of surgery for all patients, the logistics of patient schedules and their often otherwise healthy status makes this ideal impractical and, at times, unnecessary. This point is of significant concern to hospital preoperative evaluation staff who believe that resources may be inappropriately committed to patients with little need of those services to the detriment of others with more extensive medical and surgical issues and with waste of resources needed elsewhere.

The algorithm adopted by the ASA for preoperative evaluation (Fig. 14-1)[25] recognizes that there are categories of patients (healthy individuals for low-risk surgical procedures) for whom a preanesthesia assessment consisting of information being made available prior to the day of surgery for review is sufficient. Similarly, there are some individuals for whom assessment prior to the day of surgery is mandated by their medical condition and/or planned surgery. It is difficult to provide a standard recommendation as to how ambulatory surgical centers should place their patients into these categories; much depends on the ease of availability and validity of data provided prior to the day of surgery. What is uniformly recommended is that appropriate information should be made available to anesthesia staff prior to the day of surgery to allow for review and appropriate action. An example of conditions for which assessment by anesthesia directed staff prior to the day of surgery is provided in Fig. 14-2.

▶ Personnel performing the evaluation

One of the most controversial topics in preanesthesia evaluation is that of who is best able to perform the evaluation. It is often asserted that anesthesiologists should retain all preanesthesia interview responsibilities. The logic of this position is derived from the need to have anesthesiology viewed as a specialty by the patient directly involved with their care and to ensure that appropriate information is provided. This goal is laudable but, in fact, may not be practical or necessary. This perspective evolved at a time when the concept of preoperative assessment was relatively new and anesthesia staff in more plentiful supply. The issues of appropriate patient selection, testing, and consultation were less well defined, and the experience of nonanesthesiologists was limited. At this time, anesthesia staffs of all varieties are in short supply and their displacement from the operating room should be done only with clear indication of benefit.

As with many other aspects of this field, there is much in the way of common practice that, while not subjected to the rigors of scientific comparison, has been found to be successful. One is the use of physician extenders such as physician assistants, advanced clinical nurses, and nurse practitioners. Operating under the supervision of anesthesiology staff, these individuals are frequently able to effectively screen patients in a manner that is efficient and effective. Over time, they also serve as excellent professional representatives of the specialty and can enhance the public perception of the specialty.

When not performed by anesthesiologists or their associates, the assessment of patients with significant medical problems should be provided by the patient's primary care provider as the person most familiar with the patient's medical condition. The availability of facsimile (FAX) transmission permits information to be sent to preoperative evaluation centers in time for review. In order to prevent the occasional brief note on a prescription pad, a standard form for review should be provided that allows the anesthesiologist to identify those patients for whom additional intervention might be necessary.

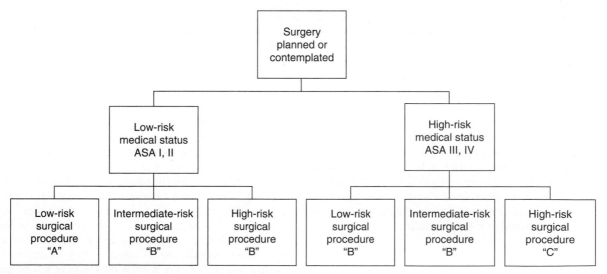

FIGURE 14-1 Illustrative algorithm for preanesthesia evaluation. *Source:* Adapted from Ref. 25.
Low-risk procedure: pose minimal physiologic stress and risk to the patient independent of medical condition (e.g., office-based, minor surgery)
Intermediate-risk procedure: moderate physiologic stress and risk with minimal blood loss, fluid shift, or postoperative change in normal physiology
High-risk procedure: significant perioperative and postoperative physiologic stress
A: patient may have preanesthesia assessment on the day of surgery on the basis of available preoperative data
B: patient may require preanesthesia consultation based on the nature of the patient's medical condition and planned procedure
C: patient should have preanesthesia consultation with anesthesia staff prior to the day of surgery.

General
Medical condition inhibiting ability to engage in normal daily activity
Medical conditions necessitating continual assistance or monitoring at home within the past 6 months
Admission within the past 2 months for acute or exacerbation of chronic condition

Cardiocirculatory
History of angina, coronary artery disease, myocardial infarction
Symptomatic arrhythmias
Poorly controlled hypertension (diastolic > 110, systolic > 160)
History of congestive heart failure

Respiratory
Asthma/COPD requiring chronic medication or with acute exacerbation and progression within past 6 months
History of major airway surgery or unusual airway anatomy
Upper and/or lower airway tumor or obstruction
History of chronic respiratory distress requiring home ventilatory assistance or monitoring

Endocrine
Insulin-dependent diabetes mellitus
Adrenal disorders
Active thyroid disease

Neuromuscular
History of seizure disorder or other significant CNS disease (e.g., multiple sclerosis)
History of myopathy or other muscle disorders

Hepatic
Any active hepatobiliary disease or compromise

Musculoskeletal
Kyphosis and/or scoliosis causing functional compromise
Temporomandibular joint disorder
Cervical or thoracic spine injury

Oncology
Patients receiving chemotherapy
Other oncology process with significant physiologic residual or compromise

Gastrointestinal
Massive obesity (>140% ideal body weight)
Hiatal hernia
Symptomatic gastroesophageal reflux

FIGURE 14-2 Conditions for which preoperative evaluation may be recommended prior to the day of surgery.

In all instances, clearance for anesthesia and selection of the appropriate technique is the responsibility of the anesthesiologist, using whatever information may be provided by others as a guide in the decision process.

Using these suggestions, a significant majority of outpatient procedures and substantial patients may be managed with evaluation on the day of surgery. A major consideration in developing such systems is the unique aspect of the health-care system in different regions of the country and, sometimes, the same city. The recommended algorithm should be modified to reflect the appropriate relationships between clinicians, their patients, and their health systems.

► Laboratory testing

Laboratory and other diagnostic tests associated with preoperative evaluations represent one of the most costly issues associated with surgery. It is difficult to attach a precise dollar cost on this activity. However, it is conservatively estimated that at least 10% of the over $30 billion spent on laboratory testing each year is for preoperative evaluation. The traditional system of the protocol "battery of tests" evolved from a lack of clear definition of their role in preoperative screening, insufficient information on their utility, and a mistaken belief that voluminous information, no matter how irrelevant, enhanced the safety of care and reduced physician liability for adverse events. Protocol testing relieved physicians and their associates of the responsibility of decision making as an easier, though more costly, alternative to selective tests based on patients' individual health profiles.

At a time when the cost of care and the convenience of patients is a major concern, the role of tests as a screening device is rightfully diminishing. The patient history, physical examination, and judgment of the physician are replacing protocols as the basis for testing. While information about other aspects of the preoperative evaluation may be ambiguous, there is extensive literature and experience to support the selective use of testing, which also confirms that the use of broad testing panels has a strong tendency to result in excessive testing. Laboratory testing, like all areas of medical intervention, should be undertaken on a "value-added" basis: a reasonable expectation that a potential issue exists that is relevant to anesthesia.

The utility of the preanesthesia test is based on several key considerations. The first issue is *relevance*. While some abnormalities are clearly of concern (e.g., cardiac and respiratory), others may have little or no effect on anesthetic plan and outcome, and thus do not warrant thorough investigation in this format. The second issue is the *prevalence* of the condition in both symptomatic and asymptotic patients. A low prevalence in asymptotic patients would indicate that screening would be of little use. The third issue is that of *test sensitivity and specificity*. Low sensitivity permits false negative results and patients at risk undergo anesthesia without appropriate preparation. Low specificity causes a large number of false positives with patients being subjected to additional testing, with their coincident inconvenience, costs, and potential morbidity. Testing should therefore be done for conditions that are medically relevant using tests of high sensitivity and specificity. A final consideration is cost. Selection of alternative testing modalities should also take into consideration the financial and nonfinancial costs of testing with selection of the less costly approach where it does not compromise the quality of the information desired. Testing in the asymptomatic population should only be done in patients for whom the potential condition is significant and of reasonable prevalence with tests of reasonable sensitivity and specificity.

Attaching precise numbers to the above caveats is difficult and is the subject of cost-benefit and cost-effectiveness analysis for each of the tests concerned. While this has not been established for many of the routine diagnostic tests that we employ, it has been established in the medical, surgical, and anesthesia literature that the use of screening tests without specific indication is not appropriate. In a study of 19,980 tests on 1000 patients, Korvin et al.[26] encountered 2223 abnormal values of which 993 were initially considered to be unanticipated. Of these, 223 led to further evaluation and new diagnoses, and in only one case was the diagnosis unrelated to other known medical issues and resulted in new patient care. Interestingly, this involved elevated liver function studies in a male who had received halothane anesthesia and for whom the recommendation was made that this agent be avoided. Robbins and Mushlin,[27] in evaluating preoperative testing from a medical perspective, provide an excellent review of the sensitivity, specificity, and consequent utility of a wide range of tests. Kaplan et al.[28] reviewed the records of 2000 patients undergoing elective surgery who received a routine battery of complete blood cell count, differential cell count, prothrombin time, partial thromboplastin time, platelet count, glucose level, and six channel chemistries. They found that 60% of these tests would not have been performed had they been done only on the basis of clinical indication and that of these only. Twenty-two percent revealed abnormalities that might have affected perioperative management. These findings were replicated by Turnbull and Buck[29] in a review of 1010 otherwise healthy patients undergoing cholecystectomy. They discovered 225 abnormal results in 5003 tests of which 104 were judged to be important and only four patients might have derived some benefit.

In addition to protocols lacking critical review, another reason for excess testing often relates to a lack of communication between medical colleagues. A retrospective study by Kitz et al.[30] compared the use of chest x-rays, electrocardiograms, and chemistry panels in patients undergoing knee arthroscopy and diagnostic laparoscopy or laparoscopic tubal ligation. The groups were divided into patients electively admitted prior to the day of surgery and those who were outpatients. Both patient groups were healthy ASA I and II with tests ordered in the first group by the admitting surgeon and in the second by the anesthesiologist. Though medically similar, the groups had significantly different rates of testing with the higher surgical rate attributable to their desire to not have cases canceled and lack of information from anesthesia staff about test indications.

Additional studies of specific tests have also confirmed the use of the history and physical as a basis for specific tests. Urinalysis, long a mainstay of testing and still required by law in some states, has been found to be of extremely limited use in patients without preexisting medical condition or positive physical findings.[31] Their use for prevention of postoperative surgical problems outside the realm of genitourinary surgery was addressed by Lawrence et al.[32] In a classic application of cost-benefit analysis, it was determined that routine urinalysis for all knee replacement surgery in the United States would cost $1,500,000 per wound infection prevented and not add to the safety or effectiveness of the surgery. Rucker et al.,[33] in a review of 905 routine chest x-rays for elective surgical procedures, determined that 368 had no risk factors by history and physical, and that only one had an abnormality, with even that being minor in nature. Of the remaining 504 remaining patients, 22% (114) had serious abnormalities, virtually all of which would have been anticipated by the history and physical examination. Charpak et al.,[34] in a retrospective review of postoperative complications, found no circumstances in which absence of a chest x-ray in patients without prior pulmonary disease would have altered outcome or management, even when the complications were respiratory in nature. In both studies, no correlation was established between age and occurrence of positive chest x-rays in patients independent of coexisting positive history or physical examination. Similar findings are available for hemoglobin determinations,[35,36] serum chemistries,[37] and pulmonary function testing.[38]

In accordance with the philosophy that a test is undertaken because of a realistic possibility of adding valuable information, protocol screening without specific indication is not appropriate. In addition to lack of utility for the physician, such testing may in fact do harm to patients through unnecessary and potentially invasive interventions, heightened anxieties, and markedly increased costs that may place the physician in a position of having to explain proceeding with surgery in the face of incomplete or irrelevant data. As observed in the literature, there is little rationale for testing other than on the basis of specific indicators. Testing should be done only on an expectation of a finding that might have reasonable relevance for anesthesia and surgery based on:

▶ presence of a positive finding on the history and physical examination

▶ need of the surgeon or other clinician for baseline values in anticipation of significant changes due to surgery or other medical interventions (e.g., chemotherapy)

▶ patient's inclusion in a population at higher risk for the presence of a relevant condition even though they may exhibit no individual signs of that condition themselves

The associated recommendations are noted in Fig. 14-3. By this standard, patients less than 50 years of age without coexisting medical disease would require no preoperative testing, while patients greater than 50 years of age an electrocardiogram as per the anesthesiologist. Further testing is done on an individualized basis as per the history, physical, and nature of the surgical procedure. It is conservatively estimated that such testing at our institution could reduce preoperative testing by 70%.

▶ Consultations

Specialty consultations should not be obtained on an automatic basis because of organ-specific problems but because there is a specific

(These tests are those required for administration of anesthesia and are not intended to limit those required by surgeons for issues specific to their surgical management)

Electrocardiogram
Age 50 or older
Diabetes mellitus (age 30 or older)
Hypertension
Current or past significant cardiac disease
Current or past circulatory disease
Renal, thyroid, or other metabolic disease

Chest x-ray
Asthma or COPD that is debilitating or with change of symptoms or acute episode within past 6 months
Cardiothoracic procedure

Serum Chemistries
Renal disease
Adrenal or thyroid disorders
Diuretic therapy
Chemotherapy

Urinalysis
Diabetes mellitus
Renal disease
Genitourologic procedure
Recent genitourinary infection
Metabolic disorder involving renal function

Complete Blood Count
Hematological disorder
Vascular procedure
Chemotherapy

Coagulation Studies
Anticoagulation therapy
Vascular procedure

Pregnancy Testing
Patients for whom pregnancy might complicate the surgery
Patients of uncertain status by history

FIGURE 14-3 Recommended laboratory testing.

issue that remains to be addressed. For example, in some centers it is routine to require all patients with any cardiac risk factor to be seen by a cardiologist prior to surgery. These consultations often provide no new information or insight other than that which can be obtained by a review of existing records and a basic history and physical examination. At worst, these requests for consultation are at times taken as a request for suggestions concerning the perioperative management with recommendations made that are based on erroneous assumptions concerning the risks associated with anesthetic techniques. When indicated, requests for consultations should be specifically and narrowly worded to request the specialist's evaluation of the patient's clinical condition, and not to "clear for anesthesia."

SUMMARY

The older patient undergoing elective surgical procedures is not at risk so much from age alone but from discrete medical conditions that pose risks to patients of all ages. In assessing these patients, risk and management of that risk should be designed to address the optimal

reasonable management of those conditions in a coherent, comprehensive fashion.

KEY POINTS

▶ The literature on the utility of preoperative evaluation prior to the day of surgery is scant and at best inconclusive. The requirement for a preoperative evaluation prior to the day of surgery should be based on the need to obtain appropriate information and provide instructions in a manner that cannot be done without this direct personal contact.

▶ While information about other aspects of the preoperative evaluation may be ambiguous, there is extensive literature and experience to support the selective use of testing which also confirms that the use of broad testing panels has a strong tendency to result in excessive testing.

▶ The utility of the preanesthesia test is based on several key considerations, including relevance, the prevalence of the condition in both symptomatic and asymptotic patients, test sensitivity and specificity, and cost.

▶ Additional studies of specific tests have also confirmed the use of the history and physical as a basis for specific tests.

▶ In accordance with the philosophy that a test is undertaken because of a realistic possibility of adding valuable information, protocol screening without specific indication is not appropriate. Testing should be done only on an expectation of a finding that might have reasonable relevance for anesthesia and surgery based on presence of a positive finding on the history and physical examination, need of the surgeon or other clinician for baseline values in anticipation of significant changes due to surgery or other medical interventions (e.g., chemotherapy), patient's inclusion in a population at higher risk for the presence of a relevant condition even though they may exhibit no individual signs of that condition themselves.

▶ Patients less than 50 years of age without coexisting medical disease require no preoperative testing while patients greater than 50 years of age an electrocardiogram as per the anesthesiologist. Further testing is done on an individualized basis as per the history, physical, and nature of the surgical procedure.

KEY ARTICLE

▶ American Society of Anesthesiologists Task Force on Preanesthesia Evaluation. Practice advisory for preanesthesia evaluation. *Anesthesiology.* 2002;96:485–496.

REFERENCES

1. National Center for Health Statistics (NCHS). Health, United States, 2002, with Chartbook on Trends in the Health of Americans. Table 96. Hyattsville, Maryland; 2002. http://www.cdc.gov/nchs.
2. Fleisher LF, Pasternak LR, Lyles A. A novel index of elevated risk of inpatient hospital admission immediately following outpatient surgery. *Arch Surg,* in press.
3. Wachtel RE, Dexter F. Differentiating among hospitals performing physiologically complex operative procedures in the elderly. *Anesthesiology.* 2004;100(6):1552–1561.
4. Saklad M. Grading of patients for surgical procedures. *Anesthesiology.* 1941;2:281–284.
5. Brown DL. Anesthetic risk: a historical perspective. In: Brown DL, ed. *Risk and Outcome in Anesthesia.* Philadelphia: JB Lippincott Co.; 1988.
6. Derrington MC, Smith G. A review of anesthetic risk, morbidity, and mortality. *Br J Anaesth.* 1987;59:815–833.
7. Farrow SC, Fowkes FGR, Lunn JN, et al. Epidemiology in anaesthesia II: factors affecting mortality in hospital. *Br J Anaesth.* 1982;54:811–816.
8. Fowkes SC, Fowkes FGR, Lunn JN, et al. Epidemiology in anaesthesia III: factors affecting mortality in hospitals. *Br J Anaesth.* 1982;54:811–816.
9. Goldstein A, Keats AS. The risk of anesthesia. *Anesthesiology.* 1970;33:130–143.
10. Lunn JN, Farrow SC, Fowkes FGR, et al. Epidemiology in anaesthesia I: anaesthetic practice over 20 years. *Br J Anaesth.* 1982;54:803–809.
11. Lunn JN, Hunter AR, Scott DB. Anesthesia-related surgical mortality. *Anaesthesia.* 1983;38:1090–1096.
12. Vacanti CJ, VanHouten RJ, Hill RC. A statistical analysis of the relationship of physical status to postoperative mortality in 68,388 cases. *Anesth Analg.* 1970;49:564–566.
13. Keats AS. Anesthesia mortality in perspective. *Anesth Analg.* 1990;70:113–119.
14. Rao TLK, Jacobs KH, El-Etr AA. Reinfarction following anesthesia in patients with myocardial infarction. *Anesthesiology.* 1983;59:499–505.
15. Dripps RD, Lamont A, Eckenhoff JE. The role of anesthesia in surgical mortality. *JAMA.* 1961;178:261–266.
16. Marx GF, Mateo CV, Orkin LR. Computer analysis of postanesthetic deaths. *Anesthesiology.* 1973;39:54–58.
17. Carter DC, Campbell D. Evaluation of the risks of surgery. *Br Med Bull.* 1988;44:322–340.
18. Apfelbaum JL. Preoperative evaluation, laboratory screening, and selection of adult surgical outpatients in the 1990s. *Anesthesiol Rev.* 1990;17:4–12.
19. Meridy HW. Criteria for selection of ambulatory surgical patients and guidelines for anesthetic management: a retrospective study of 1553 cases. *Anesth Analg.* 1982;61:921–926.
20. Fleisher LA. Applying the new AHA/ACC perioperative cardiovascular evaluation guidelines to the elderly outpatient. SAMBA. 2002.
21. Fischer SP. Development and effectiveness of an anesthesia preoperative evaluation clinic in a teaching hospital. *Anesthesiology.* 1996;85:196–206.
22. Arellano R, Cruise C, Chung F. Timing of the anesthetist's preoperative outpatient interview. *Anesth Analg.* 1989;68:645–648.
23. Rosenblatt MA, Bradford C, Miller R, Zahl K. A preoperative interview by an anesthesiologist does not lower preoperative anxiety in outpatients. *Anesthesiology.* 1989;71:A926.
24. Twersky RS, Frank D, Lebovits A. Timing of preoperative evaluation for surgical outpatients—does it matter? Part II. *Anesthesiology.* 1990;73:A1.
25. American Society of Anesthesiologists Task Force on Preanesthesia Evaluation. Practice advisory for preanesthesia evaluation. *Anesthesiology.* 2002;96:485–496.
26. Korvin CC, Pearce RH, Stanley J. Admissions screening: clinical benefits. *Ann Intern Med.* 1975;83:197–203.
27. Robbins JA, Mushlin AI. Preoperative evaluation of the healthy patient. *Med Clin N Am.* 1979;63:1145–1156.
28. Kaplan EB, Sheiner LB, Boeckman AJ, et al. The usefulness of preoperative laboratory testing. *JAMA.* 1985;253:3576–3581.
29. Turnbull JM, Buck C. The value of preoperative screening investigations in otherwise health individuals. *Arch Intern Med.* 1987;147:1101–1105.
30. Kitz DS, Slusarz-Ladden C, Lecky JH. Hospital resources used for inpatient and ambulatory surgery. *Anesthesiology.* 1988;69:383–386.
31. Zilva JF. Is unselective urine biochemical urine testing cost effective? *Br Med J.* 1985;291:323–325.
32. Lawrence VA, Gafni A, Gross M. The unproven utility of the preoperative urinalysis: economic evaluation. *J Clin Epidemiol.* 1989;42:1185–1191.
33. Rucker L, Frye BD, Staten MA. Usefulness of chest roentgenograms in preoperative patients. *JAMA.* 1983;250:3209–3211.
34. Charpak Y, Blery C, Chastang C, et al. Prospective assessment of a protocol for selective ordering of preoperative chest x-rays. *Can J Anaesth.* 1988;35:259–264.
35. Hackman T, Steward DJ. What is the value of preoperative hemoglobin determinations in pediatric outpatients? *Anesthesiology.* 1989;71:A1168.
36. O'Conner ME, Drasner K. Preoperative laboratory testing of children undergoing elective surgery. *Anesth Analg.* 1990;70:176–180.
37. Bold AM, Currin B. Use and abuse of clinical chemistry in surgery. *Br Med J.* 1965;2:1051–1052.
38. Zibrak JD, O'Donnell CR, Marton K. Indications for pulmonary function testing. *Ann Intern Med.* 1990;112:763–771.

Geriatric Trauma

Mahmood Jaberi

INTRODUCTION

In the United States, injuries lead to more than 800,000 hospital admissions and 28% of all deaths in the geriatric population.[1] In patients above 65 years of age, trauma ranks seventh as the cause of death and consumes about 25% of trauma care dollars in the United States. The heterogeneity in this segment of the population with respect to their physical health, along with complexities related to social, cultural, and economic diversity mandate special considerations in strategic planning of their treatment.

Degenerative changes in structure and reduced reserve function of different organ systems are universal in the elderly. Although these changes may not be readily apparent in normal daily life, following trauma, this diminution in reserve function plays a critical role in the outcome and survival of these patients. Presence of significant comorbidities particularly of the cardiopulmonary, hepatic, or renal systems affects the intensity of medical care, length of hospital stay, and health-care costs.

The trauma management of geriatric patient should be directed toward a favorable, cost-effective, functionally independent outcome. This goal can be reached by collaborative and systematic efforts incorporated between different specialties including geriatrics, surgery, anesthesiology, and intensive care, along with nursing personnel, respiratory therapy, rehabilitation medicine, nutrition, physiotherapy, psychiatry, social work, and the emergency medical service (EMS) system. Evidently, ideal outcome results are more attainable if the trauma care is managed in a well-organized trauma system. The dedicated trauma specialists, state-of-the-art diagnostic and therapeutic facilities, and comprehensive medical care from admission to rehabilitation improve outcome.

In spite of abundant literature in the field of geriatric trauma and anesthetic management, most of the studies are retrospective without proper standardization and firm recommendations.[2] To improve the standard of care and achieve desirable outcomes, well-designed, prospective controlled studies are needed.

▶ Why is the geriatric trauma mortality rate high?

Overall, 28% of all trauma deaths occur in the elderly. Although the mortality rate has dropped from 20% in the 1960s to about 8% in the past decade, emergency procedures continue to carry a higher risk of morbidity and mortality. Furthermore, elderly patients who survive trauma may have poor functional outcomes. In a study of more than 38,000 trauma patients older than 65 years, it was found that 50% were discharged home and 25% were discharged to a skilled nursing facility. Inaba et al. reported a significant decline in independent function (98% down to 68%) at 2.8 years after injury in elderly patients and 25% required home care.[3] However, the risk to life due to complications of prolonged bed rest in most cases makes surgical intervention preferable to conservative treatment.

The following factors contribute to the high incidence of morbidity and mortality in geriatric patients: inadequate information about the premorbid functional status; insufficient time for pre-op preparation; personnel and facility availability; optimization of cardiopulmonary status; impact of trauma on different organ function; diminished reserve and increased demands of different organ systems. In addition, the factors of age, gender, comorbidities, and severity of injury have been investigated and evaluated in different studies focused on morbidity and mortality in geriatric patients.

Age

The American College of Surgery Committee on Trauma compared the survival rate of 3833 patients above 65 years of age versus 42,944 patients under 65. They found that the mortality rate rose sharply between the ages of 45 and 55 years and was doubled at age 75. This age-dependent survival decrement occurred at all injury severity scores and body regions involved. Increased trauma mortality rate begins at age 45 and there is 2.46-fold increase in early mortality and 4.64-fold increase in late mortality (death after 24 hours) in injured patients.[4] For each year increase in age beyond 65 years, the odds of geriatric patients dying after trauma increases 6.8%.

Taylor et al. retrospectively studied the outcome of 37,762 trauma patients. They excluded 6509 young patients under 18 years of age, 4062 patients with penetrating injuries, 807 burn patients, and 10,927 patients with minor injuries whose length of stay was less than 24 hours or patients with early nonpreventable death due to hemorrhagic shock and severe traumatic brain injury and they found that the mortality rate in 15,457 patients, age between 18 and 64 years, was 1.8% and in 7117 patients above 65 years of age raised to 6.7%. They found that age was an independent predictor of outcome for mortality and length of stay.[5] The senile degenerative changes and impaired functional reserve noted in every major organ system played a role for higher morbidity and mortality in geriatric trauma patients.

Despite these findings, Jacobs et al., in developing management guidelines for geriatric trauma, recommend "other factors being equal, advanced age, in and of itself, is not predictive of poor outcome after trauma, and therefore, should not be used as the sole criterion for denying or limiting care in this patient population."[2]

Table 15-1

Mortality Rate

Age	Without Preexisting Disease	With Preexisting Disease
65–74	11.1%	13.9%
>75	27.9%	30.1%

Gender

Trauma mortality rate is higher in males than females. In the United States, for patients under 65 years of age, the incidence of motor vehicular death is higher in men than women. The incidence of fall and related mortality increases with advancing age, especially in females after menopause.

Comorbidities

The comorbidities associated with organ dysfunction usually determine the outcome. Preexisting conditions such as hepatic disease, renal disease, and cancer affect the length of hospital stay, morbidity, and mortality rates. Jacobs and coworkers demonstrated that preexisting disease adversely affects the outcome. However, in very old patients, the degenerative functional changes of aging have a more negative effect on survival than preexisting conditions.[2] Miltzman et al., in a study of 7798 multiple trauma patients, found that the effect of preexisting conditions on mortality is independent of age and Injury Severity Score (Table 15-1). This effect becomes progressively less important above age 55 and/or Injury Severity Score >20.[6]

COMMON TRAUMAS IN GERIATRIC POPULATIONS

▶ Type and mechanism of injury

Types of injury are classically divided into blunt and penetrating injuries. Blunt trauma is much more prevalent in elderly trauma patients. Penetrating injuries due to stab wounds or gunshot wounds also occur in the elderly, though at a much lower rate. Overall, the vast majority of injury-related hospital admissions in the geriatric population are due to falls, motor vehicle accidents (MVAs), assaults, and suicidal attempts. Thermal injury occurs less frequently in elderly patients. Other types of injuries resulting from biologic, nuclear, chemical, or environmental hazards are also possible but go beyond the scope of this chapter and are not discussed.

Falls

Falls are the most common cause of trauma in the elderly population. Its incidence as well as the severity of injury rises significantly with advancing age and after menopause.[7] The elderly trauma patient sustaining falls should be evaluated for the risk factors listed in Table 15-2. In the elderly, falls predominantly occur from a standing position, a chair, a wheelchair, a commode, on a sidewalk, or after slipping and tripping. Though multilevel falls, such as a fall down the stairs, occur less frequently, they carry a much higher risk of morbidity and mortality. About 90% of fractures, including pelvis, hip, and forearm fractures, are due to falls, and 40% of the patients residing in nursing homes are admitted with fall injuries.

In a retrospective study of 43,297 patients 65 years and older admitted to Pennsylvania hospitals between 1988 and 2000, Grossman et al. found that 40.9% were above 80 years with a female preponderance. Trauma falls occurred in 64.5% of the patients. Overall, 98% of admissions were in blunt trauma categories.[8]

Table 15-2

Risk Factors for Falls

1. Visual impairment
2. Gait and balance abnormality
3. Cognitive impairment
4. Use of sedatives and antidepressants
5. Lower extremity disability
6. Foot problems
7. Use of assistant device
8. Lack of safety awareness

Sterling et al., in a retrospective study of 1512 trauma patients, found that the incidence of severe injury is higher in geriatric patients[7] (Table 15-3). They recommend "having a higher index of suspicion for potential serious injury, even after simple same level falls, and it is necessary to diagnose and treat them in a timely fashion."

Motor vehicle accident

The mechanism of injury in older-age patients is somehow different than in younger age groups. In teenage patients, MVAs are usually due to reckless driving and irresponsible behavior. In elderly patients, the common causes are erratic driving, passing through stop signs, T-bone accidents, and pedestrian struck. These constitute 24.5% of elderly traumatic injuries. Alcohol use has been noted in about 20% of elderly patients involved in falls and MVAs, but this ratio is higher in younger patients.[9]

The majority of patients are admitted to level 1 trauma centers secondary to MVAs. Older persons may be involved in the accident as driver, passenger, or pedestrian. According to the U.S. National Center for Health Statistics, elderly males (White, Black, or Hispanic) above the age of 65 are two to three times more likely to die in a MVA compared to females of the corresponding race. This difference is higher among American Indians and Alaskan natives.[1] The risk factors for MVAs in geriatric patients are demonstrated in Table 15-4. Clark and his coworkers showed that MVA crash fatalities more likely happen in intersections in urban areas. Alcohol use and illicit drug use were noted in 50% and 12% of patients, respectively.[10]

The mechanism of MVAs in geriatric patients falls into one of the following categories: rear impact, head-on collision, side impact, ejection injuries, and pedestrian injuries.

Rear Impact This type of collision often happens to drivers who travel at lower speeds as compared to other vehicles. In an unrestrained

Table 15-3

Trauma in Old versus Young Patients

	Age >65	Age <65
Number of patients	333	1149
Falls	48%	7%
Serious injury	30%	4%
Head and neck	47%	23%
Chest injury	23%	9%
Pelvic and extremity injuries	27%	15%

Table 15-4

Risk Factors Contributing to Motor Vehicle Accidents in the Elderly

1. Slow response
2. Poor eyesight
3. Confusion
4. Transient ischemic attacks (TIA)
5. Myocardial infarction
6. Drugs and alcohol
7. Hypoglycemia

driver, a rear impact collision usually causes abrupt extension-flexion injuries (whiplash) with manifestation of stretching, straining, and tearing of the cervical ligaments and muscles. In more severe cases, cervical spine fractures with possible neurological injuries may occur.

Head-On Collision Head-on collisions, which result in additive forces during impact, often cause serious injuries with high morbidity and mortality. Confusion, transient ischemic attacks, driving under the influence of drugs, and alcohol may play a contributory factor in the accident. Depending on the speed and the energy at impact, this type of trauma may cause multiple injuries including head injury, facial fractures, spine injuries, chest wall fractures, pulmonary lacerations, major vascular tears, intra-abdominal injuries, pelvic fractures, extremity fractures, and even death at the scene of the accident. Moran et al., in a retrospective study of front seat passengers involved in frontal collisions during 1995–2000, found that the risk of lower extremity fracture started to rise from fourth decade and was significantly higher by the seventh decade.[11]

Side Impact Side impact occurs at intersections when an elderly person fails to stop at a stop sign or is hit from the side when pulling out of a driveway. Depending on the speed and make of car and the energy dissipated at impact, the intrusion of the body of the car can cause severe blunt trauma to the head, neck, chest wall, abdominal contents, spinal column, long bones, and pelvic areas. Lateral compression fracture of the hip joint is frequently noted with side impact injuries.

Ejection Injuries Although this injury is more common in younger drivers with rollovers, it may happen to the elderly while as a passenger, or after a severe side impact. It may cause partial body damage, such as crushed arm out of the window, or total body ejection, with multiple severe injuries.

Pedestrian injuries Poor peripheral vision, kyphotic changes of the spinal column, and slow movement in crossing the road are counted as the preinjury factors in pedestrian trauma patients. The massive soft tissue injury resulting from shearing forces on different organs causes severe physical damage and biochemical changes in the patient. The motor vehicle may have passed over the body causing muscle tears, swelling, ischemia, and necrosis of the soft tissues. This massive injury may compromise the circulation resulting in ischemic compartmental syndromes. Delay in surgical diagnosis and improper resuscitation measures are common causes of loss of limb, rhabdomyolysis, myoglobulinuria, metabolic acidosis, and multiple organ failure in these patients. At the time of admission, attention

should be focused on presence of peripheral pulses, especially those distal to the fracture, dislocation sites, and evaluation of neurological function and peripheral perfusion of the extremity.

Crush injuries

Multiple fractures and soft tissue injuries are caused by natural disasters, sports, suicidal attempts, and MVAs. In geriatric trauma patients with severe multiple injuries, the association of acute respiratory insufficiency, massive blood loss, and head injury leads to a deterioration in hemodynamic function and renders the patient in imminent danger of death. These types of patients should be managed in a trauma center with a skillful trauma team, fully functioning operating system, and specialized intensive care units (ICUs).

Penetrating injuries

In the elderly population, the incidence of penetrating injuries is less than 10% of all trauma injuries. These injuries should be individually examined and properly treated.

Stab Wounds The characteristics of the tissues involved, the type of wounding instrument, velocity and depth of penetration, in accordance with clinical and diagnostic findings, dictate the strategy and urgency of the treatment.

Gunshot Wounds The type of firearm, shape of the bullet, velocity of impact, trajectory within the body, degree of fragmentation, and body regions involved are important to ascertain for evaluation and treatment. Gunshot wounds, strangulation, and other means of suicide attempts occur in the elderly. The U.S. Census report of 1999 documents that elderly male patients above 65 years of age are much more likely to commit suicide than their female counterparts.[1] White males have the highest suicidal rates among the elderly and usually are attributed to unemployment and other emotional factors. Other penetrating or blunt trauma injuries may occur in the elderly during muggings, burglaries, and fights. Alcohol intake is common in assault victims.

TRAUMA INJURY ASSESSMENT

▶ General considerations

At the scene of the accident, emergency medical care providers should match the patient's needs with available resources. Factors like trauma severity, resource availability, the patient's desire, and functional survival outcome should be considered in the triage and treatment plan. Operative procedures, invasive and expensive critical care therapies will be used in patients who are expected to have a good long-term outcome. The activity needs to be coordinated with the physicians in receiving facilities. It is the responsibility of prehospital personnel and the medical director to transport the patient to an appropriate facility capable of delivering the best care to the trauma patient. If the number of patients involved in the accident is more than the capacity of the receiving center or if the available facility and staff are unable to deliver proper urgent care to the trauma patients, then patients with the best chance of survival with the least expenditure of time and supplies should be prepared first to be transported to the medical center. Pertinent information about type and mechanism of injury, related events, patient history, physical findings, vital signs, and rendered treatments should be conveyed to the receiving hospital for imminent emergency treatment plans.

The assessment of elderly trauma patients and the resuscitative measures follow the established protocols of Advanced Trauma Life Support (ATLS) and guidelines of the American Society of Anesthesiologists (ASA).[12,13] In the field, cervical spine precautions with application of cervical collars prevent excessive movement of cervical spine. Placement of the patient on a backboard and stabilization of the head and neck during transport prevent further unintentional movement and possible damage to the spinal cord. The EMS protocols, trauma skills, and the management of the medical director of the team dictate establishment of intravenous access for fluid resuscitation, endotracheal intubation, and other emergency measures. Assessment of the severity of injury at the scene of accident or in the emergency department can be accomplished by following statistical scoring systems. These different trauma scores with their ability to predict outcome can assist the trauma team leader in patient management.

▶ Trauma scores

The statistical trauma scores are valuable in predicting trauma patient outcome during the course of injury management. The impact of trauma on different organ systems and evaluation of severity of injury is a basic part of trauma management. The trauma scores take into consideration the impact of trauma on anatomical organs, physiologic parameters, and/or a combination of both. These scores meet several objectives: 1) they allow for evaluation of severity of injury using a unique criterion; 2) they objectively guide triage and the use of resources; 3) they allow for documentation of progress and evaluation of trauma care; and 4) they provide objective measures that can be used to predict morbidity and mortality. Most of the trauma scores and statistical models are presented in Table 15-5.

Anatomical scores

Abbreviated Injury Scale This simple anatomical score has been used since 1971. The entire body is divided into six different regions, including head, neck, chest, abdomen, extremities, and general surface of body regions. The severity of injury is coded from 1 to 6 (Table 15-6). Since its inception, the Abbreviated Injury Scale (AIS) has undergone modifications in 1980 and 1985 to define injuries and increase the predictability, especially in penetrating injuries. There is no age factor involved in its calculations and there is no specific prospective study concerning its specificity of outcome prediction in geriatric trauma patients.

Injury Severity Score This anatomical scoring system is based on AIS calculation. It represents the sum of the squares of the highest AIS scores (maximum = 5) in each of the three most severely injured body regions. Most of the studies in geriatric trauma patients have found a positive correlation between the Injury Severity Score (ISS) and outcome. Usually an ISS of 15 and above favors severe trauma and above 35 favors the very severe category. Van der Sluis et al., in a study of 121 geriatric trauma patients with ISS scores equal or above 16, found that no patient with ISS above 50 survived the injury.[14]

Measurement of the ISS at the accident scene is not an easy task because it needs radiological and diagnostic tools for identifying the injuries. The ISS statistical score is more applicable in blunt trauma patients. Torreta et al., in studying survival outcome in significantly traumatized elderly patients (excluding slip and falls) managed in multicenter, level 1 trauma centers, found no positive correlation between ISS and survival rate.[15]

Physiologic statistical scores

Glasgow Coma Scale Glasgow Coma Scale (GCS) is universally used to evaluate central nervous system injuries. GCS has three components: verbal, visual, and motor, with the additive scores ranging from 3 to 15 (Table 15-7).

Paramedics at the field to evaluate the severity of head injury routinely use GCS. Sometime assessment of the GCS score at the scene of accident varies quickly with sudden changes in level of consciousness or the impact of hemodynamic parameters on central nervous system function. Vollmer et al. studied 661 patients older than 15 years with head injury and found 38% mortality for the entire group. In the subgroup of patients older than 55 years, the mortality rate was 80%. They found that GCS <8 in patients above 45 years of age is a significant independent predictor of death and vegetative outcome.[16] Kotowica and Jakubowski found 90% mortality in patients above 70 years old with a GCS <9 who required craniotomy and 76% mortality in nonsurgical patients.[17] Tamjoom et al. found an 86% mortality rate in a study of 66 patients above 65 years old with GCS 4 who underwent craniotomy for evacuation of hematoma.[18] Ross et al. reported 100% mortality 6 months post

Table 15-5

Trauma Statistical Scores

Type	Abbreviation	Name/Definition
Anatomical scores	AIS	Abbreviated Injury Scale
	ISS	Injury Severity Score
Physiologic scores	GCS	Glasgow Coma Scale
	TS	Trauma Score
	RTS	Revised Trauma Score
	SIRS	Systemic Inflammatory Response Syndrome Scoring System
	PTS	Physiologic Trauma Score
Combination	TRISS	Trauma Injury Severity Score
	ASCOT	A Severity Characterization of Trauma
	CRAMS	Circulation, Respiration, Abdomen, Motor, Speech

Table 15-6

Abbreviated Injury Scale

1. No injury
2. Minimal injury
3. Moderate injury
4. Severe injury (non life-threatening)
5. Severe life-threatening injury
6. Critical injury with low probability of survival (maximal fatal untreatable injury)

Table 15-7

Glasgow Coma Scale

Best verbal response	
Oriented	5
Confused	4
Inappropriate words	3
Incomprehensible sounds	2
None	1
Eye opening	
Spontaneous	4
To speech	3
To pain	2
None	1
Best motor response	
Obeys commands	6
Localizes	5
Withdraws	4
Abnormal flexion	3
Abnormal extension	2
None	1
Total GCS 3–15	

Table 15-8

Trauma Score

			Score
a.	Respiratory rate (per minute)	10–24	4
		25–35	3
		>35	2
		<10	1
		0	0
b.	Respiratory effort	Normal	1
		Shallow or retracted	0
c.	Systolic BP	>90 torr	4
		70–90	3
		50–69	2
		<50	1
		No pulse	0
d.	Capillary refill	Normal	2
		Delayed	1
		None	0
e.	Glasgow Coma Scale	14–15	5
		11–13	4
		8–10	3
		5–7	2
		3–4	1

Total points = (a + b + c + d + e)

Best score = 16

trauma in those who were above 65 years old with a persistent GCS <8 for 72 h after injury.[19]

Trauma Score The trauma score (TS) is summation of five different parameters as illustrated in Table 15-8. The range is 1–16. Osler et al., in a case-matched review of 100 patients above 65 years, found that no elderly patients with TS <9 survived and no elderly patients with a TS <7 survived long enough to reach the hospital.[20] Kudson supported this finding in 852 elderly patients with the same TS. Aggressive treatment is likely to be futile if the admission trauma score is less than 7. Pellicane et al., in a study of 374 trauma patients above 65 years old, reported 5% mortality with a TS 15–16, 25% with a TS 12–14, and 65% with TS <12.[21]

Revised Trauma Score Because of subject variability and environmental factors, the respiratory effort and capillary refill components were removed from the TS. The Revised Trauma Score (RTS) is widely used by paramedics at the field and has good correlation with morbidity and mortality. The score ranges between 0 and 8 (Table 15-9). These objective physiological scores are readily available to prehospital providers as well as to the trauma resuscitation team.

Systemic Inflammatory Response Syndrome Scoring System Because trauma triggers the inflammatory response, Systemic Inflammatory Response Syndrome (SIRS) Scoring System has been developed to predict hospital admission and outcome prediction[22] (Table 15-10). Hypothermia is the best predictor of mortality, hospital length of stay, and ICU admission. Neutrophil count >12,000 is the best predictor of total hospital length of stay.

Physiologic Trauma Score Physiologic Trauma Score (PTS) is the cumulative number of SIRS, GCS, and age. PTS predictability of

mortality is comparable to Trauma Injury Severity Score (TRISS). It can easily be calculated in ICU patients.[23]

Anatomical and physiological combination scales

Trauma Injury Severity Score Trauma Injury Severity Score (TRISS) was devised to calculate survival based on various patient characteristics, taking both anatomical as well as physiological determinants into account, and uses scores from both ISS and GCS, respectively, along with age. This methodology also takes into account the type of trauma as related to blunt or penetrating injuries.

Table 15-9

Revised Trauma Score

GCS	Systolic Blood Pressure	Respiratory Rate	Coded Value
13–15	>89	10–29	4
9–12	76–89	>29	3
6–8	50–57	6–9	2
4–5	<49	1–5	1
3	0	0	0

Table 15-10

SIRS Scoring System

SIRS Scoring System includes:

a. Fever (temp >38°C) or hypothermia (temp <36°C)

b. Tachycardia

c. Tachypnea

d. Abnormal white blood cell count (neutrophil >12,000 or <4000)

(Each component represents one point.)

Scoring 0–4

A Severity Characterization of Trauma Score Champion and his coworkers introduced this anatomic-physiologic scoring system to predict mortality rate in trauma patients. A Severity Characterization of Trauma (ASCOT) Score is calculated by summation of squares of AIS (3, 4, or 5) lesions in three categories of organ systems (brain and spinal cord, thorax and front of neck, and injury in all other body organs) plus RTS points. Different coefficients are considered for blunt versus penetrating injuries. The age factor is included in calculation of the ASCOT score. ASCOT has a good predictive ability, but its calculation is feasible only after the patient's admission to a trauma center. For a complete description of the ASCOT scoring system, the reader is referred to one of several excellent Web sites (http://www.sfar.org/scores2/ascot2.html).

CRAMS Scale This anatomic-physiological scale is readily available to paramedics and emergency care physicians (Table 15-11). If Circulation, Respiration, Abdomen, Motor, Speech (CRAMS) score is equal or less than 8, major trauma has occurred. The total score of 9 is mild trauma, so there is a fairly narrow range for triage of the patient. The sensitivity and specifity of CRAMS score is above 0.9 and predictive value is above 0.5. Application of this scoring system in geriatric trauma needs to be determined.

Table 15-11

CRAMS Scale

Circulation	Normal capillary refill and BP >100	2
	Delayed capillary refill and BP <85	1
	No capillary refill or BP <85	0
Respiration	Normal	2
	Abnormal	1
	Absent	0
Abdomen	Abdomen and thorax tender	2
	Abdomen or thorax tender	1
	Abdomen rigid in flail chest	0
Motor	Normal	2
	Responds to pain	1
	No response or decreased	0
Speech	Normal	2
	Confused	1
	No intelligible words	0

Applicability of trauma scoring systems

In spite of availability and development of different trauma scales, there is no one system with adequate sensitivity and predictability to be universally applied to all types of geriatric trauma patients. The RTS and GCS have been widely applied by prehospital care providers for triage of trauma patients. These physiological scales are easy to determine in the field, but their sensitivity is lower than anatomic-based scoring, especially in multiple trauma patients.

The TRISS, as a combination of anatomic and physiologic scoring systems, has shown promise in determining severity of injury. Required calculations make complex scoring systems difficult to use at initial patient assessment, and their use in triage and prioritizing admission treatments is limited. SIRS criteria are readily available in the trauma admitting area and are an independent predictor of mortality, ICU admission, and length of hospital stay.

The PTS (combination of SIRS, GCS, and age) has considerably higher discriminating power than SIRS score alone and is comparable with TRISS and superior to ISS.[23]

Trauma versus nontrauma centers

The elderly patient with multiple trauma, ISS >15, moderately low GCS, and/or systolic blood pressure below 90 mm Hg should be directed to a trauma center with capability of trauma intensive care management. Mann et al. demonstrated that geriatric patients who were treated in an organized statewide trauma system had a 5.1% higher survival rate than counterparts who were managed in nontrauma centers.[24] Demetriades believes that care of the elderly patient above age 70 should be restricted to trauma centers.[25] However, the functional outcomes for such a recommendation require further evaluation.

Unfortunately, trauma center treatment is not as accessible to the elderly compared to young patients who have a similar severity of injury.[26]

GERIATRIC TRAUMA EVALUATION

General considerations

The basic guidelines of ATLS, including primary survey, resuscitation, and secondary survey, are applicable during trauma patient assessment and resuscitation. As the cardiopulmonary reserve of the elderly is compromised secondary to senile degenerative changes, the hemodynamic response of the geriatric trauma patient may be different than young adults. For instance, the sympathetic nervous system response to hypovolemia is blunted by cardiac degenerative changes and current medication taken for other comorbidities. Aggressive resuscitation measures need to be managed in ICUs. Continuous physiological monitoring should be applied during resuscitation, diagnostic radiological procedures, operating rooms interventions, and intensive care.

Measurement of cardiac index, O_2 consumption, and base deficit guide management of resuscitation. In a study of 274 trauma patients, age greater than 55 years, a significant correlation was found between base deficit, ICU length of stay, and mortality. Elderly patients with severe base deficit (<−10) had an 80% mortality.[27] Scalea et al., using the selection criteria of multiple fractures, pedestrian struck, head injury, ISS >18, and acidosis showed that maintaining cardiac index above 4 L/min and oxygen consumption index above 170 mL/min/m² decreased mortality from 54% to 34% in the elderly population.[28] Dune et al., in a prospective study of 15,179 patients admitted to a level 1 trauma center, demonstrated that admission blood lactate and base deficit are significant independent predictors of mortality, ICU, and hospital length of stay in trauma patients.[29] The benefit of invasive monitoring in improving the outcome of elderly trauma patients is not universally accepted and further prospective research is needed to resolve this controversial issue.

The incidence of cardiac morbidity is higher with congestive heart failure (CHF), but finding the incidence of CHF is difficult because one-third of the elderly patients will have a normal systolic function with CHF. The cause of their diastolic dysfunction can be attributed to ventricular hypertrophy, intrinsic myocardial disease, ischemic myocardium, and accelerated hypertension. Patients above 80 years with history of CHF have 4.3-fold increased cardiac events and 3.3-fold risk of developing cardiac arrhythmias. Prevention and treatment of these complications is feasible in ICUs with invasive monitoring capabilities.

▶ Resuscitation

The geriatric trauma patient may seem to be stable, yet be suffering from hypoperfusion states and respiratory insufficiency. Aggressive and timely resuscitative measures should be executed without delay. The resuscitative measures should focus on airway management, ventilatory, and cardiovascular issues.

Airway management

In the elderly population, upper airway evaluation deserves specific attention to the presence of loose teeth and soft tissue injuries, broken or displaced dentures, mandible and maxillary fractures, vomitus and other foreign bodies, nasal and oral bleeding, and temporomandibular joint dislocation. The loose redundant pharyngeal tissues easily obstruct the upper airway and jeopardize its patency. As the pharyngeal reflexes are diminished with advancing age, the elderly patient carries a higher risk of regurgitation and aspiration, especially if obtunded.

The presence of arthritis, ankylosis, spondylosis, premorbid conditions, and prior surgeries for stabilization of cervical spine mandate extra skill in airway management of the elderly.

Supplemental oxygen via nonrebreathing mask is recommended in spontaneously breathing patients.[30] Fitting of the mask for positive pressure ventilation in edentulous patients with mandible atrophy sometime requires filling the buccal area with gauze prior to positive pressure ventilation.

In-line stabilization of the head and neck, cricoid pressure, rapid sequence induction with hypnotics and muscle relaxants, and oral endotracheal intubation are recommended during emergency airway management.[31] Other routes for intubation should be considered if clinically indicated. The selection of larger size endotracheal tubes may facilitate pulmonary toilet in the ICU. In the trauma setting, it is critical to maintain cricoid pressure until proper confirmation of endotracheal tube position and obtaining a stable end-tidal CO_2 tracing.

It is important to be aware that subluxation of cervical spine may occur during laryngoscopy and intubation. Lennarson et al. studied cervical spine motion in fresh human cadavers while intact and after C4–5 posterior ligamentous injury. During laryngoscopy for intubation, videofluoroscopy was used to detect motion. The greatest motion (extension) was noted at the atlanto-occipital joint followed by the C1–C2 junction. After creation of C4–5 injury, the direction of motion at C4–5 was changed from extension to flexion. Traction with Gardner-Wells traction limited but did not prevent motion at the atlanto-occipital joint. Therefore, traction and/or in-line cervical immobilization did not significantly reduce the motion at the subaxial site of injury.[32]

The thinned mucosa of the oropharynx may be abraded during harsh laryngoscopy generating bleeding and hematoma formation. Awake intubation may be considered in situations where immediate evaluation of spinal cord function is necessary after intubation. The technique of fiber-optic intubation is not feasible in uncooperative patients or in the presence of active upper airway bleeding. In semi-emergent situations, lubricating local anesthetics may be applied to the mucosa of nasal airways with serial nasal dilatators and/or topical application to the pharyngeal area. Preparation and immediate availability of difficult airway equipment and adherence to the difficult airway algorithm advised by the ASA reduces the risks of untoward events. Surgical airway via cricothyroidotomy under local anesthesia may be applied as the technique of choice in massive maxillofacial injuries and in situations when hypnotic and muscle relaxant administration may lose control of the airway.

Ventilatory issues

There are key structural and physiologic differences in the elderly that should be noted when providing ventilation and oxygenation. The degenerative changes of laryngeal cartilages and the trachea make the patient vulnerable to laryngeal and tracheal fracture dislocations. The osteoporotic changes of the chest wall make the brittle ribs susceptible to rib fractures during closed chest compressions, causing hemothorax, pneumothorax, and lung lacerations. Increased chest wall rigidity, decreased muscle power, and decreased recoil of the lung make the lungs less expandable. Airway resistance does not increase significantly, but there is a measurable increase in dead space and closing volumes. The dilatation of alveolar ducts and degeneration of alveolar walls increase the dead space and contribute to poor gas exchange. High peak airway pressure ventilation may cause rupture of peripheral alveoli and tension pneumothorax. Chest wall pain and inability to cough and take deep breaths are accentuated by decreased contractile power of respiratory muscles, leading to atelectasis and hypoxemia. Gradual degeneration of the lung elastic tissues, decrease in surface area for gas exchange, and increased alveolar-capillary membrane thickness decreases the lung compliance and lung volumes (except functional residual capacity). This makes the elderly patient more vulnerable to rapid oxygen desaturation. The dilatation of alveolar ducts and degeneration of alveolar walls increase the dead space and alters ventilation/perfusion (V/Q) mismatch.

The barotrauma of positive pressure ventilation, with overdistention of alveoli and high peak inspiratory pressure, predisposes the patient to alveolar rupture and pneumothorax during resuscitation. Pulmonary aspiration, contusion, and chest wall pain contribute to lobar atelectasis, pulmonary shunts, and hypoxemic conditions.

Cardiovascular issues

There are key features of the aging cardiovascular system that play an important role in circulation of the geriatric trauma patient. Hypoperfusion may be manifested with pale skin, weak pulse, delayed capillary refill, and change in level of mentation. The formation of atherosclerotic plaques reduces the regional blood flow to vital organs, predisposing the elderly population to cellular hypoxia and circulatory collapse. Baroreceptor reflex impairment and inability to raise the heart rate in the hypovolemic patient lead to inadequate cardiac output, vital organ ischemia, peripheral hypoperfusion, and metabolic acidosis. The degenerative changes of cardiac myofibrils, valves, and conductive system of the heart, in association with increased vascular resistance and hypertrophy of ventricles, make the heart vulnerable to arrhythmia, ischemia, and heart failure. Alterations in the autonomic nervous system and decreased sensitivity of adrenergic receptors lead to a gradual decrease of heart rate and make the cardiac output more dependent to preload volume. Increased arterial rigidity and intensified sympathetic activity in the presence of hypovolemia and hypoxemia make the hypertrophic cardiac muscles vulnerable to ischemia, arrhythmia, infarction, and cardiac arrest.

GENERAL CONSIDERATIONS IN TRAUMA MANAGEMENT

▶ Laboratory tests and imaging

Obtaining blood samples for complete blood count, electrolytes, type and crossmatch, coagulation profile, toxicology, and urinalysis are part of standard protocol during trauma resuscitation. Obtaining an electrocardiogram in men above 40 years and women above 50 years is a routine test that should be performed on admission. Determination of arterial blood gases as a baseline measure in the cardiopulmonary-compromised patient as well as measurement of base deficit and lactate level to evaluate peripheral perfusion are required during resuscitation. Patients with multiple injuries need cervical spine, chest and pelvic x-ray, or computed tomography (CT) as diagnostic measures. Depending on the type and severity of injury, other diagnostic measures such as angiography, magnetic resonance imaging (MRI), Doppler studies, ultrasound techniques, transthoracic and transesophageal echocardiography are indicated for proper diagnosis. In acute emergency situations, evaluation of pathophysiological changes in cardiac, pulmonary, hepatic, renal, and other organ systems are not feasible, and the likelihood that the results of these tests will dramatically change the perioperative care are minimal.

▶ Nutrition—NPO status

Every trauma patient is considered to have a full stomach. The time interval between last oral intake and time of trauma may correlate with retained stomach content. Decreased pharyngeal reflexes make these patients amenable to aspiration and regurgitation. Delayed gastric emptying increases the aspiration risk. Use of antacids prior to intubation is not feasible all the time and its benefits are not well documented. The technique of rapid sequence induction with cricoid pressure is assumed to lower the risk of aspiration during tracheal intubation. The placement of an orogastric or nasogastric tube immediately after intubation in emergency cases reduces the postextubation aspiration risk. Postoperatively, resuming enteral or parenteral feeding in a timely manner diminishes the catabolic response to trauma and reduces the complications related to drug metabolism and infection.

▶ Temperature control

Perioperative hypothermia is more common in elderly patients. Studies have shown that the thermoregulatory responses are initiated 1.2°C lower in elderly compared to young adults. Patients undergoing spinal anesthesia are susceptible to hypothermia because of peripheral vasodilatation and heat loss. As the general anesthetics and sedatives impair thermoregulatory response, it is not unusual for the elderly to become hypothermic during surgery. During resuscitation and massive transfusion, hypothermia is associated with hypoxemic metabolic acidosis, platelet dysfunction, and coagulopathy. Warming the operating room ambient temperature, warming blankets, fluid warmers, and warm irrigation fluids during prolonged surgeries help to protect the patient against hypothermic complications.

▶ Pain control

Proper pain relief facilitates chest physiotherapy, rehabilitation, and early ambulation. Administration of nonsteroidal anti-inflammatory drugs and opioids is the currently used mainstays of treatment for pain control. Increased gastric pH, decreased gastric motility, and decreased hepatic and renal blood flow affects the bioavailability of the medications in elderly patients.

Patient-controlled analgesia (PCA) in a patient who can use the device is safe for geriatric patient. Other methods of pain relief such as patient-controlled epidural analgesia (PCEA) effectively reduce chest wall pain and improve outcome. Continuous nerve blocks are being increasingly used for postoperative pain relief.

▶ Deep venous thrombosis prophylaxis

Patients with hip fracture are at high risk for development of venous thromboembolism. Geriatric patients, especially those with previous history of deep venous thrombosis (DVT), need to be closely scrutinized for thromboprophylaxis treatment. The risk of hospital-acquired DVT in geriatric orthopedic patients without prophylaxis is 40–60%. The in-hospital fatality rate is about 12% and case fatality rate in 1 year is 29–34%.[33] Obesity, smoking history, presence of varicose veins, and central venous catheters increase the incidence of venous thromboembolism. Placement of mechanical devices such as intermittent pneumatic impulse boots, prophylactic use of heparin, low-molecular-weight heparin, and other medications in the preoperative period diminish this risk.

▶ Infection control/prevention—immunity

The incidence of nosocomial infection in the elderly is twofold that of young patients (39% versus 17.9%).[34] Butcher et al. studied the postoperative infection complication in hip-fractured patients and found that superoxide production and phagocyte function declined up to 5 weeks after trauma.[35] The effects of hypothermia on the immune response along with an increased incidence of infection has been shown in elective surgical cases and is more problematic in emergency surgeries.

Kotani et al. showed that use of 100% oxygen during surgery in the elderly improves the proinflammatory response of alveolar macrophages and lowers the incidence of wound infection.[29]

▶ Positioning

Prolonged positioning of geriatric trauma patients on the rigid backboard for spine protection, and use of other protective devices for stabilization of injured limbs may cause skin blisters, sloughing, and wound infection. Chronic degenerative changes in joints and muscle contractures demand precautions to avoid pressure sores and peripheral nerve injury during prolonged procedures.

ORGAN-SPECIFIC MANAGEMENT OF GERIATRIC TRAUMA

▶ Traumatic brain injuries

The incidence of head injury is highest in teenage groups and gradually declines with advancing age, but begins to rise again after 70 years of age. The effect of head injury in the elderly is disproportionately severe.[36] Atrophy and shrinkage of the brain mass, accompanied by fragility of the cerebral vessels and stretching of bridging veins after trauma, play a major role in the development of subdural or intracerebral hematomas. The incidence of intracranial bleeding can increase up to 7% in elderly patients who receive anticoagulant therapy. After blunt trauma, their mortality rate can reach 50%. Reversal of anticoagulants in the warfarin group should be accomplished with fresh frozen plasma and/or coagulation factors. Vitamin K is advisable but it takes hours to become effective. Reversal of anticoagulation is required prior to any neurosurgical intervention. The incidence of traumatic intracranial hematoma is 9.4% at age 65 and 4% in younger patients. Epidural hematoma is not common in old age, as the dura mater adheres more firmly to the inner table of the skull in older patients.

Initial assessment and management of traumatic brain injury is based on the patient's history, GCS score, neurological exam, and CT findings. The prevalence of mild (GCS 13–15), moderate (GCS 9–12), and severe (GCS <8) head injuries is the same in young and old patients. It is around 84% mild, 10–11% moderate, and 5–6% severe head injury. The mortality rate in patients above 80 years of age after minor head injury is about 12%. This is seven times higher than younger patients. In other words, the mild head injury in an older patient is equivalent to severe head injury in younger patients.[37] Conventional neurological findings such as increased intracranial pressure signs may not be readily apparent in the elderly due to reduced brain mass. As brain mass is reduced in the elderly, the classic signs and symptoms of increased intracranial pressure are missing with small volume intracranial hematomas. Subdural hematoma is the most common intracranial space-occupying lesion in geriatric trauma patients.

A CT is recommended in elderly patients with minimal head injury and should be repeated after 6 h if the patient has been receiving anticoagulants. In CT scans of geriatric patients with mild head injury (GCS 13–15), demonstrable head injury was found in 14% and surgical intervention required in 20%.[38]

Other than moribund conditions at arrival, aggressive treatment may be initiated in geriatric trauma patients for 72 h and the treatment selectively continued in patients who respond favorably to aggressive treatment. Ninety-five percent probability of death has been used as a cutoff point during intensive management.

The aging brain has a limited capacity to recover after injury.[39] In a retrospective study of 694 trauma patients with isolated brain injury (22% of which were elderly patients above 65 years), Mosenthal et al. found that the mortality rate and poor functional outcomes were 30% and 13% in the elderly as compared to 14% and 5% in younger patients, respectively. Age was an independent predictor of mortality and long-term disability in severe head injury patients.[40]

Spine injuries

Two types of spine injuries are common in the elderly: odontoid fracture of C2 and compression fracture in the thoracolumbar spine. Ninety-five percent of odontoid fractures are secondary to falls and carry a high morbidity and mortality.[41] Lateral cervical spine x-ray films have 53% sensitivity in identifying fractures. Spiral computed tomography (SCT) can identify 99% of spine fractures.[42] Osteoporosis may be the underlying cause for thoracic-lumbar fractures.

Muller et al. recommend an aggressive approach to detecting unstable fractures and to stabilize the fracture area by internal fixation or the use of a halo device.[43] Type 2 fractures are unstable in extension. Operative repair using anterior screw fixation may be performed in selected patients. Halo fixation is frequently used but entails the possibility of developing pseudoarthrosis. As the conservative approach has a high failure rate, anterior stabilization may have a more favorable outcome. The issue of conservative management in patients with high surgical risk versus surgical immobilization via posterior approach has been investigated in the past and the issue has not yet been resolved.

Compression fracture in the thoracic-lumbar area is frequently hidden. Occasionally, it may be revealed on x-ray films as an incidental finding. Sometimes the acute lesion is not distinguishable from old injuries or bone tumors. Neurological deficit is rare. If compression fracture is present, unstable components should be surgically repaired. Dorsal stabilization of the spine should include more than the injured vertebra, and vertebral replacement may be needed.

Gardner-Wells tongs placement for cervical spine immobilization and reduction of dislocated vertebrae may be accomplished with local anesthesia and intravenous sedation. General anesthesia with in-line stabilization of cervical spine is the treatment of choice in uncooperative or head-injured patients[31] with the caveat that repeat neurological exam after intubation will not be feasible.

The acute cervical spine fracture patient, with neurological deficit and unstable hemodynamic condition, should have full invasive monitoring with capability to measure cardiac output and peripheral vascular resistance. Somatosensory-evoked potential (SSEP) and motor-evoked potential monitoring may facilitate nerve injury detection during neurosurgical correction of spine injury.

Thoracic injuries

Chest wall injury and rib fractures are a common finding after multiple traumas in elderly patients. The rate of morbidity and mortality proportionally rise with the number of rib fractures and with bilateral versus unilateral chest wall injury. Presence of flail chest wall, hemothorax, pneumothorax, lung lacerations, pulmonary contusion, tracheobronchial rupture, aortic tear, and major vascular injuries contribute to a higher incidence of morbidity and mortality.

Pape et al. in early evaluation of blunt chest trauma found that age >70 years had an increased risk of rib fracture rather than pulmonary contusions.[44] Bergeron et al. noted 20% mortality in geriatrics compared with 9% in nongeriatric rib fracture patients despite a lower ISS and higher GCS. For each rib fracture, the mortality rate increases by 19% and the risk of pneumonia increases by 27%.[45] Holcomb studied the impact of age and the number of rib fractures on ventilator days, ICU stay, and total hospital days and found that patients older than 45 years with more than four rib fractures had poor outcome compared to younger patients.[46] Bulger et al. compared the outcome of 277 patients age above 65 years with younger counterparts who were admitted to a level 1 trauma center with rib fractures and found that the incidence of pneumonia, length of hospital stay, and mortality is higher in elderly patients (Table 15-12). Thoracic epidural catheter placement for pain control

Table 15-12		
Thoracic Injury Outcome in Old versus Young Patients		
	Age >65	Age <65
Mean ventilator days	4.3	3.1
ICU days	6.1	4.0
Length of stay (days)	15.4	10.7
Pneumonia	31%	17%
Mortality rate	22%	10%

was associated with a significant decrease in the mortality rate in both groups.[47]

Abdominal injuries

About 30% of geriatric trauma patients may suffer from intra-abdominal injuries. In multiple trauma patients, both long bone injuries and intra-abdominal trauma are usually observed. Peritoneal signs and localization of pain in the elderly are not often distinctive as in younger patients. Delayed diagnosis and poor management of hemorrhage are the major causes of increased morbidity and high mortality in this patient population. The mortality rate of intra-abdominal injury in elderly is four- to sevenfold higher than younger patients. The bedside use of ultrasound, available to physicians at the time of trauma admission, facilitates the diagnosis of intra-abdominal bleeding. Depending on the stability of vital signs and other concomitant injuries, the patient may undergo CT scan of the abdomen, and the grades of solid organ injury can be accurately diagnosed prior to surgical intervention. Dehydration, hypovolemia, poor perfusion, and decreased glomerular filtration rate may make diagnostic x-rays with intravenous contrast dye inaccurate and misleading.

For hemodynamically unstable head injury patients with intra-abdominal injuries, emergency craniotomy for evacuation of hematoma can proceed while the trauma team surgeon performs diagnostic peritoneal lavage (DPL) to assess for intra-abdominal injuries.

Anesthetic management of intraperitoneal injuries comprise rapid sequence induction, endotracheal intubation, gastric tube placement, fluid and blood resuscitation, correction of coagulopathy, and prevention of hypothermic complications.

Until recently, nonoperative management of splenic injury was not recommended in patients above 55 years of age. Multiple studies have shown a similar success rate of nonoperative management in the elderly as in younger patients. Patients with grade 4 or 5 splenic injuries with large hemoperitoneum and ISS >17 require immediate surgery.[48] Albrecht et al. reported a nonoperative failure rate of 33% in geriatric patients, which was significantly higher than previous studies.[49]

Pelvic injuries

More than 95% of hip fractures are due to falls. Its incidence varies worldwide from 5.6/100,000 in South Africa to 80/100,000 in the United States. The incidence doubles each decade after age 50 with a white female preponderance. Hip fracture in the elderly usually occurs when the patient falls sideways on the femoral trochanter. In the United States, more than 350,000 hip fractures occur each year. The lifetime risk of hip fracture at 50 years of age is highest in White women (17%) and lowest in African-American men (3%).

Coopers et al. in 1990 reported that 72% of hip fractures occurred in female patients. The female/male ratio in the White population above age 65 is 2/1, but 1/1 in Black populations of the United States and South Africa. Lower bone density and higher rate of falling may contribute to this ratio in White patients.[50]

The risk factors for hip fracture are tabulated in Table 15-13. Different ethnic groups may have the combination of these factors, which make them unique regarding character, prevalence, type, and outcome results.[51] One-year mortality is 24% and the mortality rate of males is approximately double that of females.[52] Comorbidity does affect outcome. In a study of hip fracture patients, there was a 33% mortality rate at 1 year and the breakdown of ASA status was: ASA 1 = 0%, ASA 2 = 4.3%, ASA 3 = 21.3%, and ASA 4 = 42%. Patients who live with family have a lower mortality rate (26.5%)

Table 15-13

Risk Factors for Hip Fracture

Osteoporosis and osteopenia affecting the bone density

Bone geometry (size of the bone and length of the femoral neck)

Microdamage accumulation

Genetics (the genes which are associated with osteoporosis)

Gender (preponderance of females after menopause)

Race (different between races)

Age (risk increases exponentially with advanced age)

Cigarette smoking (50% increase lifetime risk of hip fracture)

Weight (increased incidence in low weight)

Medications (benzodiazepines, anticonvulsants, corticosteroids)

Physical activity (low quadriceps strength and limited physical activity)

than institutionalized patients (43.8%). Mortality rate of hip fracture may increase to 80% by the ninth decade and 100% in the tenth decade.

The three most common anatomic types of hip fractures are femoral neck fracture, intertrochanteric fracture, and subtrochanteric fracture.

- ► Intertrochanteric fracture: This type of extracapsular fracture is more prevalent in the elderly dependent female. The fracture is located in a well-vascularized metaphyseal area, and usually there is no interference of blood supply to the femoral head. Malunion and shortening of the limb are complications of this type of fracture.

- ► Femoral neck fracture: This intracapsular hip fracture is more common in the active elderly and carries a risk of disruption of blood supply to the femoral head. Anesthetic administration may urgently be needed for relocation or closed reduction of the femoral head to prevent femoral head necrosis and nonunion of the fracture.

- ► Subtrochanteric fracture: Accounts for 5–10% of hip fractures and is located distal to the lesser trochanter.[53]

MVAs, especially side impacts, may cause lateral compression fracture in the hip joint area in the elderly. Henry et al., in a study of traumatic pelvic fracture patients, found that the incidence of lateral compression fracture occurred 4.6 times more frequently in older patients than anteroposterior compression fracture.[54] This type of fracture requires less blood transfusion in comparison with other types of fracture, but the transfusion requirement is nine times higher in geriatric versus young patients. Severe pelvic fractures are more common in younger age groups and usually they are due to MVAs. Other types of pelvic bone fractures associated with genitourinary tract and intra-abdominal injuries may occur in the elderly following multilevel falls and MVAs.

Pre-op evaluation

The general measures of trauma care, diagnosis of other injuries, treatment of comorbidities, and blood and fluid resuscitation are considered standard of care in geriatric trauma patients. Hemostasis in massive pelvic injuries, in selected cases, can be accomplished by angiographic thromboembolization of the pelvic vessels. Acute cerebrovascular accident and myocardial infarction as the underlying cause of trauma should be treated prior to surgical intervention. For the anticoagulated patient whose anticoagulant therapy cannot be discontinued for 48 h, or in high-risk ASA physical status patients, the option of nonsurgical treatment should be considered. Among important preoperative laboratory values, serum albumin <3.5 g/dL or lymphocyte count <1500/mL are predictors of increased length of stay and mortality.[55]

It is best to establish clinical pathways when managing elderly hip fracture patients. Koval et al. proposed and tested a clinical pathway to reduce hospital length of stay and lower in-hospital mortality rate in elderly hip fracture patients. When comparing 380 patients without application of a clinical pathway protocol prior to 1990 with 747 patients adhering to the clinical pathway after 1990, there was a significant decrease in hospital length of stay (21.6 vs. 13.7 days, p <0.001), in-hospital mortality (5.3% vs. 1.5%), and 1-year mortality (14.1% vs. 8.8%) rates. There was no difference in rate of revision of hip surgery, discharge status, or recovery of ambulation between groups.[56]

The controversial issue of timing of surgery for hip fracture and its effects on morbidity and mortality has been the subject of different studies. The time period of 24–48 h post injury usually is adequate to address medical problems and prepare the patient for surgery. Zuckerman showed that 3 days delay for surgery doubled the mortality rate at the end of 1 year.[57] In contrast, Orosz et al., in a prospective study of 1206 hip fracture patients older than 50 years, compared the function and outcome of patients who had surgical repair within 24 h post admission with those after 24 h and found that early surgery was not associated with improved function or decreased mortality. However, in medically stable patients early surgery resulted in shorter length of stay, less pain, and probably less major complications.[58]

Anesthesia for hip fracture

General anesthesia, spinal anesthesia, epidural anesthesia, and peripheral nerve blocks have been used with success. General anesthesia facilitates patient positioning in the operating room and is less traumatic for the disturbed individual. Spinal anesthesia has been safely administered via single shot or with placement of an intrathecal catheter for continuous spinal anesthesia. In examining the two techniques, Favarel-garrigues et al. prospectively compared the hemodynamic changes after single-shot versus continuous spinal anesthesia in 60 patients undergoing hip fracture repair. They found decreases in mean arterial pressure, and need for ephedrine treatment was significantly less frequent in the continuous group compared to the single-shot spinal anesthesia group.[59] Epidural block with or without catheter placement is another option. A continuous epidural catheter may be used for postoperative pain relief and contribute to a lower incidence of DVT. Lumbar-sciatic nerve block provides adequate analgesia during surgery and into the postoperative period with catheter placement. The affected side is selectively blocked and hemodynamic changes, urinary tract infection (due to indwelling Foley catheter), and inability to ambulate the patient postoperatively are less frequent in this technique. De Visme et al, in a prospective study of 29 elderly hip fracture patients, compared spinal anesthesia to combined lumbar and sacral plexus block and found that hypotension was equally induced by both techniques but lasted longer with spinal anesthesia.[60]

Multiple studies have compared general versus regional anesthesia in terms of postoperative morbidity and mortality. O'Hara et al., in a retrospective study of elderly hip fracture patients undergoing general anesthesia (96,206 patients) versus regional anesthesia (3219 patients) during 1983–1993, performed in 20 U.S. hospitals, was not able to demonstrate a better outcome at 7 days or 30 days postoperatively with

regional anesthetic techniques.[61] Gilbert et al., in an observational study of 741 hip fracture patients, compared general versus spinal anesthesia on outcomes up to 24 months postoperatively. A total of 430 patients received spinal anesthesia and 311 received general anesthesia. Multivariate analysis showed that general anesthesia was at least as efficacious as spinal anesthesia and possibly better, in affording good long-term outcome.[62] Koval et al. prospectively studied 1-year morbidity and mortality of 642 hip fracture patients undergoing general (56.4%) or spinal (43.6%) anesthesia. The 1-year mortality was 12.1% and was not different between the two groups[63] (Table 15-14). Davis et al. compared general versus spinal anesthesia for emergency hip surgery in 132 elderly patients. They found the incidence of DVT and blood loss was lower in spinal anesthesia group.[64]

▶ Extremity injury

Upper extremity injury is more prevalent than lower extremity injury. Distal radius and ulna fracture are frequently noted in the elderly after falls. Humerus fracture may occur in an osteopenic elderly person while lifting a heavy object from the shelf or falling on the side. Loss of muscle strength affects the lower extremity more than the back and upper extremities. In addition, osteoarthritis and other joint diseases predispose patients to falls. Multilevel falls and MVAs cause multiple upper and lower extremity fractures.

Open fractures need to undergo irrigation and debridement followed by open reduction and internal fixation of the injured area. Open reduction with anatomic joint restoration in periarticular fractures enhances early range of motion and mobilization of the geriatric patient. Unfortunately, results are less predictable in the elderly and up to 72% of patients sustaining tibial plateau fracture are dissatisfied with the results. Application of external fixators in unstable patients is another alternative mode of treatment to achieve early mobilization and to prevent complications.

Anesthesia requirements for treatment of lower extremity fractures vary and include general anesthesia, local anesthesia with intravenous sedation, or regional anesthesia and nerve blocks. In selected patients, continuous administration of local anesthetic and narcotics can be applied via epidural catheters or intrathecal blocks.

Soft-tissue trauma

Penetrating injuries such as stab wounds and gunshot wounds may affect the vascular tissues with interruption of blood supply to the musculoskeletal system, as well as damage to the peripheral nerves

Table 15-14

General versus Regional Anesthesia for Hip Fracture Repair

	General Anesthesia	Spinal Anesthesia
Number of patients	362 (56.4%)	280 (43.6%)
Average age	78	81
Number of deaths during hospitalizations	13	7
Inpatient complication rate	11.3%	11.4%
Mortality	3.6%	2.5%
Death within 1 year	46 (13.3%)	28 (10.4%)

Source: Adapted from Ref. 63.

and other soft tissues. Evaluation of distal pulses in injured extremities, clinical evaluation of peripheral nerve function, and determination of the extent and depth of muscle and tendon injuries will help to choose the proper anesthetic technique. Irrigation and debridement of soft-tissue injury and protection of the skeleton occasionally requires prolonged, repeated, and extensive reconstructive surgeries.

Crush injuries and pedestrian struck patients may present with massive soft-tissue swelling and compromised blood supply due to compartmental injuries. Emergency fasciotomy and establishment of blood supply are the initial steps of surgical treatment in these cases. Prolonged tissue healing is expected in geriatric patients.

▶ Complications

It goes without saying that the outcome of geriatric trauma patients is adversely affected by complications occurring during hospitalization. Routine therapeutic measures must be aggressively undertaken to decrease common complications in the elderly. These include early mobilization, especially after pelvic and lower extremity injuries; prevention of skin breakdown; thromboembolic prophylaxis as pulmonary embolism is the most common complication; attention to nutritional status and correction of hypoalbuminemia; psychological support; and early rehabilitation. Prevention and management of the common pulmonary, cardiovascular, and neurological complications observed in the elderly trauma patient are discussed elsewhere within this textbook.

SUMMARY WITH KEY POINTS

▶ Health care administration is concerned about the escalating cost of geriatric trauma care. To improve the quality of care in this growing segment of society, collaborative efforts are needed between different specialties to improve favorable functional outcome. In the United States, the heterogeneity and diversity of the geriatric patient poses new challenges for delivery of the health care.

▶ The diminished functional reserve of organ systems challenges the anesthesiologist in hemodynamic stabilization of emergency trauma patients. Understanding the senile pathophysiological changes and correction of comorbid conditions lower the incidence of morbidity and mortality in these high-risk patients.

▶ The risk factors and type of trauma in the elderly are different than young adults. The preinjury risk factors, mechanism of injury, and use of trauma scoring scales assist the clinician in strategic planning of treatment and prediction of the outcome. Aggressive management and intensive care should be applied in patients who are expected to have a favorable functional outcome.

▶ Patients with multiple trauma, head injury, unstable hemodynamics, and severe injury should be cared for in an organized trauma system with availability of ICUs as well as rehabilitation facilities.

▶ Anesthetic administration is tailored according to the patient's needs. Control of hemodynamic parameters regarding perfusion of different organ systems, especially the brain, is critical in the elderly and requires diligent monitoring.

▶ Prevention of secondary injuries during prolonged procedures and intensive care shortens the length of stay and decreases mortality rates.

▶ The majority of acute emergency trauma patients require general anesthesia with definitive airway management. In selected trauma

patients with cardiovascular and pulmonary compromise, aggressive resuscitation and optimization of hemodynamic parameters reduce morbidity and mortality rates.

▶ Blunt trauma, especially falls, supercedes the other injuries in advanced age patients.

▶ General anesthesia and regional block have been used in older trauma patients with similar outcomes.

▶ In spite of an abundant volume of literature concerning the elderly trauma patient, controlled, prospective studies in geriatric trauma anesthesia are required to improve the health care of these fragile patients.

KEY REFERENCES

▶ Jacobs DG, Plisier BR, Barie PS, et al. Practice management guidelines for geriatric trauma: the EAST Practice Management Guidelines Work Group. *J Trauma Inj Infect Crit Care.* 2003;54(2):391–416.

▶ Nirula R, Gentilello LM. Futility of resuscitation criteria for the "young" old and the "old" old trauma patient: a national trauma data bank analysis. *J Trauma Inj Infect Crit Care.* 2004;57(1):37–41.

▶ Mosenthal AC, Lavery RF, Addis M, et al. Isolated traumatic brain injury: age is an independent predictor of mortality and early outcome. *J Trauma Inj Infect Crit Care.* 2002;52(5):907–911.

▶ Kuhls DA, Malone DL, McCarter RJ, et al. Predictors of mortality in adult trauma patients: the physiologic trauma score is equivalent to the trauma and Injury Severity Score. *J Am Coll Surg.* 2002; 194(6):695–704.

REFERENCES

1. Hobbs FB, Damon BL. 65+ in the United States. U.S. Census Bureau April 1999. http://www.census.gov/prod/1/pop/p23-190.html.
2. Jacobs DG, Plisier BR, Barie PS, et al. Practice management guidelines for geriatric trauma: the EAST Practice Management Guidelines Work Group. *J Trauma Inj Infect Crit Care.* 2003;54(2):391–416.
3. Inaba K, Goecke M, Sharkey P. Long-term outcomes after injury in the elderly trauma. *J Trauma.* 2003;54:486–491.
4. American College of Surgeons Committee on Trauma. *Resources for Optimal Care of the Injured Patient: 1999.* Chicago, IL: American College of Surgeons; 1998.
5. Taylor MD, Tracy JK, Meyer W, et al. Trauma in the elderly: intensive care resource use and outcome. *J Trauma.* 2002;53(3):407–414.
6. Miltzman DP, Boulanger BR, Rodriguez A, et al. Pre-existing disease in trauma patients: a predictor of fate independent of age and injury severity score. *J Trauma.* 1992;32:236–243.
7. Sterling D, O'Connor J, Bonadies J. Geriatric falls: Injury Severity is high and disproportionate to mechanism. *J Trauma Inj Infect Crit Care.* 2001;50(1):116–119.
8. Grossman M, Scaff D, Miller D, et al. Functional outcome in octogenarian trauma. *J Trauma Inj Infect Crit Care.* 2003;55(1):26–32.
9. Zautcke J, Coker S, Morris R. Geriatric trauma in the state of Illinois: substance use injury pattern. *Am J Emerg Med.* 2002;20(1):14–17.
10. Clark DE. Motor vehicle crash fatalities in the elderly rural vs. urban. *J Trauma.* 2001;51:896–900.
11. Moran SG, McGwin GJ, Metzger JS, et al. Relationship between age and lower extremity fracture in frontal motor vehicle collisions. *J Trauma.* 2003;54(2):261–265.
12. American College of Surgeons Committee on Trauma. Advanced Trauma Life Support Program for Physicians. Chicago, IL: American College of Surgeons; 1999.
13. Wilson WC. Trauma: airway management, American Society of Anesthesiologists Newsletter. Nov 2005, vol 69 #11, p9-16
14. Van der sulis CK, Timmer HW, Eisma WH, et al. Outcome in elderly injured patients: Injury Severity versus host factors. *Injury.* 1997;28:588–592.

15. Torreta P, Mostafavi H, Riina J, et al. Morbidity and mortality in elderly trauma patients. *J Trauma*. 1999;46:702–706.

16. Vollmer DG. Age and outcome following traumatic coma: why older patients fair worse? *J Neurosurg*. 1991;75:S37–S49.

17. Kotowica Z, Jakubowski JK. Acute head injuries in the elderly: an analysis of 136 consecutive patients. *Acta Neurochir (Wien)*. 1992;118:98–102.

18. Tomjoom A, Nelson R, Stranjalis G, et al. Outcome following surgical evacuation of traumatic intracranial hematomas in the elderly. *Br J Neurosurg*. 1992;6:27–32.

19. Ross AM, Pitts LH, Kobayashi S. Prognosticators of outcome after major head injury in the elderly. *J Neurosci Nurs*. 1992;24(2):88–93.

20. Osler T, Hales K, Baack B, et al. Trauma in the elderly. *Am J Surg*. 1988; 156:537–543.

21. Pellicane JV, Byrne K, DeMaria EJ. Preventable complications and death from multiple organ failure among geriatric trauma victims. *J Trauma*. 1992;33:440–444.

22. Assayama K, Aikawa N. Evaluation of systemic inflammatory response syndrome as a predictor of mortality in emergency patients transported by ambulance. *Keio J Med*. 1998;47:19–27.

23. Kuhls DA, Malone DL, McCarter RJ, et al. Predictors of mortality in adult trauma patients: the physiologic trauma score is equivalent to the trauma and Injury Severity Score. *J Am Coll Surg*. 2002;194(6):695–704.

24. Mann NC, Cahn RN, Mullins RG, et al. Survival among injured geriatric patients during construction of a statewide trauma system. *J Trauma*. 2001;(50):1111–1116.

25. Demetriades D, Karaiskakis MV, Elmahos G, et al. Effect on outcome of early intensive management of geriatric trauma patients. *Br J Surg*. 2002; 89:1319–1322.

26. Lane P, Sorondo B, Kelly J. Elderly trauma patients: are they accessing trauma center care? *Acad Emerg Med*. 2000;7(5):654.

27. Davis JW, Kapus KL. Base deficit in the elderly. A marker of severe injury and death. *J Trauma*. 1998;45:873–877.

28. Scalea TM, Simon HM, Duncan AO, et al. Geriatric blunt trauma: improved survival with early intensive monitoring. *J Trauma*. 1990;30:129–134.

29. Dune JR, Tracy JK, Scalea TM, et al. Lactate and base deficit in trauma: does alcohol or drug use impair their predictive accuracy? *J Trauma Inj Infect Crit Care*. 2005;58(5):959–966.

30. Kotani N, Hashimoto H, Sessler D, et al. Supplemental interaoperative oxygen augments antimicrobial and proinflammatory response of alveolar macrophages. *Anesthesiology*. 2000;93:15–25.

31. Criswell JC, Parr MJ, Nolan JP. Emergency airway management in patients with cervical spine injuries. *Anesthesia*. 1994;49(10):900–903.

32. Lennarson PJ, Smith DW, Sawin PD, et al. Cervical spine motion during intubation. *J Neurosurg*. 2000;94(Suppl. 2):265–272.

33. Geerts WH, Pineo GF, Heit JA. The seventh ACCP conference on antithrombotic and thrombolytic therapy: evidence based guidelines. *Chest*. 2004;126(3): 2297–2299.

34. Buchicchio GV, Joshi M, Knorr KM, et al. Impact of nosocomial infection in trauma: does age make a difference? *J Trauma*. 2001;50:612–617.

35. Butcher SK, Killampalli V, Chahal H, et al. Effect of age on susceptibility to post traumatic infection in the elderly. *Biochem Soc Trans*. 2003;31:449–451.

36. Lennarson PJ, Smith D, Todd MM, et al. Segmental cervical spine motion during orotracheal intubation of the intact and injured spine with and without external stabilization. *J Neurosurg*. 2000;92(Suppl. 2):201–206.

37. Amacher AL, Bybee DE. Toleration of head injury by the elderly. *Neurosurgery*. 1987;20:954–958.

38. Maurice-Williams RS. Head injury in the elderly. *Br J Neurosurg*. 1999;13(1):5–8.

39. Boczko W. Cranial surgery among Medicare beneficiaries. *J Trauma Inj Infect Crit Care*. 2005;58:40–46.

40. Mosenthal AC, Lavery RF, Addis M, et al. Isolated traumatic brain injury: age is an independent predictor of mortality and early outcome. *J Trauma Inj Infect Crit Care*. 2002;52(5):907–911.

41. Lomoschitz FM, Blackmore CC, Mirza SK, et al. Cervical spine injuries in patients 65 years old and older: epidemiologic analysis regarding the effect of age and injury mechanism on distribution, type, and stability of injuries. *AJR Am J Roentgenol*. 2002;178:573–577.

42. Brown CV, Anteril JL, Sise MJ, et al. Spiral computed tomography for the diagnosis of cervical, thoracic, and lumbar spine fractures: its time has come. *J Trauma Inj Infect Crit Care*. 2005;58(5):890–896.

43. Muller EJ, Wick M, Russe O. et al. Management of odontoid fracture in the elderly. *Eur Spine J*. 1999;8(5):360–365.

44. Pape HC, Remmers D, Rice J. Appraisal of early evaluation of blunt chest trauma: development of a standardized screening system for initial clinical decision making. *J Trauma Inj Infect Crit Care*. 2000;49(3): 496–504.

45. Bergeron E, Lavoie A, Clas D, et al. Elderly trauma patients with rib fractures are at great risk of death and pneumonia. *J Trauma Inj Infect Crit Care*. 2003;5433:478–485.

46. Holcomb JB, McMullin NR, Kozar RA, et al. Morbidity from rib fracture increases after age 45. *J Am Coll Surg*. 2003;196:549–555.

47. Bulger EM, Arenson MA, Mock CN, Jurkowich GI. Rib fractures in the elderly. *J Trauma Inj Infect Crit Care*. 2000;48(6):1040–1047.

48. Ochsner MG. Factors of failure for nonoperative management of blunt liver and splenic injury. *J Surg*. 2001;25:1393–1396.

49. Albrecht RM, Schermer CR, Morris A. Nonoperative management of blunt splenic injuries: factors influencing success in age >55 y. *Am Surg*. 2002;68(3):227–230.

50. Cooper C, Barker D, Morris J, et al. Osteoporosis, falls, and age in fracture of the proximal femur. *Br Med J*. 1987;306:1506–1509.

51. Dubey A, Koval KJ, Zuckerman JD. Hip fracture epidemiology: a review. *Am J Orthop*. 1999;Sept:497–506.

52. Wehren LE, Magaziner J. Hip fracture: risk factors and outcomes. *Curr Osteoporos Rep*. 2003;1:78–85.

53. Zuckerman JD. Hip fracture. *N Engl J Med*. 1996;334(23):1519–1525.

54. Henry SM, Pollak AN, Jones AL, et al. Pelvic in geriatric patients: a distinct clinical entity. *J Trauma Inj Infect Crit Care*. 2002;53(1):15–21.

55. Koval KJ, Maurer SG, Su ET, et al. The effect of nutritional status on outcome after hip fracture. *J Orthop Trauma*. 1999;13(3):164–169.

56. Koval KJ, Chen AL, Aharonoff GB, et al. Clinical pathway for hip fractures in the elderly: the Hospital for Joint Diseases experience. *Clin Orthop Relat Res*. 2004425:72–81.

57. Zuckerman JD, Skovron ML, Koval KJ, et al. Post operative complications and mortality associated with operative delay in old patients who have fracture of the hip. *J Bone Joint Surg*. 1995;77A:1551–1556.

58. Orosz GM, Magaziner J, Hannan EL, et al. Association of timing of surgery for hip fracture and patient outcomes. *JAMA*. 2004;291(14): 1738–1743.

59. Favarel-garrigues JF, Sztark F, Petitjean ME, et al. Hemodynamic effects of spinal anesthesia in the elderly: single dose versus titration through a catheter. *Anesth Analg*. 1996;82(2):312–316.

60. De Visme V, Picart F, Le Jouan R, et al. Combined lumbar and sacral plexus block compared with plain bupivacaine spinal anesthesia for hip fractures in the elderly. *Reg Anesth Pain Med*. 2000;25(2):158–162.

61. O'Hara DA, Duff AM, Berlin JA, et al. The effect of anesthetic technique on postoperative outcome in hip fracture repair. *Anesthesiology*. 2000; 92(4):947–957.

62. Gilbert TB, Hawkes WG, Hebel JR, et al. Spinal anesthesia versus general anesthesia for hip fracture repair: a longitudinal observation of 741 elderly patients during 2-year follow-up. *Am J Orthop*. 2000;29(i): 25–35.

63. Koval K, Aharonoff GB, Schmigelski C, et al. Hip fracture in the elderly: the effect of anesthetic technique. *Orthopedics*. 1999;22(1):31–34.

64. Davis FM, Laurenson VG. Spinal anesthesia or general anesthesia for emergency hip surgery in elderly patients. *Anaesth Intensive Care*. 1981; 9(4):352–358.

Diastolic Heart Function and the Elderly

Jochen Steppan
Dan E. Berkowitz
Elizabeth Martinez
Daniel Nyhan

INTRODUCTION

Over the last 15 years, the recognition of the importance of abnormal ventricular filling as an important potential cause of the symptoms of heart failure has emerged. This delay in recognition was due to the widely held view that the sole problem in heart failure was impaired systolic function (reduced ejection). It remained for cardiologists to develop more sophisticated noninvasive (primarily echocardiographic/Doppler) techniques to describe diastolic function and its abnormalities associated with symptoms of heart failure in patients with preserved systolic function. A perusal of the cardiac literature of the last several years might have one conclude that diastolic dysfunction and its more severe clinical counterpart, diastolic heart failure, are common.[1–5] The pendulum may, however, have swung too far. Not everyone agrees that diastolic dysfunction and diastolic heart failure are as common as purported or that perturbations in diastolic performance represent the primary abnormality, even in patients with diastolic heart failure.[6] Undoubtedly, disturbances in diastolic indices are present in patients with heart failure, but this does not necessarily mean that the underlying mechanisms represented by these indices are primarily responsible for the clinical syndrome. Moreover, diastolic abnormalities can be demonstrated in all patients with systolic heart failure.[2] It is likely that primary diastolic heart failure, while not uncommon, may not be as prevalent as some have suggested, and that diastolic heart failure occurs most frequently in elderly, hypertensive females[1,4,7] (Table 16-1). To understand these incongruities requires some knowledge of normal diastolic performance. Thus, we begin with a brief description of overall physiology and a discussion of relevant molecular and biophysical mechanisms.

THE CARDIAC CYCLE

The changes during the cardiac cycle are summarized in the classic Wiggers diagram (Fig. 16-1). The precise duration or definitions of systole and diastole depend on whether one is using a physiological or clinical definition. Physiological diastole begins once active contraction ceases, and occurs while intraventricular pressure is still high and well before aortic valve closure. Similarly, physiological diastole ends when contraction begins and, strictly speaking, before mitral valve closure (it is what causes left ventricular pressure to increase above left atrial pressure and precipitate mitral valve closure). The term protodiastole (early diastole) is used physiologically to refer to that period of diastole beginning

with decreases in forward aortic flow (and decreases in the aortic and left ventricular pressures) and ending with aortic valve closure (panel D, Fig. 16-1). Clinical diastole occupies that period of the cycle between aortic valve closure and mitral valve closure (Fig. 16-1). Clinical systole begins with the mitral valve closure and ends with aortic valve closure.

Overall, systolic function describes the ability of the heart to empty and is influenced by heart rate, loading conditions (pre- and afterload), and contractility. Diastolic function denotes the overall ability of the heart to fill, and is influenced by both active and passive characteristics of the myocardium and the vasculature, that is, by *vascular-ventricular (V-V) coupling* (vide infra). Either systolic or diastolic dysfunction can independently impair forward flow, and thus at least in theory, cause congestion proximal to the heart with the attendant symptoms and signs of heart failure.

Table 16-1

Comparison between SHF and DHF: Demographic and Prognostic Features

Characteristics	SHF	DHF
Demographics		
Age (years) (mean)	61	72
Sex (% female)	35	66
Hypertension (%)	62	85
CAD (%)	86	45
Symptoms and signs		
Exercise duration	↓	↓
Systolic BP	N-↓	↑
Pulse pressure	↓	↑
VO$_2$	↓	↓
BNP	↑ ↑	↑
Morbidity	↑ ↑	↑ ↑
Mortality	↑ ↑	↑

Abbreviations: CAD = coronary artery disease; N = no change; BP = blood pressure; ↓ = decreased; VO$_2$ = maximum oxygen consumption; ↑ = increased; BNP = brain natriuretic peptide.
Source: With permission from Ref. 1.

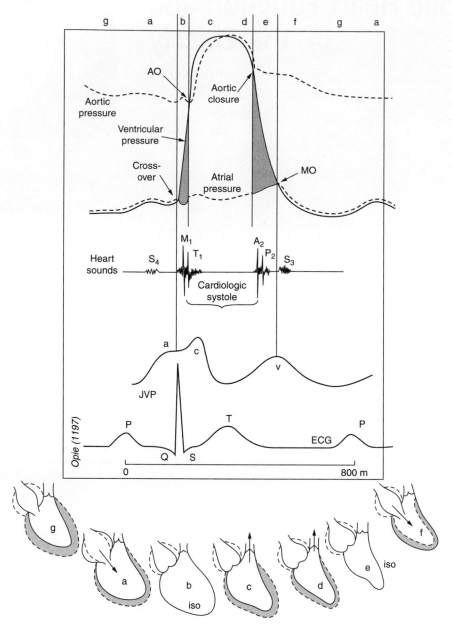

FIGURE 16-1 The cardiac cycle (Wiggers diagram) showing eight phases of left ventricular systole. By convention, the cycle begins with contraction of the ventricle, so that atrial systole is placed at the end of ventricle diastole. The top three curves represent aortic pressure (upper dashed line), left ventricular pressure (solid line), and left atrial pressure (lower dashed line). Units of pressure are millimeters of mercury. The solid line below these pressure curves is left ventricular volume, below which are the heart sounds: A, atrial (or fourth) sound; I, first heart sound; II, second heart sound; III, third heart sound. The bottom line shows the timing of the electrocardiogram which is a recording of the electrical events during the cardiac cycle. *(With permission from Ref. 14.)*

DIASTOLE

Clinical diastole (from aortic valve closure to mitral valve closure) is classically divided into isovolumic relaxation and the "auxotonic" left ventricular filling phases of diastole. The latter include early, rapid left ventricular filling; a second middle phase termed *diastasis*; and a late phase associated with atrial augmentation of ventricular filling. Several lines of investigation[8,9] suggest that early diastolic filling is not just pre-load-dependent, that is, a gradient between a positive left atrial pressure and a left ventricular pressure of zero does not fully explain early diastolic filling. The collagen matrix of the myocardium (including endo-, peri-, and epimysial fibers) is important not only in myocyte orientation but also contributes to diastolic function and ventricular

filling. Robinson was the first to suggest that the energy of contraction during systole is subsequently utilized as potential energy to effect early diastolic suction and a negative left ventricular pressure.[10] In effect, the collagen network forms a deformable type of elastic "sponge."[11] Left ventricular filling is profoundly influenced by passive stiffness characteristics of the ventricle. Indices of diastolic function (vide infra) can be categorized into those that assess the process of relaxation and those that measure features of ventricular stiffness (i.e., ventricular filling). The distinction is somewhat arbitrary since relaxation mechanisms extend into the filling phase and are not confined to protodiastole and isovolumic relaxation.

Clinically, diastole encompasses that period during the cardiac cycle following aortic valve closure. However, relaxation mechanisms are activated before aortic valve closure and prior to isovolumic relaxation, and are initiated at the point when peak pressures are achieved, that is, at the beginning of decreases in left ventricular and aortic pressures (Fig. 16-1). Relaxation is an active, energy-dependent multistep process requiring calcium release from the contractile elements, detachment of cross-bridges between the contractile elements, a decrease in cytosolic concentrations affected by reuptake of calcium by the sarcoplasmic reticulum (sarcoplasmic/endoplasmic reticulum calcium adenosine triphosphatase [SERCA]-dependent), extrusion of calcium across the sarcolemma (sodium/calcium exchange-dependent), and slowing of the cross-bridge cycling rate with a return to resting sarcomere lengths. Each of these steps can be modulated by regulatory mechanisms. For example, sarcoplasmic reticulum calcium reuptake is dependent on inhibition (by phosphorylation) of the inhibitory protein, phospholamban. This phosphorylation is mediated by protein kinase A, the downstream effects of beta-adrenergic signaling. This signaling cascade therefore represents the primary mechanism by which adrenergic activation enhances lusitropy (and couples inotropy and lusitropy). Active relaxation is an early diastolic event. The inference that subsequent diastolic events (i.e., the stress/strain relationship) are exclusively a function of passive phenomena and not influenced by active events, is overly simplistic. For example, titin, a structurally critical intrasarcomeric macromolecule, contributes significantly to diastolic muscle stiffness. However, titin, in addition to occurring in different isoforms, can also be posttranslationally modified by phosphorylation and by calcium. Protein kinase A-induced phosphorylation of titin enhances diastolic compliance.[6,12]

Measurements purported to reflect specific features of diastolic performance have multiple shortfalls[6] (vide infra). Assessments of isovolumic relaxation require invasive measurements with high-fidelity manometers to determine negative dp/dt (rate of decrease in pressure) and the time constant for isovolumic relaxation, tau (i.e., the time required for peak left ventricular pressure to decrease by two-thirds). Echocardiographic-dependent noninvasive measurements made during the auxotonic phases of diastole reflect volume transients during ventricular filling but are subject to many confounding variables including load dependency and prior systolic performance. Moreover, these measurements reflect both active relaxation and passive stiffness characteristics of the ventricle.

Diastolic dysfunction can be caused by multiple mechanisms, including myocardial and extramyocardial factors (Fig. 16-2). Clearly, the myocardium is ultimately where diastolic dysfunction is effected but may not be where the primary causal factors lie. Myocardial properties are still critical in this process. Intrinsic properties of the heart can be assessed by measuring its pressure/volume relationship. The maximum and minimum stiffness characteristics of the heart are reflected by the end-systolic and end-diastolic elastances, respectively; that is, by the slopes of the end-systolic pressure-volume relationship (ESPVR) and the end-diastolic pressure-volume relationship (EDPVR) (Fig. 16-3). The influence of systolic performance (e.g., Anrep, Bowditch effects) on subsequent diastolic behavior is beyond the scope of this discussion. The interested reader is referred to monographs by Opie[13] and Katz.[14] The slope and position of the EDPVR are modulated by the stiffness characteristics of the ventricle (an increase in slope is thought to reflect alterations in relaxation mechanisms, while an upward parallel shift is thought to reflect changes in intrinsic stiffness (Fig. 16-3). The measurements used to determine intrinsic stiffness can be influenced by external forces (e.g., pericardial and intrapleural pressures). Notwithstanding, intrinsic myocardial stiffness is thought to be a pivotal determinant of diastolic function, and is modulated by both myocyte and extracellular

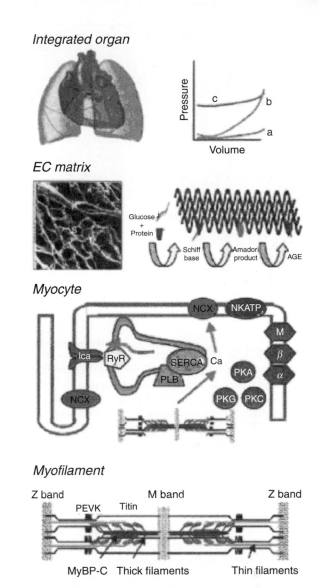

FIGURE 16-2 Mechanisms of diastolic dysfunction from the sarcomere through to the intact heart coupled with the vasculature. At the level of the myofilament, abnormal stiffness and relaxation can occur by modifications of proteins within the contractile thick and thin filaments, myosin-binding protein C (MyBP-C), and the linkage protein titin. Changes in the PEVK region of titin among its isoforms can confer differential stiffness and elastic recoil to the myocardium. At the myocyte level, calcium signaling and interaction with myofilaments play an important role. Expression and posttranslation modifications of the sarcoplasmic reticular channel (RyR, Ca2+ uptake proteins [PLB, SERCA], sarcolemmal exchanger [NCX], and ion pumps [sodium/potassium ATPase, NKATP]) by kinases all participate in this interaction. At the next level of integration, diastolic properties are coupled with an EC matrix that surrounds each myocyte and forms bundles among muscle fibers. The scanning electron micrograph (left) shows the connective tissue skeleton from a human heart, with perimysial fibers (P) enveloping groups of myocytes, smaller endomysial fibers supporting the connecting individual cells, and endomysial weave (W) enveloping individual myocytes, with cells linked to adjacent cells by lateral struts (S). Collagen is also posttranslationally cross-linked to alter its properties (including generation of advanced glycation cross-links AGE) from protein/glucose interaction. At the integrated organ level, properties of the heart are impacted by the vascular loads imposed, by geometric factors, and external constraints (pericardium/right heart). Measured diastolic pressure-volume relationships (DPVRs) shifted upward in parallel (a vs. c, top right) more commonly reflect such extrinsic influences, whereas intrinsic stiffness appears as a steeper relation (a vs. b). *(With permission from Ref. 6.)*

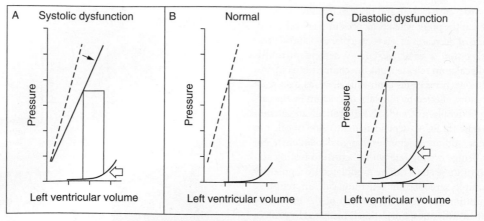

FIGURE 16-3 Left ventricular pressure-volume loops in systolic and diastolic dysfunction. In systolic dysfunction, left ventricular contractility is depressed, and the end-systolic pressure-volume line is displaced downward and to the right (panel A, black arrow); as a result, there is a diminished capacity to eject blood into the high-pressure aorta. In diastolic dysfunction, the diastolic pressure-volume line is displaced upward and to the left (panel C, black arrow); there is diminished capacity to fill at low left atrial pressures. In systolic dysfunction, the ejection fraction is depressed, and the end-diastolic pressure is normal (panel A, open arrow); in diastolic dysfunction, the ejection fraction is normal and the end-diastolic pressure is elevated (panel C, open arrow). *(With permission from Ref. 1.)*

matrix characteristics. Intrinsic myocardial properties can be altered by changes in the structural and physiological properties of these elements. For example, the macromolecule, titin, is the most important intrasarcomeric contributor to myocardial stiffness, at least at normal sarcomere lengths. Titin can be expressed in two primary isoforms which have differential effects on stiffness.[15] Moreover, and as referred to above, titin can be posttranslationally modulated and these changes can also alter stiffness characteristics conferred by titin. Myocardial collagen, especially what is referred to as *perimysial* collagen fibers which connect adjacent muscle bundles, is also an important contributor to myocardial stiffness, especially at longer sarcomere lengths. Though controversial, the ratio of soluble to insoluble collagen (increases in the ratio of type I to type III collagen) with fibrosis development may be a contributor to altered stiffness characteristics in disease states. Collagen can also be posttranslationally modified. There is now abundant evidence to indicate that the renin-angiotensin aldosterone system (RAAS) may mediate part of its adverse myocardial effects via its influence on collagen and fibrosis development.[16,17]

Finally, the formation of stable and, with age, escalating levels of advanced glycation endproducts (AGE) contributes to myocardial changes, including stiffness changes. AGE are formed by a nonenzymatic reaction between reducing sugars and proteins, including collagen[18,19] (Fig. 16-4). AGE-related cross-link formation is increasingly recognized to be important in many senescence-related changes in the cardiovascular system, for example, endothelial dysfunction, atherosclerosis, diastolic dysfunction as implied above, and hypertension. The interaction

between the vasculature and the ventricle (V-V coupling) and the changes induced in that relationship with hypertension are central to one's understanding of diastolic dysfunction and whether the latter exists as a primary abnormality, or develops as a secondary event, or perhaps both. Moreover, the V-V relationship provides a basis for understanding the clinical evolution of diastolic dysfunction and may allow one to identify specific targeted treatments.

VASCULAR-VENTRICULAR COUPLING

Teleologically, we would predict that the interaction between the vasculature and the ventricle is such that one achieves maximum, or near maximal, myocardial efficiencies in terms of work and power. Moreover, we might predict that dysregulation in V-V coupling, as might occur with increased vascular and myocardial stiffness, could contribute to the cardiovascular pathology observed in the elderly. However, attempts to quantitate the coupled relationship between the vasculature and the heart are rendered problematic partly because indices of cardiac performance are best assessed in a time domain (measure pressure, volume, and flow), while indices of vascular function are best evaluated in a frequency domain because of the contribution of pulsatile elements to arterial properties.

In addition to the inertial load of blood, the total arterial load imposed on the ventricle is not only a function of mean vascular resistance, which is the primary determinant of stroke volume, but also of pulsatile elements related to arterial compliance and wave reflections.

A number of approaches have been described, which attempt to characterize the V-V relationship. Among the most frequently used is that which was originally outlined by Sunugawa et al.[20–22] These investigators suggested that total arterial impedance could be quantified by measuring the ratio of the pressure generated over the stroke volume ejected. This approach, depicted in Fig. 16-5, in effect characterizes the total arterial load as an *effective elastance* (E_a). E_a encompasses all factors that contribute to arterial load. If, as occurs under physiological circumstances, arterial resistance is the main determinant of load, then it will be the main determinant of E_a. Critically, however, this measurement also encompasses phasic elements (compliance-related changes in the arterial wall and wave reflections) that contribute to arterial load.[23] Moreover, at least in a controlled experimental setting, E_a measurements have the capacity to segregate the individual contributions of each determinant of total arterial load including pulsatile elements.[24]

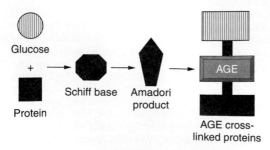

FIGURE 16-4 Nonenzymatic protein glycation to form irreversible advanced glycation endproduct (AGE) cross-linked proteins. *(With permission from Ref. 18.)*

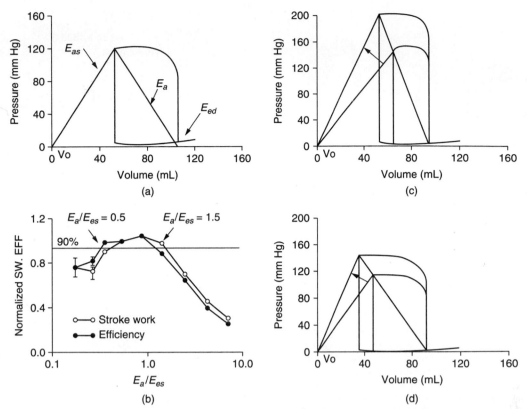

FIGURE 16-5 (A) Schematic diagram of pressure-volume loop for ventricle, with ventricular systolic (E_{es}) and diastolic (E_{ed}) elastances, and effective arterial elastance (E_a). E_{es} defines chamber systolic stiffness, while E_{ed} is the diastolic stiffness. E_a equals the ratio of Pes/SV, and reflects arterial loading. The intersection point of the E_a and E_{es} lines is the ventricular-arterial equilibrium set point. The ratio of E_a/E_{es} is used to index relative coupling between the heart and vascular systems. (B) Influence of varying ventricular-arterial coupling ratio on ventricular external work (SW) and efficiency (EFF). Both parameters reach optimal values between E_a/E_{es} ratios spanning from 0.3 to 1.3. (C) Influence of varying vascular load on the net effect of higher contraction function on blood pressure and output. Upper panel displays example with high arterial resistance. With the increase in contractility (arrow), the systolic pressure rises markedly for a given change in stroke volume. Lower panels display the identical contractility change, but at a lower arterial load. (D) In this instance, the pressure risk is much less relative to a slightly greater stroke volume increase. Thus, the net effects of systolic reserve critically depend upon the interaction of the heart and arterial systems. *(With permission from Ref. 25.)*

Finally, because the arterial E_a measurement is in effect a pressure-volume relationship (pressure developed/stroke volume), one can characterize its relationship with any adjacent component of the cardiovascular system if the latter too can be quantitated in pressure-volume terms. Thus, one can characterize the vasculature's relationship with the heart and the latter's pressure-volume relationship.[25] Therein lies the basis for quantitating V-V coupling and its perturbations in disease states.

Age, per se, is now recognized as the dominant cardiovascular risk factor,[26] and is associated with both structural and functional alterations in the arterial tree. The specific mechanisms underlying these arterial wall changes are multiple and include protean pertubations. However, the net result is an increase in arterial stiffness and the induction of perturbations in myocardial stiffness characteristics (as assessed by alterations in V-V coupling characteristics) (Fig. 16-6). The clinical manifestations can include the development of diastolic dysfunction and even diastolic heart failure.

CONSEQUENCES OF ARTERIAL WALL CHANGES WITH AGE

Changes in the arterial tree with age, including the development of endothelial dysfunction and the formation of AGE (Fig. 16-4), result in an increase in vascular stiffness and specifically an increase in arterial stiffness (Fig. 16-6). The latter is associated with augmented pulse wave velocity, including reflected waves, resulting in increased systolic blood pressure, increased pulse pressure, and increased late systolic load on the heart. In effect, reflected arterial waves return to the central circulation in late systole as opposed to early diastole as occurs in a younger, healthy cardiovascular system where pulse wave velocity is normal and slower. Indeed, increased pulse pressure is now well recognized as a specific risk factor for the development of both coronary artery disease and stroke[27-29] and for the development of heart failure.[30] Increased arterial stiffness and altered myocardial loading conditions result in a coupled increase in myocardial stiffness characteristics, including increases in both systolic stiffness and diastolic stiffness (Fig. 16-6; panel B, Fig. 16-7). Ultimately, myocardial structural changes, which may or may not include ventricular hypertrophy, develop. Importantly, age-related increases in arterial stiffness (increases in E_a) correlate with both diastolic stiffness (E_{ed}) (panel B, Fig. 16-6), and with systolic stiffness (E_{es}), and both with each other (panel B, Fig. 16-7), maintaining optimum efficiency as loading conditions change (panel B, Fig. 16-5). In contrast, indices of contractility do not correlate with age (panel A, Fig. 16-7), suggesting that arterial stiffness, and by inference structural elements in the myocardium, may be important factors in age-related diastolic changes. In addition to its influence on diastolic performance, V-V coupling of stiffer vessels with a stiffer heart has an overall deleterious effect on pressure and flow regulation (including coronary blood flow) resulting in decreased cardiovascular reserve and a lower threshold for the development of cardiovascular disease.[25,31]

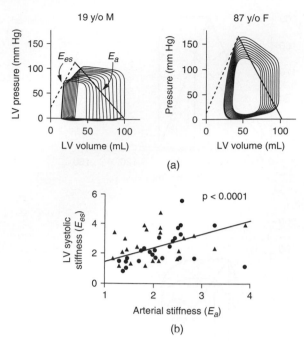

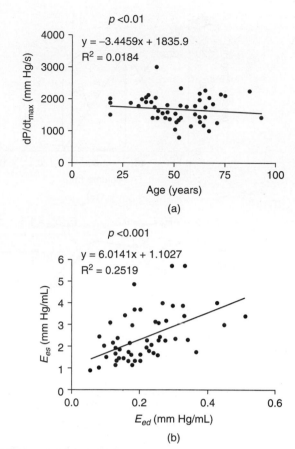

FIGURE 16-6 (A) Example pressure-volume loops and E_{es}/E_a relations for a young versus old patient. In both instances, the E_a and E_{es} values are similar to each other, coupling with a relative ratio near 1.0. However, in the elderly subject, both parameters are increased, consistent with both vascular stiffening and ventricular systolic stiffening. (B) Group data from 57 patients. There is a significant relation between a rise in effective arterial stiffness reflected by E_a and ventricular systolic stiffness as reflected by E_{es}. Tandem increases in both characterize aging. *(With permission from Ref. 25.)*

FIGURE 16-7 (A) Plot of maximal dP/dt versus age from the same patients shown in Fig. 16-6(B). Unlike E_{es}, there is no relation between this systolic contractile parameter and age. This suggests that the rise in E_{es} is due to more structural than contractile changes. (B) E_{es} does significantly correlate with diastolic chamber stiffness (E_{ed}), supporting the notion that intrinsic chamber stiffening affects both diastole and systole in the aging heart. *(With permission from Ref. 25.)*

DEFINITION OF DIASTOLIC DYSFUNCTION AND DIASTOLIC HEART FAILURE

The concept of diastolic heart failure was initially described as recently as the late 1980s.[32] Subsequent investigators described patients in whom systolic properties seemed normal, but who exhibited concentric hypertrophy, normal left ventricular dimensions, evidence of delayed relaxation, and increased ventricular stiffness.[33–35] Notwithstanding controversies related to the incidence of diastolic dysfunction and diastolic heart failure, and what represents the primary underlying pathophysiology (vascular vs. myocardial), both diastolic dysfunction and diastolic heart failure are increasingly recognized, especially in elderly hypertensive females.[1,4,7]

Diastolic dysfunction implies abnormalities in indices (prolongation, delay, or incomplete) that reflect the ventricle's ability to relax and fill in the setting of normal systolic function, and in the absence of the clinical symptoms and signs of heart failure. Indices of relaxation depend on the onset, rate, and extent of decline in left ventricular pressure and filling, while ventricular stiffness characteristics are assessed by determining the pressure-volume (stress/strain) relationship.

Diastolic heart failure is distinguished from diastolic dysfunction by the presence of symptoms and signs of heart failure. Diastolic heart failure is characterized by the clinical syndrome of heart failure in the setting of a preserved ejection fraction (Table 16-2). As with systolic heart failure, diastolic heart failure can produce symptoms at rest (New York Heart Association [NYHA], Class IV), with less than ordinary activity (NYHA, Class III) or with ordinary activity (NYHA, Class II).[2]

Ideally, a diagnosis of diastolic dysfunction or diastolic heart failure depends on the confident documentation of an increase in left ventricular end-diastolic pressure in the setting of normal systolic function, a normal or decreased left ventricular volume (accurately assessed, noninvasively only by magnetic resonance imaging [MRI] or three-dimensional [3-D] echocardiography), and the absence of ischemia and lung disease.

DIAGNOSIS

Although diastolic dysfunction and diastolic heart failure developing as a result of primary myocardial disease may be uncommon, diastolic dysfunction and diastolic heart failure are not uncommon in patients with coronary artery disease, and in those with abnormal loading conditions, for example, aortic stenosis and hypertension. As already discussed, diastolic heart failure is distinguished from diastolic dysfunction by the presence of the symptoms and signs of heart failure. While the diagnosis of heart failure can be made at the bedside, the distinction between diastolic heart failure and systolic heart failure cannot. The clinical application of the criteria used to diagnose diastolic function is limited because of the reasons outlined above.[2,36,37] However, some workers have suggested that the diagnosis

Table 16-2

Prevalence of Specific Symptoms and Signs in Systolic versus Diastolic Heart Failure

	Diastolic Heart Failure (EF >50%)	Systolic Heart Failure (EF <50%)
Symptoms		
Dyspnea on exertion	85	96
Paroxysmal nocturnal dyspnea	55	50
Orthopnea	60	73
Physical examination		
Jugular venous distension	35	46
Rales	72	70
Displaced apical impulse	50	60
S3	45	65
S4	45	66
Hepatomegaly	15	16
Edema	30	40
Chest radiograph		
Cardiomegaly	90	96
Pulmonary venous hypertension	75	80

Note. Data are presented as percent of patients in each group with the listed symptom or sign of heart failure. There were no statistically significant differences between patients with an EF >50% versus <50%.
Source: With permission from Ref. 2.

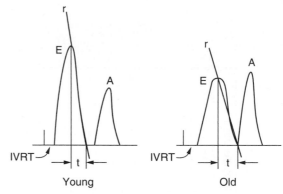

FIGURE 16-8 Doppler assessment of diastolic dysfunction. Schematic representing Doppler time-velocity plot of left ventricular diastolic inflow. Record on left represents normal state; record on right is seen in diastolic dysfunction of the elderly. E = peak velocity of early filling wave; A = peak velocity of atrial transport wave; t = E-wave deceleration time; line r = E-wave deceleration slope; IVRT = isovolumic relaxation time. *(With permission from Ref. 11.)*

CONFOUNDING ISSUES IN THE DIAGNOSIS OF DIASTOLIC DYSFUNCTION AND DIASTOLIC HEART FAILURE

Much of the controversy regarding the diagnosis of diastolic dysfunction and diastolic heart failure is related to: failure to recognize that acute heart failure is often paroxysmal; specificity of indices used to determine systolic function; and difficulty in clinically determining diastolic function.

Acute heart failure may indeed result from primary diastolic mechanisms. However, in addition to diastolic heart failure, there are other important causes of acute heart failure with preserved systolic function (Table 16-3).[41] The inherent nature of the clinical syndrome is such that subsequent workup, following effective treatment and resolution of the acute event, may not necessarily readily identify the inciting cause. Since the diagnosis of heart failure may be unreliable, the conclusion that patients with dyspneic symptoms, who have a normal ejection fraction and normal valves, have diastole heart failure may be perilous because their symptoms may have a noncardiac origin.[41] Moreover, following diuresis of patients with volume overload or acute mitral regurgitation, the acute heart failure may be erroneously ascribed to diastolic heart failure with preserved systolic function.[42] Gandhi and coworkers attempted to answer this question directly by measuring ejection fraction both during and after acute hypertension-associated pulmonary edema. Using two-dimensional (2-D) transthoracic echocardiography, they demonstrated that the ejection fraction, both during and after resolution of the acute pulmonary edema, were similar (Fig. 16-10). They concluded that the pulmonary edema was likely due to hypertension-induced exacerbation of diastolic dysfunction.[43]

A diagnosis of diastolic heart failure implies normal systolic function. Systolic function is most frequently determined clinically by measuring the ejection fraction, simply because it is a relatively easy measure to determine. Yet, ejection fraction (depending on one's cutoff, e.g., 40% vs. 50%) may be "normal" in systolic heart failure depending on the left ventricular end-diastolic volume.[2,44] A decrease in cardiac output resulting in inadequate tissue oxygenation is the

of diastolic heart failure can be made without measurements of diastolic function.[33] Zile and coworkers subjected patients with heart failure, who had an ejection fraction greater than 50%, to left heart catheterization and Doppler echocardiography. 100% of these patients, who were devoid of significant coronary artery disease, demonstrated abnormalities in either Doppler or pressure-derived indices of diastolic function leading to the conclusion that in patients with clinical heart failure, who have an ejection fraction of greater than 50%, indices of diastolic function serve to confirm rather than establish the diagnosis of diastolic heart failure.

The circumstances surrounding diastolic dysfunction are more problematic, because there are no symptoms or signs of heart failure, and the diagnosis does depend on determining indices of diastolic function. Many of the noninvasive echocardiographic indices of diastolic function can be misinterpreted, especially if viewed in isolation. For example, the E to A ratio can be normal in the setting of diastolic dysfunction and elevated left atrial pressures. Moreover, isovolumic relaxation time may be prolonged in diastolic dysfunction, but can return to normal as dysfunction becomes more severe and left atrial pressures increase. E-wave deceleration rate (half-time) and E-wave deceleration time are other indices that have been used to further the diagnosis of diastolic dysfunction (Fig. 16-8).[11] The diagnosis of diastolic dysfunction should not be based on any one noninvasive echocardiographic measurement. Rather, the diagnosis of same should be based on multiple structural and Doppler-derived flow parameters (Fig. 16-9), including tissue imaging[38–40] in patients in whom there is equal confidence that systolic function is normal. Some of the pitfalls in confirming the latter are discussed in the next section.

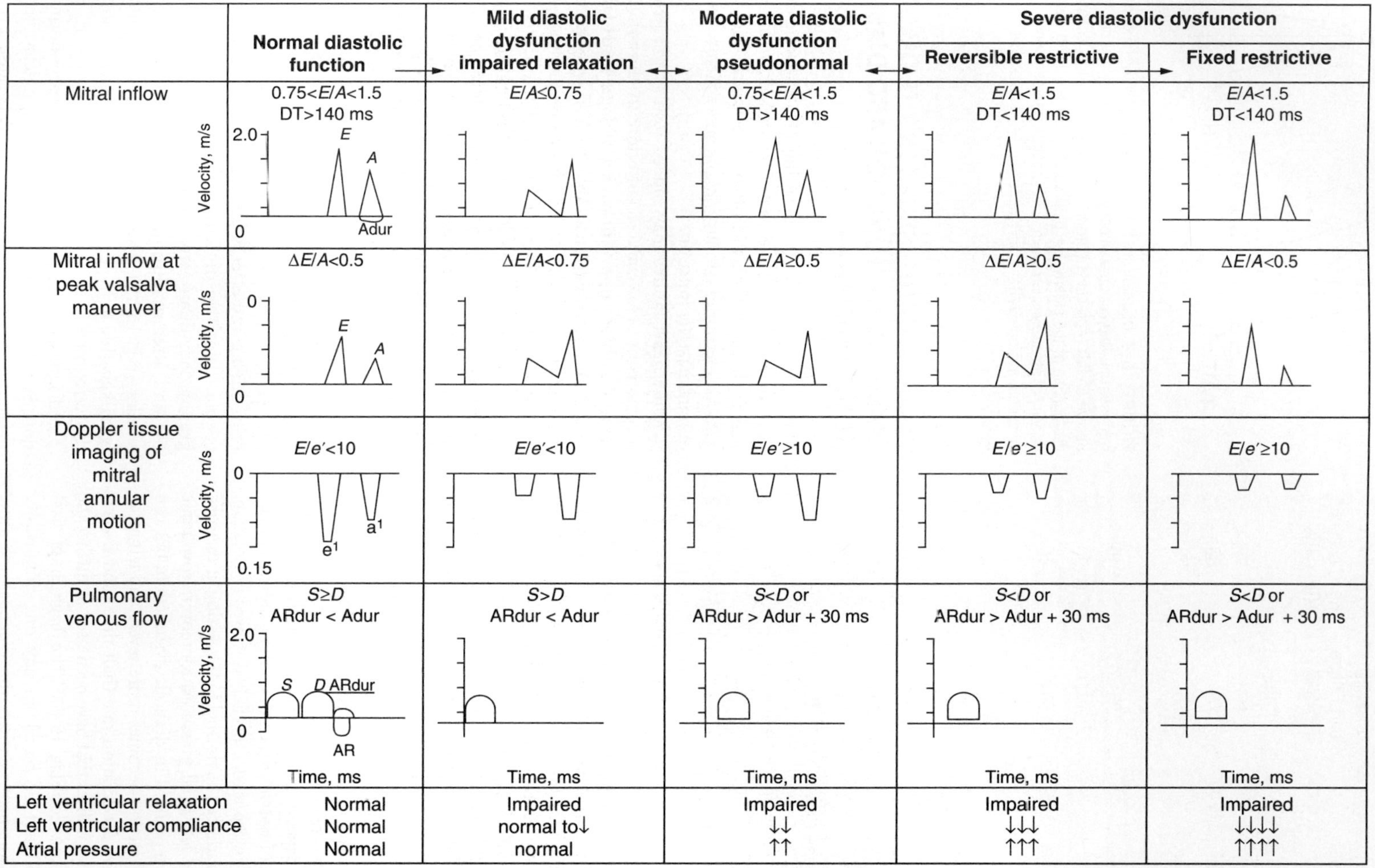

	Normal diastolic function	Mild diastolic dysfunction impaired relaxation	Moderate diastolic dysfunction pseudonormal	Severe diastolic dysfunction Reversible restrictive	Severe diastolic dysfunction Fixed restrictive
Mitral inflow	$0.75 < E/A < 1.5$ DT>140 ms	$E/A \leq 0.75$	$0.75 < E/A < 1.5$ DT>140 ms	$E/A < 1.5$ DT<140 ms	$E/A < 1.5$ DT<140 ms
Mitral inflow at peak valsalva maneuver	$\Delta E/A < 0.5$	$\Delta E/A < 0.75$	$\Delta E/A \geq 0.5$	$\Delta E/A \geq 0.5$	$\Delta E/A < 0.5$
Doppler tissue imaging of mitral annular motion	$E/e' < 10$	$E/e' < 10$	$E/e' \geq 10$	$E/e' \geq 10$	$E/e' \geq 10$
Pulmonary venous flow	$S \geq D$ ARdur < Adur	$S > D$ ARdur < Adur	$S < D$ or ARdur > Adur + 30 ms	$S < D$ or ARdur > Adur + 30 ms	$S < D$ or ARdur > Adur + 30 ms
Left ventricular relaxation	Normal	Impaired	Impaired	Impaired	Impaired
Left ventricular compliance	Normal	normal to↓	↓↓	↓↓↓	↓↓↓↓
Atrial pressure	Normal	normal	↑↑	↑↑↑	↑↑↑↑

FIGURE 16-9 Comprehensive Doppler echocardiographic assessment of diastolic function. To adequately assess diastolic function and filling pressures using Doppler echocardiography, the comprehensive assessment of a number of parameters is needed. No single parameter provides adequate information, and the more variables consistent with a certain stage of diastolic dysfunction, the more certain the diagnosis. *(With permission from Ref. 3.)*

Table 16-3

Causes of Acute Heart Failure with Preserved LV Systolic Function

Diastolic heart failure (e.g., acute global myocardial ischemia)

Acute transient left ventricular systolic dysfunction

Transient mitral regurgitation

Acute pressure or volume overload

Tachyarrhythmia

Source: With permission from Ref. 4.

seminal feature of heart failure. The ejection fraction measurement (a ratio) may not accurately reflect cardiac output if one does not take into account the left ventricular end-diastolic volume and the left ventricular end-systolic volume (both absolute measures).[44] Moreover, recent echocardiographic studies indicate that routine, 2-D and M-mode studies may not be sensitive enough to detect abnormalities in systolic function in the setting of left ventricular hypertrophy.[45,46] Thus, patients could be erroneously assigned a diagnosis of diastolic heart failure when in fact they had perturbations in systolic function, as determined by tissue Doppler imaging of the left ventricular long axis.

Precise and specific noninvasive indices of diastolic function do not exist. This is simply because all measured noninvasive indices are integrated measurements that also represent the modulating effects of loading conditions, myocardial blood flow, ventricular chamber geometry, and altered myocardial matrix. As a corollary, there is no single clinical definition of diastolic dysfunction, since indices of pressure and volume decay, indices of lengthening, measures of tissue velocity, and even increased end-diastolic pressures with altered filling are nonspecific. Not only are relaxation delays in pressure or cell lengthening nonspecific, but the monoexponential fit used to calculate and interpret the decay waveforms may yield artificially prolonged values, especially in the setting of heart failure.[6,47–49] Thus, the contribution of relaxation delay could be inadvertently exaggerated. This may, in part,

explain one of the challenges of studying diastolic dysfunction and diastolic heart failure; that is, two observations may both be true, but not causally related. Thus, while delayed relaxation does occur in diastolic heart failure, it likely has little influence on late diastolic filling and end-diastolic pressures. Similarly, while preload can influence relaxation, it is not thought to be quantitatively important, and active diastolic tone, while present, has little impact on diastolic properties, at least physiologically.[6] Moreover, there exists no animal model of diastolic heart failure, and there are few specific treatments distinct from those also used to treat systolic heart failure. Finally, diastolic dysfunction and heart failure are not amenable to an experimental approach whereby one can identify and investigate the various contributing factors in isolation.[6]

In the context of the above limitations and in the clinical setting, the absence of invasive measurements, the diagnosis of diastolic dysfunction (and if symptomatic, diastolic heart failure) should be made with caution and not be dependent on one or just a few abnormal indices. The more complete the approach, the greater the potential accuracy of the diagnosis (Fig. 16-9).

PREVALENCE, PROGNOSIS, AND THE INFLUENCE OF AGE

The prevalence of diastolic dysfunction without diastolic heart failure and the prevalence of mild diastolic dysfunction are not known.[2] However, some reports[3] suggest a prevalence of 14.1% in patients with cardiovascular risk factors. The segregation of patients with heart failure into those with diastolic heart failure versus systolic heart failure is, as discussed, dependent on an evaluation of cardiac output and ejection fraction. Moreover, while gender has an influence on the frequency and type of heart failure development (Table 16-1), age has emerged as the variable with the greatest influence not only on diastolic heart failure prevalence, but also on prognosis (Table 16-4).[2,50–53] The annual mortality for all patients with diastolic heart failure is 5–8%. This contrasts with an annual mortality of 10–15% for systolic heart failure. However, the mortality for both systolic and diastolic heart failure is greater than for matched controls (Fig. 16-11). Most importantly, in patients over 70, the annual mortality for systolic and diastolic heart failure is similar.[2,54] Based on multiple studies, 50% of patients greater than 70 who present with heart failure have diastolic heart failure, and these patients exhibit a 50% five-year mortality rate (Table 16-4).

MANAGEMENT OF PATIENTS WITH DIASTOLIC DISEASE

▶ Chronic therapy

The recommendations for treatment of diastolic heart failure are based on clinical investigations of small numbers of patients. There are no large randomized, double-blind, placebo-controlled trials. It is entirely unknown if the treatment of asymptomatic diastolic dysfunction confers any long-term benefit.

Strategies used to treat diastolic heart failure are outlined in Table 16-5. These approaches can be categorized into three groups: (1) those that target attenuation of symptoms in patients with failure; (2) those that attempt to address the underlying cause, for example, coronary artery disease, aortic stenosis, hypertension; and (3) those that target fundamental mechanisms. For example, candesartan or

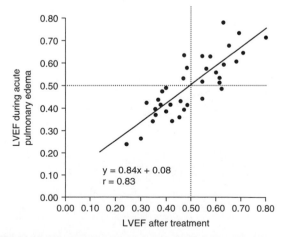

FIGURE 16-10 Left ventricular ejection fraction (LVEF) during acute pulmonary edema and 1–3 days later, after treatment. The solid line is the regression line. The dotted lines indicate normal values for the ejection fraction. *(With permission from Ref. 43.)*

Table 16-4

Diastolic Heart Failure: Effects of Age on Prevalence and Prognosis

	Age (years)		
	<50	50–70	>70
Prevalence	15	33	50
Mortality	15	33	50
Morbidity	25	50	50

Note: All values are percentages. Prevalence indicates percentage of all heart failure patients presenting with diastolic heart failure; Mortality, 5-year mortality rate; and Morbidity, 1-year rate of hospital admission for heart failure. The percentage values given in this table are approximate and rounded figures based on multiple studies.
Source: With permission from Ref. 2.

losartan target the RAAS, while NCC-135 accentuates calcium reuptake by the sarcoplasmic reticulum. All of these latter drugs are in the clinical trials phase. Some therapeutic strategies fall into more than one category, for example, interruption of the RAAS modulates not only fundamental underlying mechanisms when used long-term, but can also be important in the acute treatment of patients with diastolic heart failure (Table 16-5). By inference, most of the differing treatments for diastolic failure versus systolic heart failure reside in category C. However, although many of the agents used to treat diastolic heart failure are identical to those used to manage systolic failure, the rationale for their use, the initiation of therapy, the rate at which therapy is escalated, and the consequences of inappropriate use of these therapies are profoundly different (see below).

▶ Acute therapy (including perioperatively)

Many of the treatment strategies used chronically to manage diastolic heart failure can also be used acutely. These include strategies used to attenuate pulmonary vascular and left ventricular volume, maintenance of sinus rhythm and prevention of tachycardia, fluid and diuretic management, and the use of pharmacological adjuncts, for example, nitrates, beta-blockers, calcium antagonists, and perhaps blockade of the RAAS. Inotropes should be used cautiously, if at all, in patients with diastolic heart failure.

Heart rate and rhythm

Intuitively, one would predict that the absence of sinus rhythm (e.g., in patients with atrial fibrillation) or tachycardia will compromise ventricular filling with a decrease in forward flow and proximal congestion in the setting of decreased ventricular compliance. Indeed, tachycardia and the absence of sinus rhythm are poorly tolerated in these patients. Tachycardia adversely affects myocardial oxygen supply-demand determinants, may compromise complete relaxation because diastole is preferentially shortened, and may slow relaxation rate. A heart rate of 60–70 bpm has been suggested as a reasonable target. However, surgical stimulation in the perioperative setting may require a more aggressive and flexible approach with additional pharmacological blockade. Although V-V coupling may be maintained in patients with increases in vascular and ventricular chamber stiffness, these result in an exaggerated systolic blood pressure response to changes in heart rate. Thus, for any given change in heart rate, the resulting change in blood pressure will be greater in patients with a noncompliant (stiff) vasculature and ventricle. This effect of heart rate on blood pressure is in addition to, but independent of, directionally similar effects of changes in preload (see below) and

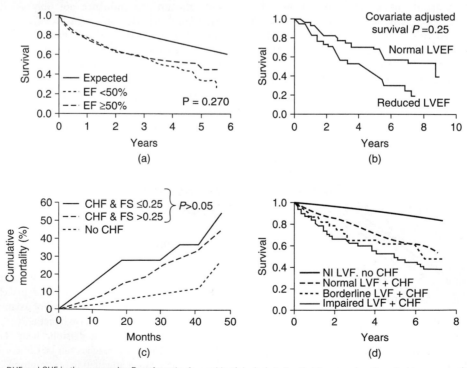

FIGURE 16-11 Survival in DHF and SHF in the community. Data from the four epidemiological studies that have compared survival in persons with SHF and DHF. Data from (A) the Olmsted County, Minn., study, (B) the Framingham Heart Study, and (C) the Helsinki Aging Study (presented as mortality) suggest similar prognosis in those with SHF or DHF. However, data from (D) the Cardiovascular Health Study suggest that survival may be slightly better in those with DHF as compared with those with SHF. *(With permission from Ref. 3.)*

Table 16-5

Diastolic Heart Failure: Treatment

Symptom-targeted treatment

    Decrease pulmonary venous pressure

    Reduce LV volume

    Maintain atrial contraction

    Prevent tachycardia

    Improve exercise tolerance

    Use positive inotropic agents with caution

Nonpharmacological treatment

    Restrict sodium to prevent volume overload

    Restrict fluid to prevent volume overload

    Perform moderate aerobic exercise to improve cardiovascular conditioning, decrease heart rate, and maintain skeletal muscle function

Pharmacological treatment

    Diuretics, including loop diuretics, thiazides, and spironolactone

    Long-acting nitrates

    Beta-adrenergic blockers

    Calcium channel blockers

    Renin-angiotensin-aldosterone antagonists, including ACE inhibitors, angiotensin II receptor blockers, and aldosterone antagonists

Disease-targeted treatment

    Prevent/treat myocardial ischemia

    Prevent/regress ventricular hypertrophy

Mechanism-targeted treatment

    Modify myocardial and extramyocardial mechanisms

    Modify intracellular and extracellular mechanisms

Source: With permission from Ref. 2.

Fluid management, diuretics

A consequence of decreased ventricular compliance (increased E_{es}) and decreased vascular compliance (increased E_a) is that one will observe greater changes in blood pressure for any given change in volume. Thus, for the heart, even small changes in preload (left ventricular end-diastolic volume and filling) will result in relatively larger increases in blood pressure. For the vasculature, the same ejected stroke volume will result in greater increases in blood pressure in stiff vessels. When combined, these result in exaggerated hemodynamic lability when venous return changes. This influence of compliance-stiffness on blood pressure was exquisitely illustrated by Chen and coworkers,[55] who demonstrated the preload sensitivity of systolic blood pressure and the influence of age thereon (Fig. 16-12).[6,55] Thus, one would predict and one should anticipate enhanced cardiovascular lability following intravascular fluid shifts (e.g., generous fluid administration, deficits in fluid resuscitation, surgical bleeding, third spacing, diuretic administration) in these patients. Conceptually, it is not difficult to recognize these concepts and their clinical implications. However, the effective clinical management of patients with diastolic heart failure, diastolic dysfunction, and increased chamber and vascular stiffness requires: a) that one can accurately determine the preload necessary to generate a target blood pressure; and b) that the compliance characteristics remain stable even in the acute perioperative setting. The former is difficult and moreover the compliance characteristics are subject to acute as well as chronic influences. The

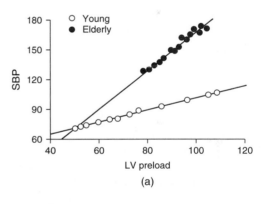

(a)

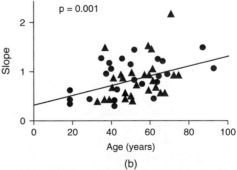

(b)

FIGURE 16-12 (A) Influence of varying cardiac preload volume on systolic blood pressure (SBP) in young versus elderly patients. In the young individual, there is a shallow slope of this relationship, reflecting the compliant arterial and ventricular systems. In contrast, the aged subject has a steeper relation, reflecting ventricular-vascular stiffening. (B) Group data showing the slope of relations as depicted in panel A as a function of age. With age, there is a gradual increase in the preload sensitivity of arterial pressure. This is related to the combination of both ventricular and arterial stiffness. *(With permission from Ref. 25.)*

---

vasomotor tone on blood pressure. Therein lies the basis for the hemodynamic lability observed in elderly patients with a noncompliant vasculature and ventricle. It is not unreasonable to invoke whatever pharmacological or electrical therapy necessary to treat patients not in sinus rhythm (e.g., atrial fibrillation, supraventricular tachycardia), especially if the abnormal rhythm is paroxysmal or of recent onset. In general, pharmacological approaches can be divided into those that promote conversion to sinus rhythm, for example, amiodarone, or those that aid in rate control following conversion to sinus rhythm, for example, beta-blockers (although these latter may also play a role in prophylaxis, either per se or of relapse). Chronic atrial dysrhythmias are likely to be relatively intractable and not amenable to conversion. Moreover, one runs the risk of precipitating thromboembolic phenomena in patients with chronic atrial fibrillation (and atrial flutter), all of whom have the potential to develop left atrial thrombi.

In addition to the principles delineated in Table 16-5 and to the extent that they apply perioperatively, there are additional management nuances that are important in the acute management of these patients. These include fluid management, use of inotropes, and the administration of beta-blockers, diuretics, and calcium antagonists.

better indices of ventricular preload (and left ventricular preload specifically) include echocardiographic (transesophageal echocardiography) assessment of left ventricular volume and pressure measurements, (left ventricular end-diastolic pressure/left atrial pressure surrogates, i.e., pulmonary artery occlusion pressure or pulmonary artery diastolic pressure [if pulmonary vascular resistance is normal and the patient is not tachycardic]). Right-sided filling pressures are a poor indicator of left-sided preload for multiple reasons, especially in patients with diastolic heart failure and diastolic dysfunction. In addition to diastolic chamber stiffness and relaxation changes in these patients, a combination of vascular and ventricular stiffening may indeed explain sudden onset pulmonary edema as a result of acute shifts in intravascular fluid from a stiff ventricle and vasculature to a relatively less stiff venous, right heart, and pulmonary vascular bed.[25] It has been suggested that diastolic heart failure represents the forgotten manifestation of hypertensive heart disease.[4] Clearly, transesophageal echocardiography and pulmonary artery catheter assessments of left ventricular preload must be customized to the specific patient. However, even in the same patient, V-V stiffness characteristics can be modulated acutely by, for example, activation of the autonomic nervous system. Sympathetic activation can not only have direct effects on the vasculature and the ventricle, but can further influence hemodynamic behavior indirectly by modulating venous tone (and thus, preload) and heart rate (see above). Neurohumoral activation of the RAAS acutely modulates salt and water fluxes and vasomotor tone, and chronically mediates fundamental mechanisms intrinsic to cellular changes that underlie the increased vascular and ventricular stiffness characteristics which develop with age. Though not currently available, acute interrogation of the RAAS may represent a future potent target for perioperative intervention.

Role of nitrates, RAAS interruption, beta-blockers, and calcium antagonists in diastolic heart failure

The immediate management objectives in patients with diastolic heart failure (including that which develop perioperatively) are similar to those in patients with systolic heart failure, that is, to decrease pulmonary congestion and central blood volume. Clearly, discretion regarding fluid management is central to this objective. Diuretics are also appropriate in these circumstances. The venodilator effects of nitrates also attenuate central blood volume. However, nitrates at the usual clinical doses also exert salutary effects on large conduit arteries, which may be especially significant in patients with increased vascular stiffness. Moreover, in patients in whom ischemia is a significant contributor to their diastolic failure, nitrates have the additional benefit of improving myocardial oxygen supply-demand balance—increasing supply and decreasing demand. The increased endocardial-to-epicardial myocardial blood-flow ratios following nitrate administration likely reflect decreased left ventricular intracavitary pressures secondary to venodilatation rather than a direct coronary influence of nitrates. Only at higher doses do nitrates exert an influence on arterial resistance vessels, and then only on coronary vessels greater than 200 μm in diameter. As already discussed, the blood pressure responses to any of these interventions (fluid manipulation, diuretics, nitrates) will be amplified in these patients. Thus, caution and prudent titration are required, because one is operating on the steep component of the left ventricular diastolic pressure-volume relationship (Fig. 16-3).

Activation of the RAAS is an important underlying mechanism in this disease process. Acutely, RAAS activation causes salt and water retention with central blood volume expansion. Chronic RAAS activation contributes to altered fibroblast activity and myocardial stiffness development.[50] Thus, at least as chronic therapy, angiotensin-converting enzyme inhibition, angiotensin-1 receptor antagonism, and aldosterone antagonism are logical therapeutic strategies in patients with diastolic heart failure.

Beta-blockers are indicated in these patients for heart rate control and for prophylaxis of atrial dysrhythmias. If ischemia is an important underlying cause of diastolic heart failure, beta-blockers have the added benefit of favorably influencing myocardial oxygen supply-demand variables and modulating endothelial function,[56] the redox milieu,[57] and nitric oxide bioavailability.[58] Beta blockade has clearly been shown to improve outcome in circumstances where ischemia may be an important underlying issue (e.g., in patients with post-myocardial infarction,[59] and perioperatively, in patients undergoing noncardiac surgery.[60–62]

Calcium antagonists are another group of drugs that represent rational therapy in diastolic disease. Mechanistically, their benefits are mediated by modulation of heart rate as well as their cardiac and vascular effects.

The role of phosphodiesterase inhibition (e.g., milrinone) has been assessed in at least one study in patients with diastolic heart failure.[63] Although the direct myocardial effects of milrinone (positive inotropy) suggest caution, their effects on the vasculature, including the pulmonary vasculature, may be of benefit in patients with acute pulmonary congestion secondary to diastolic heart failure.

Role of inotropes

These are not usually used in patients with diastolic heart failure because left ventricular function is preserved. In addition, these agents have the capacity to accentuate diastolic heart failure by adversely modulating underlying mechanisms, for example, inducing tachycardia, promoting disequilibrium in myocardial oxygen supply-demand, lowering dysrhythmia thresholds, and negatively impacting myocardial energetics. However, as with milrinone, some authors have suggested that the judicious use of sympathicomimetics may have a role to play in the management of acute pulmonary edema secondary to diastolic heart failure.[38,64,65] Any benefits of sympathicomimetics in these circumstances may be related to their lusitropic effects.

▶ Differences in treating diastolic versus systolic heart failure

The influence of ventricular and vascular stiffness on the blood pressure response to changes in preload is discussed above. This principle also applies to diuretic use. Thus, in patients with diastolic heart failure, one should use doses of diuretics that are lower than used in systolic heart failure.

The rationale for beta-blockers in systolic and diastolic heart failure are entirely different. In systolic failure, beta-blockers are used to increase inotropy by modulating beta-adrenoreceptor sensitivity and number, and in the long-term by altering ventricular remodeling. It is critical that the initial dose of beta-blockers in systolic heart failure is low, and that they are titrated carefully to avoid exacerbating the primary disease, that is, contractile dysfunction. In contrast, in diastolic heart failure, beta-blockers are used for heart rate control and modulation of the diastolic interval. Moreover, the dose used can be more liberal because contractile function is preserved.

Although the above agents are used differently in systolic and diastolic heart failure, other drugs are appropriate in one, but contraindicated in the other. The rationale for calcium antagonists in diastolic heart failure is discussed above. However, these agents (nifedipine, diltiazem, verapamil) may exacerbate contractile dysfunction in systolic heart failure and are contraindicated.

SUMMARY

Diastolic heart failure is distinguished from diastolic dysfunction by the presence of the symptoms and signs of heart failure. The clinical manifestations of both diastolic and systolic heart failure are similar. The distinction between these two causes of heart failure is dependent upon the documentation of normal systolic function, and the documentation of the multiple indices of abnormal diastolic function and of normal or reduced ventricular volumes in patients with diastolic heart failure. The presence of diastolic dysfunction implies the absence of a clinical syndrome, that is, the absence of the symptoms and signs of heart failure. The diagnosis of diastolic dysfunction can be difficult because many of the indices used to assess diastolic dysfunction are subject to multiple confounding variables. Thus, one is obligated to look at the totality of the information available, including multiple echocardiographic parameters.

Diastolic heart failure (and likely diastolic dysfunction) developed most frequently in patients with abnormal ventricular loading. In clinical terms, diastolic heart failure occurs most frequently in elderly hypertensive females. Although many of the treatment strategies for patients with diastolic heart failure are similar to those used in systolic heart failure, there are important subtleties in terms of how these therapeutic strategies are executed. Diastolic heart failure is a common and important cause of heart failure in patients over 70, and its presence is associated with a poor prognosis (50% five-year mortality rates).

KEY POINTS

▶ Both diastolic dysfunction and diastolic heart failure are not easily diagnosed conditions.

▶ Diastolic heart failure is characterized by the clinical symptoms and signs of heart failure in the setting of normal systolic function.

▶ Diastolic dysfunction by definition denotes patients who do not have symptoms of failure but do exhibit echocardiographic indices of diastolic dysfunction.

▶ There is no one echocardiographic diagnostic index of diastolic dysfunction, and this diagnosis depends on the interpretation of the totality of the echocardiographic information.

▶ Diastolic heart failure occurs most frequently in elderly hypertensive females who have abnormal myocardial loading conditions.

▶ Abnormal loading conditions modulate myocardial performance via vascular-ventricular coupling.

▶ Diastolic heart failure is an important cause of heart failure in the elderly, and is associated with a poor prognosis (50% five-year mortality).

▶ Many of the pharmacological therapies for diastolic heart failure are similar to those used in systolic heart failure. However, there are important differences in how these are initiated and escalated.

▶ A seminal feature of diastolic heart failure is decreased compliance in characteristics of both the myocardium and vasculature. Thus, a relatively small shift in fluid volume gives rise to relatively large changes in hemodynamic indices.

▶ An understanding of the preceding concept is fundamental for effective fluid/diuretic therapy in patients with diastolic dysfunction.

KEY ARTICLES

▶ Zile MR, Brutsaert DL. New concepts in diastolic dysfunction and diastolic heart failure: Part I. *Circulation.* 2002;105:1387–1393.

▶ Kass DA, Bronzwaer JGF, Paulus WJ. What mechanisms underlie diastolic dysfunction in heart failure? *Circ Res.* 2004;94:1533–1542.

▶ Opie LH. *The Heart: Physiology from Cell to Circulation.* 3rd ed. Philadelphia: Lippincott Williams & Wilkins; 1998.

▶ Katz AM. *Physiology of the Heart.* 3rd ed. Philadelphia: Lippincott Williams & Wilkins; 2001.

▶ Kass DA. Age-related changes in ventricular-arterial coupling: pathophysiologic implications. *Heart Fail Rev.* 2002;7:51–62.

▶ Najjar SS, Scuteri A, Lakatta EG. Arterial aging: is it an immutable cardiovascular risk factor? *Hypertension.* 2005;46:454–462.

▶ Sorrell V, Nanda N. Role of echocardiography in the diagnosis and management of heart failure in the elderly. *Clin Geriatr Med.* 2000;16:457–476.

▶ Appleton C, Firstenberg M, Garcia M, et al. The echo-Doppler evaluation of left ventricular diastolic function. *Cardiol Clin.* 2000;18:513–546.

▶ Zile MR, Brutsaert DL. New concepts in diastolic dysfunction and diastolic heart failure: Part II: Causal mechanisms and treatment. *Circulation.* 2002;105:1053–1058.

REFERENCES

1. Zile MR, Baicu CF, Bonnema DD. Diastolic heart failure: definitions and terminology. *Prog Cardiovasc Dis.* 2005;47:307–313.
2. Zile MR, Brutsaert DL. New concepts in diastolic dysfunction and diastolic heart failure: Part I. *Circulation.* 2002;105:1387–1393.
3. Owan TE, Redfield MM. Epidemiology of diastolic heart failure. *Prog Cardiovasc Dis.* 2005;47:320–332.
4. Lapu-Bula R, Ofili E. Diastolic heart failure: the forgotten manifestation of hypertensive heart disease. *Curr Cardiol Rep.* 2004;6:164–170.
5. Banerjee P, Banerjee T, Khand A, et al. Diastolic heart failure: neglected or misdiagnosed? *J Am Coll Cardiol.* 2002;39:138–141.
6. Kass DA, Bronzwaer JGF, Paulus WJ. What mechanisms underlie diastolic dysfunction in heart failure? *Circ Res.* 2004;94:1533–1542.
7. Aurigemma GP, Gaasch WH. Diastolic heart failure. *N Engl J Med.* 2004;351:1097–1105.
8. Nikolic S, Yellin E, Tamura K, et al. Passive properties of canine left ventricle: diastolic stiffness and restoring forces. *Circ Res.* 1988;62:1210–1222.
9. Nakatani S, Beppu S, Seiki N, et al. Diastolic suction in the human ventricle: observation during balloon mitral valvuloplasty with a single balloon. *Am Heart J.* 1994;127:143–147.
10. Robinson TF, Factor SM, Sonnenblick EH. The heart as a suction pump. *Sci Am.* 1986;254:84–91.
11. Burlew BS. Diastolic dysfunction in the elderly—the interstitial issue. *Am J Geriatric Cardiol.* 2004;13:29–38.
12. Yamasaki R, Wu Y, McNabb M, et al. Protein kinase A phosphorylates titin's cardiac-specific N2B domain and reduces passive tension in rat cardiac myocytes. *Circ Res.* 2002;90:1181–1188.
13. Opie LH. *The Heart: Physiology from Cell to Circulation.* 3rd ed. Philadelphia: Lippincott Williams & Wilkins; 1998.
14. Katz AM. *Physiology of the Heart.* 3rd ed. Philadelphia: Lippincott Williams & Wilkins; 2001.
15. Wu Y, Cazorla O, Labiet D, et al. Changes in titin and collagen underlie diastolic stiffness diversity of cardiac muscle. *J Mol Cell Cardiol.* 2000;32: 2151–2162.
16. Rossi MA. Pathologic fibrosis and connective tissue matrix in left ventricular hypertrophy due to chronic arterial hypertension in human. *J Hypertens.* 1998;16:1031–1041.
17. Weber KT, Brilla CC. Pathological hypertrophy and cardiac interstitium: fibrosis and renin-angiotensin-aldosterone system. *Circulation.* 1991;83: 1849–1865.
18. Zieman SJ, Kass DA. Advanced glycation end product cross-linking: pathophysiologic role and therapeutic target in cardiovascular disease. *Congest Heart Fail.* 2004;10:144–151.
19. Zieman SJ, Kass DA. Advanced glycation endproduct crosslinking in the cardiovascular system. *Drugs.* 2004;64:459–470.

20. Sunagawa K, Maughan WL, Burkhoff D, et al. Left ventricular interaction with arterial load studied in isolated canine ventricle. *Am J Physiol.* 1983; 245:H773–H780.

21. Sunagawa K, Maughan WL, Sagawa K. Optimal arterial resistance for the maximal stroke work studied in isolated canine left ventricle. *Circ Res.* 1985;56:586–595.

22. Sunagawa K, Sagawa K, Maughan WL. Ventricular interaction with the vascular system in terms of pressure-volume relationships. In: Yin FCP, ed. *Ventricular/Vascular Coupling: Clinical, Physiologic, and Engineering Aspects.* New York: Springer Verlag; 1987:210–239.

23. Kelly RP, Ting CT, Yang TM, et al. Effective arterial elastance as index of arterial vascular load in humans. *Circulation.* 1992;86:513–521.

24. Kelly RP, Tunin R, Kass DA. Effect of reduced aortic compliance on cardiac efficiency and contractile function of in situ canine left ventricle. *Circ Res.* 1992;71:490–502.

25. Kass DA. Age-related changes in ventricular-arterial coupling: pathophysiologic implications. *Heart Fail Rev.* 2002;7:51–62.

26. Najjar SS, Scuteri A, Lakatta EG. Arterial aging: is it an immutable cardiovascular risk factor? *Hypertension.* 2005;46:454–462.

27. Vaccarino V, Holford TR, Krumholz HM. Pulse pressure and risk for myocardial infarction and heart failure in the elderly. *J Am Coll Cardiol.* 2000;36:130–138.

28. Benetos A, Rudnichi A, Safar M, et al. Pulse pressure and cardiovascular mortality in normotensive and hypertensive subjects. *Hypertension.* 1998;32:560–564.

29. Franklin SS, Khan Sa, Wong MD, et al. Is pulse pressure useful in predicting risk for coronary heart disease? The Framingham heart study. *Circulation.* 1999;100:354–360.

30. Chae CU, Pfeffer MA, Glynn RJ, et al. Increased pulse pressure and risk of heart failure in the elderly. *JAMA.* 1999;281:634–639.

31. Kass DA, Saeki A, Tunin RS, et al. Adverse influence of systemic vascular stiffening on cardiac dysfunction and adaptation to acute coronary occlusion. *Circulation.* 1996;93:1533–1541.

32. Kessler KM. Diastolic heart failure: diagnosis and management. *Hosp Pract.* 1989;24:111–138.

33. Zile MR, Gaasch WH, Carroll JD, et al. Heart failure with a normal ejection fraction: is measurement of diastolic function necessary to make the diagnosis of diastolic heart failure? *Circulation.* 2001;104:779–782.

34. Zile MR, Baicu CF, Gaasch WH. Diastolic heart failure—abnormalities in active relaxation and passive stiffness of the left ventricle. *N Engl J Med.* 2004;350:1953–1959.

35. Baicu CF, Zile MR, Aurigemma GP, et al. Left ventricular systolic performance, function, and contractility in patients with diastolic heart failure. *Circulation.* 2005;111:2306–2312.

36. European Study Group of Diastolic Heart Failure. How to diagnose diastolic heart failure. *Eur Heart J.* 1998;19:990–1003.

37. Vasan RS, Levy D. Defining diastolic heart failure: a call for standardized diagnostic criteria. *Circulation.* 2000;101:2118–2121.

38. Sorrell V, Nanda N. Role of echocardiography in the diagnosis and management of heart failure in the elderly. *Clin Geriatr Med.* 2000;16: 457–476.

39. Appleton C, Firstenberg M, Garcia M, et al. The echo-Doppler evaluation of left ventricular diastolic function. *Cardiol Clin.* 2000;18:513–546.

40. Tokushima T, Reid CL, Gardin JM. Left ventricular diastolic function in the elderly. *Am J Geriatr Cardiol.* 2001;10:20–29.

41. Banerjee P, Clark AL, Cleland JG. Diastolic heart failure: a difficult problem in the elderly. *Am J Geriatr Cardiol.* 2004;13:16–21.

42. Banerjee P, Clark AL, Nikitin N, et al. Diastolic heart failure. Paroxysmal or chronic? *Eur J Heart Fail.* 2004;6:427–431.

43. Gandhi SK, Powers JC, Nomeir A-M, et al. The pathogenesis of acute pulmonary edema associated with hypertension. *N Engl J Med.* 2001;344: 17–22.

44. Andrew P. Diastolic heart failure demystified. *Chest.* 2003;124: 744–753.

45. Nikitin NP, Witte KKA, Clark AL, et al. Color tissue Doppler-derived long-axis left ventricular function in heart failure with preserved global systolic function. *Am J Cardiol.* 2002;90:1174–1177.

46. Yip G, Wang M, Zhang Y, et al. Left ventricular long axis function in diastolic heart failure is reduced in both systole and diastole: time for a redefinition? *Heart.* 2002;87:121–125.

47. Frank KF, Bolck B, Brixius K, et al. Modulation of SERCA: implications for the failing human heart. *Basic Res Cardiol.* 2002;97(Suppl. 1):172–178.

48. Senzaki H, Fetics BJ, Chen CH, et al. Comparison of ventricular pressure relaxation assessments in human heart failure: quantitative influence on load and drug sensitivity analysis. *J Am Coll Cardiol.* 1994;34:1529–1536.

49. Matsubara H, Takaki M, Yasuhara S, et al. Logistic time constant of isovolumic relaxation pressure-time curve in the canine left ventricle. Better alternative to exponential time constant. *Circulation.* 1995;92:2318–2326.

50. Zile MR, Brustsaert DL. New concepts in diastolic dysfunction and diastolic heart failure: Part II: Causal mechanisms and treatment. *Circulation.* 2002;105:1053–1058.

51. Kitzman DW, Gardin JM, Gottdiener JS, et al. Importance of heart failure with preserved systolic function in patients >65 years of age. *Am J Cardiol.* 2001;87:413–419.

52. Gottdiener JS, Arnold AM, Aurigemma GP, et al. Predictors of congestive heart failure in the elderly: the Cardiovascular Health Study. *J Am Coll Cardiol.* 2000;35:1628–1637.

53. Aurigemma GP, Gottdiener JS, Shemanski L, et al. Predictive value of systolic and diastolic function for incident congestive heart failure in the elderly: the cardiovascular health study. *J Am Coll Cardiol.* 2001;37: 1042–1048.

54. O'Connor CM, Gattis WA, Shaw L, et al. Clinical characteristics and long-term outcomes of patients with heart failure and preserved systolic function. *Am J Cardiol.* 2000;86:863–867.

55. Chen C-H, Nakayama M, Nevo E, et al. Coupled systolic-ventricular and vascular stiffening with age implications for pressure regulation and cardiac reserve in the elderly. *J Am Coll Cardiol.* 1998;32:1221–1227.

56. Garlichs CD, Ahang H, Mugge A, et al. Beta-blockers reduce the release and synthesis of endothelin-1 in human endothelial cells. *Eur J Clin Invest.* 1999;29:12–16.

57. Dunzendorfer S, Wiedermann CJ. Modulation of neutrophil migration and superoxide anion release by metoprolol. *J Mol Cell Cardiol.* 2000;32:915–924.

58. Hijmering ML, Stroes ES, Olijhoek J, et al. Sympathetic activation markedly reduces endothelium-dependent, flow-mediated vasodilation. *J Am Coll Cardiol.* 2002;39:683–688.

59. Held PH, Yusuf S. Effects of beta-blockers and calcium channel blockers in acute myocardial infarction. *Eur Heart J.* 1993;14:18–25.

60. Wallace A, Layug B, Tateo I, et al. Prophylactic atenolol reduces postoperative myocardial ischemia. McSPI Research Group. *Anesthesiology.* 1998;88:7–17.

61. Mangano DT, Layug EL, Wallace A, et al. Effect of atenolol on mortality and cardiovascular morbidity after noncardiac surgery. Multicenter Study of Perioperative Ischemia Research Group. *N Engl J Med.* 1996;335:1713–1720.

62. Poldermans D, Boersma E, Bax JJ, et al. The effect of bisoprolol on perioperative mortality and myocardial infarction in high-risk patients undergoing vascular surgery. *N Engl J Med.* 1999;341:1789–1794.

63. Monrad ES, McKay R, Baim DS, et al. Improvement in indexes of diastolic performance in patients with congestive heart failure treated with milrinone. *Circulation.* 1984;70:1030–1037.

64. Udelson JE, Cannon RO, Bacharach SL, et al. Beta adrenergic stimulation with isoproterenol enhances left ventricular diastolic performance in hypertrophic cardiomyopathy despite potentiation of myocardial ischemia: comparison to rapid atrial pacing. *Circulation.* 1989;79: 371–382.

65. Lang RM, Carroll JD, Nakamura S, et al. Role of adrenoceptors and dopamine receptors in modulating left ventricular diastolic function. *Circ Res.* 1988; 63:126–134.

SECTION

5

CONTROVERSIES IN INTRAOPERATIVE MANAGEMENT

Body Temperature Management in the Elderly Surgical Patient

Steven M. Frank

The perioperative management of elderly patients can be most challenging, given the high incidence of coexisting disease, and the age-related impairment of basic homeostatic function such as thermoregulation. Since perioperative morbidity in elderly patients is greater than in younger patients, the prevention and treatment of perioperative stress is critical in elderly patients. This includes optimal management of stressors including preoperative anxiety, hemodynamic aberrations, pain, and body temperature abnormalities. Although hypothermia protects against ischemia during periods of decreased organ perfusion, in awake postoperative patients, hypothermia triggers a sympathetic nervous system response, which increases plasma levels of catecholamines and can precipitate myocardial ischemia and cardiac morbidity. Since cardiac morbidity is the number one cause of death in the perioperative period, it is important to prevent postoperative hypothermia in the elderly patient. Maintenance of body temperature in the elderly is beneficial since as little as 1 or 2°C decrease in body temperature significantly impairs coagulation. This chapter covers the effects of anesthetics on thermoregulation to illustrate why hypothermia occurs so commonly in the elderly. The physiologic effects of hypothermia are discussed with specific focus on the sympathetic nervous system and cardiovascular outcomes. Methods for monitoring and controlling body temperature are also covered to provide practical information on caring for the elderly patient.

THERMOREGULATION

An understanding of perioperative heat balance requires basic knowledge on thermoregulation. The anterior hypothalamus is the center of thermoregulatory control.[1] There are three general components of the thermoregulatory system: the afferent input of thermal information; central processing of this information; and the efferent responses that control heat loss and production (Fig. 17-1).[2] Afferent information is taken from thermoreceptors in the hypothalamus itself, other parts of the brain and spinal cord, deep visceral tissues, and from the skin surface. The relative contribution of thermal information to the central thermoregulatory system is 80% from the core and deep body tissues, and 20% from the skin surface.[3] In the hypothalamus, this information is compared to an internal set point temperature which is analogous to the setting on a thermostat. When body temperature is above or below this set point, the first response to correct the body's temperature is a behavioral one that involves changing the ambient temperature to which the person is exposed or altering one's clothing to optimize heat balance. When

behavioral thermoregulation is inadequate, and temperature exceeds the set point, vasodilation and sweating are triggered to release heat to the atmosphere. When temperature is below the set point, vasoconstriction is triggered to conserve heat, and shivering and nonshivering thermogenesis are triggered to produce heat. Nonshivering thermogenesis is not thought to occur in adult humans.

ANESTHETICS AND HEAT BALANCE

Drugs can modify heat balance by altering one or more of the three components of the thermoregulatory system: the afferent pathway; the central control mechanism; or the efferent paths. Atropine, for example, may result in hyperthermia by blocking the efferent sympathetic diaphoresis response to warm environments. General anesthetics impair all three components while regional anesthesia (major conduction blockade) impairs the afferent and efferent, but not the central pathways. Over the past decade, numerous studies have characterized the effects of different anesthetic drugs and techniques on thermoregulatory function. The results of these studies show that virtually all anesthetics (regional and general) impair thermoregulation, rendering patients poikilothermic during surgery.[4,5] The overall effects of anesthesia on thermoregulation are illustrated in Fig. 17-2. Considering the cold operating room environment, hypothermia occurs in approximately 50% of patients when defined as a core temperature <36°C, and in 33% of patients when defined as a core temperature <35°C.[6]

▶ Sedatives

Direct cerebral application of barbiturates induces an increase in skin blood flow with resultant radiant heat loss to the environment.[7] Benzodiazepines lower the thresholds for sweating, vasoconstriction, and shivering but only minimally compared to other anesthetic drugs.[8] Propofol has little effect on sweating, but significantly inhibits responses to cold (vasoconstriction and shivering) in a dose-dependent fashion, thus predisposing to hypothermia.[9]

▶ Opioids

Intracerebral morphine decreases body heat production.[10] All opioids in high doses given systemically cause hypothermia.[11] Meperidine is most effective in treating postoperative shivering when compared to fentanyl and morphine, an effect related to the kappa-receptor agonist properties of the drug.[12] Alfentanil (a mu-agonist) causes a linear

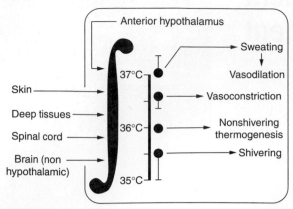

FIGURE 17-1 A model of thermoregulatory control. Afferent input of thermal information is derived from tissues throughout the body, including the brain, skin surface, spinal cord, and deep tissues. A mean body temperature below the set point initiates cold responses (vasoconstriction, shivering and nonshivering thermogenesis). A mean body temperature above the set point triggers the warm responses (vasodilation and sweating). *(From Ref. 2.)*

dose-dependent inhibition of vasoconstriction and shivering, but has little effect on sweating.[13] In general, opioids predispose to hypothermia due to significant impairment of thermoregulation.

Inhaled anesthetics

The volatile anesthetics as well as nitrous oxide inhibit all thermoregulatory responses in a dose-dependent fashion.[14,15] There is a sudden redistribution of heat within the body after induction of general anesthesia, which is characterized by a 1°C decrease in core temperature in the first 30-60 min of general anesthesia.[2] This represents heat flow from the core to the peripheral thermal compartment from vasodilation.[16] At typical doses of volatile anesthetics, the interthreshold range is expanded tenfold and vasoconstriction is not triggered until core temperature is near 34°C. Thus, core temperature continues to decrease over the first 2-3 h of general anesthesia. At this time, the core temperature

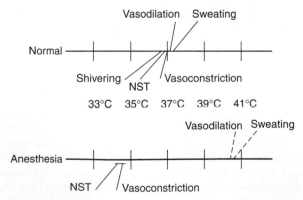

FIGURE 17-2 A schematic illustrating thresholds and gains for thermoregulatory responses in awake and anesthetized humans. The X-axis represents mean body temperature. For each individual thermoregulatory response, the threshold is indicated by the intersection with the X-axis and the gain is represented by the slope of the line that intersects. The interthreshold range is shown as the range of temperatures that do not trigger a response. This range (between sweating and vasoconstriction) is expanded approximately tenfold by anesthesia. This effect of anesthesia renders patients poikilothermic and body temperature drifts toward environmental temperature. *(From Sessler DI. Temperature monitoring. In: Miller HD, ed. Anesthesia, 3rd ed. New York: Churchill Livingstone; 1990:1227–1242.)*

often plateaus due to activation of vasoconstriction. Upon emergence, active vasoconstriction and shivering are frequently observed as the anesthetic is discontinued in the hypothermic patient.[5,17]

Regional anesthesia

In contrast to general anesthetics, epidural or spinal anesthesia does not modify central thermoregulatory activity. However, major conduction blockade is associated with approximately the same magnitude of hypothermia as occurs during general anesthesia when all other factors are the same.[4] In a controlled randomized trial comparing epidural and general anesthesia in patients undergoing radical prostatectomy, mean core temperature was identical at the end of the surgical procedure.[5] Thus, when all factors are taken into consideration, the risks of hypothermia appear to be similar with regional and general anesthetics; however, this risk is increased in the elderly.

The effects of regional anesthesia on afferent thermal signals are such that the hypothalamus is fooled by apparent warm signals from the lower body as the dominant cold signals are blocked.[18] The efferent responses are also blocked as vasoconstriction and shivering cannot occur below the level of the block, and heat loss continues without the plateau phase as with general anesthesia. There is evidence that higher block levels predispose to more hypothermia, an effect which is increased with advanced age.[19,20] It also may be that core temperature is slower to recover in the postoperative period with regional than with general anesthesia due to residual sympathectomy and the resultant heat loss.[5] Shivering occurs but with less heat production since only the upper body contributes.

Despite the risks and consequences (see below) of hypothermia, body temperature is largely ignored during regional anesthesia, and hypothermia is often neither recognized, nor prevented or treated.[21] Body temperature monitoring sites typically used during general anesthesia (nasopharynx, esophagus, and oropharynx) are not tolerated in awake or sedated patients, and thus some clinicians feel it is not convenient to monitor temperature during regional anesthesia. Historically, temperature monitoring became popular in the early 1960s when malignant hyperthermia (MH) was first described. Since regional anesthesia is not associated with MH, temperature monitoring was initially not thought to be important. We now recognize that hypothermia occurs frequently during regional anesthesia, and that temperature should be monitored and controlled.

Combined regional and general anesthesia

Vasoconstriction thresholds are reduced and core cooling rates are increased in patients receiving combined regional/general anesthesia compared to those receiving only general anesthesia.[2] This appears to be related to lower extremity heat loss in the complete absence of vasomotor tone during regional anesthesia in addition to the central thermoregulatory inhibition from general anesthesia. For this reason, core temperature should be carefully monitored and active warming used to maintain body temperature when combined regional/general anesthesia is employed.

BODY TEMPERATURE MONITORING

There are, as Dubois described, "many different temperatures of the human body and its parts."[22] In the simplest model, the body is divided into two thermal compartments, the core and the periphery. The core has a relatively constant internal temperature that is protected by the insulation from the peripheral compartment. The chest, abdomen, pelvis, and head make up the core compartment. The extremities and skin surface make up the peripheral compartment. Mean body temperature lies somewhere in between the two and is defined as 0.66•(core temperature) + 0.34•(mean skin-surface temperature).[23]

For the purposes of temperature monitoring during anesthesia and surgery, the best monitoring sites are those that are closest to blood temperature which is considered the "true" core temperature.[24] The various sites for core temperature monitoring are listed in Table 17-1 in order from most to least accurate for correlation with blood temperature.

Besides blood temperature in the pulmonary artery, nasopharyngeal and esophageal temperatures are the most accurate estimates of core temperature. Esophageal measurements, however, must be from the lower third of the esophagus. If the probe is placed in the upper or middle third, then the respiratory gases will heat or cool the temperature probe.[25] The distal third can be reached by going 10 cm beyond the point of maximum heart sounds with an esophageal stethoscope. Tympanic measurements are an excellent representation of core temperature since the internal carotid artery passes near the tympanic membrane.[24] When body temperature is changing (i.e., during anesthesia and surgery) bladder and rectal temperatures are the slowest to change, and are likely to underestimate the magnitude of alteration in body temperature. In some clinical situations (i.e., cardiac surgery), these sites are deliberately monitored since the "slow to change" characteristic is helpful to assess the "completeness" of cooling and warming on cardiopulmonary bypass.[26] The skin surface is usually 2-3°C lower than core temperature, but the core to skin gradient depends on ambient temperature and vasomotor tone.[27] For this reason, skin-surface temperature monitoring can be misleading in the perioperative period by underestimating true core temperature.[28] The relative changes in body temperature from various monitoring sites are shown during cooling and rewarming on cardiopulmonary bypass in Fig. 17-3.

The definition of normal core temperature varies since there is a circadian rhythm of ≈1°C with a nadir in the morning and a peak in the afternoon. There is also a monthly variation in menstruating women with a sudden increase in core temperature (≈0.5°C) at the onset of the luteal phase in response to increasing progesterone levels. There is no change in basal core temperature related to age.[29] Taking all variables into account, including differences among measurement

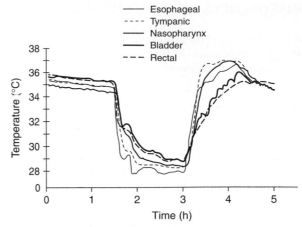

FIGURE 17-3 Body temperature monitoring in a patient on cardiopulmonary bypass. The relative ability of each monitoring site to reflect core temperature is shown. Arterial blood temperature coming from the bypass pump into the ascending aorta is shown along with various sites that are used to monitor "core" temperature. The fastest temperature sites to show change during cooling and warming (other than arterial blood) are those measured at the nasopharynx, tympanic membrane, and esophagus. Temperatures in urinary bladder and rectum area are slower to change and are considered to be "intermediate" temperatures rather than core temperatures. These sites are helpful in assessing the completeness of cooling and warming during cardiac surgery. Although skin-surface temperature is not shown, changes in skin temperature occur even more slowly than those measured in the rectum or urinary bladder.

sites, it is difficult to define a "normal" core temperature, but 36.5–37.5°C is within the normal range.

BENEFITS OF HYPOTHERMIA

▶ Neurologic protection

As little as 2°C of cooling provides significant protection for the brain and spinal cord during periods of interrupted blood flow.[30] Thus, mild hypothermia can be used for brain protection during carotid endarterectomy or procedures with high aortic cross clamps where the spinal cord is at risk from ischemia. Paraplegia is a well-recognized complication of aortic surgery, especially when aortic cross clamps are placed high on the aorta. The incidence of paraplegia is as high as 20-40% in some series where aortic cross clamp is prolonged or the aneurysm is dissecting. In a series of patients cooled to 30°C on partial cardiopulmonary bypass, we found no neurologic deficits in 20 patients.[31] Certainly, there are multiple variables that contribute to spinal cord injury, but even mild hypothermia appears to be protective. Animal studies have shown a twofold prolongation in the duration of aortic cross clamp required to produce paraplegia at 35°C versus 37°C,[32] thus supporting the findings in brain protection studies of the benefits of mild hypothermia for neurologic protection.

▶ Renal protection

Suprarenal aortic cross clamping renders the kidneys ischemic, and prolonged ischemia (>1 h) can precipitate renal failure, especially in those patients with preexisting renal insufficiency. Mild hypothermia (as little as 2°C cooling) provides significant renal protection during aortic cross clamp. Although the kidneys can be locally cooled with topical ice or slush, whole body cooling is the usual method of renal protection during thoracic and high aortic surgery, since spinal cord protection is also achieved.

Table 17-1

Accuracy of Temperature Monitoring Sites

Ability to Represent Core Temperature	Monitoring Site
Most accurate	Pulmonary artery
	Esophagus (distal one-third)
	Tympanic membrane
	Nasopharynx
	Oropharynx
Intermediate	Urinary bladder
	Rectum
	Axilla
Least accurate	Skin surface

CONSEQUENCES OF HYPOTHERMIA

Table 17-2 summarizes the physiological effects of hypothermia, and Table 17-3 gives the results of randomized outcome studies on perioperative thermal management.

▶ Shivering and metabolism

One of the most commonly recognized effects of hypothermia is postoperative shivering. Despite earlier suggestions that inhalational anesthetics cause shivering by disassociation of spinal reflexes from cortical centers in the brain, it is now believed that most perioperative shivering (with general or regional anesthesia) is thermoregulatory in origin.[33]

Based on studies from 20–30 years ago with small numbers of patients and questionable methods, the myth has been perpetuated that shivering dramatically increases total body oxygen consumption by ≈400% above baseline. In these earlier studies, there were single patients that reportedly increased their metabolic rates by >400%,[12,34] but the methods used to measure oxygen consumption were inferior and the average increase with shivering was ≈100%. In general, these

Table 17-2

Physiological Effects of Hypothermia

System	Effect
Metabolism	Postoperative shivering increases total body oxygen consumption (average increase is ≈40%, maximum is ≈100%)
Respiratory	Blunted ventilatory response to CO_2
	5% decrease in tissue oxygen requirements for each °C of cooling
	Increased oxygen solubility in blood
	Increased affinity of hemoglobin for oxygen (left shift in Hgb-O_2 curve)
Adrenergic	Activation of sympathetic nervous system
	100–500% increase in norepinephrine
	Little or no adrenomedullary or adrenocortical response (epinephrine and cortisol unchanged)
Cardiovascular	Systemic and pulmonary vasoconstriction
	Increased arterial blood pressure
	Increased risk of ventricular dysrhythmias
	Increased risk of myocardial ischemia and cardiac morbidity
Coagulation	Impaired platelet function
	Impaired coagulation cascade
	Enhanced fibrinolysis
Immunologic	Impaired neutrophil and macrophage function
	Decreased tissue partial pressure for oxygen
	Increased risk of bacterial wound infection
Pharmacokinetics	Increased effect of neuromuscular blockers
	Prolonged duration of neuromuscular blockers
	Decreased MAC for inhaled anesthetics

Table 17-3

Summary of Randomized Trials of Thermal Management and Outcome

Publication	Surgical Procedure	Outcome	Average Score	Outcome Difference
Kurz A, et al.[52]	Colon resection	Wound infection	34.7	Threefold
Schmeid H, et al.[51]	Hip arthroplasty	Bleeding	35.0	20% increase
Frank SM, et al.[45]	Abdominal, thoracic with cardiac risk factors, and vascular	Cardiac morbidity	35.3	55% relative risk reduction
Leihardt R, et al.[56]	Major abdominal	PACU length of stay	34.8	40 min increase
Fleisher LA, et al.[68]	Gynecologic	PACU length of stay	35.4	No difference
Kurz A, et al.[36]	Major abdominal	Thermal comfort	34.4	40 points on a 100-point scale
Krenzischeck DA, et al.[37]	Abdominal, thoracic, vascular	Thermal comfort	35.3	2 points on a 10-point scale

were young patients receiving little or no opioid analgesia. Recent more carefully conducted studies have shown that shivering increases oxygen consumption, but the average increase is ≈40%, with a maximum increase of ≈100%.[17] Other predictors of increased oxygen consumption were male gender and increased core temperature (Fig. 17-4). Although shivering is uncomfortable for most patients, it is unlikely that this relatively small increase in total body oxygen consumption in the average shivering patient is associated with perioperative morbidity.

It is common for patients to complain that their worst memory from the recovery room is the intense cold sensation and uncontrollable shivering. Shivering can be attenuated by relatively small doses of opioids. Although all opioids reduce shivering, meperidine is most effective (12.5–25 mg) due to the increased activity at the kappa receptor.[12,35] Other drugs that are effective in the treatment of shivering include Clonidine, neostigmine, and ketanserine (a serotonin antagonist). Thermal comfort is significantly improved and shivering can be virtually eliminated with the use of cutaneous warming during or following surgery with forced air warming.[36,37] For every 1°C of core hypothermia, approximately 4°C of skin-surface warming is required to attenuate the shivering response.[4]

▶ Hypothermia and the respiratory system

Hypothermia blunts the ventilatory response to CO_2. The slope of the CO_2 response curve decreases from 0.38 L/min/mm Hg at 37°C to 0.10 L/min/mm Hg at 28°C.[38] The respiratory quotient, or ratio of CO_2 production to oxygen utilization, does not change with hypothermia. Thus, oxygen utilization decreases at the same rate as CO_2 production. Like CO_2 content, oxygen content does not change.

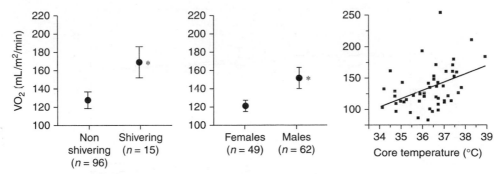

FIGURE 17-4 Total body oxygen consumption in the early postoperative period and the effects of shivering, gender, and core temperature. Oxygen consumption was increased in shivering vs. nonshivering patients but the magnitude of increase was only 40%. Males had a 25% greater metabolic response compared to females due to a greater lean body mass. Core temperature was directly proportional to oxygen consumption. These findings indicate that even when shivering is accounted for, hypothermia is associated with a decrease in metabolism not the increase that one would expect if all hypothermic patients shivered, and all shivering was associated with a large increase in metabolism.*, $P < 0.05$ vs. Nonshivering and vs. Females. *(Modified from Ref. 17.)*

An increase of oxygen solubility in blood occurs along with an overall 7.5% per °C increase in oxygen affinity of hemoglobin, the latter decreasing unloading of oxygen from hemoglobin at the level of the tissues. Even mild hypothermia induces pulmonary vasoconstriction, which interferes with hypoxic pulmonary vasoconstriction.[39]

▶ Hypothermia and sympathetic activation

The adrenergic response to hypothermia in the awake patient is significant. Although this response is not manifested during anesthesia, norepinephrine is significantly increased postoperatively in awake mildly hypothermic patients. A core temperature of <35.5°C following surgery triggers a twofold increase in norepinephrine, vasoconstriction, and increased arterial blood pressure.[40] When young, awake human volunteers are cooled to a core temperature of 35.2°C, a 500% increase in norepinephrine is induced, along with vasoconstriction and increased arterial blood pressure.[41] This response appears to be primarily from the peripheral sympathetic nervous system, with little or no adrenal response, since epinephrine and cortisol are unchanged with core hypothermia (Fig. 17-5). The adrenergic response is of greater magnitude in younger individuals, which may explain the decreased ability for the elderly to protect their core temperature through sympathetically-mediated vasoconstriction during cold challenge.[29]

▶ Hypothermia and the cardiovascular system

It is well recognized that cold stress adversely affects the cardiovascular system by triggering myocardial ischemia. For more than 50 years, a seasonal variation in death rate from myocardial infarction has been recognized with increased morbidity during the winter months.[42,43] This effect appears to be temperature-related and independent of snowfall or other climatic changes. In high-risk patients (those with risk factors for coronary disease), a core temperature less than 35°C is associated with a two- to threefold increase in the incidence of early postoperative myocardial ischemia.[44] This "cold-induced" myocardial ischemia is independent of anesthetic technique (regional or general) and age (median age was 65 years). In a prospective randomized trial, we demonstrated a 55% reduction of the relative risk for early postoperative cardiac morbidity in patients who were warmed to normothermia during and after surgery.[45] The incidence of postoperative ventricular tachycardia and morbid cardiac events was reduced in the normothermic group (core temperature = 36.7°C) compared to the hypothermic group (core = 35.3°C) (Fig. 17-6). Of interest is that intraoperatively, cardiac outcomes occurred with similar frequency in the two groups. This suggests that cold-induced perioperative cardiovascular morbidity is likely to be mediated by the adrenergic response since the effect of temperature on outcome is significant in the postoperative period after emergence, not during anesthesia when the adrenergic response to hypothermia is attenuated. Since perioperative cardiac morbidity is 10 times more likely after vascular compared to nonvascular surgery,[46] it is of utmost importance to prevent the stress of postoperative hypothermia in such high-risk patients.

▶ Hypothermia and coagulation

The coagulation system is significantly influenced by hypothermia through three different mechanisms: platelet function, the coagulation cascade, and fibrinolysis. The function of platelets is impaired by hypothermia due to reduced levels of thromboxane B2 at the site of tissue injury.[47] There is also reduced activity of coagulation factors in the coagulation cascade since the enzymes involved in the cascade, like all enzymes, are temperature-dependent.[48] Since the prothrombin time (PT) and partial thromboplastin time (PTT) tests are routinely performed at a temperature of 37°C in most laboratories, it is likely that most temperature-related coagulopathies are missed in the clinical setting. Fibrinolysis is enhanced with hypothermia which destabilizes clot and predisposes to increased bleeding.[49] Platelet sequestration is also thought to contribute to hypothermia-related coagulopathy. Sequestration, however, has only been shown in severely hypothermic dogs (20°C)[50] and is unlikely to be significant in the perioperative setting. A recently completed study in patients undergoing total hip arthroplasty showed a significant reduction in blood loss and reduced requirements for allogeneic blood transfusion in patients maintained normothermic compared to those with mild hypothermia (35°C).[51]

▶ Body temperature, wound healing, and infection

There is evidence that wound healing is impaired and that patients are more susceptible to wound infection when hypothermia (core <35°C) occurs during surgery.[52] Mild hypothermia (34.7°C) increased the incidence of wound infection threefold (19% vs. 6%) compared to

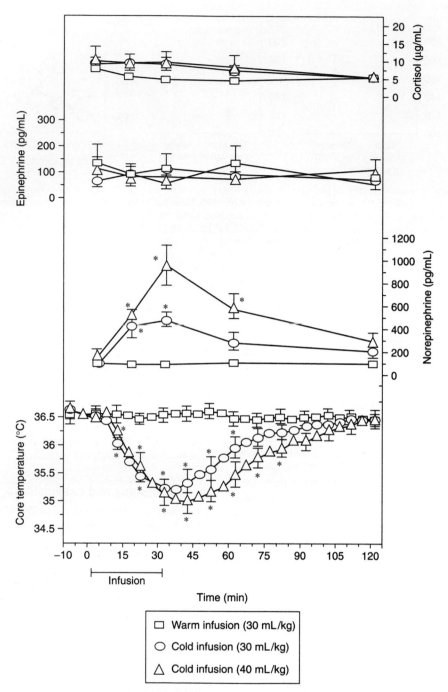

FIGURE 17-5 The adrenergic response to core cooling. Mild core hypothermia (35.0–33.5°C) was induced by infusion of cold intravenous fluids. Norepinephrine increased 500% while epinephrine and cortisol were unchanged. Thus, a peripheral sympathetic response is activated by core hypothermia but the adrenal response is absent. The norepinephrine response is associated with increased vasomotor tone and increased arterial blood pressure. *, $P < 0.05$ vs. preinfusion baseline. *(Modified from Ref. 41.)*

normothermic patients (36.6°C) undergoing colon surgery. This effect is presumably related to impaired macrophage function and reduced tissue oxygen tension secondary to thermoregulatory vaso-constriction. Collagen deposition in the wound has also been shown to be impaired with hypothermia. Increased susceptibility to infection with hypothermia at the time of introduction of bacteria into the skin has also been shown in animal models.[53,54] The "window of opportunity" for infection to become established is reportedly in the first 3 h following inoculation. If hypothermia occurs at this critical time, then infection occurs more frequently.

▶ Altered pharmacokinetics and pharmacodynamics in hypothermic patients

The minimum alveolar concentration (MAC) for potent inhaled anesthetics is reduced by ≈5% for each °C of reduction in body temperature.[55] In addition, the blood/gas solubility for inhaled anes-thetics is increased with hypothermia. In combination, these effects contribute to the slow emergence from general anesthesia in hypothermic patients. In a recently completed blinded randomized trial, the duration of time in the post anesthesia care unit (PACU)

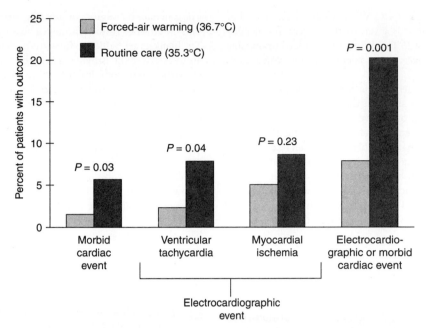

FIGURE 17-6 The incidence of early postoperative cardiac morbidity (<24 h following surgery) in patients who were randomized to receive active warming with a forced-air system (normothermic), or to receive no exogenous warming (hypothermic). Morbid cardiac events (unstable angina, myocardial infarction, or cardiac arrest), ventricular tachycardia (>5-beat runs), and myocardial ischemia occurred more frequently in the hypothermic patients. *(Modified from Ref. 45.)*

required to be ready for discharge was prolonged by an average of 40 min in hypothermic (34.8°C) versus normothermic (36.7°C) patients.[56] These findings suggest that substantial cost savings can be achieved by maintaining normothermia and expediting recovery from general anesthesia.

Mild hypothermia increases the duration of action of nondepolarizing neuromuscular blockers. At 34°C, the duration of vecuronium is doubled.[57] This effect is thought to be a pharmacokinetic one and not pharmacodynamic. Atracurium is also prolonged but somewhat less—a 60% increase in duration occurs at 34°C.[58] When added to the changes in MAC and solubility for inhaled anesthetics, this prolongation of neuromuscular blockade can delay or prevent emergence from general anesthesia, especially in the elderly who already have a reduced MAC and are especially susceptible to hypothermia.

METHODS OF CONTROLLING BODY TEMPERATURE

Ambient operating room temperature

Anesthesia induces poikilothermia whereby patients tend to equilibrate body temperature with ambient temperature. At the turn of the century, there were reports of heat stroke during surgery which occurred in anesthetized patients in hot operating rooms prior to air conditioning.[59] Operating rooms are now maintained at temperatures between 65 and 70°F, primarily for the comfort of the staff. At these temperatures, patients are predisposed to hypothermia especially with the high rate of air exchange which creates a "windchill" effect. When ambient temperature is >23°C (≈73°F), unintentional hypothermia occurs less frequently during surgery,[4,60,61] but this warm environment is not well tolerated by the surgical staff since surgical gowns are now impermeable to fluids and uncomfortable to wear. It is therefore preferable to warm the patient rather than the entire operating room and the surgical staff therein.

Warming the inspired gases

Active heating and humidification of the inspired gases has little or no effect on core temperature except in neonates where this method may help in maintaining normothermia.[62] Less than 10% of total heat loss during surgery occurs from the respiratory tract in adult patients, but this fraction is increased in small children. Earlier studies showing a significant effect on core temperature may have been flawed by measuring core temperature in the esophagus where direct heating of the temperature probe occurs when airway gases are warmed. Passive humidification with heat-moisture exchangers (HMEs) will increase humidity in the airway but has no effect on the patient's core temperature.[63] Current recommendations are to use an HME for any patient who would benefit from added moisture. This includes patients with chronic obstructive pulmonary disease, asthma, or significant pulmonary conditions where secretions are not well cleared. Active heating and humidification of the respiratory gases are not necessary unless other methods of warming small children (forced air warming) are unavailable. The approximate cost of an HME is $1 compared to the cost of an active-heated humidifier system which is ≈$14. Active heater/humidifier systems have been associated with inadvertent disconnects in the breathing circuit and overheating of the inspired gases.

Warming the intravenous fluid

Fluid warming can be used to help reduce the magnitude of hypothermia during surgery but cannot be used to warm patients since fluids cannot be delivered at temperatures significantly greater than 37°C. For minor procedures requiring minimal fluids (less than 2 L), it is unnecessary to warm the intravenous fluids. For procedures where fluids are given at increased flow rates or in higher volumes, it becomes necessary to warm the fluids in order to maintain normothermia. Either prewarmed fluids can be given or an in-line fluid/blood warmer may be used. When transfusion is likely, a fluid/blood warmer should be used since blood is stored at 4°C. When a unit of cold blood or room temperature crystalloid is given to the patient, mean body temperature is reduced by 0.25°C.[35] When this is added to ongoing heat loss from the skin surface, the problem with unwarmed fluids is compounded.

When fluid warmers are used, two factors must be considered in determining the temperature at which the fluid is delivered to the patient (flow rate and length of intravenous tubing).[64] At low flow rates, the fluid returns to ambient room temperature after it leaves the warmer, before it reaches the patient. This heat loss can be eliminated by a warmed fluid-filled jacket around the intravenous tubing, but heat loss from low-flow fluid administration is not significant except in pediatric patients. At high flows, fluids pass through the warmer so quickly that the fluids cannot be warmed sufficiently. Newer models of warmers are designed for delivery of warm fluids even at high flow rates.

Passive insulation

A layer of passive insulation reduces heat loss from the skin surface by 30%. The type of insulator is relatively unimportant as there is little difference between materials (plastic, cotton, paper, or reflective "space blankets").[65] The layer of air between the insulation cover and the patient's skin provides the insulation independent of the material itself. Prewarmed cotton blankets are commonly used in the operating room. Patients feel immediate warmth and comfort, but actual heat flux through the skin is virtually identical with both warmed and unwarmed cotton blankets.

Active patient warming

Although passive insulation and intravenous fluid warming can reduce heat loss from the patient, these therapies cannot be used to transfer heat into the patient. Therefore, active warming is required to maintain normothermia during the intraoperative period. Of the available warming systems, the most effective is forced air (Fig. 17-7).[63] This type of warming became available in the late 1980s and its use has increased dramatically over the last decade. Forced air was initially used to actively warm hypothermic patients in the postoperative period, but it was quickly recognized that preventing hypothermia was more desirable than treating hypothermia. The forced-air system consists of two components—the forced-air generator and the blanket.

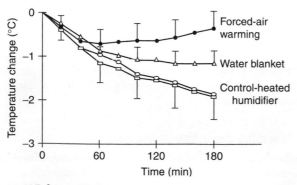

FIGURE 17-7 Core temperature was compared in patients receiving four different warming methods during renal transplant surgery. Core temperature decreased 1°C in the first hour in all patients due to redistribution of heat. In the subsequent 2 hours, heated humidification did not maintain core temperature better than control, circulating water mattresses prevented further hypothermia, but only forced-air warming increased core temperature back to baseline values. *(Modified from Ref. 63.)*

The generator blows air at various flow rates and delivery temperatures into the attached blanket through a hose that inserts into the blanket. The blankets are baffled to fill with warm air with small holes for the air to exit onto the patient's skin surface. They are designed for covering the upper body, lower body, or full body, and the appropriate design is chosen based on the location of the surgical field. Pediatric size blankets are available. Heat transfer with these systems is between 60 and 100 W,[66] making this therapy more efficient than other warming systems such as circulating water mattresses or radiant heaters.

Circulating water mattresses are also designed to actively warm patients during surgery. These mattresses are placed underneath the patient and are connected to a warm water source that circulates flow through the mattress. Heat transfer with this device is limited since cutaneous blood flow to the patient's back is limited due to pressure on the capillary beds from the body's weight. Water mattresses have been shown to be most effective in transferring heat when used over the ventral surface of the patient, which is sometimes an option in the postoperative period, but is impractical during surgery.

Radiant heater is another type of active warming system. These systems are often used during the intraoperative period and are incorporated into the beds used for neonates. Radiant heaters should be used with a skin-surface thermistor that provides thermostatic feedback to the warmer and reduces the risk of burning. Radiant heaters have also been used in the recovery room for adult patients. By warming the skin surface, shivering is immediately attenuated with radiant warming.[67] The effectiveness of radiant heating has not been compared to other active warming methods with regard to core rewarming of hypothermic patients.

CONCLUSIONS

Elderly patients are high-risk surgical candidates since significant perioperative stress is incurred in combination with a high incidence of coexisting cardiac and pulmonary disease. Hypothermia can be to the patient's advantage intraoperatively to protect from ischemic injury to the vital organs during periods of decreased perfusion. Postoperative hypothermia, however, in the awake patient, should be considered a significant contributor to perioperative stress through sympathetic activation and should be aggressively avoided and/or treated. As with the other vital signs, body temperature should be carefully monitored and controlled in the perioperative period in order to optimize outcome in the elderly patient.

KEY POINTS

▶ Virtually, all anesthetics render patients poikilothermic, and body temperature invariably decreases during surgery. The elderly patient is especially susceptible to alterations in body temperature since thermoregulatory control is impaired with age.

▶ In the postoperative setting, even mild hypothermia can exacerbate the stress response by activation of the sympathetic nervous system and increasing catecholamines, which can precipitate myocardial ischemia and cardiac morbidity.

▶ As little as 2°C of core hypothermia impairs coagulation and predisposes to increased bleeding.

▶ Hypothermia slows emergence from general anesthesia by both pharmacokinetic and pharmacodynamic mechanisms, which is especially noticeable in elderly patients who have a delayed clearance of drugs and a reduced MAC.

▶ In the elderly, body temperature should be carefully monitored and controlled with the same level of attention that is given to the other vital signs. With special attention to the control and maintenance of body temperature, perioperative outcomes can be improved and morbidity reduced in elderly patients.

KEY ARTICLES

▶ Frank SM, Fleisher LA, Breslow MJ, et al. Perioperative maintenance of normothermia reduces the incidence of morbid cardiac events: a randomized trial. JAMA. 1997;277:1127–1134.

▶ Sessler DI. Mild perioperative hypothermia. N Engl J Med. 1997; 336:1730–1737.

▶ Kurz A, Sessler DI, Lenhardt R. Perioperative normothermia to reduce the incidence of surgical-wound infection and shorten hospitalization. New Engl J Med. 1996;334:1209–1215.

▶ Lenhardt R, Marker E, Goll V, et al. Mild intraoperative hypothermia prolongs postanesthetic recovery. Anesthesiology. 1997;87:1318–1323.

REFERENCES

1. Benzinger TH. Heat regulation: homeostasis of central temperature in man. Physiol Rev. 1969;49:671–759.
2. Sessler DI. Mild perioperative hypothermia. N Engl J Med. 1997;336: 1730–1737.
3. Frank SM, Raja SN, Bulcao C, Goldstein D. Relative contribution of core and cutaneous temperatures to thermal comfort, and the autonomic response in humans. J Appl Physiol. 1999;86:1588–1593.
4. Frank SM, Beattie C, Christopherson R, et al. Epidural versus general anesthesia, ambient operating room temperature, and patient age as predictors of inadvertent hypothermia. Anesthesiology. 1992;77:252–257.
5. Frank SM, Shir Y, Raja SN, et al. Core hypothermia and skin-surface temperature gradients: epidural vs. general anesthesia and the effects of age. Anesthesiology. 1994;80:502–508.
6. Vaughan MS, Vaughan RW, Cork RC. Postoperative hypothermia in adults: relationship of age, anesthesia, and shivering in rewarming. Anesth Analg. 1981;60:746–751.
7. Lomax P. The hypothermic effect of pentobarbital in the rat: sites and mechanisms of action. Brain Res. 1966;1:296–302.
8. Kurz A, Sessler DI, Annadata R, et al. Midazolam minimally impairs thermoregulatory control. Anesth Analg. 1995;81:393–398.
9. Leslie K, Sessler DI, Bjorksten AR, et al. Propofol causes a dose-dependent decrease in the thermoregulatory threshold for vasoconstriction but has little effect on sweating. Anesthesiology. 1994;81:353–360.
10. Lotti VJ, Lomax P, George R. Temperature responses in the rat following intracerebral microinjection of morphine. J Pharmacol Exp Ther. 1965; 150:135–139.
11. Rosow CE, Miller JM, Pelikan EW, Cochin J. Opiates and thermoregulation in mice. I. Agonists. J Pharmacol Exp Ther. 1980;213:273–283.
12. MacIntyre PE, Pavlin EG, Dwersteg JF. Effect of meperidine on oxygen consumption, carbon dioxide production, and respiratory gas exchange in postanesthetic shivering. Anesth Analg. 1987;66:751–755.
13. Kurz A, Go JC, Sessler DI, et al. Alfentanil slightly increases the sweating threshold and markedly reduces the vasoconstriction and shivering thresholds. Anesthesiology. 1995;82:293–299.
14. Sessler DI, Olofsson CI, Rubinstein EH. The thermoregulatory threshold in humans during nitrous oxide-fentanyl anesthesia. Anesthesiology. 1988;69:357–364.
15. Sessler DI, Olofsson CI, Rubinstein EH, Beebe JJ. The thermoregulatory threshold in humans during halothane anesthesia. Anesthesiology. 1988; 68:836–842.
16. Matsukawa T, Sessler DI, Sessler AM, et al. Heat flow and distribution during induction of general anesthesia. Anesthesiology. 1995;82:662–673.
17. Frank SM, Fleisher LA, Olson KF, et al. Multivariate determinates of early postoperative oxygen consumption: the effects of shivering, core temperature, and gender. Anesthesiology. 1995;83:241–249.
18. Emerick TH, Ozaki M, Sessler DI, et al. Epidural anesthesia increases apparent leg temperature and decreases the shivering threshold. Anesthesiology. 1994;81:289–298.
19. Leslie K, Sessler DI. Reduction in the shivering threshold is proportional to spinal block height. Anesthesiology. 1996;84:1327–1331.
20. Frank SM, ElRahmany HK, Cattaneo CG, et al. Predictors of hypothermia during spinal anesthesia. Anesthesiology. 2000;92:1330–1334.
21. Frank SM, Nguyen JM, Garcia CM, Barnes RA. Temperature monitoring practices during regional anesthesia. Anesth Analg. 1999;88: 373–377.
22. DuBois EF. The many different temperatures of the human body and its parts. West J Surg Obstet Gynecol. 1951;59:476–490.
23. Colin J, Timbal J, Houdas Y, et al. Computation of mean body temperature from rectal and skin temperatures. J Appl Physiol. 1971;31:484–489.
24. Frank SM. Body temperature monitoring. In: Levitt R, ed. Anesthesiology Clinics of North America. Philadelphia: WB Saunders; 1994:387–407.
25. Whitby JD, Dunkin LJ. Temperature differences in the oesophagus. Br J Anaesth. 1968;40:991–995.
26. ElRahmany HK, Frank SM, Schneider G, et al. Forced-air warming decreases vasodilator requirement following coronary artery bypass surgery. Anesth Analg. 2000;90:286–291.
27. Ikeda T, Sessler DI, Marder D, Xiong J. The influence of thermoregulatory vasomotion and ambient temperature variation on the accuracy of core-temperature estimates by cutaneous liquid-crystal thermometers. Anesthesiology. 1997;86:603–612.
28. Cattaneo CG, Frank SM, Hesel TW, et al. The accuracy and precision of body temperature monitoring methods during regional and general anesthesia. Anesth Analg. 2000;90:938–945.
29. Frank SM, Raja SN, Bulcao C, Goldstein DS. Age-related thermoregulatory differences during core cooling in humans. Am J Physiol Regul Integr Comp Physiol. 2000;279:R349–R354.
30. Busto R, Dietrich WD, Globus MY, et al. Small differences in intraischemic brain temperature critically determine the extent of ischemic neuronal injury. J Cereb Blood Flow Metab. 1987;7:729–738.
31. Frank SM, Parker SD, Rock P, et al. Moderate hypothermia with partial bypass and segmental sequential repair for thoracoabdominal aortic aneurysm. J Vasc Surg. 1994;19:687–697.
32. Vacanti FX, Ames AA. Mild hypothermia and Mg++ protect against irreversible damage during CNS ischemia. Stroke. 1983;15:695–698.
33. Sessler DI. Perianesthetic thermoregulation and heat balance in humans. FASEB J. 1993;7:638–644.
34. Bay J, Nunn JF, Prys-Roberts C. Factors influencing arterial PO_2 during recovery from anaesthesia. Br J Anaesth. 1968;17:398–407.
35. Sessler DI. Consequences and treatment of perioperative hypothermia. In: Levitt RC, ed. Temperature Regulation During Anesthesia. Philadelphia: WB Saunders; 1994.
36. Kurz A, Sessler DI, Narzt E, et al. Postoperative hemodynamic and thermoregulatory consequences of intraoperative core hypothermia. J Clin Anesth. 1995;7:359–366.
37. Krenzischeck DA, Frank SM, Kelly S. Forced-air skin-surface warming vs. routine thermal care and core temperature monitoring sites. J Postanesth Nurs. 1995;10:69–78.
38. Regan MJ, Eger EI. Ventilatory responses to hypercapnia and hypoxia at normothermia and moderate hypothermia during constant-depth halothane anesthesia. Anesthesiology. 1966;27:624–633.
39. Benumof JL, Wahrenbrock EA. Dependency of hypoxic pulmonary vasoconstriction on temperature. J Appl Physiol. 1977;42:56–58.
40. Frank SM, Higgins MS, Breslow MJ, et al. The catecholamine, cortisol, and hemodynamic responses to mild perioperative hypothermia: a randomized clinical trial. Anesthesiology. 1995;82:83–93.
41. Frank SM, Higgins MS, Fleisher LA, et al. The adrenergic, respiratory, and cardiovascular effects of core cooling in humans. Am J Physiol. 1997;272: R557–R562.
42. Bainton D, Moore F, Sweetnam P. Temperature and deaths from ischemic heart disease. Br J Prev Soc Med. 1977;31:49–53.
43. Rose G. Cold weather and ischemic heart disease. Br J Prev Soc Med. 1966;20:97–100.
44. Frank SM, Beattie C, Christopherson R, et al. Unintentional hypothermia is associated with postoperative myocardial ischemia. Anesthesiology. 1993;78:468–476.

45. Frank SM, Fleisher LA, Breslow MJ, et al. Perioperative maintenance of normothermia reduces the incidence of morbid cardiac events: a randomized trial. *JAMA*. 1997;277:1127–1134.

46. Mangano DT. Perioperative cardiac morbidity. *Anesthesiology*. 1990;72: 153–184.

47. Valeri CR, Feingold H, Cassidy G, et al. Hypothermia-induced reversible platelet dysfunction. *Ann Surg*. 1987;205:175–181.

48. Rohrer MJ, Natale AM. Effect of hypothermia on the coagulation cascade. *Crit Care Med*. 1992;20:1402–1405.

49. Yoshihara H, Yamamoto T, Mihara H. Changes in coagulation and fibrinolysis occurring in dogs during hypothermia. *Thromb Res*. 1985;37:503–512.

50. Hessel EA, Schmer G, Dillard DH. Platelet kinetics during deep hypothermia. *J Surg Res*. 1980;28:23–34.

51. Schmied H, Kurz A, Sessler DI, et al. Mild hypothermia increases blood loss and transfusion requirements during total hip arthroplasty. *Lancet*. 1996;347:289–292.

52. Kurz A, Sessler DI, Lenhardt R. Perioperative normothermia to reduce the incidence of surgical-wound infection and shorten hospitalization. *New Engl J Med*. 1996;334:1209–1215.

53. Sheffield CW, Sessler DI, Hunt TK. Mild hypothermia during isoflurane anesthesia decreases resistance to E. Coli dermal infection in guinea pigs. *Acta Anaesthesiol Scand*. 1994;38:201–205.

54. Sheffield CW, Sessler DI, Hunt TK, Scheuenstuhl H. Mild hypothermia during halothane anesthesia decreases resistance to S. Aureus dermal infection in guinea pigs. *Wound Repair Regen*. 1994;2:48–56.

55. Vitez TS, White PF, Eger EI. Effects of hypothermia of halothane MAC and isoflurane MAC in the rat. 1974;41:80–81.

56. Lenhardt R, Marker E, Goll V, et al. Mild intraoperative hypothermia prolongs postanesthetic recovery. *Anesthesiology*. 1997;87:1318–1323.

57. Heier T, Caldwell JE, Sessler DI, Miller RD. Mild intraoperative hypothermia increases duration of action and spontaneous recovery of vecuronium blockade during nitrous oxide-isoflurane anesthesia in humans. *Anesthesiology*. 1991;74:815–819.

58. Leslie K, Sessler DI, Bjorksten AR, Moayeri A. Mild hypothermia prolongs the duration of action of atracurium. *Anesth Analg*. 1995;80:1007–1014.

59. Moschcowitz AV. Post-operative heat stroke. *Surg Gynecol Obstet*. 1916;23:443–451.

60. Morris RH. Operating room temperature and the anesthetized paralyzed patient. *Arch Surg*. 1971;103:95–97.

61. El-Gamal N, El-Kassabany N, Frank SM, et al. Age-related thermoregulatory differences in a warm operating room environment (approximately 26°C). *Anesth Analg*. 2000;90:694–698.

62. Bissonnette B, Sessler DI. Passive or active inspired gas humidification increases thermal steady-state temperatures in anesthetized infants. *Anesth Analg*. 1989;69:783–787.

63. Hynson JM, Sessler DI. Intraoperative warming therapies: a comparison of three devices. *J Clin Anesth*. 1992;4:194–199.

64. Faries G, Johnston C, Pruitt KM, Plouff RT. Temperature relationship to distance and flow rate of warmed IV fluids. *Ann Emerg Med*. 1991;20:1198–1200.

65. Sessler DI, McGuire J, Sessler AM. Perioperative thermal insulation. *Anesthesiology*. 1991;74:875–879.

66. Giesbrecht GG, Ducharme MB, McGuire JP. Comparison of forced-air patient warming systems for perioperative use. *Anesthesiology*. 1994;80: 671–679.

67. Sharkey A, Lipton JM, Murphy MT, Giesecke AH. Inhibition of postanesthetic shivering with radiant heat. *Anesthesiology*. 1987;66:249–252.

Hemodilution

Robert William Thomsen

BLOOD CONSERVATION STRATEGIES IN THE ELDERLY

▶ Complications of homologous blood transfusions

Introduction

Physiologic changes associated with aging predispose the elderly to increased morbidity and mortality during the perioperative period. Anemia may be poorly tolerated in these patients secondary to the effects of ageing on the cardiovascular and cerebrovascular systems. Many comorbidities prevalent in the geriatric population affect oxygen delivery to vital organs, and maintenance of oxygen-carrying hemoglobin should logically decrease the risk of ischemia.

The diminished functional capacity created by anemia can have profound implications for longevity and independence. We must strive to limit the severity of anemia and maintain sufficient reserves for both safe hospitalization and rapid convalescence. Allogenic blood transfusion, however, is associated with a multitude of complications and can be responsible for morbidity and mortality itself.

Transfusion reaction

Exposure to foreign proteins present in allogenic blood may precipitate an immune response ranging in severity from fever to anaphylaxis.

The most common cause of hyperpyrexia during a transfusion is the febrile, nonhemolytic transfusion reaction. Associated symptoms include headache, nausea, and malaise. This reaction is caused by an immunologic response to donor plasma which contains pyrogenic cytokines. Febrile, nonhemolytic transfusion reactions occur in approximately 1% of red cell transfusions and up to 30% of platelet transfusions. Leukocyte-reduced preparations of red cells dramatically reduce the likelihood of this reaction. Under anesthesia, hyperthermia is the most significant finding and should alert the anesthesiologist to the possibility of even more significant pathology.

Back pain, rigors, flushing, tachycardia, hypotension, disseminated intravascular coagulation, or hemoglobinuria may herald the appearance of a hemolytic transfusion reaction. Antibodies directed against donor red cells cause hemolysis and activation of the compliment system. Hemoglobinuria can precipitate acute renal failure, further complicating management. This reaction is rare, occurring in 1 per 250,000 to 1 per 1,000,000 units transfused, but mortality is estimated between 20% and 60%. Clerical errors during administration of transfusions are responsible for a significant portion of these cases.

The small population of patients with immunoglobulin A (IgA) deficiency is susceptible to true anaphylaxis during allogenic transfusion. This type 1 immediate hypersensitivity reaction may manifest as urticaria, bronchospasm, mucosal edema, and circulatory collapse.

Transfusion-related acute lung injury

Fever associated with hypoxemia, tachycardia, and acute bilateral infiltrates on chest radiographs may be the result of donor leukocyte-antibody complex deposition in the pulmonary vasculature. An extremely rare condition, transfusion-related acute lung injury (TRALI) may have a brief course lasting less than 48 hours but with mortality up to 14%.[1]

Infection

A major psychological aversion to blood transfusion is the risk of disease transmission (Fig. 18-1). Despite exceedingly rare transfusion-associated infections, public perception stemming from transfusion-related acquired immunodeficiency syndrome (AIDS) cases during the 1980s is difficult to alter. The indolent natural history of some of these diseases may not result in significantly reduced longevity in the geriatric population (Table 18-1).

Weakened immunity associated with aging, however, may place older patients at risk for significant infections[2] from less virulent pathogens found in the blood supply, including cytomegalovirus, Epstein-Barr virus, West Nile virus, and human herpes viruses 6, 7, and 8.

Bacterial contamination of the blood supply may also result in fever, tachycardia, disseminated intravascular coagulation (DIC), and septic shock. Platelet transfusions are particularly susceptible to contamination as they are stored at room temperature. A study of 9598 elderly patients undergoing hip fracture repair demonstrated a 35% higher risk of bacterial infection and a 52% higher risk of pneumonia in the cohort that received a transfusion.[3]

Successful screening programs have greatly improved the safety of the blood supply. We should not forget that currently unknown pathogens may produce clinically significant infections in the future. Less than 30 years ago, human immunodeficiency virus (HIV) did not exist. Potential pathogens such as the transfusion transmitted (TT) virus and the SEN virus are appearing in recipients of blood products, although their clinical significance is not yet known.

Immunomodulation

In the 1970s, the observation that renal transplant patients who received allogenic blood transfusions had improved allograft survival revolutionized the transplant surgery world. Allogenic transfusions

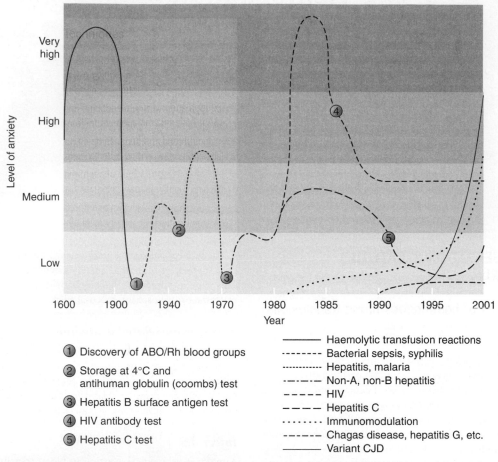

① Discovery of ABO/Rh blood groups
② Storage at 4°C and antihuman globulin (coombs) test
③ Hepatitis B surface antigen test
④ HIV antibody test
⑤ Hepatitis C test

——— Haemolytic transfusion reactions
- - - - - - - Bacterial sepsis, syphilis
·············· Hepatitis, malaria
—·—·—·— Non-A, non-B hepatitis
– – – – – HIV
— — — — Hepatitis C
············ Immunomodulation
- - - - - Chagas disease, hepatitis G, etc.
——— Variant CJD

FIGURE 18-1 The degree of anxiety and concern about the safety of blood transfusion over the centuries. *(From Vanderlinde ES, Heal JM, Blumberg N. Autologous transfusion. Br Med J. 2002;324:772–775, with permission from BMJ Publishing Group.)*

were actively administered to induce a state of immune suppression and decrease the risk of transplant rejection. The advent of pharmacologically mediated immunosuppression has eliminated this practice, given the competing consideration of HLA alloimmunization.

In the 1980s, additional evidence of the immunosuppressive effects of allogenic transfusion was found in several retrospective and observational reports of cancer patients who appeared to have increased tumor recurrence if they had received a transfusion.

Postoperative infection appears to be higher in patients who have received a transfusion compared to their matched cohorts in multiple series. This risk increases with the total number of units transfused.

The true relationship between transfusions and postoperative infections, cancer recurrence, and the development of autoimmune diseases remains controversial. The associations are strong but clear evidence is lacking. A mechanism known as microchimerism has been advanced as an explanation for these effects. Microchimerism occurs when there is HLA compatibility between donor and recipient blood. Donor leukocytes are not recognized as foreign proteins and persist in the host where they stimulate release of anti-inflammatory cytokines and cause host T-cell hyporeactivity.

Alloimmunization

Allogenic transfusion exposes patients to foreign HLA antigens and results in the development of antibodies against these proteins. The number of transfusions given to an individual is directly proportional

to their degree of sensitization. These antibodies may limit the availability of future transfusions by making properly crossmatched blood difficult to obtain, and may limit the potential donor pool in the event that a living donor organ transplant is required.

Volume overload

Transfusion of blood products precipitates acute congestive heart failure in 1–8% of all transfusions to young children and patients older than 60. Evidence of circulatory overload may include hypoxia, cyanosis, dyspnea, widened pulse pressure, tachycardia, and hypertension. These patients may require longer intensive care unit (ICU) and total hospital length of stays, and the associated mortality rate has been estimated at nearly 4%.

Storage lesion

The storage lesion refers to morphologic and physiologic changes that occur in blood between donation and administration, resulting in decreased red cell viability and reduced ability to transport oxygen.

Adenosine triphosphate (ATP) is associated with maintenance of erythrocyte discoid shape, cellular flexibility, and membrane lipid levels. At the end of its storage life, ATP levels are less than half of their original amounts, resulting in more spherical and rigid erythrocytes that may sludge in the microcirculation and reduce oxygen delivery.

The oxygen dissociation curve of stored blood is left shifted due to reduced 2,3-diphosphoglycerate (2,3-DPG) levels and results in

Table 18-1

Risks of Blood Transfusion

Risk Factor	Estimated Frequency		No. of Deaths per Million Units	Reference
	Per Million Units	Per Actual Unit		
Infection				
Viral*				
Hepatitis A	1	1/1,000,000	0	Dodd[35]
Hepatitis B	7–32	1/30,000–1/250,000	0–0.14	Schreiber et al.[17]
Hepatitis C	4–36	1/30,000–1/150,000	0.5–17	Schreiber et al.[17]
HIV	0.4–5	1/200,000–1/2,000,000	0.5–5	Schreiber et al.,[17] Lackritz et al.[18]
HTLV types I and II	0.5–4	1/250,000–1/2,000,000	0	Schreiber et al.[17]
Parvovirus B19	100	1/10,000	0	Dodd[35]
Bacterial contamination				
Red cells	2	1/500,000	0.1–0.25	Dodd,[35] Sazama[54]
Platelets	83	1/12,000	21	Dodd[35]
Acute hemolytic reactions	1–4	1/250,000–1/1,000,000	0.67	Sazama,[54] Linden et al.[55]
Delayed hemolytic reactions	1000	1/1000	0.4	Sazama,[54] Linden et al.,[55] Ness et al.,[59] Shulman[60]
Transfusion-related acute lung injury	200	1/5000	0.2	Linden et al.,[55] Popovsky and Moore[70]

*HIV denotes human immunodeficiency virus, and HTLV human T-cell lymphotropic virus.
(From Goodnough LT, Brecher ME, Kanter MH, et al. Transfusion medicine. First of two parts. N Engl J Med. 1999;340:438–447, with permission from the Massachusetts Medical Society.)

impaired oxygen release from hemoglobin. After 35 days of storage, 2,3-DPG levels are less than 10% of baseline. After transfusion, however, 2,3-DPG is rapidly regenerated, reaching 50% of normal after 4 hours and returning to baseline after 24 hours.

Packed red cell preparations are stored at 4°C to reduce metabolism and limit bacterial growth. At this temperature, the sodium-potassium ATPase is essentially nonfunctional, resulting in equilibration of sodium and potassium between intracellular and extracellular compartments. Furthermore, spontaneous red cell lysis or enhanced lysis during irradiation of the specimen will further elevate plasma potassium concentration, which may result in significant hyperkalemia during massive transfusion or in patients with end-stage renal disease.

▶ Blood conservation techniques

Preoperative autologous donation

In preparation for a surgery where transfusion is likely, patients may deposit whole blood for reinfusion if anemia develops. The clear advantage to autologous blood is avoidance of the viruses, immunomodulation, and alloimmunization associated with allogenic blood. Patients who have rare blood phenotypes or are known to have multiple antibodies are especially good candidates for autologous donation. The restrictions for participation in a preoperative autologous blood donation (PAD) program are significantly more liberal than for altruistic donors to the general blood supply. The American Association of Blood Bank's guidelines state that patients may donate autologous blood if their hemoglobin is 11 g/dL or greater. Patients with

active infections or bacteremia should not donate as well as those patients whose underlying medical conditions would be exacerbated by sudden fluid shifts. In contrast to allogenic donors, there are no criteria for minimum age or weight. Patients with coronary artery disease have safely donated autologous blood in a monitored setting with no apparent adverse outcomes. The first unit donated by all individuals is screened for potential pathogens so that appropriate precautions or possible exclusion from the PAD program may be undertaken. Additional units, however, may not undergo this testing process with associated cost savings. Patients may begin donation weeks in advance of their surgery, but the last donation should occur no less than 72 hours before surgery to allow appropriate volume expansion.

PAD is appropriate in surgeries where significant blood loss is likely and the patient wishes to limit exposure to allogenic blood. It usually provides 1-3 units of refrigerated whole blood for reinfusion as indicated during the perioperative and immediate postoperative periods. The availability of PAD blood during the postoperative period where additional transfusions may be required is a distinct advantage over other autologous transfusion techniques.

Although it is an effective technique for reducing exposure to allogenic products, there are several limitations. There is an extensive planning component to PAD where a patient must know several weeks in advance of their surgery to initiate PAD. It is unavailable for patients undergoing urgent or emergent operations. There is significant cost associated with collection and storage of the blood that is compounded by extensive waste. Up to 50% of donated PAD units are not utilized and are inappropriate for crossover into the general blood supply.[4] The platelet component of PAD whole blood has been inactivated by refrigerated storage. The risk of viral infection should be eliminated but the possibility of bacterial infection is unchanged. Clerical errors are the cause of the majority of transfusion-associated complications in a PAD program whereby patients are inadvertently given allogenic blood when autologous blood is available. New York State Department of Health data identified clerical error as the cause of transfusion reaction in 1 of every 19,000 units.[5] This exposes the patient to all of the attendant risks of an allogenic transfusion, including viral infection and hemolytic transfusion reaction.

Acute normovolemic hemodilution

Acute normovolemic hemodilution (ANH) is the perioperative process of phlebotomizing a patient with concurrent volume expansion using crystalloids, colloids, or both. Blood is collected at the time of surgery and stored in standard anticoagulant bags for reinfusion after the majority of blood loss has occurred or significant anemia has developed. This technique may be considered when surgical blood loss is expected to exceed 20% of the patient's blood volume, and the starting hemoglobin is greater than 10 g/dL. Anemia is well tolerated, provided adequate volume expansion is provided. Tissue oxygen delivery is maintained through a combination of improved hemorheology, increased cardiac output, and increased tissue oxygen extraction

(Fig. 18-2). By inducing a normovolemic anemia, total red cell loss is reduced for an equivalent surgical blood loss. Reinfusing collected blood restores red cell mass and reduces the likelihood of allogenic transfusion (Fig. 18-3).

There are multiple advantages to ANH. ANH is the only source of fresh, whole, autologous blood available in the operating room and, as such, is replete with erythrocytes, clotting factors, fibrinogen, and functional platelets. ANH blood may be reinfused up to 8 h after collection when stored at room temperature. There is minimal cost associated with collection of ANH blood and no storage fee as all blood is reinfused before conclusion of the surgery. It is available in emergency surgeries with no additional preparation, provided the starting hemoglobin level is adequate. Furthermore, creation of anemia occurs under the constant supervision and monitoring of the anesthesiologist and may be terminated if adverse physiologic derangements occur. There is no risk of clerical error as all blood collected remains with the patient until reinfusion.

The primary disadvantage of ANH is minimal savings of red cell mass unless sufficiently large volumes of blood are collected, resulting in severe anemia (Fig. 18-4). ANH is effective when a hematocrit of 28% is used, but this level of anemia may not be tolerated by some patients and does not allow a large buffer in the event of sudden, massive hemorrhage.

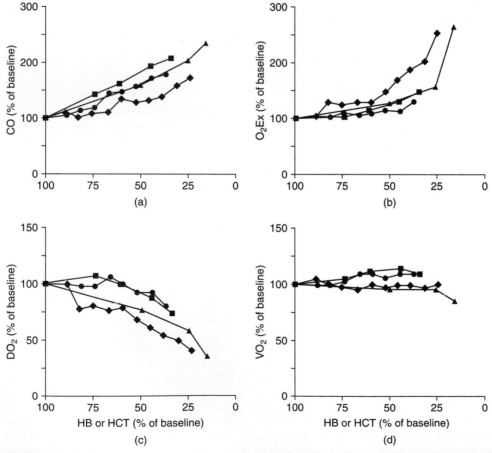

FIGURE 18-2 Relative changes of (A) cardiac output (CO, % of baseline), (B) O_2 extraction (O_2Ex, % of baseline), (C) O_2 delivery (DO_2, % of baseline), and (D) O_2 consumption (VO$_2$, % of baseline) during progressive ANH in pigs (squares), dogs (diamonds), baboons (triangles), and man (circles). Note that the combined increases of CO and O_2 extraction allow maintenance of VO$_2$ even at low hemoglobin levels. *(Modified according to Moss et al., Weiskopf et al., van der Linden et al., and van Woerkens et al.; from Jamnicki M, Kocian R, van der Linden P, et al. Acute normovolemic hemodilution: physiology, limitations, and clinical use. J Cardiothorac Vasc Anesth. 2003;17:747–754, with permission from Elsevier Science.)*

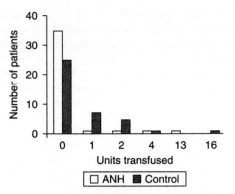

FIGURE 18-3 The number of units of allogenic blood transfused for the acute normovolemic hemodilution and control groups. *(From Matot I, Scheinin O, Jurim O, et al. Effectiveness of acute normovolemic hemodilution to minimize allogenic blood transfusion in major liver resections. Anesthesiology. 2002;97:794–800, with permission from Lippincott Williams & Wilkins.)*

Intraoperative cell salvage

Intraoperative cell salvage (ICS) is another blood conservation technique that is readily available and may limit exposure to allogenic blood products. ICS utilizes a special surgical suction device that collects blood from the surgical field and holds it in a heparinized storage facility until processing. After a sufficient volume of blood has been recovered from the surgical field, it is washed to reduce nonerythrocyte particulate matter, including fat, bone, and contaminants, and then reinfused when clinically appropriate. ICS can provide the equivalent of 10 units of packed red blood cells per hour during periods of massive blood loss.

Like ANH, ICS is available for emergency operations. It can be used regardless of the hemoglobin level and does not require advance collection time. It is the only technique that can be used continuously throughout an operation to limit red cell loss.

Equipment and operator costs are higher than for ANH. It is inappropriate in grossly contaminated operations such as bowel perforations and most cancer operations. Small studies have examined their use in conjunction with leukocyte depletion filters and observed a reduction in viable tumor cells if the filters were employed, but the clinical significance of this finding is unknown.[6,7]

ICS recovers erythrocytes but platelets and clotting factors are largely eliminated during the washing process.

TRANSFUSION TRIGGERS IN THE ELDERLY

▶ Anemia and the elderly

Anemia is a prevalent disease in the geriatric population. An age-related decline in hemoglobin level has been observed in healthy elderly patients.[8] Chronic disease and malnutrition accentuate this decreased hemoglobin level, and many patients who present for surgery are acutely anemic secondary to hemoptysis, hematuria, or gastrointestinal bleeding. Defining a transfusion trigger in this population is a complex problem, given the competing interests of preservation of tissue oxygenation and avoidance of transfusion-associated complications. An echocardiographic study of elderly patients with severe but chronic anemia (mean hemoglobin 6.3) demonstrated that oxygen delivery could be maintained with increased cardiac output achieved mainly by increased stroke volume.[9] The decision to transfuse allogenic blood should be based on the severity of anemia, the duration of anemia, the presence of continued blood loss, coexisting medical conditions, and the risks of transfusion. Additional considerations unique to this group are the duration of hospitalization, as they are especially vulnerable to nosocomial infections, and the convalescent period where faster recovery may provide greater chance of return to normal function.

Multiple observational studies have examined the effects of anemia and transfusion on clinical outcomes. Limiting exposure to morbidities associated with inactivity and improving psychological outlook are major benefits to early recovery of function. Exercise tolerance improved in patients with hemoglobin levels less than 10 after treatment with erythropoietin.[10] A retrospective study of 5793 patients demonstrated that higher postoperative hemoglobin levels were independently associated with the ability to walk greater distances after hip surgery. Figure 18-5 represents unadjusted univariate data.[11] A prospective study of 550 hip fracture patients suggested that higher postoperative hemoglobin levels were associated with shorter hospital stay and lower readmission rates but no differences in mortality or measures of functionality.[12] A subgroup analysis of this study population identified the group of patients transfused at

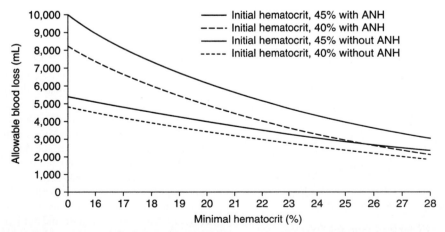

FIGURE 18-4 Maximal allowable blood loss in a patient with a blood volume of 5000 mL and an initial hematocrit of 45% or 40% in the presence and absence of ANH. *(From Goodnough LT, Brecher ME, Kanter MH, et al. Transfusion medicine. Second of two parts. N Engl J Med. 1999;340:525–533, with permission from the Massachusetts Medical Society.)*

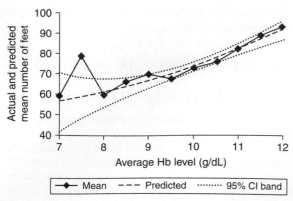

FIGURE 18-5 Postoperative Hb level and distance walked at discharge. *(From Ref. 11, with permission from Blackwell Publishing.)*

a trigger hemoglobin less than 10 as the population that benefited from reduced readmission rates.[13]

An observational study examining the duration of hospitalization in 444 hip fracture patients identified perioperative transfusion as a risk factor for wound healing disturbances and significantly increased length of hospital stay.[14] The Orthopedic Surgery Transfusion Hemoglobin European Overview (OSTHEO) study found that wound infection rates were higher in hip fracture patients who received an allogenic transfusion compared with those receiving autologous blood products.[15] Perioperative transfusion was also identified as an independent predictor of increased length of hospitalization in an observational study of 1095 patients who underwent colorectal surgery.[16]

An analysis of 1958 patients who refused transfusion for religious reasons provides insight into the effect of anemia on mortality. The adjusted odds ratio for mortality increased as preoperative hemoglobin decreased, but this was especially pronounced for patients with cardiovascular disease[17] (Fig. 18-6).

Houge et al. identified a hematocrit less than 28%, intraoperative tachycardia, and risk factors for coronary artery disease as independent predictors of perioperative myocardial ischemia.[18]

Our avoidance of allogenic blood transfusion has increased in the last decade based on several large studies of ICU patients. A prospective observational study of 4892 patients found that a nadir hemoglobin level less than 9 g/dL was associated with increased mortality and length of stay, but patients who received transfusions were more likely to experience a complication, and that this risk increased with the number of transfusions received[19] (Fig. 18-7).

In their prospective observational study, Vincent et al. found both ICU and overall mortality rates were significantly higher in those patients who received a transfusion compared with a matched cohort.[20]

In a retrospective study of Medicare patients admitted for treatment of acute myocardial infarction, Wu et al. found a reduction in 30-day mortality in patients who received a transfusion if their hematocrit on admission was less than 33%. However, an increase in mortality was seen in patients who received a transfusion and had an admission hematocrit greater than 36.1%.[21]

Carson et al. specifically addressed the perioperative period in their retrospective study of 8787 hip fracture patients. Despite a median patient age of 80.3 years, they found no difference in 30- or 90-day mortality in patients with a hemoglobin count of 8 g/dL who received a perioperative transfusion compared with those who did not.[22]

In the Transfusion Requirements in Critical Care (TRICC) study, investigators redefined transfusion practice in the critically ill with a randomized controlled study of 838 ICU patients. Patients with Acute Physiology and Chronic Health Evaluation II (APACHEII) scores less than 20 or age younger than 55 had significantly lower 30-day mortality if a restrictive transfusion practice was used (hemoglobin less than 7 g/dL vs. 10 g/dL for the liberal transfusion group). The authors concluded that, excepting patients with acute myocardial infarction and unstable angina, a restrictive transfusion practice was at least as effective as the standard practice.[23]

A subgroup analysis of the TRICC study addressed the issue of a restrictive transfusion practice for patients with cardiovascular disease. In 357 critically ill patients with cardiovascular disease there was no significant difference in 30-day mortality, but patients in the liberal transfusion group had significantly more changes in multiple organ dysfunction measures. There was a nonsignificant trend toward increased mortality in the 257 patients with severe ischemic heart disease who received the restrictive transfusion strategy[24] (Fig. 18-8).

In spite of the growing body of evidence that restrictive transfusion strategies preserve resources and may confer a survival advantage in critically ill patients, the perioperative period is replete with physiologic stressors including catecholamine surges, fluid shifts, and the potential for massive, acute hemorrhage. Anesthesia may reduce metabolic demands but emergence from anesthesia can precipitate myocardial ischemia as myocardial oxygen demand abruptly increases. Table 18-2 delineates objective parameters for initiating transfusion in patients with cardiovascular disease (Table 18-2). A rational perioperative blood conservation strategy is to limit exposure to allogenic blood products by enhancing hemoglobin preoperatively, ensuring meticulous surgical hemostasis, maintaining normothermia, and conserving autologous erythrocytes.

▶ Autologous transfusion in the elderly

Of the three currently available autologous transfusion techniques, intraoperative cell salvage provides the greatest capacity to limit allogenic exposure as surgical bleeding is collected and reinfused as needed. The high capital cost of machinery and disposables is minimized as blood loss increases. Multiple studies have demonstrated the safety and efficacy of PAD in the elderly. In a retrospective study of 879 elderly patients undergoing hip arthroplasty, knee arthroplasty, or spine surgery, 87.8% of patients avoided allogenic transfusion by participation in a preoperative donation program. Despite 73 patients with known cardiovascular disease, only 2 patients experienced a cardiac complication and both cases were brief episodes of atrial fibrillation.[25] In healthy elderly blood donors, there was no effect on exercise tolerance and similar cardiovascular compensatory mechanisms as their younger cohorts after donation[26] (Fig. 18-9).

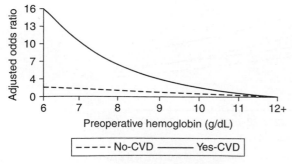

FIGURE 18-6 Adjusted odds ratio for mortality by cardiovascular disease and preoperative hemoglobin. *(From Ref. 17, with permission from Elsevier Science.)*

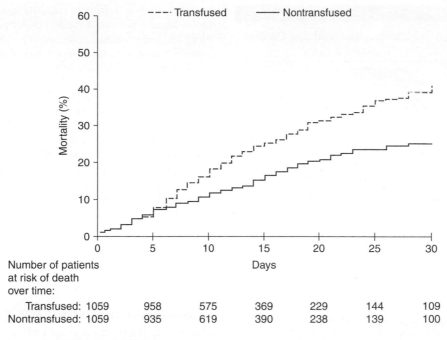

Number of patients
at risk of death
over time:

Transfused: 1059	958	575	369	229	144	109
Nontransfused: 1059	935	619	390	238	139	100

Log rank = 24.02; $p < 0.0001$.

FIGURE 18-7 Mortality by transfusion status for propensity-matched patients. *(From Ref. 19, with permission from Lippincott Williams & Wilkins.)*

No alterations in cutaneous microcirculation were found in a study of healthy elderly patients after donation of 1 unit of blood.[27] Studies of isovolumic blood donation in patients with cardiovascular disease demonstrated stable hemodynamics which supports other evidence that isovolumic anemia is well tolerated.[28,29] A pilot study of 50 patients scheduled for coronary artery bypass demonstrated no difference in myocardial ischemic events in patients who participated in an autologous blood donation program compared to controls.[30] The safety and efficacy of preoperative donation by patients with end-stage heart or lung disease was further supported by a small study of patients awaiting heart or lung transplantation where no significant complications were observed after a total donation of 1–8 units.[31] However, many elderly patients are limited in their donations due to preexisting anemia.

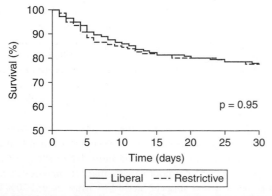

FIGURE 18-8 Survival of >30 days in all cardiac patients in the restrictive and liberal allogenic red blood cell transfusion groups. This graph illustrates Kaplan-Meier survival curves for all cardiac patients in both study groups. There was no difference in mortality in patients in the restrictive group compared with the liberal group ($p = 0.95$). *(From Ref. 24, with permission from Lippincott Williams & Wilkins.)*

Several studies of oral and intravenous iron supplementation have been performed to examine the effect on erythropoiesis. Non-iron-deficient patients do not appear to benefit from iron supplementation as the erythropoietic response to donation is not sufficiently strong to deplete endogenous iron stores.[32] A small study of elderly patients admitted for hip fracture repair suggested a benefit from iron supplementation if admission hemoglobin was greater than 12. Interestingly, a reduction in the postoperative infection rate was also seen in the treatment group.[33] Iron supplementation is important to maximize the erythropoietic response when recombinant human erythropoietin is used to augment erythropoiesis.[34]

Even with enhanced erythropoiesis, many elderly patients are ineligible for preoperative donation programs, given the urgency of their surgical interventions or persistent anemia. Multiple studies have compared the efficacy of PAD programs to acute normovolemic hemodilution and found no difference in allogenic exposure.[35–38] Given the potential waste associated with preoperative autologous donation, hemodilution may offer cost savings in addition to improved hemorheology, lack of storage lesion, zero clerical error rate, preserved coagulation factors, and functional platelets. There is a growing body of evidence examining the effect of hemodilution in the elderly.

A preliminary study of hemodilution in elderly patients without known cardiac disease found a hemoglobin of 8.8 g/dL to be well tolerated and fully compensated by increased oxygen extraction and cardiac output without evidence of myocardial ischemia.[39] Anesthesia reduced the increase in cardiac index of hemodilution patients but tissue oxygenation was maintained through increased oxygen extraction. Cardiac output was reduced primarily through a blunting of the tachycardic response with preservation of increased stroke index.[40] This observation is reminiscent of the adaptation to severe, chronic anemia presented earlier. Anesthesia decreases metabolic requirements but a study of anesthetic depth in animals demonstrated increased critical hemoglobin level in more deeply anesthetized animals. Cardiac depression with reduction in oxygen delivery was the primary mechanism.[41]

Table 18-2

Transfusion Indication in Patients with Coexisting Cardiac Diseases

	Evidence-Based/ Scientific	Realizable in Public/Teaching Hospitals	
		Intraoperatively and ICU	Postoperatively General Ward
New ST-segment depression >0.1 mV	Yes	Yes	Yes
New ST-segment elevation >0.2 mV	Yes	Yes	Yes
New wall motion abnormality in TEE	Yes	Yes	Yes
Oxygen extraction rate	>50%	>40%	Not applicable
SvO$_2$	<50%	<60%	Not applicable
Decrease in oxygen consumption	>10–50%	>10%	Not applicable
Hemoglobin transfusion triggers*			
All patients	6 g/dL	7 g/dL	7–8 g/dL
Patients >80 years		7–8 g/dL	8–9 g/dL
Patients with severe CAD		8 g/dL	8–9 g/dL
Patients with signs of CHF		8 g/dL	8–9 g/dL
Patients with >1 catecholamine		8 g/dL	Not applicable
Patients with SaO$_2$ <90%		8–9 g/dL	9 g/dL

Note: The listed parameters are only an indication for blood transfusion after correction of hypovolemia, optimization of anesthesia, and ventilation and the correction of a tachycardia (if any).

Abbreviations: CAD = coronary artery disease; CHF = congestive heart failure; SvO$_2$ = mixed venous oxygen saturation; TEE = transesophageal echocardiography.

*A blood transfusion is allowed at hemoglobin levels below the indicated threshold without specific sign of inadequate oxygenation. Blood transfusions, however, are not mandatory in each case.

(From Spahn DR, Dettori N, Kocian R, et al. Transfusion in the cardiac patient. Crit Care Clin. 2004;20:269–249, with permission from Elsevier Science.)

the effect of severe anemia on cognitive function, and hemodilution to this degree is rarely undertaken. Furthermore, improved hemorheology and increased cardiac output in patients with internal carotid artery occlusion resulted in increased cerebral perfusion.[43] Hemodilution has been proposed as an adjunctive treatment for some cases of cerebrovascular disease.

Limited data exist regarding the effect of hemodilution on the pulmonary system. One small study of 47 patients undergoing anesthesia with one lung ventilation demonstrated impaired gas exchange in patients with chronic obstructive pulmonary disease (COPD) but not in control subjects. A positive effect of hemoglobin on the hypoxic pulmonary vasoconstrictive response was postulated as a possible mechanism for this observation.[44]

Oxygen extraction by the myocardium is already high, resulting in a precarious supply and demand relationship. Patients with coronary artery disease would be expected to be at high risk of myocardial ischemia during periods of anemia. Data previously presented have demonstrated the safety of restrictive transfusion strategies in critically ill patients with cardiac disease. Additional evidence specifically evaluating effect of hemodilution in the surgical setting is amassing.

Spahn et al. found that modest hemodilution (mean hemoglobin 9.9 g/dL) was well tolerated in patients with coronary artery disease. Despite beta-blocker therapy and a left ventricular ejection fraction between 26% and 83%, compensatory mechanisms to anemia remained intact.[45] The supply and demand relationship is favorably altered during hemodilution as transstenotic blood flow is increased in an animal model.[46] Furthermore, the normal tachycardic response to hemodilution is blunted by anesthesia, thereby minimizing increased demand.

Licker et al. examined the cardiovascular response to moderate hemodilution in patients with coronary artery disease using echocardiography. Decreased blood viscosity associated with hemodilution resulted in increased stroke volume, which was primarily related to increased venous return and greater preload. Additionally, left ventricular diastolic dysfunction remained constant in 4 of 15 patients and improved after hemodilution in 11.[47]

A small, randomized controlled trial of hemodilution in addition to standard myocardial preservation techniques during cardiopulmonary bypass demonstrated significantly lower myocardial enzyme levels, lower levels of inotropic support, and fewer arrhythmias in the group with hemodilution to a hematocrit of 28%.[48]

As technologic advances in fluid replacement therapy occur, hemodilution may become more efficient and easier to manage. An animal model of profound hemodilution (hematocrit 10%) suggests better preservation of cardiac myocytes by hydroxyethyl starch (HES) compared with lactated Ringer (LR) solution and a functionally significant decline in left ventricular function noted on echocardiography in the LR group.[49] A study comparing hypertonic saline and HES with HES alone demonstrated increased cardiac index and right ventricular ejection fraction with significantly less volume when hypertonic saline was added to HES.[50]

Existing evidence supports the safety of moderate hemodilution in the elderly but questions remain about its efficacy. Casati et al. found no efficacy of low volume hemodilution in 204 patients undergoing open heart surgery.[51] Weiskopf's mathematical analysis of hemodilution concluded that surgical blood loss must exceed 70% of the patient's blood volume to save 1 unit of erythrocytes.[52] A meta-analysis of 42 trials found that hemodilution only reduced allogenic exposure by 1–2 units.[53] Conversely, Karakaya et al. found acute normovolemic hemodilution to be more effective than nitroglycerin-induced hypotension in reducing allogenic transfusion in a small group of

Currently available evidence does not suggest increased morbidity from anemia in patients with cerebrovascular disease. Although young, healthy volunteers subjected to acute, profound isovolumic anemia (mean hemoglobin 5.7) exhibited tachycardia and cognitive deficits, these deficits improved after administration of supplemental oxygen[42] (Fig. 18-10). Maintenance of high PaO$_2$ appears to mitigate

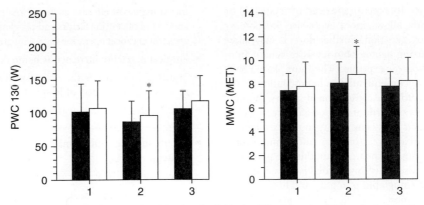

FIGURE 18-9 Treadmill exercise testing the day before (black bars) and the day after (white bars) blood donation. PWC = physical working capacity; MWC = maximal working capacity. Values are given for the PWC at a heart rate of 130/min (PWC 130) and MWC. 1 = mean age 65 years; 2 = mean age 58 years; 3 = control group (mean age 65 years). Mean ± SD. *, $p < 0.05$ vs. the day before donation. *(From Ref. 26, with permission from Blackwell Publishing.)*

patients undergoing total hip arthroplasty.[54] Preexisting anemia that may limit participation in a preoperative autologous donation program may also prevent clinically relevant erythrocyte savings with hemodilution. Furthermore, hemodilution is substantially more

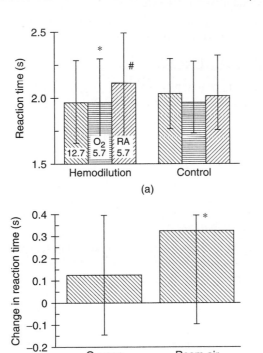

FIGURE 18-10 (A) Reaction time for the digit-symbol substitution test (DSST) increased at hemoglobin concentration of 5.7 g/dL when breathing room air compared with the reaction time at hemoglobin concentration of 12.7 g/dL (#, $P < 0.05$). Increasing PaO_2 to 406 mm Hg by breathing oxygen decreased the reaction time (*, $P < 0.02$ vs. breathing room air at hemoglobin 5.7 g/dL) to a value not different from that at hemoglobin concentration of 12.7 g/dL ($P = 0.96$). Data are mean ± SD. Hemodilution data are from 31 volunteers, and control data from 10 volunteers. (B) Comparison of DSST data from the 10 volunteers who were studied on hemodilution and control days. Reaction time increased at hemoglobin concentration of 5.7 g/dL when breathing room air, but not oxygen, compared with the reaction time at hemoglobin concentration of 12.7 g/dL. *, $P < 0.05$ for comparison of the difference between experimental and control days for the difference between the value at the hemoglobin concentration of 5.7 g/dL and the baseline hemoglobin concentration of 12.7 g/dL. Data are mean ± SD, n = 10. *(From Ref. 42, with permission from Lippincott Williams & Wilkins.)*

efficacious with moderate to severe degrees of induced anemia. There are no studies at this time confirming the safety of severe hemodilution in the geriatric population.

▶ Augmented hemodilution

In an effort to obviate the need for allogenic blood transfusion, oxygen-carrying compounds composed of modified human or bovine hemoglobin and synthetic halogenated chemicals are under investigation. These compounds are designed to maintain tissue oxygenation in spite of profound anemia. Clinical trials demonstrate efficacy of these products but there are multiple limitations to their widespread use.

Cell-free hemoglobin is rapidly oxidized and cleared by the kidney. Hemoglobin must, therefore, be modified to enhance stability and prevent nephrotoxicity that occurs when the kidney is exposed to high concentrations of free hemoglobin. Multiple products are currently available in which the hemoglobin has been surface-modified, cross-linked, or polymerized. These modifications reduce clearance rates but the longest plasma half-lives are still no longer than 72 h. In many products, the hemoglobin molecules are still able to scavenge nitric oxide. This results in clinically relevant vasoconstriction, hypertension, and decreased cardiac indices. The effect is so pronounced with some preparations that they are being developed, not as oxygen therapeutics, but as vasopressors for the treatment of septic shock. The risk of viral transmission is nearly eliminated with processing but transmissibility of the organism that causes bovine spongiform encephalitis from bovine preparations is unknown. Many of the human preparations are derived from expired, banked blood which may become a limited commodity as blood bank resources are more efficiently administered.

An alternative to the biologically derived hemoglobin solutions is perfluorocarbon. This inexpensive, inert, synthetic compound is able to dissolve large amounts of gasses. It has a long shelf life and the potential for unlimited production. Notable side effects include fever, a flu-like syndrome, and a dose-related thrombocytopenia.[55] In contrast to hemoglobin, the oxygen-carrying capacity of perfluorocarbons is substantially lower. The oxygen-carrying capacity, however, is linearly related to PaO_2 and may not be saturable. Hundred grams of perfluorocarbon emulsion exposed to a PaO_2 of 600 mm Hg results in an oxygen-carrying ability similar to 1 unit of whole blood.

Given their current limitations, oxygen therapeutics have minimal utility in the treatment of anemia. However, they are ideally situated to augment the harvest of autologous blood for isovolumic hemodilution. Use of oxygen therapeutics instead of crystalloid or colloid during hemodilution allows more aggressive phlebotomy while maintaining tissue oxygenation. Furthermore, it may allow patients with marginal starting hemoglobin levels to benefit from hemodilution and avoid allogenic exposure. The short plasma half-lives of these products are inconsequential to hemodilution as the collected blood is reinfused before the completion of surgery. Multiple phase II and III clinical trials of perfluorocarbons and hemoglobin compounds have verified their safety and ability to reduce allogenic exposure.[56,57] A case report of a 78-year-old man undergoing a complex aortic reconstruction with augmented hemodilution permitted stable hemodynamics and absence of myocardial ischemia, despite posthemodilution cellular hemoglobin of 6 g/dL and nadir cellular hemoglobin of 3 g/dL. Furthermore, allogenic transfusion was avoided even after a 4000 mL blood loss.[58]

CONCLUSIONS

Anemia is a prevalent disease in the elderly. Evidence continues to accumulate that allogenic blood transfusion produces significant, clinically relevant increases in morbidity and mortality. Multiple studies have demonstrated the safety of preoperative autologous donation, acute normovolemic hemodilution, and intraoperative cell salvage in a myriad of elderly and critically ill patients. All of these techniques have limitations that preclude their use in specific populations, and their overall effectiveness is still controversial. A comprehensive blood conservation plan combining multiple modalities, including pharmacologic enhancement of erythropoiesis, and oxygen-carrying capacity may provide the greatest opportunity to avoid allogenic blood transfusion while maintaining adequate hemoglobin levels and promoting rapid convalescence and return to function.

KEY POINTS

▶ Risk of transmission of currently known viruses is extremely small but bacterial contamination may cause sepsis.

▶ Febrile reactions to transfusion are extremely common.

▶ Transfusions may produce clinically relevant lung injury and increase ICU and overall duration of hospitalization.

▶ Allogenic transfusion may induce a state of immunosuppression or stimulate production of alloantibodies.

▶ Wound infections are more common in patients receiving a transfusion.

▶ Storage of blood decreases its ability to deliver oxygen, reduces red cell viability, and produces metabolic derangements.

▶ Preoperative autologous donation provides refrigerated, whole blood for the entire perioperative period. However, platelets are functionally inactive. It requires advanced planning and may create anemia prior to surgery. There is a high cost of acquisition and storage compounded by large amount of wasted units. Clerical error may result in allogenic exposure.

▶ Acute normovolemic hemodilution provides a source of fresh, whole blood. Phlebotomy is performed under monitored conditions with physician supervision. It is inexpensive and available for emergency procedures. There is no chance for clerical error. However, there is limited red cell mass savings unless severe anemia created intraoperatively.

▶ Intraoperative cell salvage has the greatest potential for erythrocyte recovery. It is available for emergency procedures and becomes

increasingly cost effective as blood loss rises. Processed erythrocytes are devoid of clotting factors and platelets. Cell salvage is inappropriate in most cancer operations and with grossly contaminated wounds.

▶ Surgical mortality increases as hemoglobin level decreases.

▶ Transfusion increases the risk of postoperative wound infection and increases duration of hospital stay.

▶ A restrictive transfusion strategy is safe in ICU patients with cardiovascular disease.

▶ Elderly surgical patients may benefit from a restrictive transfusion strategy.

▶ Elderly patients may participate in an autologous donation program.

▶ Patients with cardiovascular disease tolerate modest hemodilution.

▶ Hemodilution improves perfusion in patients with cerebrovascular disease.

▶ Hemodilution is well tolerated by healthy elderly patients.

▶ Modified hemoglobin solutions and perfluorochemicals are under investigation as oxygen therapeutics.

▶ Hemoglobin solutions are expensive with half-lives less than 72 h.

▶ Perfluorocarbon emulsions contain small quantities of dissolved oxygen unless PaO_2 is high.

▶ Oxygen therapeutics allow extreme anemia during hemodilution with maintenance of tissue oxygenation.

KEY REFERENCES

▶ Carson JL, Duff A, Poses RM, et al. Effect of anaemia and cardiovascular disease on surgical mortality and morbidity. *Lancet.* 1996;348:1055–1060.

▶ Rosencher N, Kerkkamp HEM, Macheras G, et al. Orthopedic Surgery Transfusion Hemoglobin European Overview (OSTHEO) study: blood management in elective knee and hip arthroplasty in Europe. *Transfusion.* 2003;43:459–469.

▶ Hébert PC, Yetisir E, Martin CF, et al. Is a low transfusion threshold safe in critically ill patients with cardiovascular diseases? *Crit Care Med.* 2001;29:227–234.

▶ Carson JL, Duff AMHS, Berlin JA, et al. Perioperative blood transfusion and postoperative mortality. *JAMA.* 1998;279:199–205.

▶ Spahn DR, Schmid ER, Seifert B, Pasch T. Hemodilution tolerance in patients with coronary artery disease who are receiving chronic beta-adrenergic blocker therapy. *Anesth Analg.* 1996;82:687–694.

▶ Yamauchi H, Fukuyama H, Ogawa M, et al. Hemodilution improves cerebral hemodynamics in internal carotid artery occlusion. *Stroke.* 1993;24:1885–1890.

▶ Spahn DR, Zollinger A, Schlumpf RB, et al. Hemodilution tolerance in elderly patients without known cardiac disease. *Anesth Analg.* 1996;82:681–686.

REFERENCES

1. Popovsky MA. Transfusion and the lung: circulatory overload and acute lung injury. *Vox Sang.* 2004;87:62–65.

2. Saxena AK, Panhotra BR. The vulnerability of middle-aged and elderly patients to hepatitis C virus infection in a high-prevalence hospital-based hemodialysis setting. *J Am Geriatr Soc.* 2004;52:242–246.

3. Carson JL, Altman DG, Duff A, et al. Risk of bacterial infection associated with allogeneic blood transfusion among patients undergoing hip fracture repair. *Transfusion.* 1999;39:694–700.

4. Renner SW, Howanitz PJ, Bachner P. Preoperative autologous blood donation in 612 hospitals: a College of American Pathologists' Q-Probe

study of quality issues in transfusion practice. *Arch Pathol Lab Med.* 1992; 116:613–619.

5. Linden JV, Wagner K, Voytovich AE, Sheehan J. Transfusion errors in New York State: an analysis of 10 years' experience. *Transfusion.* 2000;40: 1207–1213.

6. Edelman MJ, Potter P, Mahaffey KG, et al. The potential for reintroduction of tumor cells during intraoperative blood salvage: reduction of risk with use of the RC-400 leukocyte depletion filter. *Urology.* 1996;47:179–181.

7. Gray CL, Amling CL, Polston GR, et al. Intraoperative cell salvage in radical retropubic prostatectomy. *Urology.* 2001;58:740–745.

8. Nilsson-Ehle H, Jagenburg R, Landahl S, Svanborg A. Blood haemoglobin declines in the elderly: implications for reference intervals from age 70 to 88. *Eur J Haematol.* 2000;65:297–305.

9. Aessopos A, Deftereos S, Farmakis D, et al. Cardiovascular adaptation to chronic anemia in the elderly: an echocardiographic study. *Clin Invest Med.* 2004;27:265–273.

10. Clyne N, Jogestrand T. Effect of erythropoietin treatment on physical exercise capacity and on renal function in predialytic uremic patients. *Nephron.* 1992;60:390–396.

11. Lawrence VA, Silverstein JH, Cornell JE, et al. Higher Hb level is associated with better early functional recovery after hip fracture repair. *Transfusion.* 2003;43:1717–1722.

12. Halm EA, Wang JJ, Boockvar K, et al. The effect of perioperative anemia on clinical and functional outcomes in patients with hip fracture. *J Orthop Trauma.* 2004;18:369–374.

13. Halm EA, Wang JJ, Boockvar K, et al. Effects of blood transfusion on clinical and functional outcomes in patients with hip fracture. *Transfusion.* 2003;43:1358–1365.

14. Weber EW, Slappendel R, Prins MH, et al. Perioperative blood transfusions and delayed wound healing after hip replacement surgery: effects on duration of hospitalization. *Anesth Analg.* 2005;100:1416–1421.

15. Rosencher N, Kerkkamp HEM, Macheras G, et al. Orthopedic Surgery Transfusion Hemoglobin European Overview (OSTHEO) study: blood management in elective knee and hip arthroplasty in Europe. *Transfusion.* 2003;43:459–469.

16. Rickard MJFX, Dent OF, Sinclair G, et al. Background and perioperative risk factors for prolonged hospital stay after resection of colorectal cancer. *ANZ J Surg.* 2004;74:4–9.

17. Carson JL, Duff A, Poses RM, et al. Effect of anaemia and cardiovascular disease on surgical mortality and morbidity. *Lancet.* 1996;348:1055–1060.

18. Hogue C, Goodnough L, Monk T. Perioperative myocardial ischemic episodes are related to hematocrit level in patients undergoing radical prostatectomy. *Transfusion.* 1998;38:924–931.

19. Corwin HL, Gettinger A, Pearl RG, et al. The CRIT study: anemia and blood transfusion in the critically ill—current clinical practice in the United States. *Crit Care Med.* 2004;32:39–52.

20. Vincent JL, Baron J, Reinhart K, et al. Anemia and blood transfusion in critically ill patients. *JAMA.* 2002;288:1499–1507.

21. Wu W, Rathore SS, Wang Y, et al. Blood transfusion in elderly patients with acute myocardial infarction. *N Engl J Med.* 2001;345:1230–1236.

22. Carson JL, Duff AMHS, Berlin JA, et al. Perioperative blood transfusion and postoperative mortality. *JAMA.* 1998;279:199–205.

23. Hébert PC, Wells G, Blajchman MA, et al. A multicenter, randomized, controlled clinical trial of transfusion requirements in critical care. *N Engl J Med.* 1999;340:409–417.

24. Hébert PC, Yetisir E, Martin CF, et al. Is a low transfusion threshold safe in critically ill patients with cardiovascular diseases? *Crit Care Med.* 2001; 29:227–234.

25. Gandini G, Franchini M, de Gironcoli M, et al. Preoperative autologous blood donation by elderly patients undergoing orthopaedic surgery. *Vox Sang.* 2001;80:95–100.

26. Janetzko K, Bocher R, Klotz KF, et al. Effects of blood donation on the physical fitness and hemorheology of healthy elderly donors. *Vox Sang.* 1998;75:7–11.

27. Janetzko K, Kluter H, Kirchner H, Klotz K. The effect of moderate hypovolaemia on microcirculation in healthy older blood donors. *Anaesthesia.* 2001;56:103–107.

28. Kasper S, Dahlmann H, Mellinghoff H, et al. Lactated Ringer solution versus hydroxyethyl starch for volume replacement in autologous blood donors with cardiovascular disease: a controlled, randomized trial. *Vox Sang.* 1998;75:26–31.

29. Kasper S, Weimbs G, Sabatowski R, Wassmer G. A randomized crossover trial of IV fluid replacement versus no fluid replacement in autologous blood donors with cardiovascular disease. *Transfusion.* 2002;42:226–231.

30. Kasper S, Baumann M, Radbruch L, et al. A pilot study of continuous ambulatory electrocardiography in patients donating blood for autologous use in elective coronary artery bypass grafting. *Transfusion.* 1997; 37:829–835.

31. Goldfinger D, Capon S, Czer L, et al. Safety and efficacy of preoperative donation of blood for autologous use by patients with end-stage heart or lung disease who are awaiting organ transplantation. *Transfusion.* 1993;33:336–340.

32. Weisbach V, Skoda P, Rippel R, et al. Oral or intravenous iron as an adjuvant to autologous blood donation in elective surgery: a randomized, controlled study. *Transfusion.* 1999;39:465–472.

33. Cuenca J, Garcia-Erce JA, Munoz M, et al. Patients with pertrochanteric hip fracture may benefit from preoperative intravenous iron therapy: a pilot study. *Transfusion.* 2004;44:1447–1452.

34. Mercuriali F, Zanella A, Barosi G, et al. Use of erythropoietin to increase the volume of autologous blood donated by orthopedic patients. *Transfusion.* 1993;33:55–60.

35. Monk TG, Goodnough LT, Brecher ME, et al. A prospective randomized comparison of three blood conservation strategies for radical prostatectomy. *Anesthesiology.* 1999;91:24–33.

36. Monk TG, Goodnough LT, Brecher ME, et al. Acute normovolemic hemodilution can replace preoperative autologous blood donation as a standard of care for autologous blood procurement in radical prostatectomy. *Anesth Analg.* 1997;85:953–958.

37. Goodnough LT, Despotis GJ, Merkel K, Monk TG. A randomized trial comparing acute normovolemic hemodilution and preoperative autologous blood donation in total hip arthroplasty. *Transfusion.* 2000;40:1054–1057.

38. Goodnough LT, Monk TG, Despotis GJ, Merkel K. A randomized trial of acute normovolemic hemodilution compared to preoperative autologous blood donation in total knee arthroplasty. *Vox Sang.* 1999;77: 11–16.

39. Spahn DR, Zollinger A, Schlumpf RB, et al. Hemodilution tolerance in elderly patients without known cardiac disease. *Anesth Analg.* 1996;82:681–686.

40. Ickx BE, Rigolet M, van der Linden P. Cardiovascular and metabolic response to acute normovolemic anemia: effects of anesthesia. *Anesthesiology.* 2000; 93:1011–1016.

41. Van der Linden P, De Hert S, Mathieu N, et al. Tolerance to acute isovolemic hemodilution: effect of anesthetic depth. *Anesthesiology.* 2003;99: 97–104.

42. Weiskopf RB, Feiner J, Hopf HW, et al. Oxygen reverses deficits of cognitive function and memory and increased heart rate induced by acute severe isovolemic anemia. *Anesthesiology.* 2002;96:871–877.

43. Yamauchi H, Fukuyama H, Ogawa M, et al. Hemodilution improves cerebral hemodynamics in internal carotid artery occlusion. *Stroke.* 1993;24: 1885–1890.

44. Szegedi LL, van der Linden P, Ducart A, et al. The effects of acute isovolemic hemodilution on oxygenation during one-lung ventilation. *Anesth Analg.* 2005;100:15–20.

45. Spahn DR, Schmid ER, Seifert B, Pasch T. Hemodilution tolerance in patients with coronary artery disease who are receiving chronic beta-adrenergic blocker therapy. *Anesth Analg.* 1996;82:687–694.

46. Spahn DR, Smith LR, Schell RM, et al. Importance of severity of coronary artery disease for the tolerance to normovolemic hemodilution. Comparison of single-vessel versus multivessel stenoses in a canine model. *J Thorac Cardiovasc Surg.* 1994;108:231–239.

47. Licker M, Ellenberger C, Sierra J, et al. Cardiovascular response to acute normovolemic hemodilution in patients with coronary artery diseases: assessment with transesophageal echocardiography. *Crit Care Med.* 2005; 33:591–597.

48. Licker M, Ellenberger C, Sierra J, et al. Cardioprotective effects of acute normovolemic hemodilution in patients undergoing coronary artery bypass surgery. *Chest.* 2005;128:838–847.

49. Fraga AdO, Fantoni DT, Otsuki DA, et al. Evidence for myocardial defects under extreme acute normovolemic hemodilution with hydroxyethyl starch and lactated Ringer's solution. *Shock.* 2005;24:388–395.

50. Boldt J, Kling D, Weidler B, et al. Acute preoperative hemodilution in cardiac surgery: volume replacement with a hypertonic saline-hydroxyethyl starch solution. *J Cardiothorac Vasc Anesth.* 1991;5:23–28.

51. Casati VMD, Speziali GMD, D'Alessandro CMD, et al. Intraoperative low-volume acute normovolemic hemodilution in adult open-heart surgery. *Anesthesiology*. 2002;97:367–373.

52. Weiskopf RB. Efficacy of acute normovolemic hemodilution assessed as a function of fraction of blood volume lost. *Anesthesiology*. 2001;94:439–446.

53. Segal JB, Blasco-Colmenares E, Norris EJ, Guallar E. Preoperative acute normovolemic hemodilution: a meta-analysis. *Transfusion*. 2004;44:632–644.

54. Karakaya D, Ustun E, Tur A, et al. Acute normovolemic hemodilution and nitroglycerin-induced hypotension: comparative effects on tissue oxygenation and allogeneic blood transfusion requirement in total hip arthroplasty. *J Clin Anesth*. 1999;11:368–374.

55. Winslow RM. Blood substitutes: refocusing an elusive goal. Review. *Br J Haematol*. 2000;111:387–396.

56. Greenburg AG, Kim HW. Use of an oxygen therapeutic as an adjunct to intraoperative autologous donation to reduce transfusion requirements in patients undergoing coronary artery bypass graft surgery. *J Am Coll Surg*. 2004;198:373–383.

57. Hill SE, Leone BJ, Faithfull NS, et al. Perflubron emulsion (AF0144) augments harvesting of autologous blood: a phase II study in cardiac surgery. *J Cardiothorac Vasc Anesth*. 2002;16:555–560.

58. Norris EJ, Ness PM, Williams GM. Use of a human polymerized hemoglobin solution as an adjunct to acute normovolemic hemodilution during complex abdominal aortic reconstruction. *J Clin Anesth*. 2003;15:220–223.

Beta Blockade

William Vernick
Lee A. Fleisher

INTRODUCTION

Cardiac complications resulting in morbidity and mortality are some of the greatest risks associated with the perioperative care of the approximately 30 million people undergoing noncardiac surgery in the United States each year. Most of these complications are related to underlying preexisting coronary artery disease (CAD). It has been found that 1–5% of patients sustain a perioperative cardiac event, with an estimated cost of $20 billion annually.[1] Hospital stays are extended by a mean of 11 days due to these complications,[2] with an increase in charges of $15,000 per perioperative myocardial infarction (PMI).[3] The incidence should not be expected to decline despite newer technologies and medications, given the increasing age of patients undergoing elective surgery today. Patients undergoing vascular surgery are at an even higher risk. The 30-day mortality for elective vascular surgery ranges from 2.1% to 8%.[4–6] The incidence of postoperative cardiac events may be as high as 16%.[7] It is estimated that less than 10% of vascular patients present without any CAD, while 50–60% have significant CAD.[8] The incidence of CAD rises considerably with increasing age (Fig. 19-1). It is estimated that 40% of men over the age of 60 have an intermediate (10–20%) risk of coronary heart disease, and that 83% of those who die from coronary heart disease are older than 65.[9]

CORONARY REVASCULARIZATION

For much of the 1980s, there was a focus on determining the presence and extent of CAD in order to risk stratify patients. This led to the development of guidelines in order to identify those patients who would warrant further diagnostic testing. The focus has now shifted to strategies that might result in a reduction in perioperative morbidity and mortality. For those considered at increased perioperative cardiac risk, the options for risk reduction are either coronary revascularization or the implementation of pharmacologic strategies that might reduce cardiac risk.[10] Prior to the recently published Coronary Artery Revascularization Prophylaxis (CARP) trial,[11] there were no prospective randomized controlled trials evaluating the efficacy of coronary revascularization prior to noncardiac surgery. Using data from multiple retrospective studies, in 1997 the American College of Physicians (ACP) concluded that while some improvement in perioperative cardiac outcome with revascularization may be gained, when the morbidity and mortality of the revascularization itself are added, there is no benefit to prophylactic revascularization

prior to noncardiac surgery.[12] The current American College of Cardiology/American Heart Association (ACC/AHA) guidelines recommend coronary revascularization only for patients who would benefit from revascularization independent of the proposed noncardiac surgery.[13]

The CARP study was the first randomized trial which addressed the question of revascularization before noncardiac surgery.[11] This trial involved patients presenting for repair of abdominal aortic aneurysms (AAAs) or for lower extremity revascularization. Patients with a coronary stenosis of 70% or greater in at least one major coronary vessel that was deemed suitable for revascularization were eligible for the study, and a total of 510 patients were randomized to either revascularization or intensive medical therapy perioperatively. Of the 316 patients enrolled in the study who had undergone nuclear stress imaging as part of their workup, 72% had moderate to large reversible defects. This means that a large percentage of these patients would have qualified for revascularization before noncardiac surgery based on the ACC/AHA guidelines. The incidence of death or myocardial infarction (MI) within 30 days of the vascular procedure was high but similar: 14.7% versus 17.7% for revascularization and medical therapy, respectively. Perioperative medical therapy was similar in both groups and included beta-blockers (85%), aspirin (72%), statins (53%), IV nitroglycerin (33%), and heparin (93%). Long-term mortality at a median follow-up of 2.7 years was also high but similar between the groups, averaging 22.5%. The results of this study suggest that that the indications for preoperative coronary revascularization are even more limited, and that optimal medical therapy is critical.

However, there were some limitations with this trial. There was no subgroup analysis of outcome within the revascularization group based on the type of revascularization performed. In the revascularization arm, 59% received a percutaneous coronary intervention (PCI), and 41% had a coronary artery bypass graft (CABG). Patients undergoing CABG had on average 3 vessels revascularized versus 1.3 in the PCI group, with the completeness of revascularization reported as 61.9% for PCI versus 98% for CABG. There was no information regarding the type of PCI received; whether it was an angioplasty or if a bare metal stent was placed. The study was concluded before the introduction of drug-eluding stents. Thus, the question remains: how applicable are the results of the study today? If the study evaluated patients just receiving CABG or patients receiving drug-eluding stents, would the results have been different? Other questions revolve around the timing of surgery after PCI and the use of antiplatelet therapy after PCI. The paper stated that the median time to vascular

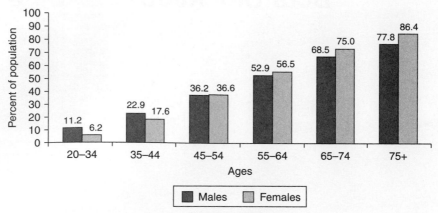

FIGURE 19-1 Prevalence of cardiovascular diseases in Americans aged 20 and older by age and sex.

surgery after PCI was 48 days, but the study design called for patients to have vascular surgery within 14 days of PCI. The current recommendations contraindicate surgery within 6 weeks of the placement of a bare-metal stent, and stipulate that patients should remain on antiplatelet therapy, beyond just aspirin, during this time frame. The study provided no information regarding the length or the type of antiplatelet therapy beyond the administration of aspirin after the PCI was performed and before vascular surgery or its use through the perioperative period. In a letter to the editor responding to these questions, the authors of the CARP study stated that only 72 patients underwent surgery within 6 weeks of PCI, and of these, there were only 4 deaths (5%) and 1 PMI.[14] They did not, however, address the issue of antiplatelet therapy. Thus, it is not known what percentage of the postoperative complications represent patients who had received inadequate antiplatelet therapy after stent placement.

THE DEBATE CONCERNING PERIOPERATIVE BETA BLOCKADE

As far as pharmacologic strategies, several small randomized trials demonstrated no benefit to either intraoperative calcium channel blockers or IV nitroglycerin in the prevention of perioperative myocardial ischemia or the incidence of PMI.[15] The results of small observational studies of perioperative beta-blockers (PBB) in the 1980s were more encouraging.[16,17] The use of beta-blockers for CAD in the ambulatory setting is strongly supported in the cardiology literature, and follows 40 years of research documenting their cardioprotective effects.[18] In the ACC/AHA practice guidelines, beta-blockers are first line therapy for the pharmacologic treatment of chronic stable angina.[19] Beta-blockers are considered as having class I evidence (defined as conditions in which there is evidence and/or general agreement that a given procedure or treatment is useful and effective) in ST elevation MI with or without thrombolysis, and in non-ST elevation MI.[20,21] Given the success of beta-blockers in the cardiology setting and the positive findings from observational studies on PBB, excitement for PBB soon grew in the mid 1990s.

PMI has long been thought to be associated with sustained elevations of heart rate and prolonged episodes of ST-segment depressions.[22] Beta-blockers can improve myocardial oxygen balance by slowing the heart rate and reducing contractility. Decreasing the heart rate not only promotes improved diastolic coronary filling, but it also decreases myocardial oxygen consumption. Beta-blockers may

also have an effect on coronary plaque stability by decreasing shear forces.[18] This may result in a lower incidence of atherosclerotic plaque rupture in the coronary arteries and a smaller probability of coronary thrombosis. Finally, in the setting of ischemia-induced arrhythmias, beta-blockers have a membrane-stabilizing effect.

The first randomized controlled trial of perioperative beta blockade was published in 1996 by Mangano and the Multicenter Study of Perioperative Ischemia Research Group (McSPI group).[23] The group found improved long-term outcomes up to 2 years after PBB in patients with or at risk for CAD undergoing major noncardiac surgery. On the basis of this trial alone, in an addendum to a consensus statement regarding the perioperative care of patients at risk for CAD, in 1997 the ACP recommended perioperative atenolol for all patients with CAD or risk factors for CAD.[12] The next influential randomized controlled trial was the Dutch Echocardiographic Cardiac Risk Evaluation Applying Stress Echocardiography (DECREASE) trial in 1999 from Poldermans and colleagues.[24] They found a significant improvement in 30-day cardiac morbidity and mortality with PBB for high-risk vascular patients who had demonstrated mild to moderate ischemia on a dobutamine stress echo (DSE). Based primarily on the results of these two trials, in 2002 the ACC/AHA made recommendations regarding the use of PBB.[13] They defined class I indications for PBB to be for use in vascular patients with ischemia on stress testing, or in patients who recently required beta-blockers to control symptoms of angina, arrhythmia, or hypertension. Class IIa indications for PBB include patients with known CAD or major risk factors for CAD, or in patients with untreated hypertension. Class II evidence is defined as conditions where there is conflicting evidence and/or divergence of opinion about the usefulness/efficacy of a procedure or treatment; however, with class IIa evidence the weight of evidence/opinion is in favor of their usefulness/efficacy.

Despite the recommendations from two important sources, the ACP and the ACC/AHA, many questions remain regarding PBB. In a quantitative systematic review of the literature from 1980 to 2000, Stevens et al. found 11 randomized trials of PBB that assessed myocardial ischemia, PMI, or 30-day cardiac mortality.[15] These trials involved 866 patients. PBB reduced the incidence of postoperative ischemia from 27.9% to 15.2%, PMI from 5.2% to 0.9%, and 30-day cardiac mortality from 3.9% to 0.8%. However, the data included only 15 cardiac deaths and 18 nonfatal MIs, with the majority of events coming from the control group in the DECREASE trial. If the DECREASE trial was excluded from analysis, statistical significance was no longer achieved for either a reduction in

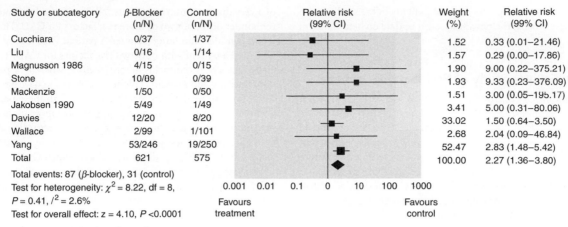

Study or subcategory	β-Blocker (n/N)	Control (n/N)	Relative risk (99% CI)	Weight (%)	Relative risk (99% CI)
Cucchiara	0/37	1/37		1.52	0.33 (0.01–21.46)
Liu	0/16	1/14		1.57	0.29 (0.00–17.86)
Magnusson 1986	4/15	0/15		1.90	9.00 (0.22–375.21)
Stone	10/09	0/39		1.93	9.33 (0.23–376.09)
Mackenzie	1/50	0/50		1.51	3.00 (0.05–195.17)
Jakobsen 1990	5/49	1/49		3.41	5.00 (0.31–80.06)
Davies	12/20	8/20		33.02	1.50 (0.64–3.50)
Wallace	2/99	1/101		2.68	2.04 (0.09–46.84)
Yang	53/246	19/250		52.47	2.83 (1.48–5.42)
Total	621	575		100.00	2.27 (1.36–3.80)

Total events: 87 (β-blocker), 31 (control)
Test for heterogeneity: $\chi^2 = 8.22$, df = 8, $P = 0.41$, $I^2 = 2.6\%$
Test for overall effect: z = 4.10, P <0.0001

FIGURE 19-2 Relative risks for bradycardia needing treatment.

PMI or cardiac death. Another literature review and meta-analysis was published in 2005 by Devereaux et al. regarding PBB, which evaluated similar perioperative cardiac outcomes (Figs. 19-2 and 19-3)[25]. A total of 22 randomized controlled trials involving 2437 patients between 1980 and 2004 were included. However, major cardiovascular events were reported in only eight trials, involving only 1152 patients. The group found a relative risk reduction of 0.44 (95% confidence interval [CI] 0.20 to 0.97, 99% CI 0.16 to 1.24) for major cardiovascular events with the use of PBB, but they cautioned that the number of patients involved and the number of events included were too small to reliably detect a difference. The group had calculated that a total of 6124 patients would be needed to reach "optimal information size." Furthermore, without taking the DECREASE trial (with its large number of events in the control group) into consideration, the beneficial effect of PBB loses significance. In their 2002 executive summary paper, the ACC/AHA even stated that the data from the few randomized trials was too limited to draw firm recommendations.[13] Currently, the PeriOperative Ischemic Evaluation (POISE) trial is ongoing; this will be the first large scale randomized trial of PBB. The study is designed to evaluate the effect of metoprolol XL (sustained release) administered 4 hours preoperatively and perioperatively in patients with intermediate and high cardiac risk undergoing major surgery, including major vascular surgery. The outcome measures to be determined are cardiac morbidity and mortality at 30 days and mortality at 1 year. The study involves 11 countries and 100 medical centers, and plans to enroll 10,000 patients.

Given the current state of the literature, the debate regarding PBB has left most clinicians confused in their attempts to determine the correct approach. Some may be withholding PBB for fear of complications associated with their use in the perioperative period. Others may be unconvinced that the literature has demonstrated evidence of efficacy. Regardless of the reason, perioperative beta blockade has not taken on widespread use in clinical practice. In a survey of Canadian anesthesiologists,[26] 93% of responders agreed that beta-blockers were beneficial in patients with CAD, but only 57% stated that they usually used them in their practice and only 34% used them beyond the early postoperative period. Furthermore, only 9% reported that a formal protocol existed at their institution. In a similar survey study in 2004 of 62 Veterans Affairs Medical Centers,[27] 71% reported frequent use of PBB in their practice, but most believed that the use was largely informal and rarely guided by a formal clinical pathway. In addition, only 30% were convinced that PBB should be used outside vascular surgery.

In this chapter, the evidence for PBB will be further reviewed with a especially close look at the above-mentioned DECREASE and McSPI trials. While the majority of data involving PBB is not specific to the

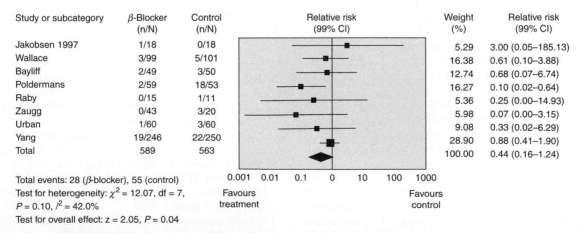

Study or subcategory	β-Blocker (n/N)	Control (n/N)	Relative risk (99% CI)	Weight (%)	Relative risk (99% CI)
Jakobsen 1997	1/18	0/18		5.29	3.00 (0.05–185.13)
Wallace	3/99	5/101		16.38	0.61 (0.10–3.88)
Bayliff	2/49	3/50		12.74	0.68 (0.07–6.74)
Poldermans	2/59	18/53		16.27	0.10 (0.02–0.64)
Raby	0/15	1/11		5.36	0.25 (0.00–14.93)
Zaugg	0/43	3/20		5.98	0.07 (0.00–3.15)
Urban	1/60	3/60		9.08	0.33 (0.02–6.29)
Yang	19/246	22/250		28.90	0.88 (0.41–1.90)
Total	589	563		100.00	0.44 (0.16–1.24)

Total events: 28 (β-blocker), 55 (control)
Test for heterogeneity: $\chi^2 = 12.07$, df = 7, $P = 0.10$, $I^2 = 42.0\%$
Test for overall effect: z = 2.05, P = 0.04

FIGURE 19-3 Relative risks for perioperative cardiovascular events (cardiovascular death, nonfatal myocardial infarction, or nonfatal cardiac arrest).

geriatric population, a large majority of patients in the studies were of geriatric age. Finally, the newest focused update on beta-blockers is discussed.

▶ The Multicenter Study of Perioperative Ischemia

The first randomized controlled trial of PBB was performed by the McSPI group; it appeared in the *New England Journal of Medicine (NEJM)* in 1996.[23] This study looked at the effects of PBB on cardiac outcome up to 2 years after major elective noncardiac surgery in patients with CAD or risk factors for CAD. The inclusion criteria were males with a history of MI, typical angina, or a positive stress test, or the presence of two or more risk factors for CAD. The considered risk factors were age >65, hypertension, current tobacco use, serum cholesterol >240 mg/dL, or diabetes mellitus. A total of 200 patients were randomized to receive either perioperative atenolol or placebo. The average age of participants was 67–68 years. Study group patients were given 5 or 10 mg of intravenous (IV) atenolol based on the hemodynamic effect of the initial 5-mg dose 30 minutes before entering the operating room, and then either 5–10 mg IV or 50–100 mg orally, starting on postoperative day 1. The medication was continued until postoperative day 7 or hospital discharge, whichever came first.

The clinical characteristics were similar between groups, except for preoperative medications. In the study group, 19.4% were already on beta-blockers and 23.7% were on an angiotensin-converting enzyme (ACE) inhibitor. In the control group, 8.2% were on beta-blockers and 8.2% were on an ACE inhibitor. All preoperative cardiovascular medications were continued throughout the perioperative period, except for beta-blockers. Those in the study group on a beta-blocker were switched to atenolol, while those in the control had preoperative beta-blockers discontinued altogether. All patients underwent general anesthesia, but modes of postoperative pain control were not mentioned. Major vascular surgery represented 40.5% of the cases.

The primary endpoint was cardiac mortality, and the secondary endpoint was cardiac events, defined as MI, unstable angina, congestive heart failure (CHF), or the requirement for coronary revascularization. There was no difference in cardiac outcome during the 7-day perioperative period. Three patients died from PMI, two in the control and one in the study group. With reference to nonfatal cardiac events, 16 patients developed CHF and 5 had an episode of ventricular tachycardia, with the distribution of events occurring similarly between groups. Therefore, PBB did not significantly impact the incidence of perioperative cardiac events. Follow-up occurred at 6 months and then at year 1, and again at year 2 postoperatively. At 6-month follow-up, there were no additional nonfatal cardiac events or cardiac deaths after the initial 7-day perioperative period in the study group, versus 12 nonfatal events and 7 cardiac deaths in the control group. After the initial 6–8 month postoperative period, there was not a statistically significant difference between the groups in nonfatal cardiac events or cardiac deaths, but the results remained significant all the way out to the full 2-year follow-up.

The 15% reduction in 2-year event-free survival and the 100% reduction in cardiac events during the first 6–8 months were very impressive. However, there are several limitations with this study, as well as some issues with the study design. This was a small study involving only 200 patients who received care at a single center; there was no standardization of the surgical, anesthetic, or postoperative care plan, including postoperative pain control, therefore calling into question the generalizability of the findings. The study included a wide range of surgical procedures without any subgroup analysis. Not only were the surgical procedures varied, but also the cohort consisted

of a very diverse group of patients. While 39% had definite CAD, the remainder only had two or more risk factors for CAD. There is a difference in life expectancy between a patient with a previous MI or CHF and a patient with only two risk factors for CAD. This is especially true given the inclusion risk factors, whereby a patient with only smoking and a serum cholesterol >240 could have been enrolled. There was no further risk stratification and all these patients were grouped together, again without any subgroup analysis except for patients with diabetes. The cardiology literature regarding ambulatory beta-blocker use does not support grouping patients with only risk factors for CAD with patients with documented CAD.

While the authors were confident that there was no statistically significant difference in medication use between the study and control groups, and stated that the control group used cardiovascular medications (beta-blockers, calcium channel blockers, nitrates, and ACE inhibitors) at least as often as the study group, a closer look calls these claims into question. As mentioned above, there was a significant difference in the use of beta-blockers and ACE inhibitors preoperatively between the groups. At hospital discharge, the use of ACE inhibitors was 14.3% higher in the study group. It was not until the 6-month follow-up period that the use of ACE inhibitors was equal between the groups, the same time period when the improvement in cardiac outcomes stopped. During the 7-day study period, there was a 100% difference in the use of beta-blockers between the groups, although 8.2% of the placebo group were on these medications preoperatively. At hospital discharge, only 14% of the study group remained on beta-blockers versus 7.1% of the control group, and at 6 months, study group use was 13.8% versus 8.3% in the control. This means that during the 6–8 month postoperative period, when the improvement in cardiac outcomes with PBB were significant, there was very little difference in the use of beta-blockers, while there was no difference in 7-day postoperative outcome when the difference in beta-blocker use was 100%.

It is hard to imagine that a medication given for a 7-day perioperative period would have no effect on outcome during its administration period, but would have a significant effect during the next 6–8 months, when the majority of patients had stopped the medication altogether. As Devereaux et al.[28] point out, the magnitude of this effect seems implausible. The contention of the investigators was that plaque stabilization perioperatively was the critical event for improved long-term outcome. There is no direct evidence to support this notion, and if there was such significant plaque instability without PBB, it seems unlikely that there would have been only 2 PMIs in the control group during the 7-day perioperative period.

Wallace et al. published a secondary analysis of the incidence of myocardial ischemia that occurred during the 7-day perioperative period in the aforementioned atenolol trial by Mangano and the McSPI group.[29] Ischemia was monitored by a Holter 3-lead ECG, which was begun 24 hours preoperatively and continued during surgery, and until postoperative day 7. Automated ST-segment analysis was used and then reviewed by blinded investigators. Ischemia was defined as reversible ST-segment changes lasting at least 1 minute. Holter data was available a total of 78% of the time, but by days 6 and 7, it was available only 49% of the time. A 12-lead ECG was also performed preoperatively and daily for 7 days. During the first 48 hours, 17 patients in the study group had at least one episode of ischemia, while 34 had such episodes in the control. For the entire 7 days, there were 24 patients who experienced ischemia in the study group versus 39 in the control.

Study limitations again cloud the initially impressive findings. Despite a 30–50% reduction in ischemia, there were no differences for in-hospital cardiac events or cardiac mortality. The lack of an association between perioperative ischemia and PMI is inconsistent with the previous findings of Mangano's group, in which they reported a ninefold increase in the incidence of PMI when perioperative ischemia occurred.[1] In contrast to a threshold of 1 minute or more for defining ischemia in an analysis by Wallace et al., other studies have shown that Holter monitoring of ischemia was predictive of cardiac complications only after a cumulative ischemic time of 120 minutes or a single episode of greater than 30 minutes.[30,31] Landesberg et al. compared the incidence of PMI, defined as a cardiac troponin I (cTnI) >3.1 ng/mL, in 185 patients undergoing vascular surgery, with duration of automated ST-segment changes on continuous 12-lead ECG Holter monitoring.[32] Those who developed a PMI sustained ischemia a cumulative seven times longer than those without a PMI. The average length of the longest ischemic episode per patient who developed a PMI was 26 minutes versus 22 minutes for those without PMI. While using 1 minute or more of ST-segment changes for defining ischemia is consistent with some other studies, one has to question the significance of findings of Wallace et al. In addition, the specificity of Holter monitor-detected ischemia may be significantly lower in asymptomatic patients with only moderate risk for CAD, compared to patients at higher risk for CAD.[33] Finally, there was no mention of 12-lead ECG changes confirming the presence of ischemia found on 3-lead Holter monitoring, or the presence of any serum electrolyte or hemodynamic abnormalities at the time of Holter ST-segment changes.

If Wallace et al. were able to show subtle myocardial damage in the setting of reversible ischemic ECG changes, the findings of improved cardiac morbidity and mortality at 6–8 months would have more theoretical support. Using a cTnI as a marker for PMI in 229 patients having high-risk vascular surgery, Kim et al. were able to show an increase in 6-month mortality of 15% in those with a postoperative cTnI >1.5 ng/mL.[34] Despite a decrease of 6-month mortality associated with their use, somewhat paradoxically, PBB did not prevent the release of troponins to a level consistent with PMI. While creatinine kinase MB (CK-MB) levels are not as specific for PMI as troponins, they are still relatively sensitive.[35] In Landesberg's study, 83% of those with a PMI, defined by a troponin >3.1 ng/mL, had an elevated CK-MB. In Wallace's analysis, there was no mention of a positive CK-MB result for any patient. A recent study may, however, lend some support to the contention of Wallace, Mangano, and their colleagues. This was a follow-up study of 393 major vascular patients at a single center who survived at least 30 days, and who did not suffer a non-fatal PMI.[36] Using a troponin T level of only 0.1 ng/mL as a marker for myocardial damage, 54 patients were identified. There was an increase in mortality at a median follow-up of 4 years from 17% to 41% in these patients who were described as having asymptomatic elevations of troponin T in the postoperative period. Interestingly, only 17% of those with a troponin level greater than 0.1 had an abnormal CK-MB level, and there was no association between long-term mortality and abnormal CK-MB levels. This raises the possibility that perioperative events associated with subtle myocardial damage, which might otherwise go undetected, could lead to an increase in long-term mortality. It is not clear exactly how the investigators defined PMI or how they decided that these elevations of troponin T were all asymptomatic. The study was not designed to evaluate the effect of PBB on these low-level releases of troponin; however, the percentage of those on chronic beta-blockers was the same between those with and without troponin elevations.

Finally, there is the issue of beta-blocker withdrawal in 8.2% of the control group who were on beta-blockers preoperatively and then had them acutely stopped for the study. Beta-blocker withdrawal has long been known to lead to adrenergic hyperactivity with rebound hypertension and tachycardia. Psaty et al. found a fourfold increase in the incidence of cardiac events in patients who recently stopped their beta-blockers in the ambulatory setting.[37] An increased incidence of cardiac complications from beta-blocker withdrawal in the perioperative setting has also been found.[38,39] It is likely that withdrawal may have played at least some role in the incidence of ischemia found by Wallace et al. on Holter monitoring.

Conclusions based on the studies of Mangano, Wallace, and colleagues are limited not only by study design and data interpretation issues, a small sample size, and an absence of troponin measurements, but also by the diversity of the patient population. The lack of any significant subgroup analysis regarding patient characteristics or procedures limits the ability to discern which patients would truly benefit from PBB based on their studies.

▶ Diabetic Postoperative Mortality and Morbidity trial

The only subgroup analysis in the atenolol trial of Mangano et al. was conducted for patients with diabetes. Atenolol was found to reduce 2-year mortality by 75% in diabetics. The Diabetic Postoperative Mortality and Morbidity (DIPOM) trial sought to confirm the positive effects on PBB in patients with diabetes.[40,41] The study was a double-blind, placebo-controlled, randomized trial conducted at nine Danish hospitals. The inclusion criteria were insulin-dependent and non-insulin-dependent diabetics older than age 40 who were undergoing major surgery, defined as surgery lasting longer than 1 hour. Exclusion criteria were current beta-blocker use, contraindications to beta-blockers, class IV heart failure, and conditions indicating beta blocker treatment. The study drug was metoprolol, which was given the night before surgery and continued at a dose of 100 mg daily on the day of surgery and then for 7 days or until hospital discharge. Metoprolol 5 mg was given intravenously every 6 hours if patients could not take oral medications. The preliminary results were reported at the November 2004 AHA meeting.[40] A total of 921 patients were included in the study, and follow-up occurred at a median time of 18 months. The incidence of all-cause mortality, MI, unstable angina, and CHF were similar, 21% in the metoprolol group versus 20% in the placebo. While this study could be used to refute findings of Mangano et al. regarding PBB and diabetics, it is important to note the differences between the two studies regarding patient populations and the surgical procedures. The exclusion criteria for DIPOM included conditions for which beta-blockers would be indicated. While this is not specifically addressed in the published trial design, the reader is left to assume that this means patients with CAD. Does this also mean patients with risk factors for CAD other than diabetes? No patient underwent vascular surgery in this trial. With this in mind, the results of this trial suggest that relatively low-risk diabetic patients without obvious signs of CAD do not obtain a short- or long-term mortality or cardiac morbidity benefit from PBB when undergoing nonvascular surgery.

▶ The DECREASE trial

The strongest evidence so far for the effectiveness of PBB comes from the aforementioned DECREASE trial, published in 1999. This was a randomized multicenter trial which screened 1351 patients presenting for elective abdominal aortic or infrainguinal arterial reconstruction between 1996 and 1999.

The 1351 patients were screened for cardiac risk factors, which included age >70, angina, prior MI by history or Q wave, compensated

CHF or a history of CHF, current treatment for ventricular arrhythmia or diabetes mellitus, or a diminished exercise tolerance that caused an inability to perform activities of daily living. Patients with one risk factor or more underwent a DSE. Of the 1351 patients initially screened, 846 underwent DSE, and ischemia was found in 173. Patients were further excluded if they had extensive wall motion abnormalities or strong evidence of left main or triple vessel coronary disease, asthma, or were already on beta-blockers. This left 112 patients for randomization. The mean age was 67–68 years.

The study involved the administration of the oral beta-1 selective beta-blocker bisoprolol, on average 37 days and at least 1 week preoperatively, with the effectiveness of the initial dose checked 1 week after initiation. The dose was increased from 5 mg daily to up to a maximum of 10 mg daily if the resting heart rate remained above 60 bpm. The medication was continued for 30 days postoperatively. IV metoprolol was used if patients were unable to take oral medication. The dose of bisoprolol was not titrated postoperatively, but if patients were on IV metoprolol the dose was titrated to keep the heart rate below 80 bpm. The clinical characteristics of the study and control groups were similar, although the control group had twice the number of patients with greater than four ischemic segments (5/59 patients vs. 10/53 patients). The planned surgery and intraoperative anesthetic management, including modes of postoperative pain control, were similar.

The results were quite impressive, leading the safety committee to terminate the study early. The 30-day operative cardiac mortality decreased from 17% (9/53) in the control group to 3.4% (2/59) in the study group. Most of the cardiac events occurred during the first 7 days postoperatively. In the control group, 17% (9/53) sustained a nonfatal MI, while none occurred in the study group. Of the 53 patients with a positive DSE who were excluded because they were already on beta-blockers, the incidence of perioperative cardiac mortality was 7.6% (4/53), and none had a nonfatal MI.

Boersma et al. published a retrospective review of the entire cohort from the DECREASE trial in 2001 (Fig. 19-4).[42] The data set in Boersma's review included all 1351 patients initially screened in the DECREASE trial. In addition to the 846 patients with one or more clinical risk factors who underwent DSE as part of the screening process, an additional 245 with no risk factors had undergone a DSE at the discretion of the attending physician. A total of 360 patients received PBB; of these, 301 were being treated long-term and 59 were randomized in the DECREASE trial. For those patients with no risk factors or with a negative DSE, the incidence of cardiac mortality or nonfatal MI was 0.5% (1/216) on PBB versus 1.5% (14/913) for those not on PBB. This implies a limited benefit of PBB in those at low risk for cardiac complications. This is in contrast to the results of the DECREASE trial, where the incidence of cardiac mortality or nonfatal MI was 34% if a patient had a positive DSE and was not on PBB versus 3.4% if they were on PBB.

Using the Revised Cardiac Risk Index classification system for major noncardiac surgery devised by Lee and colleagues (1 point assigned for each clinical factor: high-risk procedure; history of CAD; history of CHF; history of CVA; insulin-dependent diabetes; and a preoperative serum creatinine >2.0 mg/dL),[43] the authors found that if a patient's risk score was less than 2 and PBB was used, the incidence of cardiac events was less than 2%, no matter what the results of the DSE were. However, those with extensive wall motion abnormalities were excluded from the study. For those with a negative DSE, PBB was only beneficial in those patients with a risk score of 3 or more. In patients with a revised cardiac risk index of 3 or more and a positive DSE, the incidence of cardiac events was greater than 6%, even with PBB. The risk was even higher for those with greater than four ischemic segments.

Kertai et al. subsequently published a long-term follow-up study of the original 1351 patients in 2003.[44] The intent was to examine the incidence of late cardiac complications in patients who continued beta-blockers throughout the postoperative period, and then through the follow-up period. A total of 1286 patients survived at least 30 days postoperatively, with the median follow-up occurring at 23 months postoperatively. The results of long-term follow-up were very similar to the results of the 30-day outcomes. For those who had no clinical risk factors or who had a negative DSE, there was no difference in cardiac complications, regardless of whether patients received long-term beta-blockers or not (4% vs. 4%). However, in patients with a positive DSE, the incidence of cardiac complications was 10.1% for those on beta-blockers versus 32.6% for those who were not. For those patients with revised cardiac risk index of 3 or more and a positive DSE, the risk of cardiac events was 20.3%, despite beta-blockers. Again, long-term beta-blockers were not protective in those with greater than four ischemic segments on DSE.

As mentioned above, the results from the DECREASE trial are impressive with few limitations. The most obvious problem with the study is its small size, with only 112 patients randomized. Critics have contended that the incidence of complications in the control group was extremely high, thus shedding some doubt on the significance of the results. However, this subset of patients with documented ischemia undergoing vascular surgery is at very high risk for cardiac complications. Poldermans and colleagues had previously found that a positive DSE result in patients scheduled for major vascular surgery resulted in a 38% positive predictive value for perioperative cardiac events.[45]

A relative risk reduction of 100% for nonfatal MI and 80% for cardiac mortality is significantly better than that found for beta-blockers in the cardiology literature regarding acute MI and chronic CHF.[46,47] While the perioperative setting is different, such a drastic difference does prompt some suspicion. However, even if the magnitude of the results was halved, the authors would still have had a statistically significant positive study. The trial was also criticized because physicians were unblinded to which group their patient was in. It seems unlikely that this would have had such a profound impact on the outcome of the study. Patients in the control group were allowed to receive a beta-blocker if they developed ischemia or a PMI. The patients who received PBB were started on bisoprolol an average of 37 days preoperatively, and were continued on them for 30 days with some titration to heart rate. This long treatment time frame was not used in most other trials, and might also account for the high efficacy of the study.

When looking at the results from the DECREASE trial, it is very important to keep this information in perspective, as the results pertain to a very specific group of patients, in contrast to the atenolol study conducted by Mangano et al. It involved patients undergoing high-risk vascular surgery with a positive DSE. Patients with a negative DSE or with no risk factors did not benefit from PBB at either 30 days or approximately 23 months. PBB was also not protective in patients with a revised cardiac risk index of 3 or more, or in those with extensive regional wall motion abnormalities (RWMA). It should be kept in mind that the clinical risk factors in the Revised Cardiac Risk Index and those for inclusion in the DECREASE trial were generally more severe than those for inclusion in the trial conducted by Mangano et al. In conclusion, the DECREASE trial, even though its results may be greater than expected, is very convincing for the positive impact PBB has in this very specific patient population.

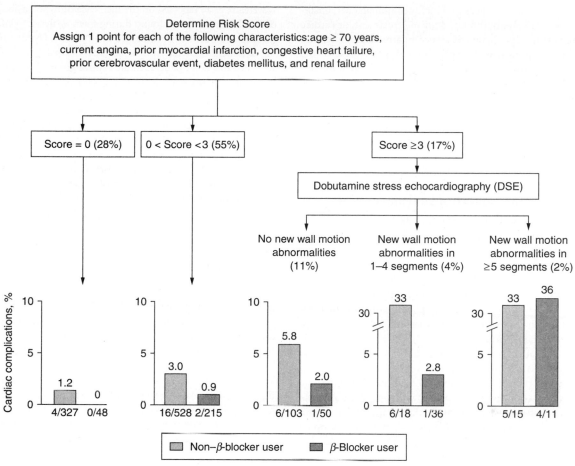

FIGURE 19-4 Results of a retrospective review of the DECREASE trial according to clinical risk score, dobutamine stress echocardiography, and receipt of β-blockers during surgery. Percentages in parentheses represent the number of patients in the target category as a proportion of the total number of 1351 patients. Numbers underneath the bars represent the actual number of events/patients in the specific category.

▶ The POBBLE trial

The difference in results between the DECREASE trial and that of the Perioperative Beta Blockade for Patients Undergoing Infrarenal Vascular Surgery (POBBLE) trial further highlights the exclusive nature of the positive findings from the DECREASE trial. The POBBLE study was a double-blind, randomized, placebo-controlled trial conducted at four UK hospitals.[5] The trial involved patients presenting for major infrarenal revascularization. Patients were excluded if they were already on beta-blockers; had contraindications to beta-blockers, such as asthma, bradycardia, or hypotension; aortic stenosis; a documented MI within 2 years of the planned surgery; unstable angina; or angina with a positive dobutamine stress test. A total of 103 patients were randomized to metoprolol or placebo between 2001 and 2004. The median age was 73 years. The study drug was administered as a test dose orally on admission, typically the day before surgery. The dose was 25 or 50 mg, depending on weight, rather than titration to effect. Patients then received an oral dose the morning of surgery, followed by a 2–4 mg IV bolus before induction of anesthesia. Twice daily oral dosing was continued for 7 days postoperatively. The study end points were 30-day cardiovascular morbidity and mortality. Morbidity was defined as MI, unstable angina, ventricular tachycardia, or stroke. Of the 103 patients randomized, 97 proceeded with surgery. Symptomatic bradycardia and hypotension were higher in the study group, with

an increased requirement of inotropic support: 64% in the control versus 92% in the study group. ST-segment depression during the 72-hour perioperative period on 3-lead Holter ECG monitoring was similar, occurring in 35% of the control group for a median duration of 33 minutes, versus 30% in the study group with a median duration of 13 minutes. The 30-day cardiovascular morbidity and mortality was also similar. Mortality was 4% (one control patient and three study patients). Morbidity was 15% (7/48) in the control group and 13% (7/55) in the study group. To reiterate, while this was a negative study for a protective effect of PBB on cardiac morbidity, it is important to keep the exclusion criteria in mind relative to the inclusion criteria for the DECREASE trial. The results of the POBBLE study again suggest that patients at lower risk for CAD did not benefit from PBB, despite undergoing high-risk vascular procedures.

▶ The Metoprolol after Vascular Surgery trial

The findings of the POBBLE study are supported by the Metoprolol after Vascular Surgery (MaVS) trial, which at this time has been reported only in abstract form.[48] This study randomized 497 patients undergoing AAA repair, infrainguinal revascularization, or extra-anatomic revascularization to receive either perioperative metoprolol or placebo. Patients were given either oral or IV metoprolol 2 hours preoperatively, and then either every 6 hours intravenously or twice a day orally for up to 5 days after surgery. Outcomes were measured at 30 days after surgery and included nonfatal MI, unstable angina, new CHF, dysrhythmias requiring treatment, or cardiac death. There was no significant difference in any of the outcomes measured between groups with events occurring in 10.1% of the metoprolol group versus 12% of the placebo group. There was a significantly higher incidence of bradycardia and hypotension requiring treatment in the metoprolol group. The cohort of patients was described by the authors as moderate to high-risk, but there is no other information provided regarding the patients' clinical histories. The study inclusion and exclusion criteria, other than the type of surgery, are also not given. Finally, the results regarding 6-month and longer outcomes have not been concluded.

▶ The retrospective cohort of Lindenauer et al.

The most recent large-scale study regarding PBB was a retrospective cohort by Lindenauer et al.[49] It was conducted by searching through a database used by 329 participating hospitals for quality assessment. The search criteria consisted of patients 18 years of age or older undergoing major noncardiac surgery, defined as procedures typically requiring a hospital stay of 2 days or more, between 2000 and 2001. Medical history was obtained by searching for the presence of secondary diagnoses in the database from ICD-9-CM codes. In-hospital use of medications was obtained from pharmacy records. A total of 663,635 patients without contraindications to beta-blockers were identified. PBB was administered to 18% of the patients, with PBB being defined as the administration of beta-blockers within the first or second day of hospitalization. Beta-blockers given after the second day were not considered prophylactic therapy. The study end point was in-hospital mortality. PBB had no effect on in-hospital mortality when evaluated for the entire cohort (2.3% vs. 2.4%). For patients with a revised cardiac risk score of 3 or more, PBB was protective. The number needed to treat with PBB to prevent one death in patients with a risk score of 4 was 33. While patients with a risk score of 1 gained no mortality benefit, those with a risk score of zero actually had an increase in mortality. While this study has several limitations, especially its reliance on claims data, as well as problems in how PBB was defined, it further supports a more limited role for PBB, with benefit for select groups of patients only.

▶ Effects of beta blockade on anesthetic requirements

The majority of the literature regarding PBB has focused on its role in the prevention of cardiac morbidity and mortality. However, PBB may have other beneficial effects. Zaug et al. conducted a study evaluating the perioperative release of norepinephrine, epinephrine, adrenocorticotropic hormone (ACTH), and cortisol in 63 patients undergoing major surgery who were greater than 65 years old.[50] Patients were randomized to receive either no beta-blockers perioperatively, pre- and postoperative atenolol, or intraoperative atenolol. There were no differences noted in the release of stress hormones. There was an improvement in hemodynamic stability during emergence from anesthesia in patients who received atenolol. Interestingly, those who received atenolol were given less intraoperative and postoperative opioids, and had a faster recovery from anesthesia while experiencing lower pain scores.

▶ Complications of perioperative beta blockade

As mentioned above, the reluctance of physicians to use PBB may be related to the fear of complications. In the clinical setting of a sympathectomy from general anesthesia, or regional anesthesia superimposed on major fluid shifts, there is concern for hypotension and cardiac insufficiency with the introduction of beta-blocker therapy.

Devereaux et al. reported on the incidence of hypotension, bradycardia, and bronchospasm found during meta-analysis.[25] Unfortunately, these events were not documented in all studies. Hypotension requiring treatment occurred in 216/986 (22%) of patients on PBB versus 147/726 (20.2%) of patients in the control group. Bradycardia requiring treatment occurred in 87/621 (14%) of the PBB group versus 31/575 (5.4%) in the control. Bronchospasm occurred in both groups in about 3% of patients. In the atenolol study conducted by Mangano et al., 85% of patients tolerated their dose of atenolol, and over 60% were able to get the full dose. While 10% had a drop of 20% or more in systolic blood pressure (SBP) or heart rate with their IV dose, none had a SBP less than 90 or a heart rate less than 40. The DECREASE trial did not disclose the incidence of hypotension or bradycardia. One concern regarding the safety of PBB is the significant underreporting in the PBB studies regarding fluid and blood product management, or the use and management of thoracic epidurals. Given the information available, PBB appears to be safe, but caution should be exercised.

▶ Focused update to the ACC/AHA guidelines

A focused update to the ACC/AHA guidelines on perioperative beta blockade was published in 2006 based upon the accumulating evidence and advocates that perioperative beta blockade is a class I indication and should be used in patients previously on beta-blockers and those with a positive stress test undergoing major vascular surgery.[51] The use of these agents in those without active CAD or undergoing less-invasive procedures is advocated as a class IIa recommendation. Based upon these newer studies, beta-blockers may not be effective if heart rate is not well-controlled, or in lower-risk patients. A complete review of the recommendations and strength of the evidence for different groups of patients can be found in Table 19-1.

Table 19-1

Recommendations for Perioperative Beta-Blockade Based Upon the Class of Recommendation and Strength of Evidence

	Low Cardiac Patient Risk	Intermediate Cardiac Patient Risk	CHD or High Cardiac Patient Risk
			Patients found to have myocardial ischemia on preoperative testing
Vascular surgery	Class IIb Level of evidence: C	Class IIb Level of evidence: C	Class I Level of evidence: B* Class IIa Level of evidence: B†
High-/ intermediate-risk surgery	‡	Class IIb Level of evidence: C	Class IIa Level of evidence: B
Low risk surgery	‡	‡	‡

*Applies to patients found to have coronary ischemia on preoperative testing.
†Applies to patients found to have coronary heart disease.
‡Indicates insufficient data. See text for further discussion.
Abbreviation: CHD = coronary heart disease.
Source: Reproduced with permission from Ref. 51.

MECHANISMS OF PERIOPERATIVE MYOCARDIAL INFARCTION

After a review of the literature on PBB, we are left with more questions than answers. Unfortunately, the questions are not limited to subjects such as how much and which drug to give or the timing of drug administration, but instead the questions that remain revolve around in whom PBB actually has efficacy. This is, in part, a reflection of the fact that the mechanism of PMI is multifactorial and not completely understood.

Traditionally, acute coronary syndromes were believed to occur secondary to intracoronary thrombosis on an acutely ruptured plaque, often associated with sympathetic surges (Fig. 19-5). It is estimated that this scenario represents 70% of fatal acute MIs and sudden cardiac death in the ambulatory setting.[22] These rupture-prone plaques are often described as *thin-cap fibroatheroma*. In other cases, a ruptured plaque cannot be identified. Rather, the intracoronary thrombosis is occurring on a de-endothelialized but intact plaque, referred to as *plaque erosion*. Other plaque characteristics that are used to help identify vulnerable plaques include active plaque inflammation, plaque fissuring, superficial calcified nodules, and intraplaque hemorrhage. Unfortunately, many of these characteristics are not readily diagnosed via standard medical diagnostic procedures, and thus vulnerable plaques are not readily discernable from nonvulnerable ones.[52]

A further distinction of coronary syndromes is that between non-Q wave MI (NQMI) and Q wave MI (QMI). Data from cardiac catheterization and autopsy studies in nonsurgical patients with MIs have shown that total coronary occlusion of the infarction-related vessel occurs in 90% of QMIs within the first 6 hours versus only 26–39% of the time in NQMIs.[53] Other studies have shown that lesions responsible for QMIs in nonsurgical patients were mostly less than 50% stenotic before the event,[54] while DeWood et al. found significant collateral flow distal to the infarction-related vessel in 85% of patients with NQMI,[55] suggesting the presence of long-standing clinically significant coronary stenosis. In addition, the clinical characteristics of those patients presenting to the hospital with NQMI had a higher prevalence of diabetes and preexisting CHF or CAD than those presenting with a QMI.[22] While there is certainly significant overlap, it would seem that QMI occurs in younger and healthier patients due to complete coronary thrombosis of previously nonsignificantly occluded vessels, involving less mature and more vulnerable plaques. NQMIs typically occur in older and sicker patients in vessels with preexisting significant coronary stenosis involving more mature plaque, with the intracoronary thrombosis likely occurring on plaque erosions rather than ruptures. These patients also have more diffuse coronary disease. The pathophysiology of NQMI is likely more complicated than that of QMI. The angiographic visualization of coronary thrombus, both forming and then dissolving during NQMI, has led to the hypothesis that coronary thrombosis may be a more dynamic process than previously thought, which would explain the finding of incomplete coronary obstructions of infarction-related vessels in the setting of NQMI.

In a review of the PMI, Landesberg summarized PMI as an entity that occurs early, and often silently, in the postoperative period, within the first 24–48 hours of surgery, and is preceded by prolonged ST depression-type ischemia, resulting in NQMI.[22] Autopsy studies of fatal PMI have supported the notion that PMI is pathophysiologically related to nonsurgical NQMIs. Dawood et al. found ruptured plaque in only 7% and intracoronary thrombosis in only 28% of patients with PMI. Cohen and Aretz found plaque rupture in 46% and coronary thrombosis in 64%.[56] As mentioned previously in this chapter, the incidence of PMI can be related to the duration of postoperative ischemia, a finding that is not suggestive of plaque rupture-type infarctions. In a study evaluating the pattern of TnI release following AAA repair, Le Manach et al. recently found two patterns of PMI.[57] In one pattern there was an early release of TnI consistent with MI within 37 hours postoperatively, and in the other there was a low level of troponin release in the early postoperative period, followed by the release of levels consistent with PMI at 74 hours postoperatively. While their time definitions were admittedly arbitrary, their work supports the notion of two general types of PMI. Acute plaque rupture is one mechanism, occurring randomly within

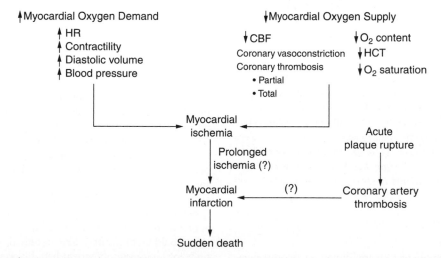

FIGURE 19-5 Pathophysiology of acute coronary syndromes during the perioperative period. In the setting of a coronary stenosis, the normal ability of vasculature to adjust flow and meet an increase in myocardial oxygen demand is limited. Even if demand is steady, acute decreases in oxygen supply can occur. Both conditions may lead to myocardial ischemia. Prolonged ischemia, in turn, may lead to infarction, although an alternative hypothesis implicates plaque rupture and thrombus formation at a noncritical stenosis. HR = heart rate; CBF = coronary blood flow; HCT = hematocrit.

the perioperative period and associated with surges in sympathetic activity. A second type of PMI is preceded by early and prolonged stress-induced ischemia, and is associated with tachycardia and early troponin release. The ischemia is felt to be related to supply-demand mismatch from postoperative tachycardia in patients with limited reserve due to fixed coronary stenosis. Patients who demonstrate a low level of troponin release with ischemia may actually benefit from aggressive control of heart rate with PBB, although this strategy has not been studied.

It is likely, however, that supply-demand mismatch is not the entire story regarding PMI. A more complex nature would explain why studies that have reduced intraoperative and postoperative ischemia with PBB have not been able to show a reduction in PMI or perioperative mortality.[23,29] Just like the dynamic angiographic nature of coronary thrombosis, noted above in nonsurgical NQMI, it is possible that PMI may be associated with a coronary thrombosis that is transient, both spontaneously dissolving and resolving. Thrombosis may be secondary to an inflammatory-related postoperative hypercoagulable state; it also may be promoted by plaque fissuring, without rupture, from sympathetic stress and inflammation. This process may be more likely in the setting of preexisting complicated plaque. In addition, there may be patient-specific factors that increase the risk of thrombosis. An elevated C-reactive protein or circulating interleukin 6 (IL-6) may be signs of increased plaque inflammation or vulnerability. Platelet polymorphisms with increased thrombogenicity may also increase the risk of coronary thrombosis.[58] The complexity of the problem helps explain why complete prevention of PMI with a single agent, such as beta-blockers, is unlikely to occur. While transient ST-segment depression ischemia may represent periods of supply-demand mismatch, it is not clear that periods of greater than 30 minutes of ischemia associated with PMI in previous studies represent the effects of prolonged supply-demand mismatch. These longer periods of ischemia could be the result of coronary thrombosis, not the cause of PMI. This would explain finding a reduction of heart rates at which ischemia occurred in patients on PBB without the prevention of ischemia. For example, in the analysis done by Wallace et al., ischemia occurred at a mean rate of 82 in the atenolol group versus 94 in the control. Prevention will require a multimodel approach, with several drugs acting on different pathways. Studies will need to evaluate the combined efficacy of drugs that act on platelets as well as plaque stabilization, such as the statin drugs, in addition to the control of sympathetic stimulation with beta-blockers. Furthermore, the lack of inclusion of either statins or antiplatelet drugs in subgroup analysis in most of the beta-blocker trials is a further limitation of these studies. This limitation is highlighted by the recent findings of improved perioperative cardiac outcomes with the use of statins. In a case-control study, Poldermans et al. found a relative risk reduction of fourfold (95% CI 0.10 to 0.47) for all-cause perioperative mortality in patients undergoing major vascular surgery who were on preoperative statins.[59] Durazzo et al. found a 68% reduction in adverse cardiovascular events during the 6-month postoperative period in vascular surgical patients randomized to atorvastatin versus placebo.[60]

CONCLUSIONS

Conclusions regarding the use of PBB are limited for reasons elucidated thoroughly throughout this chapter. The state of the literature on the subject is far from definitive, with a reliance on mostly small randomized trials with limited subgroup analysis. There does not

appear to be any significant benefit of one beta-blocker versus another, although beta-1-selective agents are preferred. Nonselective beta-blockers, such as propanolol, have been found to cause more bronchospasm than selective beta-1 agents.[61] There is also not enough information regarding dosing to make any firm recommendations. The DIPOM trial used relatively low doses, but was still able to keep an average heart rate of 75, which was on average 9 beats slower than the control group. The mean heart rate on postoperative day 1 in the DECREASE trial was 71 in the study group versus 82 in the control. It seems reasonable that the dosing should be titrated to effect based on heart rate. The ideal heart rate to titrate to is not known. In the DECREASE trial, a preoperative resting heart rate of 60 was sought and they achieved a mean preoperative heart rate of 66. Would the results of the DECREASE trial have been different if the postoperative dose of bisoprolol was titrated, and they were able to keep the postoperative heart rate closer to 60 rather than 70? This is unclear. Raby et al. titrated esmolol postoperatively to keep heart rates 20% below the ischemic threshold found on preoperative Holter monitoring in vascular surgical patients.[7] In 9 of 15 patients, they were able to keep the mean heart rate below threshold and none of those 9 developed postoperative ischemia. Ischemia occurred in 5 of the other 6 patients who had heart rates above their preoperative ischemic threshold rate. There are also questions regarding the bioavailability and efficacy of orally administered medications in the early postoperative period, but again there is not enough information to recommend the IV route for all patients over the oral route at this time.

The profound success of the DECREASE trial would suggest that administration of PBB earlier in the preoperative period is beneficial. This makes sense from a mechanistic standpoint, as a longer administration period would allow better titration with less under- and overdosing. However, this was the only study with such a long preoperative administration time frame, and there is not enough evidence to clearly conclude its superiority over immediate preoperative dosing, or even intraoperative or postoperative dosing. As far as when to discontinue PBB, most of the studies, including Mangano's atenolol study, stopped therapy after 7 days. In the DECREASE trial, PBB was continued for 30 days postoperatively. Poldermans' group later found a 20% reduction in cardiac mortality and MI in vascular surgical patients with the continuation of bisoprolol for up to 2 years postoperatively.[62] It should be noted that these patients had definite indications for ambulatory beta-blockers irrespective of their surgery, and it would be expected that they would have an improvement in long-term outcome with continuation of therapy.

▶ Recommendations

The most difficult question is that of in whom PBB should be used. Based on the current evidence, the indications are likely to be more exclusive than inclusive. PBB for patients with diabetes but without CAD has not been shown to be effective.[40] Patients undergoing minor procedures or those patients with few risk factors for CAD obtained limited benefit or potential harm from PBB. In a retrospective analysis done by Boersma et al. among patients with a negative DSE, only those who scored 3 or more on the Revised Cardiac Risk Index demonstrated benefit from PBB. The most exclusive approach, but given the current evidence, one that is not unreasonable, would be to institute PBB in only those patients with indications for long-term outpatient beta-blocker therapy, irrespective of their planned surgery. Thus, patients with known CAD who were not already on beta-blockers would be ideal candidates for PBB. Those with a revised cardiac risk index score of 3 or more could also be considered candidates. It is important to emphasize again that in those patients with 3 or more revised cardiac risk factors with positive ischemia on testing, or those patients with extensive areas of ischemia independent of risk score, were not protected by PBB alone. The ideal management strategy for these patients, especially given the results of the CARP trial, has yet to be elucidated. The underusage of outpatient beta-blocker use has been frequently reported,[63] and the perioperative period may represent an important time for the initiation of therapy. Once these patients are identified, it is not clear, as discussed above, how far in advance PBB should be started. In these patients with indications for long-term therapy, it would seem unreasonable to stop beta-blockers postoperatively. However, there are logistical issues that would likely develop regarding who would continue and who would monitor beta-blocker therapy after the postoperative period is over.

The final issue revolves around how to manage PBB in patients presenting already on beta-blockers. Giles et al. performed an analysis of the literature from 1989 to 2004 regarding the effect of chronic beta-blocker therapy on perioperative outcome for noncardiac surgery, as well as the incidence of silent ischemia.[38] A total of 18 studies were reviewed and when the results were grouped, a cardioprotective effect was not found. In fact, those on chronic beta-blockers had an increased risk of PMI. Of note, 13 of the 18 were observational studies and the rest were case-control studies, with only 2 specifically designed to evaluate the effect of chronic beta-blockers. In addition, for many of the patients, the indication for chronic beta-blocker use was hypertension, not CAD. Information on when in the postoperative period beta blockers were restarted was lacking in several of these studies as well. However, as Giles et al. point out, there is evidence from the cardiology literature in nonsurgical patients to question the cardioprotective effect of chronic beta-blockers. In a study of 3504 patients presenting with acute MI, mortality at 1 month was similar for those on chronic beta-blockers for those who were not.[64] An obvious explanation for these findings would be the upregulation of beta receptors due to chronic therapy. From previous discussion in this chapter, it is clear that chronic beta-blocker therapy should not be discontinued perioperatively. The question is should those on chronic therapy receive additional supplementation with possible titration to heart rate? There is not enough information at this time to answer this question clearly, but for those with known CAD, this approach seems appropriate. As far as patients receiving beta-blockers solely for hypertension, aggressive prophylactic supplementation and titration is likely not warranted. Finally, for patients presenting to surgery on chronic beta-blockers for the treatment of chronic heart failure, there is no information regarding a protective effect of PBB in CHF. Again, acute withdrawal is likely dangerous, but aggressive supplementation is unlikely to beneficial, as the doses typically used are lower than those for CAD and not titrated to heart rate.

In summary, PBB is beneficial in patients with known CAD undergoing major vascular surgery and other high-risk surgeries, as long as significant areas of ischemia are not found on stress testing. PBB may not be beneficial in lower-risk patients. One could argue that given the ease of administration and cost-effectiveness of PBB,[3] in the setting of a relatively good safety profile, PBB should be used broadly, even if some patients may not benefit. The findings by Lindenauer et al. of an increased in-hospital mortality with PBB for low-risk patients are an argument against more widespread use. The precise protocol and other therapeutic modalities will require further research (Fig. 19-6).

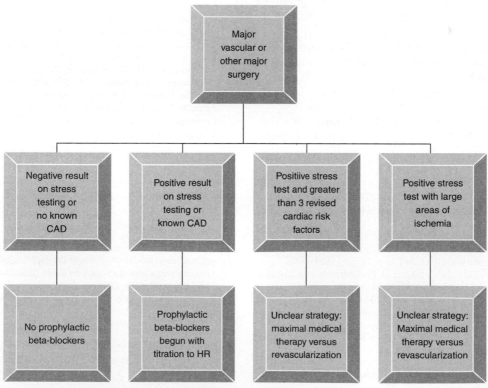

FIGURE 19-6 Algorithm.

KEY POINTS

▶ The current evidence supports the beneficial effects of perioperative beta-blockers in those patients with known CAD.

▶ There is no clear evidence to support the use of prophylactic perioperative beta-blockers in those patients with only risk factors for CAD.

▶ For those patients in whom perioperative beta-blockers are initiated, therapy should be started at least several days prior to surgery and the dose should be titrated to heart rate.

▶ Because the exact mechanism of perioperative myocardial infarction is not clearly defined and is most likely multifactorial, optimal medical management of patients at high risk should be multimodal, utilizing medications such as beta-blockers, antiplatelet drugs, alpha-2-agonists, or statins.

▶ For those patients with extensive CAD and large areas of myocardium at risk, the ideal management strategy has yet to be determined.

▶ In patients on chronic beta-blocker therapy, general consensus is that beta-blocker therapy should be continued to avoid rebound tachycardia. The benefit of further perioperative beta-blocker supplementation in patients already on chronic beta-blocker therapy is an area that requires further study.

KEY REFERENCES

▶ Mangano DT, Browner WS, Hollenberg M, et al. Effect of atenolol on mortality and cardiovascular morbidity after noncardiac surgery. *N Engl J Med.* 1996;335(23):1713–1720.

▶ Poldermans D, Boersma E, Bax JJ, et al. The effect of bisoprolol on perioperative mortality and myocardial infarction in high-risk patients undergoing vascular surgery. *N Engl J Med.* 1999; 341(24):1789–1794.

▶ Landesberg G. The pathophysiology of perioperative myocardial infarction: facts and perspectives. *J Cardiothorac Vasc Anesth.* 2003;17(1):90–100.

▶ Lindenauer PK, Pekow P, Wang K, et al. Perioperative beta-blockade therapy and mortality after major noncardiac surgery. *N Engl J Med.* 2005;353(4):349–361.

REFERENCES

1. Mangano DT, Browner WS, Hollenberg M, et al. Association of perioperative myocardial ischemia with cardiac morbidity and mortality in men undergoing noncardiac surgery. *N Engl J Med.* 1990;323:1781–1788.
2. Fleischmann KE, Goldman L, Young B, Lee TH. Association between cardiac and noncardiac complications in patients undergoing noncardiac surgery: outcomes and effects on length of stay. *Am J Med.* 2003;115:515–520.
3. Fleisher LA, Corbett W, Berry C, Poldermans D. Cost-effectiveness of differing perioperative beta-blockade strategies in vascular surgery patients. *J Cardiothorac Vasc Anesth.* 2004;18:7–13.
4. Blankensteijn JD, Lindenburg FP, Van der Graaf Y, Eikelboom BC. Influence of study design on reported mortality and morbidity rates after abdominal aortic aneurysm repair. *Br J Surg.* 1998;85:1624–1630.
5. Brady AR, Gibbs JS, Greenhalgh RM, et al. Perioperative beta-blockade (POBBLE) for patients undergoing infrarenal vascular surgery: results of a randomized double-blind controlled trial. *J Vasc Surg.* 2005;41:602–609.
6. Feinglass J, Pearce WH, Martin GJ, et al. Postoperative and amputation-free survival outcomes after femorodistal bypass grafting surgery: findings from the Department of Veterans Affairs National Surgical Quality Improvement Program. *J Vasc Surg.* 2001;34:283–290.
7. Raby KE, Brull SJ, Timimi F, et al. The effect of heart rate control on myocardial ischemia among high-risk patients after vascular surgery (see comments). *Anesth Analg.* 1999;88:477–482.
8. Eagle K, Brundage B, Chaitman B, et al. Guidelines for perioperative cardiovascular evaluation of the noncardiac surgery. A report of the American Heart Association/American College of Cardiology Task Force on Assessment of Diagnostic and Therapeutic Cardiovascular Procedures. *Circulation.* 1996;93:1278–1317.
9. American Heart Association. *Heart Disease and Stroke Statistics: 2003 Update.* Dallas, TX: American Heart Association; 2003.
10. Fleisher LA, Eagle KA. Clinical practice. Lowering cardiac risk in noncardiac surgery. *N Engl J Med.* 2001;345:1677–1682.
11. McFalls EO, Ward HB, Moritz TE, et al. Coronary-artery revascularization before elective major vascular surgery. *N Engl J Med.* 2004;351:2795–2804.
12. Palda VA, Detsky AS. Perioperative assessment and management of risk from coronary artery disease. *Ann Intern Med.* 1997;127:313–328.
13. Eagle KA, Berger PB, Calkins H, et al. ACC/AHA guideline update for perioperative cardiovascular evaluation for noncardiac surgery—executive summary: a report of the American College of Cardiology/American Heart Association Task Force on Practice Guidelines (committee to update the 1996 guidelines on Perioperative Cardiovascular Evaluation for Noncardiac Surgery). *J Am Coll Cardiol.* 2002;39: 542–553.
14. Landesberg G, Mosseri M, Fleisher LA. Coronary revascularization before vascular surgery. *N Engl J Med.* 2005;352:1492–1495; author reply 5.
15. Stevens RD, Burri H, Tramer MR. Pharmacologic myocardial protection in patients undergoing noncardiac surgery: a quantitative systematic review. *Anesth Analg.* 2003;97:623–633.
16. Pasternack PF, Grossi EA, Baumann FG, et al. Beta blockade to decrease silent myocardial ischemia during peripheral vascular surgery. *Am J Surg.* 1989;158:113–116.
17. Smulyan H, Weinberg SE, Howanitz PJ. Continuous propranolol infusion following abdominal surgery. *JAMA.* 1982;247:2539–2542.
18. London MJ, Zaugg M, Schaub MC, Spahn DR. Perioperative beta-adrenergic receptor blockade: physiologic foundations and clinical controversies. *Anesthesiology.* 2004;100:170–175.
19. Gibbons RJ, Abrams J, Chatterjee K, et al. ACC/AHA 2002 guideline update for the management of patients with chronic stable angina—summary article: a report of the American College of Cardiology/American Heart Association Task Force on practice guidelines (Committee on the Management of Patients With Chronic Stable Angina). *J Am Coll Cardiol.* 2003;41:159–168.
20. Braunwald E, Antman EM, Beasley JW, et al. ACC/AHA guideline update for the management of patients with unstable angina and non-ST-segment elevation myocardial infarction—2002: summary article: a report of the American College of Cardiology/American Heart Association Task Force on Practice Guidelines (Committee on the Management of Patients With Unstable Angina). *Circulation.* 2002;106:1893–1900.
21. Antman EM, Anbe DT, Armstrong PW, et al. ACC/AHA guidelines for the management of patients with ST-elevation myocardial infarction—executive summary: a report of the American College of Cardiology/American Heart Association Task Force on Practice Guidelines (Writing Committee to revise the 1999 guidelines for the Management of Patients With Acute Myocardial Infarction). *Circulation.* 2004;110:588–636.
22. Landesberg G. The pathophysiology of perioperative myocardial infarction: facts and perspectives. *J Cardiothorac Vasc Anesth.* 2003; 17:90–100.
23. Mangano DT, Layug EL, Wallace A, Tateo I. Effect of atenolol on mortality and cardiovascular morbidity after noncardiac surgery. Multicenter Study of Perioperative Ischemia Research Group. *N Engl J Med.* 1996; 335:1713–1720.
24. Poldermans D, Boersma E, Bax JJ, et al. The effect of bisoprolol on perioperative mortality and myocardial infarction in high-risk patients undergoing vascular surgery. Dutch Echocardiographic Cardiac Risk Evaluation Applying Stress Echocardiography Study Group (see comments). *N Engl J Med.* 1999;341:1789–1794.
25. Devereaux PJ, Beattie WS, Choi PT, et al. How strong is the evidence for the use of perioperative beta blockers in non-cardiac surgery? Systematic review and meta-analysis of randomized controlled trials. *Br Med J.* 2005;331:313–321.
26. VanDenKerkhof EG, Milne B, Parlow JL. Knowledge and practice regarding prophylactic perioperative beta blockade in patients undergoing noncardiac surgery: a survey of Canadian anesthesiologists. *Anesth Analg.* 2003;96:1558–1565; table of contents.

27. London MJ, Itani KM, Perrino AC, Jr, et al. Perioperative beta-blockade: a survey of physician attitudes in the department of Veterans Affairs. *J Cardiothorac Vasc Anesth.* 2004;18:14–24.

28. Devereaux PJ, Yusuf S, Yang H, et al. Are the recommendations to use perioperative beta-blocker therapy in patients undergoing noncardiac surgery based on reliable evidence? *CMAJ.* 2004;171:245–247.

29. Wallace A, Layug B, Tateo I, et al. Prophylactic atenolol reduces postoperative myocardial ischemia. McSPI Research Group (see comments). *Anesthesiology.* 1998;88:7–17.

30. Fleisher LA, Nelson AH, Rosenbaum SH. Postoperative myocardial ischemia: etiology of cardiac morbidity or manifestation of underlying disease. *J Clin Anesth.* 1995;7:97–102.

31. Landesberg G, Luria MH, Cotev S, et al. Importance of long-duration postoperative ST-segment depression in cardiac morbidity after vascular surgery. *Lancet.* 1993;341:715–719.

32. Landesberg G, Shatz V, Akopnik I, et al. Association of cardiac troponin, CK-MB, and postoperative myocardial ischemia with long-term survival after major vascular surgery. *J Am Coll Cardiol.* 2003;42:1547–1554.

33. Fleisher LA, Zielski MM, Schulman SP. Perioperative ST-segment depression is rare and may not indicate myocardial ischemia in moderate-risk patients undergoing noncardiac surgery. *J Cardiothorac Vasc Anesth.* 1997;11:155–159.

34. Kim LJ, Martinez EA, Faraday N, et al. Cardiac troponin I predicts short-term mortality in vascular surgery patients. *Circulation.* 2002;106:2366–2371.

35. Adams JE III, Sicard GA, Allen BT, et al. Diagnosis of perioperative myocardial infarction with measurement of cardiac troponin I. *N Engl J Med.* 1994;330:670–674.

36. Kertai MD, Boersma E, Klein J, et al. Long-term prognostic value of asymptomatic cardiac troponin T elevations in patients after major vascular surgery. *Eur J Vasc Endovasc Surg.* 2004;28:59–66.

37. Psaty BM, Koepsell TD, Wagner EH, et al. The relative risk of incident coronary heart disease associated with recently stopping the use of beta-blockers. *JAMA.* 1990;263:1653–1657.

38. Giles JW, Sear JW, Foex P. Effect of chronic beta-blockade on perioperative outcome in patients undergoing non-cardiac surgery: an analysis of observational and case control studies. *Anaesthesia.* 2004;59:574–583.

39. Shammash JB, Trost JC, Gold JM, et al. Perioperative beta-blocker withdrawal and mortality in vascular surgical patients. *Am Heart J.* 2001;141:148–153.

40. Juul AB. DIPOM American Heart Association Scientific Sessions. New Orleans, LA, 2004.

41. Juul AB, Wetterslev J, Kofoed-Enevoldsen A, et al. The Diabetic Postoperative Mortality and Morbidity (DIPOM) trial: rationale and design of a multicenter, randomized, placebo-controlled, clinical trial of metoprolol for patients with diabetes mellitus who are undergoing major noncardiac surgery. *Am Heart J.* 2004;147:677–683.

42. Boersma E, Poldermans D, Bax JJ, et al. Predictors of cardiac events after major vascular surgery: role of clinical characteristics, dobutamine echocardiography, and beta-blocker therapy. *JAMA.* 2001;285:1865–1873.

43. Lee TH, Marcantonio ER, Mangione CM, et al. Derivation and prospective validation of a simple index for prediction of cardiac risk of major noncardiac surgery. *Circulation.* 1999;100:1043–1049.

44. Kertai MD, Boersma E, Bax JJ, et al. Optimizing long-term cardiac management after major vascular surgery: role of beta-blocker therapy, clinical characteristics, and dobutamine stress echocardiography to optimize long-term cardiac management after major vascular surgery. *Arch Intern Med.* 2003;163:2230–2235.

45. Poldermans D, Arnese M, Fioretti PM, et al. Improved cardiac risk stratification in major vascular surgery with dobutamine-atropine stress echocardiography. *J Am Coll Cardiol.* 1995;26:648–653.

46. ISIS-1 (First International Study of Infarct Survival) Collaborative Group. Randomized trial of intravenous atenolol among 16,027 cases of suspected acute myocardial infarction. *Lancet.* 1986;2:57–66.

47. Leslie K, Devereaux PJ. A large trial is vital to prove perioperative beta-blockade effectiveness and safety before widespread use. *Anesthesiology.* 2004;101:803; author reply 4–6.

48. Yang H, Raymer K, Butler R, et al. Metoprolol after vascular surgery (MaVS). *Can J Anesth.* 2004;51:A7.

49. Lindenauer PK, Pekow P, Wang K, et al. Perioperative beta-blocker therapy and mortality after major noncardiac surgery. *N Engl J Med.* 2005;353:349–361.

50. Zaugg M, Tagliente T, Lucchinetti E, et al. Beneficial effects from beta-adrenergic blockade in elderly patients undergoing noncardiac surgery. *Anesthesiology.* 1999;91:1674–686.

51. Fleisher LA, Beckman JA, Brown KA, et al. ACC/AHA 2006 guideline update on perioperative cardiovascular evaluation for noncardiac surgery: focused update on perioperative beta-blocker therapy: a report of the American College of Cardiology/American Heart Association Task Force on Practice Guidelines (Writing Committee to update the 2002 guidelines on Perioperative Cardiovascular Evaluation for Noncardiac Surgery): developed in collaboration with the American Society of Echocardiography, American Society of Nuclear Cardiology, Heart Rhythm Society, Society of Cardiovascular Anesthesiologists, Society for Cardiovascular Angiography and Interventions, and Society for Vascular Medicine and Biology. *Circulation.* 2006;113: 2662–2674.

52. Naghavi M, Libby P, Falk E, et al. From vulnerable plaque to vulnerable patient: a call for new definitions and risk assessment strategies: Part I. *Circulation.* 2003;108:1664–1672.

53. Keen WD, Savage MP, Fischman DL, et al. Comparison of coronary angiographic findings during the first six hours of non-Q-wave and Q-wave myocardial infarction. *Am J Cardiol.* 1994;74:324–328.

54. Ambrose JA, Tannenbaum MA, Alexopoulos D, et al. Angiographic progression of coronary artery disease and the development of myocardial infarction. *J Am Coll Cardiol.* 1988;12:56–62.

55. DeWood MA, Spores J, Hensley GR, et al. Coronary arteriographic findings in acute transmural myocardial infarction. *Circulation.* 1983;68: I39–I49.

56. Dawood MM, Gutpa DK, Southern J, et al. Pathology of fatal perioperative myocardial infarction: implications regarding pathophysiology and prevention. *Int J Cardiol.* 1996;57:37–44.

57. Le Manach Y, Perel A, Coriat P, et al. Early and delayed myocardial infarction after abdominal aortic surgery. *Anesthesiology.* 2005;102:885–891.

58. Naghavi M, Libby P, Falk E, et al. From vulnerable plaque to vulnerable patient: a call for new definitions and risk assessment strategies: Part II. *Circulation.* 2003;108:1772–1778.

59. Poldermans D, Bax JJ, Kertai MD, et al. Statins are associated with a reduced incidence of perioperative mortality in patients undergoing major noncardiac vascular surgery. *Circulation.* 2003;107: 1848–1851.

60. Durazzo AE, Machado FS, Ikeoka DT, et al. Reduction in cardiovascular events after vascular surgery with atorvastatin: a randomized trial. *J Vasc Surg.* 2004;39:967–975.

61. Bayliff CD, Massel DR, Inculet RI, et al. Propranolol for the prevention of postoperative arrhythmias in general thoracic surgery. *Ann Thorac Surg.* 1999;67:182–186.

62. Poldermans D, Boersma E, Bax JJ, et al. Bisoprolol reduces cardiac death and myocardial infarction in high-risk patients as long as 2 years after successful major vascular surgery. *Eur Heart J.* 2001;22: 1353–1358.

63. Soumerai SB, McLaughlin TJ, Spiegelman D, et al. Adverse outcomes of underuse of beta-blockers in elderly survivors of acute myocardial infarction (see comments). *JAMA.* 1997;277:115–121.

64. Herlitz J, Karlson BW, Hjalmarson A. Prognosis in patients with acute chest pain in relation to chronic beta-blocker treatment prior to admission to hospital. *Cardiology.* 1995;86:56–59.

Consciousness Monitoring in the Elderly

CHAPTER 20

Roy G. Soto
Peter S.A. Glass

INTRODUCTION TO ELECTROENCEPHALOGRAPHY

For over 150 years, physicians have used surrogate measures of consciousness (such as respiratory pattern, pulse, blood pressure, and exhaled anesthetic concentration) to determine and adjust anesthetic depth. Certain patient populations pose a challenge to anesthetic titration including the young, old, and critically ill, and assessing level of consciousness and achieving smooth and timely emergence can be difficult.

The brain is the target organ for the hypnotic effects of anesthesia, and modern processed electroencephalography (EEG) technology allows more direct assessment of the brain's response to these medications and presumably a more accurate estimate of the level of sedation and loss of consciousness. This chapter focuses on the technologies available for consciousness monitoring, and the potential advantages and limitations of these monitors in the elderly population.

A brief history of intraoperative EEG monitoring

In 1875, Richard Caton, an English physician, was the first to discover that electric signals could be detected from the surface of the exposed brain of animals. Furthermore, he discovered that signals changed in the contralateral side if he exposed one eye or the other to light. Hans Berger, an Austrian psychiatrist, was the first to publish human data, and in 1929 he coined the phrase *electroencephalogram*, describing alpha and beta waves in detail, noting later that alpha waves changed during sleep and general anesthesia. Delta and theta waves were described by the neurophysiologist W. Grey Walter in the 1930s–1950s, with further detail made possible by improved amplification and mapping. Unfortunately, although EEG was well described by the 1950s and the effects of anesthesia on EEG were well known, its use in the operating room was impractical and difficult. Modern computing technology changed that, allowing for processing and statistical analysis of complex wave signals, and by the 1980s, processing of the EEG signal in the operating room became a reality.

The advent of processed EEG

Many attempts have been made to identify a single ideal value for interpretation of the EEG for perioperative use. Ninety-five percent spectral edge and median frequency were among the first derivatives used in clinical practice with varying degrees of success. Evoked potentials were also investigated and a commercial product utilizing audio-evoked potentials was briefly available. Following a series of experiments that confirmed the utility of a proprietary algorithm

for EEG processing in the early 1980s, Aspect Medical Systems was formed in 1987. The first literature detailing the Bispectral Index (BIS) was published in the early 1990s, with over 1 million patients monitored by 1999.[1] Physiometrix and Datex/GE followed suit, and there are currently three primary monitoring choices available.

The BIS reports a number between 100 (fully-awake) and zero (isoelectric EEG) to predict level of hypnosis, with values under 60 generally correlating with anesthetic level indicating loss of consciousness and lack of recall. Similarly, the PSA-4000 monitor manufactured by Physiometrix reports a number (known as Patient State Index, or PSI) between 100 and zero, with 50 generally representing appropriate surgical anesthetic depth.[7] The Entropy monitor (General Electric) translates the disorder in both EEG and electromyogram (EMG) into two separate measures of consciousness: state entropy (SE), which reflects cortical activity of the brain, and response entropy (RE), which reflects both cortical activity and frontalis EMG activity.[3] Technologies utilizing audio-evoked potentials have also been introduced, but are no longer available for sale in the United States.

Although frequently referred to as "depth of anesthesia" monitors, it is important to point out that of the components of anesthesia, these monitors only monitor consciousness (or hypnosis, or wakefulness, all of which are synonymous). Minimal alveolar concentration (MAC) does not equal consciousness, and indeed animals that have had their forebrains removed do not show an alteration of MAC.[4]

THE BRAIN AND ADVANCED AGE

Mental function deteriorates with age, including the abilities to concentrate and remember. Physical and chemical changes take place in the nervous system as we age, including cell death and reduction in neurotransmitter function, overall brain atrophy, and ventricular enlargement.[5,6] Many of these changes can affect the ability to effectively titrate an anesthetic in a geriatric patient.

EEG and advanced age

Although some studies have suggested a lower mean power in EEG signal in the elderly, overall EEG remains relatively normal with advanced age assuming a lack of underlying disease.[7–9] Thus, processed measures of EEG should be valid for all age populations, and indeed these devices seem to correlate appropriately with clinical signs of consciousness in the geriatric patient.

Patients with underlying neuropsychiatric disease, however, may display a significant change in EEG. Renna and others have found that the baseline awake BIS in patients with Alzheimer dementia is lower than that of normal controls. Specifically, the resting BIS in the Alzheimer group was on average five points lower,[10] while others have suggested that BIS may decrease as severity of dementia increases.[11,12] This is probably accounted for by the increase in slow-wave and decrease in fast-wave activity of the electroencephalogram in this population. The significance for patients with dementia during general anesthesia or sedation is unclear, and consciousness monitors should be used and interpreted with caution in this group.

▶ Arousal and advanced age

Sleep/wake cycles are altered in the elderly,[13] and many of the traits seen among the elderly in the recovery room such as somnolence, confusion, and delirium may be related. Stressors on the elderly patient undergoing a major operative procedure can include hypothermia, dehydration, hypo- or hyperglycemia, and anemia to name a few. Furthermore, patients receive a dizzying array of medications that can have potential postoperative effects on mental function, including premedicants, antiemetics, opiates, anticholinergics, and of course, volatile and IV anesthetics. Postoperative cognitive dysfunction and decline may or may not be related to these factors, and the topic is covered in depth elsewhere in this text. Titrating anesthetic to depth of consciousness may allow for a reduced exposure to drug, allowing for more rapid and more lucid emergence (qv).

CHALLENGES IN ESTIMATING ANESTHETIC DEPTH IN THE ELDERLY

Anesthesia providers learn to gauge anesthetic depth using end-tidal anesthetic concentrations, physical signs, and pharmacodynamic/kinetic principles derived from healthy young adults. Unfortunately, many of these assumptions are not valid, or are at least less reliable, in the elderly than in the young population.

▶ MAC requirements

MAC of volatile anesthetic represents that concentration at which 50% of patients do not move with surgical incision. The commonly published values (e.g., 2% for sevoflurane) are certainly valid for young adults, but they drop predictably in the elderly, making end-tidal gas monitoring less useful for movement prediction in this age group. If MAC is used as the primary end point for anesthetic titration, in the elderly it must be done with caution, especially when considering the significant hemodynamic effects of all potent inhaled agents.

▶ Pharmacokinetic and pharmacodynamic changes

As covered elsewhere in this text, there are significant pharmacokinetic and pharmacodynamic implications to advanced age. Alterations in drug disposition and end-organ sensitivity result in altered drug onset and duration. Volume of distribution and drug clearance are altered as are hepatic and renal function. Sensitivity to drugs that affect psychomotor function is increased, and concurrent medication use is high. As a result, "classic" measures of anesthetic depth become less reliable.

Kazama and colleagues examined the effect-site concentration of propofol in elderly and young patients while monitoring with BIS.[14] They found that BIS between groups was similar for a given propofol concentration, but that blood pressure at equivalent concentrations was lower in the elderly. The important clinical implication is that titrating anesthetic to hemodynamic effect in the elderly may result in an artificially light level of consciousness. Similarly, Katoh and colleagues examined BIS and loss of consciousness during sevoflurane inhalation in elderly and young subjects.[15] The older subjects had a reduced sevoflurane requirement for loss of response to verbal command, but BIS at that end point was similar to that in the younger population. Again, the implication is that titrating anesthetic to a presumed anesthetic level may result in an inappropriate level of consciousness. Finally, an increased brain sensitivity to opiates (as determined by EEG changes) has also been reported in the geriatric population.[16,17]

Consciousness monitoring provides a tool to aid in safe anesthetic titration in this vulnerable population. In effect, the EEG becomes a surrogate for drug effect in a population with significant physiologic variability.

▶ Beta blockade

Heart rate and blood pressure analyses have been a mainstay of anesthetic titration, with tachycardia and hypertension associated with "light" anesthesia, and the inverse true of anesthetic "overdose." With the widespread adoption of perioperative beta blockade recommendations (covered by Dr. Fleischer in this text), the utility of hemodynamic alteration interpretation in the elderly is less and less useful. A dehydrated geriatric patient that is adequately beta-blocked can represent a significant anesthetic challenge, especially when paralyzed. Is an 89-year-old-beta-blocked patient adequately anesthetized at 0.4 MAC when paralyzed and hemodynamically stable?

CONSCIOUSNESS MONITORING AND OUTCOME MEASURES

So the question becomes, can consciousness monitors improve or enhance intraoperative estimation of anesthetic adequacy? With the knowledge that drugs will potentially be more potent in the elderly, and that our geriatric patients will frequently lack a hyperdynamic response to "light" anesthetic state if beta-blocked, do these monitors tell us something that routine practice does not? A plethora of studies have explored the ability of consciousness monitors to reduce drug use, speed recovery time, aid in anesthetic titration, and potentially reduce morbidity and mortality. In effect, an attempt has been made to show that these monitors might allow for delivery of an anesthetic that is cheaper, faster, and better.

▶ Drug use

A number of well-designed studies have shown that patients receiving anesthetic titrated with consciousness monitoring received less drug, be that IV[18,19] or inhaled[20,21] without untoward consequences. It seems clear that anesthetic titrated via classical means results in a state that is "deeper" than required. Reduction of volatile and intravenous agent use potentially results in cost savings, although the cost of the monitoring equipment itself must be factored into any economic analysis.

Heck and colleagues examined the utility of BIS monitoring in patients undergoing elective coronary artery bypass grafting. Following a midazolam/sufentanil/pancuronium induction, BIS was titrated with the opiate to either 60, 50, or 40 immediately prior to intubation. In the 60 group there was an increased incidence of coughing and tearing with intubation, whereas in the 40 group there was an increased incidence of hypotension.[22] The authors suggest that to avoid intubation during "light" anesthesia and to avoid postintubation hypotension, a target BIS of 50 should be used in this elderly population. Although no systematic, large, population-based analysis of consciousness monitoring and its effect on the use of anesthetic agents in the elderly has been performed, it would seem that "less is more." That is, reduction of anesthetic delivery may result in less vasodilation, myocardial depression, respiratory depression, nausea, and all of the other commonly experienced side effects of the drugs in our armamentarium. Furthermore, an enhanced ability to titrate drug potentially will allow for better titration of drugs that have an altered pharmacodynamic profile in the geriatric population.

Recovery

Many studies have examined the effect of consciousness monitors in the younger patient population on time to awakening, orientation upon arrival in the postanesthesia care unit (PACU), length of PACU stay, and time to PACU discharge with both positive and negative results. Wong and colleagues found that isoflurane titrated to BIS in the elderly resulted in a nearly 4-minute faster time to orientation in the PACU (Fig. 20-1) as well as a more rapid time to achieve an Aldrete score >9, suggesting the potential for earlier discharge.[23] Despite a 30% reduction of isoflurane delivery in the BIS-titrated group, there were no differences in postoperative cognitive dysfunction between groups. Fredman found that when geriatric patients were monitored with BIS during short urologic procedures, there was no difference in fast-track ability (ability to facilitate PACU bypass) compared to young patients.[24] Furthermore, a European study performed using a consciousness monitor not currently available in the United States found that elderly patients could be extubated after stopping propofol infusion as quickly as younger patients.[25] It is important to remember that our geriatric patients are the highest risk of experiencing drug-induced postoperative complications due to the effects of residual anesthetics on postoperative mental and psychomotor recovery.[26,27]

Outliers

An interesting concept that is difficult to define is that of patients that are "outliers." That is, patients that do not wake up from anesthesia

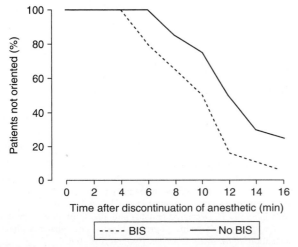

FIGURE 20-1 Time from discontinuation of general anesthetic to patient orientation. Dashed line: BIS-titrated group. Solid line: standard practice group. *(Adapted with permission from Ref. 23.)*

when they are expected to, in effect suggesting that they are more sensitive to the agents used. Gan and colleagues found that in subjects undergoing a propofol-alfentanil-nitrous oxide anesthetic, the frequency of failure to emerge within 15 minutes from anesthetic discontinuation was reduced by more than two-thirds (from 18% to 5%) if BIS was used.[18] More rapid emergence was also found, as was a reduction in propofol use, all of which may be of importance in the geriatric population.

Mortality

A retrospective chart review by Monk and colleagues examined the incidence of mortality at 1 year following major noncardiac surgery under general anesthesia.[28] The mortality rate of the 1064 patients reviewed was approximately 5% at 1 year, and slightly higher in the elderly subset. Independent predictors of increased mortality were coexisting disease, intraoperative hypotension (<80 BPs), and cumulative time of BIS <45. It was found that every hour a patient was kept below this level resulted in a 24% increased chance of mortality at 1 year. This has been repeated and presented by a separate group in abstract format,[29] but the reasons for the association remain unclear. It has long been known that mediators of inflammation increase in the perioperative period, and it has been suggested that depth of anesthetic state may alter the inflammatory cascade, affecting survival. The low BIS values may also simply be a marker of underlying disease. Multicenter randomized prospective trials are needed to determine the impact of anesthetic depth on long-term outcomes, and no conclusions can be made at this time regarding the phenomenology described.

Recall

Recent research has brought to light the incidence of intraoperative recall and the potential ability of consciousness monitors to reduce this incidence. Although no studies have yet specifically focused on the geriatric population, it has been shown by Sebel and colleagues that the incidence is high in both cardiac and ophthalmologic procedures, which specifically are performed more frequently in the elderly.[30] Nevertheless, the Sebel study found no association between age and recall during anesthesia. Similarly, there was no increased risk in the younger population, although younger age has been suggested as a risk factor for intraoperative recall on the basis of analysis of closed malpractice claims.[31]

Incidence

A number of studies have sought to determine the incidence of explicit recall following general anesthesia in the general population. Using well-constructed questionnaires and statistical methodology, it seems that the incidence is somewhere between 1 in 500 and 1 in 1000 cases.[30,32] Although most subjects recalled only auditory stimuli (rather than pain), a significant subset of patients were found to have evidence of posttraumatic stress disorder 2 years after the event.[33] As a result of this disturbing data, attempts were made to determine whether consciousness monitors could potentially reduce or eliminate this risk.

Do consciousness monitors reduce recall?

Ekman and colleagues examined the incidence of recall in a large medical center before and after introduction of BIS technology.[34] Although their incidence of recall was 0.18%, similar to what was previously published, they found a 77% reduction in this incidence when BIS technology was applied during general anesthesia. Myles and colleagues randomized nearly 2500 patients at high risk for recall to receive anesthesia titrated with either BIS or with standard practice monitoring (heart rate, end-tidal gas concentration, and so forth).[35] Similar to Ekman's findings, patients monitored with BIS had an 82% reduction in recall from the 0.9% incidence in the standard practice group.

It seems clear that the incidence of recall is higher than previously thought, that a subset of patients develop significant psychiatric sequelae from this recall, and that consciousness monitoring reduces the incidence. Studies specific to the geriatric population have not yet been performed, but the evidence in the general populace is compelling.

In part due to the findings of these studies, the BIS monitor was given an indication by the U.S. Food and Drug Administration (FDA) for recall prevention, and the Joint Commission on Accreditation of Healthcare Organizations issued a sentinel alert warning of the risk and required accredited organizations to develop a recall awareness policy at all locations performing general anesthesia. The ASA formed a task force to examine the issue, and its findings were presented at the 2005 annual meeting.

SUMMARY

Although there is a paucity of data specifically pertaining to consciousness monitoring in the elderly, it is evident that these monitors can aid in anesthetic titration, especially in geriatric patients in whom classic signs of anesthetic depth are frequently obscured. Monitors of consciousness give a glimpse into the effects of anesthetic on the brain, which is, after all, the end organ of consciousness, and as such provides insight beyond that given by hemodynamics alone.

Monitoring consciousness in the geriatric population may result in earlier recovery, reduced PACU stay, and a reduction in the incidence of intraoperative recall. Incorporating consciousness monitoring into standard practice for all patients may not be warranted, but for select patients, it may aid in providing a safer and more efficient anesthetic, allowing for adjustment of dosing of hypnotics to individual patient needs.

KEY POINTS

▶ Processed EEG monitors specifically reflect consciousness, which correlates only loosely with MAC and clinical signs of anesthetic depth.

▶ Overall EEG remains normal in the elderly, assuming a lack of underlying disease.

▶ Arousal levels, particularly in the postoperative period, may be depressed in the elderly.

▶ Classic signs of anesthetic depth can be suppressed in the elderly by beta blockade.

▶ Estimates of anesthetic onset and duration may be difficult in the elderly due to altered pharmacodynamic and pharmacokinetic characteristics.

▶ Titrating anesthetic to processed EEG results in reduced drug utilization, quicker emergence, and shorter recovery in the elderly.

▶ The incidence of intraoperative recall is approximately 0.1%, and is particularly high in patients undergoing cardiac procedures.

▶ The use of processed EEG devices reduces the risk of intraoperative recall.

KEY ARTICLES

▶ Rampil IJ, Mason P, Singh H. Anesthetic potency (MAC) is independent of forebrain structures in the rat. *Anesthesiology.* 1993;78:707–712.

▶ Duffy F, Albert M, McAnulty G, et al. Age-related differences in brain electrical activity of healthy subjects. *Ann Neurol.* 1984;16:430–438.

▶ Kazama T, Ikeda K, Morita K, et al. Comparison of the effect-site k_{eo}s of propofol for blood pressure and EEG Bispectral Index in elderly and younger patients. *Anesthesiology.* 1999;90:1517–1527.

▶ Katoh T, Bito H, Sato S. Influence of age on hypnotic requirement, Bispectral Index, and 95% spectral edge frequency associated with sedation induced with sevoflurane. *Anesthesiology.* 2000;92:55–61.

▶ Wong J, Song D, Blanshard H, et al. Titration of isoflurane using BIS index improves early recovery of elderly patients undergoing orthopedic surgeries. *Can J Anesth.* 2002;49:13–18.

▶ Fredman B, Sheffer O, Zohar E, et al. Fast-track eligibility of geriatric patients undergoing short urologic surgery procedures. *Anesth Analg.* 2002;94:560–564.

▶ Myles PS, Leslie K, McNeil J, et al. Bispectral index monitoring to prevent awareness during anaesthesia: the B-Aware randomised controlled trial. *Lancet.* 2004;363:1757–1763.

REFERENCES

1. Aspect Medical Systems, http://www.aspectms.com.
2. Prichep L, Gugino L, John E, et al. The Patient State Index as an indicator of the level of hypnosis under general anaesthesia. *Br J Anaesth.* 2004;92:393–399.
3. Ellerkmann R, Liermann V, Alves T, et al. Spectral entropy and bispectral index as measures of the electroencephalographic effects of sevoflurane. *Anesthesiology.* 2004;101:1275–1282.
4. Rampil IJ, Mason P, Singh H. Anesthetic potency (MAC) is independent of forebrain structures in the rat. *Anesthesiology.* 1993;78:707–712.
5. Akiyama H, Meyer J, Mortel K, et al. Normal human aging: factors contributing to cerebral atrophy. *J Neurol Sci.* 1997;152:39–49.
6. Bredesen D. Neural apoptosis. *Ann Neurol.* 1995;38:839–851.
7. Duffy F, Albert M, McAnulty G, et al. Age-related differences in brain electrical activity of healthy subjects. *Ann Neurol.* 1984;16:430–438.
8. Schultz A, Grouven U, Zander I, et al. Age-related effects in the EEG during propofol anaesthesia. *Acta Anaesthesiol Scand.* 2004;48:27–34.
9. Katz R, Horowitz G. Electroencephalogram in the septuagenarian: studies in a normal geriatric population. *J Am Geriatr Soc.* 1982;30:273–275.
10. Renna M, Handy J, Shah A. Low baseline Bispectral Index of the electroencephalogram in patients with dementia. *Anesth Analg.* 2003;96:1380–1385.
11. Morgan M, Cook I, Greenwald S, et al. EEG Bispectral Index Correlates with Dementia Severity. *2002 NCDEU abstracts.* II-79.
12. Sigl JC, Greenwald SD, Devlin PH, et al. Can the EEG bispectral index detect neurological decline of Alzheimer's disease? *Neurobiol Aging.* 2000;21:S1080.
13. Neubauer D. Sleep problems in the elderly. *Am Fam Physician.* 1999;59:2551–2560.
14. Kazama T, Ikeda K, Morita K, et al. Comparison of the effect-site k_{eo}s of propofol for blood pressure and EEG Bispectral Index in elderly and younger patients. *Anesthesiology.* 1999;90:1517–1527.
15. Katoh T, Bito H, Sato S. Influence of age on hypnotic requirement, Bispectral Index, and 95% spectral edge frequency associated with sedation induced with sevoflurane. *Anesthesiology.* 2000;92:55–61.
16. Scott J, Stanski D. Decreased fentanyl and alfentanil dose requirements with age: a simultaneous pharmacokinetic and pharmacodynamic evaluation. *J Pharmacol Exp Ther.* 1987;240:159–166.
17. Minto C, Schnider T, Egan T, et al. Influence of age and gender on the pharmacokinetics and pharmacodynamics of remifentanil: I. Model development. *Anesthesiology.* 1997;86:10–23.

18. Gan T, Glass P, Windsor A, et al. Bispectral index monitoring allows faster emergence and improved recovery from propofol, alfentanil, and nitrous oxide anesthesia. BIS Utility Study Group. *Anesthesiology.* 1997;87:808–815.

19. Drover D, Lemmens H, Pierce E, et al. Patient State Index: titration of delivery and recovery from propofol, alfentanil, and nitrous oxide anesthesia. *Anesthesiology.* 2002;97(1):82–89.

20. Pavlin D, Hong J, Freund P, et al. The effect of bispectral index monitoring on end-tidal gas concentration and recovery duration after outpatient anesthesia. *Anesth Analg.* 2001;93:613–619.

21. Song D, Joshi G, White P. Titration of volatile anesthetics using Bispectral Index facilitates recovery after ambulatory anesthesia. *Anesthesiology.* 1997;87:842–848.

22. Heck M, Kumle B, Boldt J, et al. Electroencephalogram Bispectral Index predicts hemodynamic and arousal reactions during induction of anesthesia in patients undergoing cardiac surgery. *J Cardiothorac Vasc Anesth.* 2000;14:693–697.

23. Wong J, Song D, Blanshard H, et al. Titration of isoflurane using BIS index improves early recovery of elderly patients undergoing orthopedic surgeries. *Can J Anesth.* 2002;49:13–18.

24. Fredman B, Sheffer O, Zohar E, et al. Fast-track eligibility of geriatric patients undergoing short urologic surgery procedures. *Anesth Analg.* 2002;94:560–564.

25. Wilhelm W, Kreuer S, Larsen R. Narcotrend Study-Group. Narcotrend EEG monitoring during total intravenous anaesthesia in 4630 patients. *Anaesthesist.* 2002;51:980–988.

26. Lauven P, Nadstawek J, Albrecht S. The safe use of anesthetics and muscle relaxants in older surgical patients. *Drugs Aging.* 1993;3:502–509.

27. Fredman B, Zohar E, Philipov A, et al. The induction, maintenance, and recovery characteristics of spinal versus general anesthesia in geriatric patients. *J Clin Anesth.* 1998;10:623–630.

28. Monk T, Saini V, Weldon C, et al. Anesthetic management and one-year mortality after noncardiac surgery. *Anesth Analg.* 2005;100:4–10.

29. Greenwald S, Sandin R, Lindholm M, et al. Duration at low intraoperative BIS levels was shorter among one-year postoperative survivors than nonsurvivors: a case controlled analysis. *Anesthesiology.* 2004;101:A383.

30. Sebel P, Bowdle T, Ghoneim M, et al. The incidence of awareness during anesthesia: a multicenter United States study. *Anesth Analg.* 2004;99: 833–839.

31. Domino K, Posner K, Caplan R, et al. Awareness during anesthesia. *Anesthesiology.* 1999;90:1053–1061.

32. Sandin RH, Enlund G, Samuelsson P, et al. Awareness during anaesthesia: a prospective case study. *Lancet.* 2000;355:707–711.

33. Lennmarken C, Bildfors K, Enlund G, et al. Victims of awareness. *Acta Anaesthesiol Scand.* 2002;46:229–231.

34. Ekman A, Lindholm M, Lennmarken C, et al. Reduction in the incidence of awareness using BIS monitoring. *Acta Anaesthesiol Scand.* 2004;48: 20–26.

35. Myles P, Leslie K, McNeil J, et al. Bispectral index monitoring to prevent awareness during anaesthesia: the B-Aware randomized controlled trial. *Lancet.* 2004;363:1757–1763.

The Controversy of Regional vs. General Anesthesia in Surgical Outcome

CHAPTER 21

Jian Hang

INTRODUCTION

There is a long-held debate among anesthesiologists as to whether regional anesthesia is safer than general anesthesia. The theoretic reasons behind the concept that regional anesthesia is safer are:

1. Regional anesthesia provides more stable cardiovascular hemodynamics.

2. Regional anesthesia and analgesia provides superior pain relief for both intraoperative and postoperative periods with a superior recovery profile and better patient satisfaction.

3. Regional anesthesia placed preoperatively may provide preemptive analgesia.

4. Regional anesthesia can avoid endotracheal intubation and mechanical ventilation, leading to less respiratory complications.

5. Regional anesthesia may also attenuate stress responses and preserve immune response.

6. Regional anesthesia and analgesia reduces opioid-related complications such as those related to the gastrointestinal system.

7. Superior pain relief may reduce unplanned hospital admission for ambulatory patients, and thus reduce costs. Although these suppositions remain controversial, increasing evidence from well-conducted clinical trials and data reviews support the notion that regional anesthesia and analgesia can improve surgical outcomes.[1-3]

The definition of regional anesthesia varies among studies. As shown in Table 21-1, there are numerous variations in anesthesia and analgesia techniques. The majority of clinical studies use regional anesthesia to mean neuraxial anesthesia, with or without postoperative neuraxial analgesia. Most studies identify peripheral nerve blocks (PNBs) as a separate entity, whereas a few studies include PNB and local anesthetic infiltration or local injection as regional anesthesia. For the purposes of this chapter, regional anesthesia refers to neuraxial anesthesia and analgesia, including spinal anesthesia, epidural anesthesia, and epidural analgesia. PNBs are considered as a separate entity, similar to most studies.

In previous studies, perioperative outcomes refer to major clinical outcomes such as mortality and cardiovascular complications. The outcomes discussed in this chapter are listed in Table 21-2 and include mortality, major morbidity, and nontraditional outcomes.[4]

This chapter does not intend to be an exhaustive review of all available data on the regional versus general debate. Instead, the focus is on data pertaining to the geriatric population, and the beneficial effects of regional anesthesia on surgical outcomes in the elderly. Table 21-3 is designed to provide a comprehensive summary of the important studies discussed below. The reader is asked to refer to this table for issues regarding individual studies.

CARDIOVASCULAR SYSTEM—PERIOPERATIVE CARDIOVASCULAR COMPLICATIONS

Most early evidence suggested little, if any, difference in overall outcome and mortality between regional and general anesthesia in the elderly.[24] Many studies conducted in the late 1970s and 1980s compared perioperative outcomes of regional anesthesia to general anesthesia: notably 12 controlled mortality studies were performed comparing regional anesthesia with general anesthesia in mostly high-risk, elderly patients undergoing acute hip surgery.[7] Only 2 of these 12 studies showed a significant benefit from regional anesthesia on short-term survival. Of interest, when data from these 12 studies were pooled and analyzed, an overall 30% reduction in early mortality in the regional anesthesia group was demonstrated. Given these results, early reviews of previously published data suggested that there appears to be no difference in cardiovascular outcomes between regional anesthesia and general anesthesia in most patient populations.[5,7,25] In contrast to other studies of that time period, in 1987 Yeager et al.[6] published a landmark study suggesting that epidural anesthesia and analgesia significantly improved postoperative outcome compared to general anesthesia.

More recent large-scale clinical trials have added controversial data (Table 21-3). A randomized controlled Veterans Affairs Cooperative Study examined 1021 patients with average age of 67.0 ± 8.8 (mean $\pm$ SD) years for general anesthesia (GA) group and 66.5 ± 8.9 years for GA combined with epidural anesthesia and analgesia (EAA) group.[10] The study found no difference in anesthetic technique in the incidence of death or major complications in a combined analysis of four types of abdominal surgeries. The analysis did show that GA + EAA provided better pain relief and improved overall outcomes depending on the type of surgery. For instance, with abdominal aortic aneurysm (AAA) the GA + EAA group had shorter length of intubation and intensive care unit (ICU) stay with lower incidence of death and major complications. Matot et al.[17] compared the effects of continuous epidural analgesia begun in the emergency room versus a systemic opioid regimen on preoperative adverse cardiac events in elderly patients with hip fracture. The results indicated that early administration of continuous epidural analgesia is associated with a

Table 21-1

Anesthesia and Analgesia Techniques

Anesthesia	
General anesthesia	General Anesthesia (inhalational agents)
	General anesthesia (intravenous agents) Or total intravenous anesthesia (TIVA)
Regional (neuraxial) anesthesia	Spinal anesthesia (subarachnoid block) (local anesthetics with or without opioids)
	Epidural anesthesia (local anesthetics with or without opioids)
Peripheral nerve block anesthesia	Peripheral nerve block anesthesia (single injection, local anesthetics)
	Continuous peripheral nerve block anesthesia (local anesthetics)
Field block anesthesia	Local anesthetic injection (infiltration)
Monitored anesthesia care (MAC)	Patient monitoring with or without sedation
Analgesia	
Systemic administered analgesia	Opioid analgesics
	Analgesics other than opioids
Neuraxial analgesia	Spinal (subarachnoid) analgesia (local anesthetics, opioid, or both)
	Continuous epidural analgesia (local anesthetics, opioid, or both)
Peripheral nerve block analgesia	Continuous epidural analgesia (local anesthetics with or without additive)

Table 21-2

Types of Perioperative Outcomes

Traditional outcomes
  Mortality
  Major morbidity
    Cerebrovascular accidents
    Cognitive dysfunction
    Cardiovascular events
    Pulmonary complications
    Gastrointestinal dysfunctions
    Coagulation complications: deep venous thrombosis, pulmonary embolism, graft patency
    Immune, endocrine, and stress response-related complications
Nontraditional outcomes
  Functional health status
  Health-related quality-of-life measurements
  Functional outcome
  Economic outcome

lower incidence of preoperative adverse cardiac events in elderly patients with hip fracture. On the other hand, a small randomized controlled trial (RCT) by Norris et al.[12] showed no outcome difference when comparing thoracic epidural anesthesia with general anesthesia versus general anesthesia alone in 168 patients undergoing abdominal aortic surgery. And, the Multicentre Australian Study of Epidural Anaesthesia (MASTER) trial showed no difference in adverse outcomes in 915 high-risk patients who underwent major abdominal surgeries, apart from the incidence of respiratory failure.[15,16]

Recent meta-analyses and reviews using previously published data from randomized clinical trials have also yielded conflicting results (Table 21-3). Rodgers et al.[9] reviewed 141 RCTs prior to January 1, 1997. A total of 9559 patients who underwent predominantly orthopedic procedures were analyzed. Rodgers et al. found an overall mortality reduction of one-third in patients receiving neuraxial blockade.[9] Beattie et al.[11] performed a meta-analysis on data obtained from 17 RCTs performed between 1966 and 1998. A total of 1173 patients were analyzed. Beattie et al. found that patients in the epidural group had fewer postoperative myocardial infarctions (MIs), and thoracic epidural analgesia lasting longer than 24 hours reduced the incidence of postoperative MI significantly.[11] However, there was no difference in overall death rate between epidural and GA groups. In a follow-up study,[19] Beattie et al. added additional data from three more recent RCTs to their original meta-analysis.[11] This brought the total number of patients to 2427. The updated meta-analysis continued to demonstrate a significant reduction in postoperative MI with the use of thoracic epidural analgesia. Wu et al.[22] performed meta-analysis on a total of 68,723 Medicare patients (age ≥65 years, younger patients on renal dialysis, or disabled) and found that the presence of postoperative epidural analgesia was associated with a significantly lower odds ratio (OR) of death at 7 days (OR, 0.52; 95% confidence interval [CI] 0.38–0.73; $p = 0.0001$) and 30 days (OR, 0.74; 95% CI 0.63–0.89; $p = 0.0005$). There was no difference in overall major morbidity, except an increase in pneumonia at 30 days for the EAA group (OR, 1.91; 95% CI 1.09–3.34; $p = 0.02$). Contrast these findings to those of Kehlet and Holte.[13] Kehlet and Holte reviewed data from RCT in which various analgesic techniques were compared. Their study found no difference between analgesic techniques in cardiac morbidity.[13]

▶ Reasons for the conflicting results

Improvement in anesthetic and surgical management results in an ongoing reduction of mortality. The continuous decline in mortality rates for modern elective surgery necessitates that studies of mortality and outcome include large numbers of patients. Sharrock et al.[26] in 1995 carried out a 10-year retrospective review of in-hospital mortality rates after elective total hip and knee arthroplasty. The overall mortality rate was 0.39% between 1981 and 1985, and 0.1% from 1987 to 1991. This improvement in perioperative mortality and morbidity makes it increasingly difficult to conduct such studies in modern surgical and anesthetic practice. Other factors including heterogeneous patient populations and diverse surgical procedures add to the complexity of conducting such studies.

Most studies did not control preoperative medication and sedation during surgeries under regional anesthesia. Deep sedation during regional anesthesia may eliminate the difference between regional anesthesia and general anesthesia.[24]

Many studies do not distinguish between different anesthetic techniques such as lower-body versus upper body procedures, lumbar

Table 21-3

Major Reviews/Meta-Analysis and Most Recent Randomized Controlled Trials (since 2000) Comparing Effects of General Anesthesia and Regional Anesthesia Perioperative Morbidity and Mortality

Authors, Year, Study Types	No. of Subjects/No. of Trials Included and Sources	Positive Results/Conclusion	Negative Results/Note
Kehlet H.[5] 1984 Review	Review of randomized clinical trials	A review of previous RCT ▸ RA with local anesthetics reduces intraoperative blood loss and postoperative thromboembolic complications after hip surgery and prostatectomy. ▸ RA probably minimizes mortality after acute hip surgery. ▸ RA may mitigate various aspects of postoperative morbidity.	No firm conclusions on ▸ Cardiac complications ▸ Pulmonary complications ▸ Mental dysfunction ▸ Infective complications ▸ Restoration of gastrointestinal function ▸ Convalescence ▸ Several pieces of evidence suggest that regional anesthesia may mitigate various aspects of postoperative morbidity.
Yeager et al.[6] 1987 RCT	N = 53	▸ EAA on postoperative morbidity high-risk patients ▸ EAA associated with a significant improvement in postoperative outcome	The study was stopped by the ethics committee after 53 patients
Atanassoff[7] 1996 Review	12 RCTs	Reviewed 12 controlled studies before 1987 ▸ Two studies showed a significant benefit from RA on short-term survival ▸ Pooled data show an overall 30% reduction in early mortality in RA group	
Ballantyne et al.[8] 1998 Meta-analysis	65 RCTs 1995–1996	Epidural opioid compared with systemic opioid ▸ A significant decreased in the incidence of atelectasis (RR = 0.53; 95% CI = 0.33–0.85) ▸ A decrease in the incidence of pulmonary infection (RR = 0.35; 95% CI = 0.21–0.65) ▸ A reduction in pulmonary complications overall (RR – 0.58; 95% CI = 0.42–0.80) ▸ A 4.56 mm Hg increase in PaO_2 (Difference = 4.56 mm Hg; 95% CI = 0.058–9.075)	Epidural opioid compared with systemic opioid (none was statistically significant): ▸ A weak tendency for decrease in infection and other pulmonary complications ▸ Intercostal block ▸ A tendency to reduce atelectasis and overall pulmonary complications ▸ No statistically significant differences in other pulmonary functions
Rodgers et al.[9] 2000 Data review	141 RCTs prior to January 1, 1997 N = 9559 predominantly orthopedic procedures	▸ An overall mortality reduction of one-third in patients who received neuraxial blockade (OR = 0.70, 95% CI = 0.54–0.90, $p = 0.006$) ▸ Reduced risks of DVT by 44%, PE 55%, pneumonia by 39%, respiratory depression by 59%, and MI by 30%; reduced transfusion requirements by 50%	No significant effects were found in other procedures (urological, abdominal, and thoracic). Most studies involved single-dose EAA regimens.
Park et al.[10] 2001 RCT	1021 VA patients 4 types abdominal surgeries: Group 1: GA + PCA Group 2: EAA* + GA	▸ Abdominal aortic surgical patients had improved overall outcomes, shorter length of intubation, and ICU stay in group 2 with lower incidence of death and major complications ▸ Overall, patients in group 2 received less analgesic medication, but had better pain relief	No difference in the incidence of death and major complications in all patients combined for four types of surgeries
Beattie et al.[11] 2001 Meta-analysis	17 out of 204 RCTs (EAA >24 h) 1966–1998 N = 1173	Epidural group had: ▸ Fewer postoperative MI ▸ Thoracic epidural analgesia >24 h reduced postoperative MI significantly ▸ Better analgesia	No difference in overall death rate

Table 21-3

Major Reviews/Meta-Analysis and Most Recent Randomized Controlled Trials (since 2000) Comparing Effects of General Anesthesia and Regional Anesthesia Perioperative Morbidity and Mortality *(Continued)*

Authors, Year, Study Types	No. of Subjects/No. of Trials Included and Sources	Positive Results/Conclusion	Negative Results/Note
Norris et al.[12] 2001 RCT	168 patients underwent AAA Group 1: EAA + GA Group 2: GA	Epidural group associated with significantly shorter time to extubation	▸ Postoperative outcomes were similar (death, MI, myocardial ischemia, pneumonia, renal failure, reoperation, length of stay, and medical costs) ▸ Postoperative pain scores were similar ▸ EAA has no major advantage or disadvantage
Kehlet and Holte[13] 2001 Review	Data from RCT of various analgesic techniques	▸ Reduced pulmonary complications in abdominal surgeries by epidural local anesthetics with or without opioid ▸ Reduced pulmonary morbidity in thoracic surgery by epidural opioid analgesia ▸ FAA with local anesthetic (≥ 24 h preferably 48 h), without opioid, led to substantial reduction in the surgical stress response and thromboembolic complications ▸ EAA with local anesthetic significantly reduced gastrointestinal complications (paralytic ileus) ▸ Integration of postoperative pain relief and rehabilitation	▸ No effects on cardiac morbidity ▸ No effect on POCD was demonstrated ▸ Effect of pain relief on postoperative morbidity remains uncertain ▸ No difference shown in hospital stay
Lien[14] 2002 Review	17 RCTs N = 2262 Prior to August 1998	▸ Significantly reduced DVT incidence in RA group (OR = 0.41, 95% CI = 0.23–0.72) ▸ Decreased O_2 saturation on first postoperative day in patients who received GA	▸ Patients who received RA tend to have a lower incidence of mortality at 1 month, but not statistically significant. ▸ No difference in PE, duration of surgery, length of hospital stay, and other perioperative outcomes
Rigg et al.[15] 2002 Multicenter trial	RCT 915 patients Major abdominal surgeries	MASTER trial ▸ Combined EAA and GA reduced respiratory failure ▸ EAA associated with better pain control	Most adverse morbid outcomes were not reduced by use of EAA
Peyton et al.[16] 2003	RCT 915 patients Major abdominal surgeries	Subgroup analysis of MASTER trial EAA associated with less respiratory failure	No difference in the incidence of any other major complications
Matot et al.[17] 2003 RCT	Preoperative epidural group (n = 34) Parenteral opioid (n = 34) Hip fracture patients	Effects of early preoperative epidural analgesia: ▸ Lowers the incidence of preoperative adverse cardiac events patients in elderly patients with hip fracture compared to conventional analgesia	
Block et al.[18] 2003 Meta-analysis	100 RCT studies (124 comparisons) 1966–4/25/2002	Efficacy of postoperative epidural analgesia compared with parenteral opioids (all $p < 0.001$) ▸ Better analgesia postthoracic surgery ▸ Better analgesia for abdominal surgery ▸ Better for both rest and incident pain ▸ Lower PONV rates with local anesthetic-based epidural analgesia	Thoracic epidural analgesia was similar to parenteral opioid

Table 21-3

Major Reviews/Meta-Analysis and Most Recent Randomized Controlled Trials (since 2000) Comparing Effects of General Anesthesia and Regional Anesthesia Perioperative Morbidity and Mortality *(Continued)*

Authors, Year, Study Types	No. of Subjects/No. of Trials Included and Sources	Positive Results/Conclusion	Negative Results/Note
Beattie et al.[19] 2003 Meta-analysis	Updated a 2001 meta-analysis with additional data from 3 more out of 4 new RCT Total 20 RCTs N = 2427	The updated meta-analysis continues to demonstrate statistically significant ▶ Reduction in postoperative MI with the use of thoracic epidural analgesia (OR = 0.60; 95% CI = 0.37–0.96; p = 0.03)	
Wu et al.[20] 2003 Meta-analysis	5% random sample of Medicare beneficiaries 1994–1999 Group 1 = GA Group 2 = GA + EA	Effect of postoperative epidural analgesia on morbidity and morality after total hip replacement surgery in Medicare patients. The unadjusted 7- and 30-day death rate was lower for GA + EA compared with GA group.	Multivariate regression analysis revealed no difference between groups in regard to major morbidity and mortality at 7 and 30 days. The use of postoperative EA was not associated with a lower incidence of mortality and major morbidity.
Parker et al.[21] 2004 Meta-analysis	22 RCTs N = 2567 patients Hip fracture surgery 1988–2004 week 10	▶ Pooled data from 8 RCTs showed RA is associated with a decreased mortality at 1 month (RR = 0.69; 95% CI = 0.50–0.95) ▶ RA associated with a reduced risk of DVT (RR = 0.64; 95% CI = 0.48–0.86) ▶ A reduced acute postoperative confusion (RR = 0.50; 95% CI = 0.26–0.95)	▶ Data pooled from 6 RCTs showed RA is not associated with any difference of 3-month mortality between groups. ▶ Insufficient evidence to draw any conclusion from 4 RCTs
Wu et al.[22] 2004 Meta-analysis	68,723 Medicare patients GA: n = 55,943 EAA: n = 12,780	Postoperative epidural analgesia is associated with ▶ A significantly lower odds of death at 7 days (OR = 0.52; 95% CI = 0.38–0.73; p = 0.0001) and ▶ A lower odds of death at 30 days (OR = 0.74; 95% CI = 0.63–0.89; p = 0.0005)	▶ No difference in overall major morbidity ▶ An increase in pneumonia at 30 days for the EAA group (OR = 1.91; 95% CI = 1.09–3.34; p = 0.02)
Liu et al.[23] 2004 Meta-analysis	15 RCTs CABG Group 1 = GA Group 2 = GA + TEA	GA + TEA (n = 1.178), compared to GA, reduced ▶ Risk of dysrhythmias (OR = 0.52) ▶ Risk of pulmonary complications (OR = 0.41) ▶ Time to extubation ▶ Pain score GA + IT (n = 668), compared to GA resulted in reduced ▶ Systemic morphine use ▶ Pain score	GA + TEA, compared to GA, resulted in ▶ No difference in mortality GA + IT resulted in no difference from GA on ▶ Mortality ▶ MI ▶ Dysrhythmia ▶ PONV ▶ Time to extubation GA + IT increases incidence of pruritus

Abbreviations:
CABG = coronary artery bypass grafting; GA = general anesthesia; CI = confidence interval; DVT = deep venous thrombosis; EA = epidural analgesia; EAA = epidural anesthesia and postoperative analgesia; ICU = intensive care unit; MI = myocardial infarction; OR = odds ratio; PCA = patient-controlled analgesia (using parenteral opioid); PE = pulmonary embolism; RA = regional anesthesia; RCT = randomized controlled trials; RR = risk ratio; TEA = thoracic epidural analgesia; IT = intrathecal analgesia; AAA = abdominal aortic aneurysm; POCD = postoperative cognitive dysfunction; PONV = postoperative nausea and vomiting
*postoperative epidural morphine analgesia.

epidural versus thoracic epidural anesthesia and analgesia, epidural anesthesia versus general combined with epidural anesthesia, epidural anesthesia versus epidural anesthesia and analgesia, or epidural local anesthetics alone versus local anesthetics combined with opioid infusion. Furthermore, the duration of postoperative analgesia is an important factor since surgical pain, stress response, and effects on cardiovascular, pulmonary, gastrointestinal, immune, endocrine systems, and central nervous system (CNS) do not subside until 2–3 days following surgery. Timing of epidural placement is another often-uncontrolled factor. However, there are only limited data available regarding its effect on surgical outcome. Parenteral use of opioids and sedatives postoperatively may also diminish the difference between regional anesthesia and general anesthesia.

RESPIRATORY SYSTEM—AIRWAY AND PULMONARY COMPLICATIONS

General anesthesia has several major effects on the respiratory system. Airway manipulation commonly occurs because patients have a high propensity to develop airway obstruction as a result of upper airway and thoracic respiratory musculature relaxation.[27] Inhalation anesthetics profoundly depress the respiratory response to both hypoxia and hypercapnea. In addition, intravenous opioids further depress the ventilatory drive. There are well-described reductions in functional residual capacity (FRC) due to diaphragmatic dysfunction, decreased chest wall compliance, and pain-limited inspiration, especially after thoracic and upper abdominal surgeries. The reduction in FRC may last until 7–10 days after surgery.[28,29] This predisposes one to atelectasis, ventilation-perfusion mismatch, and a higher risk of hypoxemia, pneumonia, and other postoperative pulmonary complications.[28]

With regional anesthesia, manipulation of the airway can be avoided, the respiratory drive is not affected, and the lung volumes are well preserved. Tidal volume, respiratory rate, and end-tidal carbon dioxide concentration are well preserved in healthy volunteers receiving spinal anesthesia.[30] Unchanged FRC has been observed after lumbar epidural anesthesia.[31] Indeed, others have observed an increased FRC during epidural anesthesia.[32] However, high thoracic[33] or cervical epidural blocks[34] as well as intercostal blocks[35] are associated with reductions in lung volumes that occur secondary to relaxation of the intercostal muscles.

Given the above, general anesthesia has greater effects on the respiratory system compared to regional anesthesia, and the choice of anesthesia may affect the degree of postoperative pulmonary dysfunctions. Catley et al.[36] showed that elderly patients had significantly fewer hypoxemic events with epidural analgesia using local anesthetics compared to systemic opioids following lower extremity orthopedic procedures. Hole et al.[37] reported that general anesthesia for total hip arthroplasty in elderly patients resulted in a significantly lower PaO_2 on postoperative day 1 compared with epidural anesthesia with local anesthetic. Rigg et al.,[15] in a randomized clinical trial of 915 patients undergoing major surgeries, found that respiratory complications were less frequent when comparing combined epidural + GA with post-op epidural analgesia versus GA with post-op IV morphine analgesia.

Several meta-analyses have demonstrated that regional anesthesia may have benefit in decreasing pulmonary complications. Patients receiving epidural analgesia were found to have decreased intubation time[21,38] and shorter ICU stay[21] compared with systemic opioid analgesia. Furthermore, another meta-analysis of 141 randomized clinical trials found that the use of thoracic epidural anesthesia and analgesia

with local anesthetics resulted in a 39% reduction in pneumonia and a 59% reduction in respiratory depression compared with the use of general anesthesia and patient-controlled anesthesia (PCA).[9].

The use of systemic and epidural opioids is associated with a higher incidence of hypoxemic events compared to epidural analgesia with a local anesthetic alone.[2] Oxygen saturation in elderly patients is higher with epidural anesthesia and analgesia without inclusion of an opioid.[36] A meta-analysis by Ballantyne et al.[8] found a decrease in the incidence of atelectasis with epidural opioid versus systemic opioid for post-op analgesia. However, there was a decrease in the incidence of pulmonary infection, overall pulmonary complications, and an increase in PaO_2 with epidural local anesthetic versus systemic opioid for post-op analgesia.[8] Kehlet and Holte[13] reanalyzed the Ballantyne data and concluded that continuous epidural local anesthetic or local anesthetic-opioid mixtures provided a reduction in postoperative pulmonary morbidity in major abdominal procedures, and epidural opioid-based regimens also reduced pulmonary morbidity in thoracic procedures.

Many randomized studies, which have failed to demonstrate a clear advantage of regional anesthetic technique in decreasing pulmonary complications,[39] have included opioid in their epidural mixtures. For example, Mann et al.[40] compared the effects of intravenous opioid PCA versus epidural PCA with local anesthetic-opioid mixture in elderly patients after major abdominal surgery and found no difference in pulmonary complications.

Using regional anesthesia and analgesia with local anesthetics for postoperative analgesia provides a greater margin of safety than systemic or epidural administration of opioid. It seems that epidural analgesia without opioid may be a more appropriate form of postoperative pain relief,[7] especially for patients with severe pulmonary impairment[41] and in the elderly population.

HEMATOLOGY AND COAGULATION—THROMBOEMBOLISM, GRAFT THROMBOSIS, AND BLOOD LOSS

A hypercoagulable state occurs following general anesthesia and surgery. Patients undergoing major orthopedic surgery are at especially high risk as they may be predisposed to thrombus formation.[42] In the 1960s and 1970s, prior to the widespread use of prophylaxis, the risk of venous thromboembolism (VTE) following major orthopedic surgery was substantial. The risk of fatal pulmonary embolism (PE) following hip fracture repair may have been as high as 7.5%.[43] Among patients who received placebo instead of anticoagulant in clinical trials, the incidence of deep venous thrombosis (DVT) was 45–57% following total hip arthroplasty, 40–84% following total knee arthroplasty (TKA), and 36–60% following hip fracture repair. Current risks after hip and knee arthroplasty appear to be about 2.5% for DVT, 1% for nonfatal PE, and a few tenths of 1% for fatal PE over a 3-month period following surgery.[43]

Anesthetic techniques are known to affect blood hemostasis. Many studies have shown that neuraxial anesthesia, as compared to general anesthesia, reduces the incidence of thromboembolic complications after surgeries associated with a high risk of postoperative DVT.[4] The exact mechanism is unclear; however, it may be related to stress response, endothelial damage with tissue factor activation, and synergism with inflammation.[44] Continuous epidural anesthesia and analgesia is associated with better fibrinolytic function and lower activation of factor VIII compared to general anesthesia + IV opioid for postoperative analgesia.[45] Many randomized trials have demonstrated that regional anesthesia decreases the incidence of DVT after orthopedic surgeries.[46–49] Sorenson et al.[50] performed a meta-analysis of 13 randomized trials comparing regional versus general anesthesia for repair of femoral neck fractures and confirmed that the incidence of DVT was 31% higher in patients receiving general anesthesia versus those receiving regional anesthesia.

Regional anesthesia decreases the incidence of graft thrombosis in vascular surgeries through attenuation of perioperative hypercoagulability.[4,51,52] Impaired fibrinolysis may be related to postoperative arterial thrombosis. Because regional anesthesia + epidural fentanyl for post-op analgesia appear to prevent the postoperative inhibition of fibrinolysis, this anesthetic technique may decrease the risk of arterial thrombotic complications in patients undergoing lower extremity revascularization.

Epidural anesthesia, especially with hypotensive technique, has the advantage of reduced blood loss in many types of surgery including orthopedic, urologic, and gynecologic procedures.[1] However, there is concern in the elderly that decreased blood pressures may be associated with compromised cerebral perfusion and potential postoperative cognitive impairment.[53] Williams-Russo et al.[54] examined postoperative cognitive function in elderly patients undergoing regional anesthesia and found no difference in hypotensive versus normotensive blood pressure management. This suggests that epidural anesthesia with hypotensive technique is safe to administer in select elderly patients.[54]

GASTROINTESTINAL SYSTEM—POSTOPERATIVE NAUSEA, VOMITING, AND GASTROINTESTINAL TRACT DYSFUNCTION (ILEUS)

Even though it does not completely abolish postoperative nausea and vomiting (PONV), regional anesthesia is thought to be associated with less PONV and offers better chance to avoid PONV compared with general anesthesia. A wide range of PONV incidences have been reported when neuraxial blockade is used.[55] An opioid-free neuraxial anesthesia regimen appears to cause less PONV after many types of surgeries.[55–58] Peripheral blocks with local anesthetic alone are generally associated with a low incidence of PONV.[55] The use of opioid-free continuous PNB with or without propofol-based general anesthesia significantly reduces PONV in most studies.[55]

The pathogenesis of postoperative gastrointestinal tract dysfunction (PGID) is clearly related to abdominal pain and surgical stress-activated reflex arcs of sympathetic activity.[2] In addition, opioid analgesics have inhibitory effects on gastrointestinal tract motility. Local anesthetics administered during epidural anesthesia and analgesia can theoretically improve bowel motility by selectively blocking the sympathetic-mediated inhibitory effects on bowel motility, resulting in an unopposed parasympathetic activity to the bowels. In addition, epidural local anesthetics can also decrease systemic use of opioids, increase gastrointestinal blood flow, and direct stimulation of gastrointestinal smooth muscle.[2,25,59] Over a dozen randomized clinical trials have demonstrated a reduced duration of postoperative ileus by thoracic epidural anesthesia and analgesia with local anesthetic.[2,59,60] There have been concerns regarding the safety of epidural anesthesia and analgesia for patients undergoing bowel resection with anastomoses. Substantial evidence in both animals and humans demonstrates that epidural with local anesthetic is not only safe for anastomoses, but also has a beneficial effect on anastomotic healing.[2]

Opioid-free neuraxial anesthesia appears to be associated with less PONV after many types of surgeries. PNBs and continuous PNBs

with local anesthetic appear to be promising alternative anesthetic techniques for many surgeries in terms of reducing incidence of PONV. Use of epidural local anesthetics appears to be the most effective means of reducing PGID. For epidural anesthesia and analgesia to be fully efficacious in reduction of postoperative ileus, it is important that epidural analgesia is begun prior to incision, the T5-L2 dermatomes are anesthetized, and postoperative epidural analgesia with local anesthetic is continued until return of bowel function.[2]

CENTRAL NERVOUS SYSTEM—POSTOPERATIVE COGNITIVE DYSFUNCTION

It has been hypothesized that regional anesthesia might reduce the incidence of postoperative cognitive dysfunction (POCD) in elderly patients.[61] However, neuraxial anesthesia has not been shown to decrease the incidence of POCD compared with general anesthesia.[62] In fact, among the 19 randomized trials examining intraoperative neuraxial anesthesia versus general anesthesia reviewed by Wu and his colleagues, only one study showed a better postoperative cognitive function with epidural anesthesia. Additionally, none of the five observational trials reviewed by Wu demonstrated a difference in cognitive function between general anesthesia and neuraxial anesthesia.[62] A significant problem in evaluating the literature is that most studies addressing this issue contain design flaws including use of benzodiazepines, sedation, only one neuropsychological test, and not being double-blinded.[62] On the other hand, spinal anesthesia without any premedication or intraoperative sedation has a reported 0% incidence of delirium in elderly patients after a high delirium risk surgery—repair of femoral neck fractures.[63]

ENDOCRINE AND IMMUNE SYSTEMS— ENDOCRINE, STRESS REDUCTION FUNCTIONS, AND IMMUNE

▶ Endocrine and stress responses

General anesthesia cannot prevent the stress response from being activated; in fact, it may even exacerbate its activation with the exception of large doses of opioids prior to incision.[39,64] Epidural anesthesia, on the other hand, can theoretically prevent the surgical stress response by blocking the somatic and sympathetic nervous systems from being activated. Thus, it may provide the most physiological anesthesia for surgery. Indeed, many studies have demonstrated that epidural anesthesia attenuates stress responses of the body to surgery and it provides more stable cardiovascular hemodynamics.[6,65]

The overall metabolic effect of the stress response is catabolism and hyperglycemia. Epidural blockade reduces postoperative hyperglycemia and improves glucose tolerance, even though plasma insulin concentration is unchanged.[66] Hyperglycemia predisposes critically ill patients to a greater complication rate of severe infection, polyneuropathy, multiple-organ failure, and death.[67] The normalization of plasma glucose and glucose tolerance with epidural anesthesia and analgesia can certainly contribute to easier management of tight glucose control with intensive insulin therapy. Epidural anesthesia and postoperative analgesia has been shown to decrease the catabolic response to surgery, improve protein economy, gastrointestinal rehabilitation, and nutritional status after surgeries, especially with abdominal surgery.[66] Whether blocking of the stress response by epidural anesthesia and analgesia leads to improved surgical outcomes remains unclear.

▶ Immune system

In absence of surgery, both general anesthesia and lumbar epidural anesthesia have only transient and minor effects on human immune function.[68] Epidural anesthesia and analgesia modestly preserves cellular and humoral immune functions, especially for surgical procedures below the umbilicus.[39] General anesthesia, on the other hand, may even exacerbate the immunosuppression that occurs following surgery.[39] Studies have suggested that use of epidural anesthesia and analgesia with local anesthetics may decrease the incidence of postoperative infectious complications.[39] The favorable effects of epidural anesthesia and analgesia on human immune functions may have implications in elderly patients, critically ill patients, and immunocompromised patients. However, there is no direct evidence to show that effects of different anesthetic techniques on human immune function have any influence on postoperative infection rate or major outcomes.

OTHER PARAMETERS—FUNCTIONAL OUTCOMES, QUALITY OF LIFE, PATIENT SATISFACTION, AND ECONOMIC OUTCOMES

▶ Functional outcomes

There is evidence suggesting that regional anesthesia and analgesia improves postoperative functional outcome and achieves rehabilitation goals earlier when compared with general anesthesia + IV opioid PCA. Williams-Russo et al.[69] showed that patients who received epidural anesthesia and analgesia achieved rehabilitative milestones earlier postoperatively than did patients who received general anesthesia + post-op systemic narcotics. Capdevila et al.[70] confirmed this finding with major knee surgery and showed that patients who received postoperative continuous femoral block analgesia had better functional prognosis as measured by the time needed to achieve target levels of knee range of motion and shorter length of hospital stay compared with patients who received intravenous morphine PCA. Other studies have indirectly supported the notion that better pain relief may translate to better functional recovery after knee replacement.[71] However, more outcome research is needed to address the role of regional anesthetic and analgesic techniques in improving functional outcome beyond its advantages of superior pain relief and decreased opioid use. With a growing interest in PNB anesthesia and continuous peripheral nerve block (CPNB) analgesia techniques, more investigations are needed to address the question of the beneficial role of PNB in multimodal analgesia techniques.

▶ Quality of life

As of this writing, quality of life as a perioperative outcome has not been used widely as a measurement to assess the effects of regional anesthesia-analgesia.

▶ Patient satisfaction

Regional anesthesia-analgesia is associated with favorable patient satisfaction. It is difficult to evaluate patient satisfaction as an outcome since adequacy of postoperative pain control has huge influence on patient satisfaction. It is also difficult to differentiate patient satisfaction from other aspects of medical care.[4] It is not clear what the impact of patient satisfaction is on other medical outcomes.

▶ Economic outcomes

There are only a few studies examining the economics of anesthesia for outpatients.[72–76] Local anesthetic infiltration under monitored anesthesia care (MAC) is probably the most cost-effective anesthesia.[72,77–79] But this modality is limited in its applications. Regional anesthesia techniques for ambulatory patients, suitable for a wider range of surgical procedures, were shown to be more cost-effective compared to general anesthesia[72,74–76] as a result of shorter time-to-home readiness, better pain control, less PONV, bypassing postanesthesia care unit (PACU), reliable same-day discharge, and lower unplanned admission. This is despite the fact that the direct cost of administering regional anesthesia may be even higher than general anesthesia.[4,78] Similarly, it is reported that PNBs may be associated with greater cost-effectiveness compared to that of general anesthesia.[74] No difference in costs between epidural and general anesthesia (GA) has been found during the intraoperative period by Schuster et al.,[60] but spinal anesthesia has intraoperative economic advantages over GA, especially for short cases. Although the cost-saving advantages of regional anesthesia in the operating room may seem insignificant, regional anesthesia could theoretically have cost-effective effects extending beyond the operating room. The advantageous effects of regional anesthesia and analgesia on decreasing postoperative complications and facilitating earlier achievement of functional rehabilitation and fulfillment of discharge criteria may have a significant impact on cost-effectiveness of patient care.

PERIOPERATIVE OUTCOMES OF PERIPHERAL NERVE BLOCKS VS. NEURAXIAL ANESTHESIA AND ANALGESIA VS. GENERAL ANESTHESIA

Hadzic et al.[80] showed that a combination of lumbar plexus and sciatic nerve blocks using short-acting local anesthetic has a superior recovery profile compared with GA in patients undergoing outpatient knee arthroscopy. The nerve blocks enabled 72% of patients to bypass phase I recovery compared with only 24% of those who received GA. There was also a significantly shorter time to discharge home. Chelly et al.[81] showed that continuous femoral nerve block (CFNB) was associated with a 90% decrease in serious complications and a 20% decrease in the length of hospitalization after TKA. The authors concluded that CFNB represents a better alternative than PCA or epidural analgesia for postoperative pain management and immediate rehabilitation after TKA. PNB provides excellent postoperative analgesia,[73] reduced PACU admission, as well as decreased unplanned hospital admission in ambulatory patients undergoing complex outpatient knee surgeries.[74] More recently, Capdevila et al.[70] showed that CPNB provides equivalent functional outcomes with fewer side effects compared to epidural analgesia following TKA.

PNBs differ from neuraxial anesthesia in terms of effects on the cardiovascular, coagulation, gastrointestinal, and urinary systems. Unfortunately, there have been few studies specifically comparing perioperative mortalities between PNB and neuraxial blocks or general anesthesia. A meta-analysis of available data from 1966 to May 21, 2004 suggests that CPNBs, regardless of catheter location, provide superior postoperative analgesia and fewer side effects when compared with opioids.[82]

Studies have shown that CPNB with local anesthetics provides excellent analgesia, good functional outcome, decreased serious complications, reduced length of hospitalization, and improved patient satisfaction.[69,70,80,81,83,84] Numerous studies demonstrate that CPNB can be safely used for ambulatory patients.[85] To date, however, there is no large clinical trial evaluating the efficacy of PNB on perioperative outcomes and potential risks.

REGIONAL VS. GENERAL ANESTHESIA IN GERIATRIC PATIENTS

As a general approach to the geriatric patient, one might consider the most common types of postoperative complications and the most common types of procedures performed to assess the benefits of regional anesthesia. The most common types of complications in the elderly are pulmonary, cardiovascular, and neurologic. Aside from opthalmologic procedures, the most common types of surgery in the elderly are orthopedic and general surgery.

The data suggest that if regional anesthesia and analgesia (EAA) is administered with local anesthetics, the respiratory response to hypoxia and hypercapnea is preserved. Most clinically significant EAA does not decrease FRC with exception of high thoracic and cervical epidural anesthesia. EAA also reduces postoperative pulmonary complications such as pneumonia and atelectasis compared with general anesthesia and systemic analgesia. It has also been shown to decrease intubation time and ICU length of stay. Whether EAA significantly reduces major perioperative cardiovascular morbidity and mortality remains controversial. The effects of PNB on cardiovascular outcomes are unclear. Unfortunately, there is no strong evidence that EAA is associated with lower POCD.

There are several advantages to the use of regional anesthesia for orthopedic procedures. Neuraxial anesthesia reduces the incidence of thromboembolic complications after surgeries, resulting in a lower incidence of DVT and PE. Epidural anesthesia also has advantages of reduced blood loss in many type procedures. Continuous epidural analgesia as well as CPNB are found to improve postoperative functional outcome and are associated with earlier achievement of rehabilitation goals compared with general anesthesia and IV PCA analgesia after major knee surgeries. In addition, CPNB is associated with fewer side effects compared to epidural analgesia. Patient satisfaction is higher in patients receiving regional anesthesia and analgesia. Besides the abovementioned pulmonary advantages, in the general surgery patient PONV occurs less with an opioid-free neuraxial anesthesia regimen. Use of preoperatively placed epidural analgesia, with a local anesthetics only regimen and with inclusion of the T5-L2 dermatomes, appears to be the most effective means of reducing PGID. In addition, use of regional anesthesia has been associated with lower incidence of graft thrombosis and a better graft patency rate for lower extremity revascularization.

Table 21-4 summarizes the benefits of regional anesthesia and analgesia. Most previous studies are based on mix-aged adult populations with a few exceptions[86] as well as mixed surgical procedures including both upper and lower body. Previous studies had different protocols of preoperative and intraoperative sedation, epidural anesthesia and analgesia with local anesthetics versus combined local anesthetics and opioid, levels of epidural blockade, and length of postoperative epidural analgesia. Previous studies had different definitions or regimens of epidural anesthesia: regional anesthesia versus combined regional and general anesthesia; epidural anesthesia only versus combined epidural anesthesia and analgesia; thoracic versus lumbar epidural. The lack of consistency between studies adds to the difficulty in making firm recommendations about the optimal anesthetic technique. However, an evidence-based approach suggests that regional anesthesia may be the optimal anesthetic in specific clinical scenarios. Geriatric patients have unique age-related changes in physiology and pharmacology. Elderly patients also may

have underlying disease with poor preoperative health status. Therefore, it is important to take into account patient age, comorbidities, and surgical procedure when deciding on the appropriate anesthetic technique.

Table 21-4

Benefits of Regional Anesthesia and Analgesia

Organ System	Benefits of Regional Anesthesia and Analgesia
Central nervous	Effects on postoperative cognitive dysfunction are unclear
Cardiovascular	May reduce myocardial infarction
	Stable hemodynamics
Respiratory	Avoid airway manipulation
	Preserved respiratory drive in response to hypoxia and hypercapnia
	Maintain functional residual capacity (FRC)
	Lower incidence of pneumonia
	Fewer hypoxemic events
	Reduced intubation time
Gastrointestinal	Lower risk of postoperative nausea and vomiting
	Reduce postoperative gastrointestinal dysfunction
Hematological	Lower incidence of venous thromboembolism
	Lower risk of deep venous thrombosis (DVT)
	Fewer pulmonary embolism (PE)
	Lower incidence of graft thrombosis
	Reduced intraoperative blood loss and transfusion requirement
Endocrine and immune	Attenuate stress responses
	Maintain glucose homeostasis and tolerance
	Decrease catabolic response and improve protein economy
	Decrease postoperative infection
	Preserve immune functions
Others	Superior pain relief
	Preemptive analgesia and postoperative analgesia
	Better recovery profile
	Better functional outcome
	Better patient satisfaction
	High PACU bypass rate
	Short home-readiness time
	Decreased length of hospital stay
	Better cost-effectiveness

KEY POINTS

► Regional anesthesia and analgesia has not consistently been associated with improvement in incidence of cardiac morbidity and mortality.

► Opioid-free regional anesthesia and analgesia has been associated with a lower incidence of postoperative pulmonary complications, shorter intubation time, and ICU stay when compared with systemic analgesia.

► Many studies suggest a lower incidence of thromboembolic events associated with the use of regional anesthesia, as compared with the use of general anesthesia. Regional anesthesia decreases graft thrombosis after lower extremity revascularization procedures.

► An opioid-free epidural anesthesia and analgesia (especially thoracic) is thought to be associated with less PONV and reduced duration of ileus.

► An evidence-based approach should be adopted in selection of optimal anesthetic and analgesic techniques for elderly patients in specific clinical scenarios by taking into account the patient's age, health status, comorbidities, and surgical procedure.

KEY REFERENCES

► Tsui BC, Wagner A, Finucane B. Regional anaesthesia in the elderly: a clinical guide. *Drugs Aging.* 2004;21(14):895–910.

► Ballantyne JC, Kupelnick B, McPeek B, Lau J. Does the evidence support the use of spinal and epidural anesthesia for surgery? *J Clin Anesth.* 2005;17(5):382–391.

REFERENCES

1. Grass JA. The role of epidural anesthesia and analgesia in postoperative outcome. *Anesthesiol Clin North America.* 2000;18(2):407–428.
2. Moraca RJ, Sheldon DG, Thirlby RC. The role of epidural anesthesia and analgesia in surgical practice. *Ann Surg.* 2003;238:663–673.
3. Tsui BC, Wagner A, Finucane B. Regional anaesthesia in the elderly: a clinical guide. *Drugs Aging.* 2004;21(14):895–910.
4. Wu CL, Fleisher LA. Outcomes research in regional anesthesia and analgesia. *Anesth Analg.* 2000;91:1232–1242.
5. Kehlet H. Influence of regional anaesthesia on postoperative morbidity. *Ann Chir Gynaecol.* 1984;73(3):171–176.
6. Yeager MP, Glass DD, Neff RK, Brinck-Johnsen T. Epidural anesthesia and analgesia in high-risk surgical patients. *Anesthesiology.* 1987;66(6):729–736.
7. Atanassoff PG. Effects of regional anesthesia on perioperative outcome. *J Clin Anesth.* 1996;8(6):446–55.
8. Ballantyne JC, Carr DB, deFerranti S, et al. The comparative effects of postoperative analgesic therapies on pulmonary outcomes: cumulative meta-analysis of randomized controlled trials. *Anesth Analg.* 1998;86:598–612.
9. Rodgers A, Walker N, Schug S, et al. Reduction of postoperative mortality and morbidity with epidural or spinal anaesthesia: results from overview of randomized trials. *Br Med J.* 2000;321(7275):1493.
10. Park WY, Thompson JS, Lee KK. Effect of epidural anesthesia and analgesia on perioperative outcome: a randomized, controlled Veterans Affairs cooperative study. *Ann Surg.* 2001;234(4):560–571.
11. Beattie WS, Badner NH, Choi P. Epidural analgesia reduces postoperative myocardial infarction: a meta-analysis. *Anesth Analg.* 2001;93(4):853–858.
12. Norris EJ, Beattie C, Perler BA, et al. Double-masked randomized trial comparing alternate combinations of intraoperative anesthesia and postoperative analgesia in abdominal aortic surgery. *Anesthesiology.* 2001;95(5):1054–1067.
13. Kehlet H, Holte K. Effect of postoperative analgesia on surgical outcome. *Br J Anaesth.* 2001;87(1):62–72.
14. Lien CA. Regional versus general anesthesia for hip surgery in older patients: does the choice affect patient outcome? *J Am Geriatr Soc.* 2002;50(1):191–194.
15. Rigg JR, Jamrozik K, Myles PS, et al. MATS: epidural anaesthesia and analgesia and outcome of major surgery: a randomized trial. *Lancet.* 2002;13:1276–1282.
16. Peyton PJ, Myles PS, Silbert BS, et al. Perioperative epidural analgesia and outcome after major abdominal surgery in high-risk patients. *Anesth Analg.* 2003;96(2):548–554.
17. Matot I, Oppenheim-Eden A, Ratrot R, et al. Preoperative cardiac events in elderly patients with hip fracture randomized to epidural or conventional analgesia. *Anesthesiology.* 2003;98(1):156–163.
18. Block BM, Liu SS, Rowlingson AJ, et al. Efficacy of postoperative epidural analgesia: a meta-analysis. *JAMA.* 2003;290(18):2455–2463.
19. Beattie WS, Badner NH, Choi PT. Meta-analysis demonstrates statistically significant reduction in postoperative myocardial infarction with the use of thoracic epidural analgesia. *Anesth Analg.* 2003;97(3):919–920.
20. Wu CL, Anderson GF, Herbert R, et al. Effect of postoperative epidural analgesia on morbidity and mortality after total hip replacement surgery in Medicare patients. *Reg Anesth Pain Med.* 2003;28(4):271–278.
21. Parker MJ, Handoll HH, Griffiths R. Anaesthesia for hip fracture surgery in adults. *Cochrane Database Syst Rev.* 2004;4:CD000521.
22. Wu CL, Hurley RW, Anderson GF, et al. Effect of postoperative epidural analgesia on morbidity and mortality following surgery in Medicare patients. *Reg Anesth Pain Med.* 2004;29(6):525–533.
23. Liu SS, Block BM, Wu CL. Effects of perioperative central neuraxial analgesia on outcome after coronary artery bypass surgery: a meta-analysis. *Anesthesiology.* 2004;101(1):153–161.
24. Roy RC. Choosing general versus regional anesthesia for the elderly. *Anesthesiol Clin North America.* 2000;18(1):91–104.
25. Breen P, Park KW. General anesthesia versus regional anesthesia. *Int Anesthesiol Clin.* 2002;40(1):61–71.
26. Sharrock NE, Cazan MG, Hargett MJ, et al. Changes in mortality after total hip and knee arthroplasty over a ten-year period. *Anesth Analg.* 1995;80(2):242–248.
27. Rassias AJ, Procopio MA. Stress response and optimization of perioperative care. *Dis Mon.* 2003;49(9):522–554.
28. Craig DB. Postoperative recovery of pulmonary function. *Anesth Analg.* 1981;60:46–52.
29. Meyers J, Lembeck L, O'Kane H, Baue A. Changes in functional residual capacity of the lung after operation. *Arch Surg.* 1975;110(5):576–583.
30. Steinbrook RA, Concepcion M. Respiratory effects of spinal anesthesia: resting ventilation and single-breath CO_2 response. *Anesth Analg.* 1991;72:182–186.
31. McCarthy GS. The effect of thoracic extradural analgesia on pulmonary gas distribution, functional residual capacity, and airway closure. *Br J Anaesth.* 1976;48:243–248.
32. Warner D, Warner M, Ritman E. Human chest wall function during epidural anesthesia. *Anesthesiology.* 1996;85(4):761–773.
33. Sundberg A, Wattwil M, Arvill A. Respiratory of high thoracic epidural anaesthesia. *Acta Anaesthesiol Scand.* 1986;30:215–217.
34. Takasak M, Takahashi T. Respiratory function during cervical and thoracic extradural analgesia in patients with normal lungs. *Br J Anaesth.* 1980;52:1271–1276.
35. Jakobson S, Ivarsson I. Effects of intercostals nerve blocks (bupivacaine 0.25% and etidocaine 0.5%) on chest wall mechanics in healthy men. *Acta Anaesthesiol Scand.* 1977;21:489–496.
36. Catley DM, Thornton C, Jordan C, et al. Pronounced, episodic oxygen desaturation in the postoperative period: its association with ventilatory pattern and analgesic regimen. *Anesthesiology.* 1985;63:20–28.
37. Hole A, Terjesen T, Breivik H. Epidural versus general anaesthesia for total hip arthroplasty in elderly patients. *Acta Anaesthesiol Scand.* 1980;24:279–287.
38. De Leoon-Casasola OA, Parker BM, Lema MJ. Epidural analgesia versus intravenous patient-controlled analgesia: differences in the postoperative course of cancer patients. *Reg Anesth.* 1994;19:307–315.
39. Liu S, Carpenter RL, Neal JM. Epidural anesthesia and analgesia: their role in postoperative outcome. *Anesthesiology.* 1995;82:1474–1506.
40. Mann C, Pouzeratte Y, Boccara G, et al. Comparison of intravenous or epidural patient-controlled analgesia in the elderly after major abdominal surgery. *Anesthesiology.* 2000;92:433–441.
41. Savas JF, Litwack R, Davis K, Miller TA. Regional anesthesia as an alternative to general anesthesia for abdominal surgery in patients with severe pulmonary impairment. *Am J Surg.* 2004;188(5):603–605.
42. Hantler C, Despotis GJ, Sinha R, Chally JE. Guidelines and alternatives for neuraxial anesthesia and venous thromboembolism prophylaxis in major orthopedic surgery. *J Arthroplasty.* 2004;19:1004–1016.

43. Edelsberg J, Ollendorf D, Oster G. Venous thromboembolism following major orthopedic surgery: review of epidemiology and economics. *Am J Health Syst Pharm.* 2001;58:S4–S13.

44. Rosenfeld BA. Benefits of regional anesthesia on thromboembolic complications following surgery. *Reg Anesth.* 1996;21(Suppl. 6):9–12.

45. Modig J, Borg T, Wegenius G, et al. Role of extradural and of general anaesthesia in fibrinolysis and coagulation after total hip replacement. *Br J Anaesth.* 1983;55:625–629.

46. Modig J, Borg T, Karlstrom G, et al. Thromboembolism after total hip replacement: role of epidural and general anesthesia. *Anesth Analg.* 1983; 62:174–180.

47. McKenie PJ, Wishart HY, Gray I, Smith G. Effects of anaesthetic technique on deep vein thrombosis. A comparison of subarachnoid and general anaesthesia. *Br J Anaesth.* 1985;57:853–857.

48. Jorgensen LN, Rasmussen LS, Nielsen PT, et al. Antithrombotic efficacy of continuous extradural analgesia after knee replacement. *Br J Anaesth.* 1991;66:8–12.

49. Hollmann MW, Wieczorek KS, Smart M, Durieux ME. Epidural anesthesia prevents hypercoagulation in patients undergoing major orthopedic surgery. *Reg Anesth Pain Med.* 2001;26:216–222.

50. Sorenson RM, Pace NL. Anesthetic techniques during surgical repair of femoral neck fractures. A meta-analysis. *Anesthesiology.* 1992;77: 1095–1104.

51. Rosenfeld BA, Beattie C, Christopherson R, et al. The effects of different anesthetic regimens on fibrinolysis and the development of postoperative arterial thrombosis. Perioperative Ischemia Randomized Anesthesia Trial Study Group. *Anesthesiology.* 1993;79(3):435–443.

52. Tuman KJ, McCarthy RJ, March RJ, et al. Effects of epidural anesthesia and analgesia on coagulation and outcome after major vascular surgery. *Anesth Analg.* 1991;73:696–704.

53. Raja SN, Haythornthwaite JA. Anesthetic management of the elderly: measuring function beyond the immediate perioperative horizon. *Anesthesiology.* 1999;91(4):909–911.

54. Williams-Russo P, Sharrock NE, Mattis S, et al. Randomized trial of hypotensive epidural anesthesia in older adults. *Anesthesiology.* 1999;91(4): 926–935.

55. Borgeat A, Ekatodramis G, Schenker CA. Postoperative nausea and vomiting in regional anesthesia: a review. *Anesthesiology.* 2003;98(2):530–547.

56. Gurlit S, Reinhardt S, Mollmann M. Continuous spinal analgesia or opioid-added continuous epidural analgesia for postoperative pain control after hip replacement. *Eur J Anaesthesiol.* 2004;21(9):708–714.

57. Jorgensen H, Wetterslev J, Moiniche S, Dahl JB. Epidural local anaesthetics versus opioid-based analgesic regimens on postoperative gastrointestinal paralysis, PONV, and pain after abdominal surgery. *Cochrane Database Syst Rev.* 2000;4:CD001893.

58. Callesen T, Schouenborg L, Nielsen D, et al. Combined epidural-spinal opioid-free anaesthesia and analgesia for hysterectomy. *Br J Anaesth.* 1999;82(6):881–885.

59. Luckey A, Livingston E, Tache Y. Mechanisms and treatment of postoperative ileus. *Arch Surg.* 2003;138:206–214.

60. Schuster M, Gottschalk A, Berger J, Standl T. A retrospective comparison of costs for regional and general anesthesia techniques. *Anesth Analg.* 2005;100(3):786–794.

61. Mackensen GB, Gelb AW. Postoperative cognitive deficits: more questions than answers. *Eur J Anaesthesiol.* 2004;21(2):85–88.

62. Wu CL, Hsu W, Richman JM, Raja SN. Postoperative cognitive function as an outcome of regional anesthesia and analgesia. *Reg Anesth Pain Med.* 2004;29(3):257–268.

63. Inouye SK, Viscoli CM, Horwitz RI, et al. A predictive model for delirium in hospitalized elderly medical patients based on admission characteristics. *Ann Intern Med.* 1993;119(6):474–481.

64. Desborough JP. The stress response to trauma and surgery. *Br J Anaesth.* 2000;85:109–117.

65. Carli F, Halliday D. Continuous epidural blockade arrests the postoperative decrease in muscle protein fractional synthetic rate in surgical patients. *Anesthesiology.* 1997;86(5):1033–1040.

66. Holte K, Kehlet H. Epidural anaesthesia and analgesia—effects on surgical stress responses and implications for postoperative nutrition. *Clin Nutr.* 2002;21:199–206.

67. Van den Berghe G, Wouters P, Weekers F, et al. Intensive insulin therapy in the critically ill patients. *N Engl J Med.* 2001;345(19):1359–1367.

68. Procopio MA, Rassias AJ, DeLeo JA, et al. The in vivo effects of general and epidural anesthesia on human immune function. *Anesth Analg.* 2001;93:460–465.

69. Williams-Russo P, Sharrock NE, Haas SB, et al. Randomized trial of epidural versus general anesthesia: outcomes after primary total knee replacement. *Clin Orthop.* 1996;331:199–208.

70. Capdevila X, Barthelet Y, Biboulet P, et al. Effects of perioperative analgesic technique on the surgical outcome and duration of rehabilitation after major knee surgery. *Anesthesiology.* 1999;91:8–15.

71. Buvanendran A, Kroin JS, Tuman KJ, et al. Effects of perioperative administration of a selective cyclooxygenase 2 inhibitor on pain management and recovery of function after knee replacement: a randomized controlled trial. *JAMA.* 2003;290(18):2411–2418.

72. Song D, Greilich NB, White PF, et al. Recovery profiles and costs of anesthesia for outpatient unilateral inguinal herniorrhaphy. *Anesth Analg.* 2000;91(4):876–881.

73. Williams BA, Kentro ML, Vogt MT, et al. Femoral-sciatic nerve blocks for complex outpatient knee surgery are associated with less postoperative pain before same-day discharge: a review of 1200 consecutive cases from the period 1996–1999. *Anesthesiology.* 2003;98:1206–1213.

74. Williams BA, Kentor ML, Vogt MT, et al. Economics of nerve block pain management after anterior cruciate ligament reconstruction: potential hospital cost savings via associated postanesthesia care unit bypass and same-day discharge. *Anesthesiology.* 2004;100(3):697–706.

75. Williams BA, Motolenich P, Kentor ML. Hospital facilities and resource management: economic impact of a high-volume regional anesthesia program for outpatients. *Int Anesthesiol Clin.* 2005;43(3):43–51.

76. Forssblad M, Jacobson E, Weidenhielm L. Knee arthroscopy with different anesthesia methods: a comparison of efficacy and cost. *Knee Surg Sports Traumatol Arthrosc.* 2004;12(5):344–349.

77. Li S, Coloma M, White PF, et al. Comparison of the costs and recovery profiles of three anesthetic techniques for ambulatory anorectal surgery. *Anesthesiology.* 2000;93(5):1225–1230.

78. Chan VW, Peng PW, Kaszas Z, et al. A comparative study of general anesthesia, intravenous regional anesthesia, and axillary block for outpatient hand surgery: clinical outcome and cost analysis. *Anesth Analg.* 2001; 93(5):1181–1184.

79. Kehlet H, Aasvang E. Groin hernia repair: anesthesia. *World J Surg.* 2005; 29(8):1058–1061.

80. Hadzic A, Karaca PE, Hobeika P, et al. Peripheral nerve blocks result in superior recovery profile compared with general anesthesia in outpatient knee arthroscopy. *Anesth Analg.* 2005;100(4):976–981.

81. Chelly JE, Greger J, Gebhard R, et al. Continuous femoral blocks improve recovery and outcome of patients undergoing total knee arthroplasty. *J Arthroplasty.* 2001;16(4):436–445.

82. Richman JM, Liu SS, Courpas G, et al. Does continuous peripheral nerve block provide superior pain control to opioids? A meta-analysis. *Anesth Analg.* 2006;102(1):248–257.

83. White PF, Issioui T, Skrivanek GD, et al. The use of a continuous popliteal sciatic nerve block after surgery involving the foot and ankle: does it improve the quality of recovery? *Anesth Analg.* 2003;97(5): 1303–1309.

84. Capdevila X, Pirat P, Bringuier S, et al. Continuous peripheral nerve blocks in hospital wards after orthopedic surgery. *Anesthesiology.* 2005; 103:1035–1045.

85. Ilfeld BM, Enneking FK. Continuous peripheral nerve blocks at home: a review. *Anesth Analg.* 2005;100(6):1822–1833.

86. Silber JH, Kennedy SK, Even-Shoshan O, et al. Anesthesiologist direction and patient outcomes. *Anesthesiology.* 2000;93(1):152–163.

SECTION

6

POSTOPERATIVE ISSUES SPECIFIC TO THE ELDERLY

Delirium and Postoperative Cognitive Dysfunction

CHAPTER 22

Christopher J. Jankowski

INTRODUCTION

The population is aging. The fastest growing segment of the population consists of those over 85 years old.[1] By 2050, there will be more than 20,000,000 U.S. residents in that age group, representing nearly 5% of the population.[2] The elderly consume health-care resources at a higher rate than younger people. For example, in the United States in 2000, those over 65 years old comprised 12% of the population, yet accounted for 20% of the surgical procedures.[2,3]

This trend has profound implications for the care of surgical patients. Several decades ago, even minor surgery was considered too risky an endeavor for patients greater than 50 years old.[4] Clearly, that is no longer the case. Anesthetic and surgical advances allow surgery to be performed on even the very old. In fact, surgery on patients greater than 90 or even 100 years old is becoming more common and is associated with good outcomes.[5–8] Although medical, surgical, and anesthetic advancements have made the perioperative care of the elderly considerably safer, the incidence of complications still increases with age.[9] Central nervous system (CNS) dysfunction is common in elderly postsurgical patients. However, traditional CNS morbidity, such as stroke, occurs relatively infrequently in the postoperative period.[10–12] Far more common are postoperative delirium (POD) and cognitive dysfunction (POCD). In fact, delirium may be the most common psychiatric condition in hospitalized patients.[13] The incidence of POD and POCD may exceed 50% in certain surgical populations.[14–21] Thus, POD and POCD are two of the most common postoperative complications in the elderly, and their incidence may be higher than that of many other major postoperative morbidities, such as myocardial infarction and respiratory failure.[22,23] This is significant because POD is associated with a variety of adverse postoperative outcomes, including death, major medical complications, increased length of hospital stay, and higher likelihood of discharge to a skilled care facility.[24–30] The economic impact of delirium is considerable. It adds $2500 to the cost of hospitalization and may be responsible for about $6.9 billion in Medicare costs per year in the United States.[31] Less is known about the long-term impact of POCD, though early POCD is associated with an increased risk of respiratory and infectious complications.[32] Clearly, postoperative cognitive changes have significant public health implications.

Although POD and POCD are common and associated with poor outcome, they have attracted little notice until recently. Thus, despite the CNS being the primary target organ for general anesthetics, understanding of *postoperative brain failure* is poor. Compared to the amount of research devoted to the cardiopulmonary implications of anesthesia and surgery, little has been dedicated to cognitive outcomes. This is unfortunate. Cognitive functioning relates directly to functional status,[33] an outcome that determines whether or not patients will be discharged to a skilled care facility instead of to home. Further, functional status is a strong predictor of mortality after hospitalization.[34] Therefore, in the elderly, functional status may be a more relevant outcome than traditional medical morbidity.

In part, the relative paucity of literature pertaining to and lack of clinical awareness of POCD and POD may be because they often are not apparent until well after patients have left the recovery room and the anesthesiologist has completed the postoperative visit. Thus, anesthesiologists may not be aware of the presence of these complications unless informed of it by the surgical team. Another issue is the lack of suitable research techniques with which to study these entities. For example, there is no universally agreed upon definition of POCD;[35–37] without a definition, it is difficult to design and interpret studies in this area. However, advances in research protocols have allowed more in-depth study of POCD and POD recently.[30,32,38–46] POD and POCD occur far more frequently in the elderly than in younger adults.[30,32,47] Given that the elderly are increasing in number and as a proportion of the population, it is critical to better understand these conditions and apply that knowledge to the care of older surgical patients.

Three issues make study of the literature concerning POD and POCD in the elderly difficult. The first is adequately defining "elderly." Although the medical literature concerning geriatric patients has arrived at a consensus concerning terminology ("older" patients being those from 55 to 64 years old; the "young-old" being 65–74 years old; the "old" being 75–84 years old; and the "oldest old" being those over 85 years old),[48,49] the anesthesia and surgical literature has not been as consistent. Clearly, there is a great deal of physiological variation between groups of patients from 55 years old to those over 85 years old. Therefore, it can be difficult to draw clinically relevant conclusions from studies of the "elderly" containing patients in all of the above categories.

Secondly, within the age-defined subgroups of the elderly, there may be significant variation in functional and physiological capacity, ranging from being fit to debilitated and frail.[48,50–53] Within an age category, there are significant differences between the fit and frail in the ability to withstand the stress of the perioperative period.

Finally, as noted above, there is inconsistency in definitions and techniques from study to study. For example, some studies use the Mini Mental State Examination (MMSE),[54] a relatively insensitive instrument designed for dementia screening, to assess patients for POCD.[55] Others use extensive neuropsychological test batteries.[32,56,57]

This chapter attempts to provide an overview of POD and POCD. First, definitions of the syndromes are discussed, an essential starting point. Next, potential mechanisms of POD and POCD are addressed. Current understanding of the predictors of POD and POCD, including pre-, intra-, and postoperative factors, are reviewed. The available data on the implications on long-term outcome of these syndromes are examined. Finally, strategies to prevent and treat the syndromes are presented.

DEFINITIONS

Before discussing POD and POCD, it is important to establish definitions of the two conditions. Without clear definitions, discussions regarding incidence, long-term outcomes, risk factors, and potential mechanisms are difficult to interpret. In order to provide context, definitions of dementia and the emerging concept of mild cognitive impairment (MCI) are also included.

▶ Dementia

Dementia consists of multiple cognitive deficits, the most prominent of which is memory impairment.[58] At least one of the following must also be present: aphasia, apraxia, agnosia, and deteriorating executive function (the ability to plan, organize, sequence, and think abstractly). For a patient to be diagnosed with dementia, these clinical findings must present significant problems with social or occupational activities and represent a decline from previous status. Personality changes and apathy often occur early. As the condition progresses, behavioral changes become more apparent.[59] Psychotic symptoms may be late signs and are difficult to control.[60] Finally, dementia does not occur exclusively during delirium. Although Alzheimer disease is the most common form,[61] a variety of other types exist, including Lewy body, Parkinson-associated, frontal lobe, and vascular dementias. A more detailed discussion of dementia is found in Chap. 27.

▶ Mild cognitive impairment

MCI is a relatively recent concept and describes a transitional level of neurocognitive impairment between that associated with normal aging and early dementia.[62–64] The presence of MCI predicts future dementia. Patients with MCI develop dementia at a rate of 12% per year.[65] Currently, its diagnosis relies on a combination of clinical observation and formal neuropsychological testing.[64,66] MCI is classified into four subtypes based on whether or not there is memory impairment and if multiple cognitive domains are affected.[67] The various subtypes are associated with different etiologies of dementia.

▶ Delirium

Delirium is a formally recognized psychiatric diagnosis.[58] It is a disturbance of fluctuating consciousness that develops over the course of hours to days. Inattention is a feature. There is altered cognition or perception not due to dementia. Also, there must be evidence that the condition is the result of a general medical condition.[58]

Emergence delirium

As its name implies, emergence delirium presents shortly after consciousness is regained following general anesthesia. It has been well-described in the pediatric population[68–71] and a clinically relevant, validated scale exists for its diagnosis in this group.[72] Less is known about the phenomenon in elderly surgical patients. No agreed upon set of diagnostic criteria exists, and it is unclear whether traditional instruments for diagnosing delirium are useful for diagnosing emergence delirium. However, it is not a trivial condition. For example, although it is generally thought to have little significance outside the recovery room, there is evidence that emergence delirium predicts traditional POD.[73] Therefore, the condition deserves further study.

Postoperative delirium

Unlike emergence delirium, POD does not present in the immediate postoperative period. Patients appear normal upon leaving the postanesthesia care unit. Typically, POD develops on postoperative days 1–3.[74] It may be sustained for more than a week. Two primary forms exist—hyperactive, the less common but easily identified variety, and the more common hypoactive type.[38,75] Unless clinicians have a high index of suspicion, hypoactive form of delirium is easily overlooked since these patients typically do not demand a great deal of attention from staff.

Clinical diagnosis of delirium can be challenging, especially for nonpsychiatrists. The Confusion Assessment Method (CAM) is a useful instrument for the diagnosis of POD.[76] It was originally developed for research and consists of a structured observation and interview that assesses for (1) the presence of an acute change in mental status with a fluctuating course, (2) inattention, (3) disorganized thinking, and (4) altered level of consciousness. Patients are diagnosed with delirium when features (1) and (2) are present along with either (3) or (4) (see Fig. 22-1). An attractive aspect of the CAM is that it can easily be administered by the staff caring for the patient. It requires little training, has a sensitivity and specificity exceeding 90%, and excellent positive and negative predictive values.[76] The CAM has also been modified for use in ventilated patients (CAM for the Intensive Care Unit).[44,45]

▶ Postoperative cognitive dysfunction

Many clinicians are aware of patients who complain after surgery of difficulties performing cognitive tasks that they were previously able to do without difficulty. Postoperative cognitive dysfunction (POCD) is the term used to describe this condition. It can consist of a variety of cognitive deficits. However, unlike patients with POD, those with POCD are generally alert and oriented. Also unlike delirium, POCD is not a formally recognized condition. In fact, some authorities doubt that it truly exists.[77] One issue is that patients' subjective complaints of POCD are often not borne out on objective testing.[78] The investigators

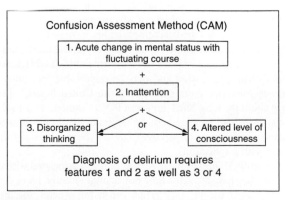

FIGURE 22-1 The Confusion Assessment Method. Features are based on a structured interview; see Ref. 76. *(Adapted and reprinted with permission from Ref. 44.)*

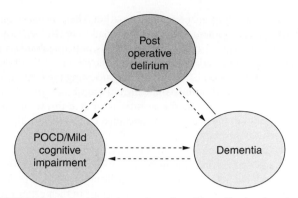

FIGURE 22-2 Relationships between dementia, mild cognitive impairment, postoperative cognitive dysfunction, and delirium. Preoperative dementia predicts postoperative delirium. The remaining associations are largely speculative.

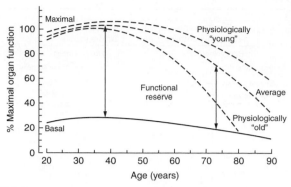

FIGURE 22-3 Age and functional reserve. Functional reserve is defined as the difference between maximal and basal organ function. Functional reserve determines the ability to compensate for physiological challenges. It decreases with age, irrespective of disease, and the rate of decrease varies from individual to individual and between organ systems within an individual. *(Reprinted with permission from Ref. 92.)*

of the International Study of Postoperative Cognitive Dysfunction (ISPOCD) group developed criteria for POCD based on changes between preoperative and postoperative scores on a set of neuropsychological tests that evaluate a broad range of cognitive domains.[32,35,42] Though this approach is not without controversy, it is the definition used in some of the most important studies on the subject.[32,35,47,56,79–81]

Another issue regarding POCD is defining the time point at which it can be said to exist. Some studies characterize POCD as cognitive dysfunction occurring in the early postoperative period.[57,82–84] Others do not consider POCD to exist unless changes are apparent at longer intervals from surgery (1 week to 1 year).[32,47,56,85] The latter approach seems more appropriate since residual effect of anesthetics and analgesics could easily influence cognitive function in the immediate postoperative period. In addition, lack of motivation may result in apparent declines in cognitive status early after an operation.[86,87]

The relationships between these four clinical entities are unclear (see Fig. 22-2). Dementia predicts delirium in both medical and surgical patients.[30,88] And there is some evidence that subtly decreased preoperative cognitive status predicts POD.[89] However, studies of POCD have excluded patients with preexisting cognitive impairment.[32,47,56] Thus, it is unclear whether such patients are likely to suffer further declines in cognitive status after surgery. Similarly, the effects of POD and POCD on long-term cognitive outcomes have not been well-defined.[13] For example, POD may predict POCD or MCI and, subsequently, dementia. Alternatively, there may be no relationship between POD and future POCD, MCI, and dementia. Data exist to support both hypotheses.[13,90,91]

MECHANISMS

The hallmark of normal aging is declining functional reserve. While basal function may be maintained, the ability to compensate for a variety of stresses is compromised. Declining functional reserve occurs across organ systems and is independent of age-associated disease.[92] (see Fig. 22-3). In the CNS, several changes are characteristic of normal aging. There is a generalized diminution in brain mass, neuron density, and complexity of neuronal interconnections.[93] The number of serotonin, acetylcholine, and dopamine receptors declines, combined with decreased production and increased postsynaptic degradation of a variety of neurotransmitters.[92–95] Perception thresholds for sensory input, including vision, touch, smell, hearing, temperature, proprioception and pain, are increased.[92] These changes, combined with the effects of age-related disease (e.g., stroke), limit the ability

of the brain to respond appropriately to a variety of stresses, including the challenges posed by anesthesia and surgery.

There are a number of putative mechanisms for POD. For example, a variety of neural pathways and neurotransmitters have been implicated. Altered metabolism of acetylcholine and dopamine, alterations in function of the γ-aminobutyric acid (GABA)ergic neurons and the thalamus, and perturbations of melatonin secretion, all may play a role.[96–99] However, the contribution of these to the development of POD is still mainly speculative. That said, the animal model of delirium is an anticholinergic one.[100,101] The association of POD with anticholinergic drugs also makes the neurotransmitter hypothesis attractive.[102]

Another possible mechanism is inflammatory. In a study of hip fracture patients, a normal preoperative white blood cell count was predictive of POD.[103] Since an increased white blood cell count would be expected as a result of injury, these results suggest that altered immune system response plays a role in the development of POD. There is evidence to support this theory. Cytokines are released as part of the surgical stress response,[104,105] and are associated with neuronal death.[106] Administration of interleukin-2 is associated with a high incidence of delirium.[107] In addition, tumor necrosis factor-α, interleukin-1 and other proinflammatory cytokines may play a role, while somatostatin and insulin-like growth factor-I may be protective. Finally, glucocorticoid excess has been implicated.[108]

Lastly, embolic brain injury may be the mechanism behind POD. Cardiac and orthopedic surgical procedures are among those most commonly associated with POD[26,83] and embolism figures prominently in both types of operations.[109–111]

Like POD, the mechanism behind POCD is not known. In vitro and animal studies suggest that inhalational and intravenous anesthetic agents alter neuronal function after exposure.[112–114] Neurons exposed to volatile anesthetics in vitro have increased oligomerization and cytoxicity of β-amyloid, the protein associated with Alzheimer disease.[114] In aged rats, exposure to anesthetic agents causes long-term declines in cognitive function.[115–117] However, the clinical relevance of these findings is unclear because studies examining the influence of regional versus general anesthesia on the incidence of POCD in humans have not found a difference between the two techniques.[56,57] One reason may be that patients who received regional anesthesia in those studies also received intravenous sedatives. Another may be that postoperative management was not controlled. Stress plays a role in cognitive

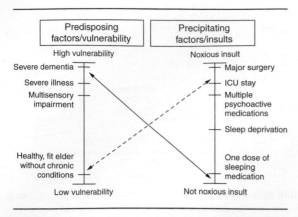

FIGURE 22-4 Patient vulnerability to postoperative cognitive dysfunction (POCD) and delirium (POD), and physiological stressors. Only minor stressors are required for POD and POCD to occur in highly vulnerable patients. Conversely, major stressors are required in patients with low vulnerability. *(Reprinted with permission from Ref. 132.)*

function.[118] Although regional anesthetic techniques attenuate the surgical stress response,[119–122] if these techniques were not continued into the postoperative period, any benefit may have been negated. Also, by not continuing regional analgesic techniques into the postoperative period, patients were exposed to higher doses of opiates, which may have influenced their cognitive outcomes.[123,124]

There may be a genetic component to POCD. The apolipoprotein E4 (apo E4) allele is associated with Alzheimer disease.[125] Investigations have not found an association between the apo E4 genotype and POCD.[126,127] However, that does not rule out the possibility of other genetic markers for POCD.

Finally, there have been efforts to identify a biochemical marker for POCD.[128,129] These sorts of studies ultimately may provide key information regarding the pathogenesis of POCD.

Though the exact mechanisms by which POD and POCD occur are not well understood, the likely cause is an acute insult in a vulnerable patient (see Fig. 22-4). The degree of surgical or physiological insult required to precipitate POD or POCD varies from patient to patient. In patients with a high degree of preoperative cognitive reserve, a substantial insult is required for POD and/or POCD to occur. Conversely, in patients with a lower degree of cognitive reserve, a relatively minor stress is all that is necessary for POD and/or POCD to develop.[130–132]

PREDICTORS

▶ Delirium

Delirium in medical (as opposed to surgical) patients is recognized as one of the *geriatric syndromes*. Thus, there has been a large amount of research concerning it. This work has lead to clinically relevant predictive models and interventional strategies.[88,133–135] Independent predictors of delirium in medical patients include vision impairment, significant cognitive dysfunction, severe illness, and dehydration.[134] In-hospital predictors include the use of physical restraints and bladder catheters, malnutrition, the addition of three or more medications, and iatrogenic events.[133] Other factors that have been implicated include age, male gender, decreased functional status, infection, depression, alcohol and drug abuse, and medications.[26,39,84,133,136,137] A wide variety of drugs are associated with delirium, many of which

are used frequently in the perioperative period. These include benzodiazepines, anticholinergics, opioids (especially meperidine, because of its atropine-like structure), corticosteroids, anticonvulsants, antidopaminergic antiemetics, and H_2 antagonists.[31,123,133,138–140] Although a recent critical review of the literature concerning the relationship of psychoactive medications and delirium found that the evidence for an association is weak, the authors attributed this to methodological issues in the studies and concluded that a relationship may indeed exist.[141]

Given the frequency with which it occurs, delirium could be considered a geriatric syndrome in surgical patients, as well. However, less research has addressed specifically delirium in surgical patients. This is significant because delirium that occurs in the postoperative period may differ from that in patients who are hospitalized for medical indications for at least two reasons.[142] First, at the time of admission, the characteristics of medical and surgical patients may differ. For example, nearly all patients hospitalized for medical reasons are either acutely ill or suffer from exacerbations of chronic disease. On the other hand, many operations are elective, and patients have been managed to ensure optimal physical status before entering the hospital. Second, the experience of anesthesia and surgery represents a significant stress not present in medical patients. For example, persistent effects of anesthetics and analgesics, as well as postsurgical pain contribute to delirium in surgical patients and are not present in medical patients. Thus, the predictors, approaches to prevention and treatment, and long-term consequences of POD may differ for delirium which occurs in medical patients. Fortunately, efforts are being made to systematically study delirium in surgical patients.

Patient factors

A number of preoperative factors are associated with POD. These include significant functional and cognitive impairment, sleep deprivation, immobility, visual and hearing impairment, dehydration, advanced age, low serum albumin, alcohol abuse, glucose and electrolyte abnormalities, comorbidity, anticholinergic drugs, polypharmacy, and benzodiazepines.[26,30,84,143–145] Type of procedure also influences the incidence of POD. Operations with a high likelihood of POD include (in descending order of frequency) hip fracture and aortic aneurysm repair, cardiac, intrathoracic, other orthopedic, intraperitoneal, and ophthalmological.[26,30] High levels of education appear to have a protective effect.[146] This may merely be indicative of a higher level baseline cognitive reserve.

Investigators have applied multivariate analysis to the study of POD risk factors. Marcantonio and colleagues performed a large, single center, prospective, cohort study with the goal of developing a clinical prediction rule for POD.[30] Patients ≥50 years old undergoing noncardiac surgery were enrolled. Independent predictors of POD were age ≥70 years, alcohol abuse, significant preexisting cognitive impairment, severely impaired physical function, type of surgery (aortic aneurysm and noncardiac thoracic), and markedly abnormal serum chemistries (K^+ <3.0 or >6.0 meq/L, Na^+ <130 or >150 meq/L, and glucose <60 or >300 mg/dL). Point values were assigned to each of the multivariate predictors and the risk of POD was determined by the number of points (see Table 22-1).

The prediction rule developed by Marcantonio et al. is clinically relevant and indicates that patients with significant impairments having high-risk surgery are likely to develop POD. However, delirium also occurs in patients with lesser degrees of illness. There are indications that even mild debility may predict POD. For example, subtle preoperative cognitive dysfunction and minimally reduced functional

Table 22-1

Independent Predictors and Clinical Prediction Rule for Postoperative Delirium Following Noncardiac Surgery

Variable	Odds Ratio (95% Confidence Interval)	Points
Age ≥70 years	3.3 (1.9–5.9)	1
Alcohol abuse	3.3 (1.4–8.3)	1
TICS score <3*	4.2 (2.4–7.3)	1
SAS class IV†	2.5 (1.2–5.2)	1
Markedly abnormal preoperative sodium, potassium, or glucose level‡	3.4 (1.3–8.7)	1
Aortic aneurysm surgery	8.3 (3.6–19.4)	2
Noncardiac thoracic surgery	3.5 (1.6–7.4)	1

Note: Patients with 0, 1–2, and ≥3 points have a 2%, 11%, and 50% risk of delirium, respectively.
*TICS indicates Telephone Interview for Cognitive Status (scores <30 suggest cognitive impairment).
†SAS indicates Specific Activity Scale (class IV represents severe physical impairment).
‡Markedly abnormal levels were defined as follows: sodium, <130 or >150 mmol/L; potassium, <3.0 or >6.0 mmol/L; and glucose, <3.3 or >16.7 mmol/L (<60 or >300 mg/dL).
Source: Reprinted with permission from Ref. 30.

status predict POD.[89] Thus, further investigations are required into the preoperative predictors of POD.

Intraoperative factors

The hypothesis that POD is the result of age-associated central cholinergic deficiency has been the driving force behind studies examining the role of intraoperative management as it relates to POD. Arguably, the most substantive decision regarding anesthetic management is whether patients should have a regional or general anesthetic. In theory, regional anesthetic techniques should be associated with reduced incidence of POD because these techniques minimize exposure to agents that influence central cholinergic activity and drugs that are associated with delirium in medical patients, such as opiates and benzodiazepines. Further, regional anesthesia deeply suppresses the neuroendocrine stress response to surgery.[119,147–150] Unfortunately, studies to date have not demonstrated that regional anesthetic techniques reduce the incidence of POD.[39,57,151]

For example, in a prospective trial of elderly patients undergoing total knee arthroplasty, Willams-Russo et al. randomized patients to either epidural or general anesthesia and found no difference in the incidence of POD related to anesthetic technique.[57] However, this study, like others[56], did not control postoperative management. It is possible that regional techniques need to be continued into the postoperative period to influence the occurrence of POD. Doing so would further attenuate the surgical stress response and minimize exposure to drugs associated with delirium.

Other intraoperative variables associated with POD include massive blood loss, the need for transfusion, and marked electrolyte or glucose abnormalities.[39] However, it is unclear whether these somehow induce POD or are merely indicators of sicker patients or more

severe surgical insult. Finally, hypoxia and hypotension may precipitate POD by decreasing oxygen delivery to the brain.[152]

Postoperative factors

Postoperative pain increases the risk of POD. But interestingly, maximum pain and pain with movement are not predictive of delirium. Only high levels of rest pain are associated with POD.[144] As a class, opiates are not associated with POD, except for meperidine.[40] This may be secondary to its atropine-like structure and influence on brain cholinergic activity. However, as noted above, opiates are associated with delirium in medical (nonsurgical) patients.[123,124] The disparity may relate to the fact that opiate use is ubiquitous in the perioperative period, and no study has been adequately powered to assess the relative contributions of the other members of the class to POD. Postoperative use of benzodiazepines has also been associated with POD.[40]

Little else is known about the postoperative risk factors for POD. However, as noted above, in-hospital predictors of delirium in medical patients include the use of physical restraints, malnutrition, the addition of three or more medications, the use of a urinary catheter, and iatrogenic events such as volume overload, urinary tract infections, and pressure ulcers.[133] Applying these principles to postoperative patients seems prudent, though maybe not possible (e.g., the addition of three or more medications is almost a given in surgical patients).

▶ Postoperative cognitive dysfunction

Less is known about the risk factors for POCD. Type of surgery certainly plays role. POCD occurs most frequently with patients who have undergone cardiac surgery.[32,153,154] To some extent, this may reflect the issues related to the stress of surgery and cardiopulmonary bypass. Intrinsic patient factors, such as atherosclerosis, may also be of significance.[155] Other operations associated with POCD include carotid endarterectomy and hip fracture repair. The ISPOCD group performed a large, well-known study whose intent was to determine whether intraoperative hypotension and hypoxemia are associated with POCD.[32] A large number of patient variables were assessed. Predictors of POCD at 1 week included increasing age and duration of anesthesia, low educational level, a second operation, postoperative infection, and respiratory complications. Only age was a predictor of POCD at 3 months. The same group performed a study to examine the effect of anesthetic management on the incidence of POCD.[56] Patients undergoing noncardiac surgery were randomized to receive either general or epidural anesthesia. Postoperative management was not controlled. There were no differences in the incidence of POCD based on type of anesthesia. Interestingly, unlike for POD, perioperative use of benzodiazepines is not associated with POCD.[32,156]

LONG-TERM OUTCOME

Delirium is associated with functional decline.[27,134,157–160] What is less clear is whether or not POD affects long-term cognitive outcome. Jackson et al. recently reviewed the issue of postdischarge cognitive outcome in patients who had had delirium, and concluded that, though weak, the available evidence suggests that there is a relationship between delirium and cognitive decline.[13] Of nine studies included in the review, only one included surgical patients exclusively[161] and it found that delirium at the time of hospital admission predicted future cognitive decline. However, delirium that developed after hospital admission did not predict future cognitive decline.

A more recent study of hip fracture patients suggests that in-hospital cognitive impairment predicts 1-year cognitive and functional impairment.[162] However, methodological issues make it difficult to determine the contribution of POD to the functional and cognitive outcomes.

Similarly, there is little information concerning the long-term implications of POCD. There is evidence that coronary artery bypass grafting is associated with a high incidence of POCD at 5 years.[154] More recent studies support the hypothesis that long-term decline is a function of illness not the bypass operation, per se. For example, the incidence of cognitive decline at 1 year is the same whether one has coronary artery bypass graft surgery or percutaneous revascularization, suggesting that atherosclerosis, not surgery, may be the culprit.[155,163]

PREVENTION AND MANAGEMENT

▶ Delirium

The first step in preventing POD is to identify those at risk. The preoperative visit should include a drug history and screening for depression, substance abuse, and cognitive decline. A recent study examined the utility of pharmacological prophylaxis for POD. Kalisvaart and colleagues randomized hip fracture patients to receive either 1.5 mg/day of haloperidol or placebo starting preoperatively and continuing for up to 3 days postoperatively.[164] Although haloperidol did not reduce the incidence of POD, it diminished the severity and duration of delirium. Further study will clarify the role of preoperative strategies to prevent POD.

Intraoperatively, the specific anesthetic technique is probably less important than the care with which it is applied. Adequate oxygenation and perfusion should be maintained. When appropriate, patients should be normocarbic. Glucose and electrolyte abnormalities should be corrected. Benzodiazepines, centrally acting anticholinergics, and meperidine are best avoided. In order to compensate for alterations in body composition, drug sensitivity, and clearance and elimination that occur with aging[165–172] (see Chap. 8), dosages should be altered and short-acting agents are preferred.

There has been little inquiry into postoperative measures for preventing POD. In medical patients, a protocolized intervention aimed at managing six risk factors for delirium (cognitive impairment, sleep deprivation, immobility, visual and auditory impairment, and dehydration) reduced the incidence of delirium.[135] In a study of hip fracture patients, geriatrics consultation, which provided recommendations to ensure optimal medical, nutritional, and rehabilitation care, decreased the incidence delirium and severe delirium.[173] Recommendations focused on the following: adequate CNS oxygen delivery, fluid and electrolyte balance, simplification of medication regimens, bowel and bladder function, nutrition, mobilization and rehabilitation, analgesia, appropriate environmental stimuli, appropriate treatment of agitated delirium and prevention, and early recognition and treatment of major complications. Although these interventions did not reduce length of stay[173] or improve long-term outcomes,[174] it is reasonable to apply this approach broadly to surgical patients. In essence, the recommendations are a formalized approach to the meticulous care required by geriatric surgical patients. With increased awareness and education, they could easily become part of routine postoperative care of the elderly.

Pain management deserves special mention. Pain should be treated aggressively while avoiding drugs associated with delirium. Thus,

there may be a role for the use of sophisticated regional analgesic techniques, such as in-dwelling perineural catheters, which are associated with reduced incidence of POD.[175]

It is important to recognize that POD may be the presenting symptom of a number of complications, including sepsis, urinary tract infections, myocardial infarction, stroke, and pneumonia.[124] Thus, the first step in managing POD is to identify and treat organic causes. After addressing possible medical causes of POD, measures should be taken to reorient the patient. If agitation is endangering the patient, haloperidol or atypical antipsychotics[176] may be used (see Table 22-2). If the delirium is due to a withdrawal syndrome, beta-blockers, clonidine, and benzodiazepines may be indicated. (This is the only instance for which benzodiazepines are considered a first-line treatment for POD.) For alcohol withdrawal, thiamine should be administered also. Finally, psychosocial and occupational and physical therapy referrals will aid in functional rehabilitation.

▶ Postoperative cognitive dysfunction

Until POCD is further defined as a clinical entity and its predictors and consequences determined, it is difficult to make recommendations for its prevention and treatment. Patients who complain of postoperative cognitive changes should be followed closely and reassured since POCD persists past 1 year in only 1–2% of cases. When appropriate, workup for other causes of cognitive decline, such as stroke or Alzheimer disease, should be pursued.

FUTURE DIRECTIONS

Although understanding of issues related to POD and POCD is improving, it should be clear from the above that current understanding of these conditions, while not rudimentary, is far from ideal. Several issues should take priority. First, a consensus needs to be reached regarding the definition of POCD that considers the timing of the dysfunction relative to surgery as well as what neuropsychological criteria constitute the condition. This will likely require longitudinal studies that consider the functional implications of postoperative cognitive impairment as well as declines in test scores. Second, well-designed studies are needed to assess the relationship between POD and long-term cognitive decline. If an association were found, it would imply that the effects of POD are even more significant than previously appreciated. It could also help direct efforts to understand the pathophysiological basis of both conditions. Studies addressing these issues should be performed in a manner that takes into account the various age subcategories of the "elderly" (from "older" to the "oldest-old") and the patients' degree of frailty.

Finally, investigations into the effect of anesthetic technique (e.g., regional vs. general) on POD and POCD are needed in which post- as well as intraoperative management is controlled and optimized.

This work will be expensive and requires much effort. However, given the enormous economic and public health implications of POD and POCD, these studies are vital.

SUMMARY

The aging population will profoundly influence the practice of perioperative medicine. POD and POCD are common sequelae in elderly surgical patients with significant public health implications that will only increase over time. The mechanisms by which POD and

Table 22-2

Pharmacologic Treatment Options for Postoperative Delirium

Class and Drug	Dose	Adverse Effects	Comments
Antipsychotic			
Haloperidol	0.5–1.0 mg twice daily orally, with additional doses every 4 h as needed (peak effect, 4–6 h) 0.5–1.0 mg intramuscularly; observe after 30–60 min and repeat if needed (peak effect, 20–40 min)	Extrapyramidal symptoms, especially if dose is >3 mg per day Prolonged corrected QT interval on electrocardiogram Avoid in patients with withdrawal syndrome, hepatic insufficiency, neuroleptic malignant syndrome	Usually agent of choice Effectiveness demonstrated in randomized, controlled trials Avoid intravenous use because of short duration of action
Atypical antipsychotic			
Risperidone Olanzapine Quetiapine	0.5 mg twice daily 2.5–5.0 mg once daily 2.5–5.0 mg once daily	Extrapyramidal effects equivalent to or slightly less than those with haloperidol Prolonged corrected QT interval on electrocardiogram	Tested only in small uncontrolled studies Associated with increased mortality rate among older patients with dementia
Benzodiazepine			
Lorazepam	0.5–1.0 mg orally, with additional doses every 4 h as needed*	Paradoxical excitation respiratory depression, oversedation	Second-line agent Associated with prolongation and worsening of delirium symptoms demonstrated in clinical trial Reserve for use in patients undergoing sedative and alcohol withdrawal, those with Parkinson disease, and those with neuroleptic malignant syndrome
Antidepressant			
Trazodone	25–150 mg orally at bedtime	Oversedation	Tested only in uncontrolled studies

*Intravenous use of lorazepam should be reserved for emergencies.
Source: Adapted and reprinted with permission from Ref. 31.

POCD occur are unknown. However, they are likely the result of an acute surgical insult in patients made vulnerable by decreased cognitive function reserve resulting from a combination of age-associated CNS changes and disease. Research into the mechanisms, predictors, and sequelae of POCD and POD as well as appropriate prevention and treatment strategies has improved understanding of these conditions; though much work remains.

KEY POINTS

- ▶ The aging population will result in ever-increasing numbers of elderly patients requiring surgery.
- ▶ POD and POCD are two of the most common complications in elderly surgical patients and are associated with poor outcome.
- ▶ Dementia, MCI, and POD and POCD may be related. However, the interactions between the four entities are not well-understood.
- ▶ The mechanisms of POD and POCD are likely multifactorial and the result of an acute insult in a vulnerable patient. In patients with a high degree of baseline cognitive reserve, a major surgical and anesthetic insult is necessary to precipitate POD and POCD. Similarly, in patients with a low degree of baseline cognitive reserve, a minor operation may lead to the conditions.

- ▶ Intraoperative management (i.e., regional vs. general anesthesia) appears to play little role in the development of POD and POCD.
- ▶ POD may be an early sign of other complications.

KEY REFERENCES

- ▶ Inouye SK, van Dyck CH, Alessi CA, et al. Clarifying confusion: the confusion assessment method. A new method for detection of delirium. *Ann Intern Med.* 1990;113(12):941–948.
- ▶ Inouye SK, Bogardus ST Jr, Charpentier PA, et al. A multicomponent intervention to prevent delirium in hospitalized older patients. *N Engl J Med.* 1999;340(9):669–676.
- ▶ Inouye SK, Viscoli CM, Horwitz RI, et al. A predictive model for delirium in hospitalized elderly medical patients based on admission characteristics. *Ann Intern Med.* 1993;119(6):474–481.
- ▶ Johnson T, Monk T, Rasmussen LS, et al. Postoperative cognitive dysfunction in middle-aged patients. *Anesthesiology.* 2002;96(6):1351–1357.
- ▶ Marcantonio ER, Juarez G, Goldman L, et al. The relationship of postoperative delirium with psychoactive medications. *JAMA.* 1994;272(19):1518–1522.

▸ Marcantonio ER, Goldman L, Mangione CM, et al. A clinical prediction rule for delirium after elective noncardiac surgery. *JAMA.* 1994;271(2):134–139.

▸ Moller JT, Cluitmans P, Rasmussen LS, et al. Long-term postoperative cognitive dysfunction in the elderly ISPOCD1 study. ISPOCD investigators. International Study of Post-Operative Cognitive Dysfunction. *Lancet.* 1998;351:857–861.

▸ Rasmussen LS, Johnson T, Kuipers HM, et al. Does anaesthesia cause postoperative cognitive dysfunction? A randomized study of regional versus general anaesthesia in 438 elderly patients. *Acta Anaesthesiol Scand.* 2003;47(3):260–266.

REFERENCES

1. Projected Population Change in the United States, by Age and Sex: 2000 to 2050. Available at http://www.census.gov/ipc/www/usinterimproj/natprojtab02b.pdf. 2004.

2. Projected Population of the United States, by Age and Sex: 2000 to 2050. Available at http://www.census.gov/ipc/www/usinterimproj/natprojtab02a.pdf. 2004.

3. Bailes BK. Perioperative care of the elderly surgical patient. *AORN J.* 2000;72:186–207.

4. Ochsner A. Is the risk of operation too great in the elderly? *Geriatrics.* 1927;22:121.

5. Hosking MP, Warner MA, Lobdell CM, et al. Outcomes of surgery in patients 90 years of age and older. *JAMA.* 1989;261:1909–1915.

6. Hosking MP, Lobdell CM, Warner MA, et al. Anaesthesia for patients over 90 years of age. Outcomes after regional and general anaesthetic techniques for two common surgical procedures. *Anaesthesia.* 1989; 44:142–147.

7. Warner MA, Hosking MP, Lobdell CM, et al. Surgical procedures among those greater than or equal to 90 years of age. A population-based study in Olmsted County, Minnesota, 1975–1985. *Ann Surg.* 1988; 207:380–386.

8. Warner MA, Saletel RA, Schroeder DR, et al. Outcomes of anesthesia and surgery in people 100 years of age and older. *J Am Geriatr Soc.* 1998; 46:988–993.

9. Tiret L, Desmonts JM, Hatton F, Vourc'h G. Complications associated with anaesthesia—a prospective survey in France. *Can Anaesth Soc J.* 1986;33:336–344.

10. Moller JT, Pedersen T, Rasmussen LS, et al. Randomized evaluation of pulse oximetry in 20,802 patients. I. Design, demography, pulse oximetry failure rate, and overall complication rate. *Anesthesiology.* 1993;78: 436–444.

11. Larsen SF, Zaric D, Boysen G. Postoperative cerebrovascular accidents in general surgery. *Acta Anaesthesiol Scand.* 1988;32:698–701.

12. Kam PC, Calcroft RM. Perioperative stroke in general surgical patients. *Anaesthesia.* 1997;52:879–883.

13. Jackson JC, Gordon SM, Hart RP, et al. The association between delirium and cognitive decline: a review of the empirical literature. *Neuropsychol Rev.* 2004;14:87–98.

14. Olofsson B, Lundstrom M, Borssen B, et al. Delirium is associated with poor rehabilitation outcome in elderly patients treated for femoral neck fractures. *Scand J Caring Sci.* 2005;19:119–127.

15. Savageau JA, Stanton BA, Jenkins CD, Frater RW. Neuropsychological dysfunction following elective cardiac operation. II. A six-month reassessment. *J Thorac Cardiovasc Surg.* 1982;84:595–600.

16. Savageau JA, Stanton BA, Jenkins CD, Klein MD. Neuropsychological dysfunction following elective cardiac operation. I. Early assessment. *J Thorac Cardiovasc Surg.* 1982;84:585–594.

17. Shaw PJ, Bates D, Cartlidge NE, et al. Early intellectual dysfunction following coronary bypass surgery. *Q J Med.* 1986;58:59–68.

18. Hammeke TA, Hastings JE. Neuropsychologic alterations after cardiac operation. *J Thorac Cardiovasc Surg.* 1988;96:326–331.

19. Shaw PJ, Bates D, Cartlidge NE, et al. Long-term intellectual dysfunction following coronary artery bypass graft surgery: a six-month follow-up study. *Q J Med.* 1987;62:259–268.

20. Treasure T, Smith PL, Newman S, et al. Impairment of cerebral function following cardiac and other major surgery. *Eur J Cardiothorac Surg.* 1989;3:216–221.

21. Murkin JM, Martzke JS, Buchan AM, et al. A randomized study of the influence of perfusion technique and pH management strategy in 316 patients undergoing coronary artery bypass surgery. II. Neurologic and cognitive outcomes. *J Thorac Cardiovasc Surg.* 1995;110:349–362.

22. Lawrence VA, Hilsenbeck SG, Mulrow CD, et al. Incidence and hospital stay for cardiac and pulmonary complications after abdominal surgery. *J Gen Intern Med.* 1995;10:671–678.

23. Ashton CM, Petersen NJ, Wray NP, et al. The incidence of perioperative myocardial infarction in men undergoing noncardiac surgery. *Ann Intern Med.* 1993;118:504–510.

24. Zakriya K, Sieber FE, Christmas C, et al. Brief postoperative delirium in hip fracture patients affects functional outcome at three months. *Anesth Analg.* 2004;98:1798–1802.

25. Roca R. Psychosocial aspects of surgical care in the elderly patient. *Surg Clin North Am.* 1994;74:223–243.

26. O'Keeffe ST, Ni Chonchubhair A. Postoperative delirium in the elderly. *Br J Anaesth.* 1994;73:673–687.

27. Gustafson Y, Berggren D, Brannstrom B, et al. Acute confusional states in elderly patients treated for femoral neck fracture. *J Am Geriatr Soc.* 1988;36:525–530.

28. Billig N, Stockton P, Cohen-Mansfield J. Cognitive and affective changes after cataract surgery in an elderly population. *Am J Geriatr Psychiatry.* 1996;4:29–38.

29. Goldstein MZ, Young BL, Fogel BS, Benedict RH. Occurrence and predictors of short-term mental and functional changes in older adults undergoing elective surgery under general anesthesia. *Am J Geriatr Psychiatry.* 1998;6:42–52.

30. Marcantonio ER, Goldman L, Mangione CM, et al. A clinical prediction rule for delirium after elective noncardiac surgery. *JAMA.* 1994;271:134–139.

31. Inouye SK. Delirium in older persons. *N Engl J Med.* 2006;354: 1157–1165.

32. Moller JT, Cluitmans P, Rasmussen LS, et al. Long-term postoperative cognitive dysfunction in the elderly ISPOCD1 study. ISPOCD investigators. International Study of Post-Operative Cognitive Dysfunction. *Lancet.* 1998;351:857–861.

33. Lee Y, Kim JH, Lee KJ, et al. Association of cognitive status with functional limitation and disability in older adults. *Aging Clin Exp Res.* 2005; 17:20–28.

34. Inouye SK, Peduzzi PN, Robison JT, et al. Importance of functional measures in predicting mortality among older hospitalized patients. *JAMA.* 1998;279:1187–1193.

35. Rasmussen LS, Larsen K, Houx P, et al. The assessment of postoperative cognitive function. *Acta Anaesthesiol Scand.* 2001;45:275–289.

36. Lewis MS, Maruff PT, Silbert BS. Examination of the use of cognitive domains in postoperative cognitive dysfunction after coronary artery bypass graft surgery. *Ann Thorac Surg.* 2005;80:910–916.

37. Lewis MS, Maruff PT, Silbert BS, et al. The sensitivity and specificity of three common statistical rules for the classification of postoperative cognitive dysfunction following coronary artery bypass surgery. *Acta Anaesthesiol Scand.* 2006;50:50–57.

38. Marcantonio E, Ta T, Duthie E, Resnick NM. Delirium severity and psychomotor types: their relationship with outcomes after hip fracture repair. *J Am Geriatr Soc.* 2002;50:850–857.

39. Marcantonio ER, Goldman L, Orav EJ, et al. The association of intraoperative factors with the development of postoperative delirium. *Am J Med.* 1998;105:380–384.

40. Marcantonio ER, Juarez G, Goldman L, et al. The relationship of postoperative delirium with psychoactive medications. *JAMA.* 1994;272: 1518–1522.

41. Marcantonio ER, Simon SE, Bergmann MA, et al. Delirium symptoms in post-acute care: prevalent, persistent, and associated with poor functional recovery. *J Am Geriatr Soc.* 2003;51:4–9.

42. Rasmussen LS, Siersma VD. Postoperative cognitive dysfunction: true deterioration versus random variation. *Acta Anaesthesiol Scand.* 2004; 48:1137–1143.

43. Ely EW, Gautam S, Margolin R, et al. The impact of delirium in the intensive care unit on hospital length of stay. *Intensive Care Med.* 2001; 27:1892–1900.

44. Ely EW, Inouye SK, Bernard GR, et al. Delirium in mechanically ventilated patients: validity and reliability of the confusion assessment method for the intensive care unit (CAM-ICU). *JAMA.* 2001;286:2703–2710.

45. Ely EW, Margolin R, Francis J, et al. Evaluation of delirium in critically ill patients: validation of the Confusion Assessment Method for the Intensive Care Unit (CAM-ICU). *Crit Care Med.* 2001;29:1370–1379.

46. Ely EW, Shintani A, Truman B, et al. Delirium as a predictor of mortality in mechanically ventilated patients in the intensive care unit. *JAMA.* 2004;291:1753–1762.

47. Johnson T, Monk T, Rasmussen LS, et al. Postoperative cognitive dysfunction in middle-aged patients. *Anesthesiology.* 2002;96:1351–1357.

48. Suzman R, Riley MW. Introducing the "oldest old." *Milbank Mem Fund Q Health Soc.* 1985;63:177–186.

49. Kinsella KV, Velkoff VA. *An Aging World.* Washington DC: U.S. Government Printing Office; 2001.

50. Cohen NH. Anesthetic depth and long-term mortality—in response. *Anesth Analg.* 2005;101:1559–1560.

51. Cohen NH. Anesthetic depth is not (yet) a predictor of mortality! *Anesth Analg.* 2005;100:1–3.

52. Rockwood K. What would make a definition of frailty successful? *Age Ageing.* 2005;34:432–434.

53. Levy WJ. Is anesthetic-related mortality a statistical illness? *Anesth Analg.* 2005;101:1238;author reply 1239–1240, 1240–1241.

54. Folstein MF, Folstein SE, McHugh PR. "Mini-mental state." A practical method for grading the cognitive state of patients for the clinician. *J Psychiatr Res.* 1975;12:189–198.

55. Folks DG, Freeman AM, III, Sokol RS, et al. Cognitive dysfunction after coronary artery bypass surgery: a case-controlled study. *South Med J.* 1988;81:202–206.

56. Rasmussen LS, Johnson T, Kuipers HM, et al. Does anaesthesia cause postoperative cognitive dysfunction? A randomized study of regional versus general anaesthesia in 438 elderly patients. *Acta Anaesthesiol Scand.* 2003;47:260–266.

57. Williams-Russo P, Sharrock NE, Mattis S, et al. Cognitive effects after epidural vs. general anesthesia in older adults. A randomized trial. *JAMA.* 1995;274:44–50.

58. American Psychiatric Association. *Diagnostic and Statistical Manual of Mental Disorders.* 4th ed. Text revision. Washington DC: American Psychiatric Association; 2000.

59. Kawas CH. Clinical practice. Early Alzheimer's disease. *N Engl J Med.* 2003;349:1056–1063.

60. Mega MS, Cummings JL, Fiorello T, Gornbein J. The spectrum of behavioral changes in Alzheimer's disease. *Neurology.* 1996;46:130–135.

61. Bachman DL, Wolf PA, Linn R, et al. Prevalence of dementia and probable senile dementia of the Alzheimer type in the Framingham Study. *Neurology.* 1992;42:115–119.

62. Petersen RC, Morris JC. Mild cognitive impairment as a clinical entity and treatment target. *Arch Neurol.* 2005;62:1160–1163; discussion 1167.

63. Petersen RC. Mild cognitive impairment: where are we? *Alzheimer Dis Assoc Disord.* 2005;19:166–169.

64. Winblad B, Palmer K, Kivipelto M, et al. Mild cognitive impairment—beyond controversies, towards a consensus: report of the International Working Group on Mild Cognitive Impairment. *J Intern Med.* 2004; 256:240–246.

65. Petersen RC, Morris JC. Clinical features. In: Petersen RC, ed. *Mild Cognitive Impairment: Aging to Alzheimer's Disease.* New York: Oxford University Press; 2003:15–40.

66. Petersen RC. Mild cognitive impairment as a diagnostic entity. *J Intern Med.* 2004;256:183–194.

67. Petersen RC. Clinical dementia rating (CDR): current version and scoring rules. In: Petersen RC, ed. *Mild Cognitive Impairment: Aging to Alzheimer's Disease.* New York: Oxford University Press; 2003:1–14.

68. Davis PJ, Cohen IT, McGowan FX, Jr, Latta K. Recovery characteristics of desflurane versus halothane for maintenance of anesthesia in pediatric ambulatory patients. *Anesthesiology.* 1994;80:298–302.

69. Welborn LG, Hannallah RS, Norden JM, et al. Comparison of emergence and recovery characteristics of sevoflurane, desflurane, and halothane in pediatric ambulatory patients. *Anesth Analg.* 1996;83:917–920.

70. Cole JW, Murray DJ, McAllister JD, Hirshberg GE. Emergence behavior in children: defining the incidence of excitement and agitation following anaesthesia. *Paediatr Anaesth.* 2002;12:442–447.

71. Mayer J, Boldt J, Rohm KD, et al. Desflurane anesthesia after sevoflurane inhaled induction reduces severity of emergence agitation in children undergoing minor ear-nose-throat surgery compared with sevoflurane induction and maintenance. *Anesth Analg.* 2006;102:400–404.

72. Sikich N, Lerman J. Development and psychometric evaluation of the pediatric anesthesia emergence delirium scale. *Anesthesiology.* 2004; 100:1138–1145.

73. Sharma PT, Sieber FE, Zakriya KJ, et al. Recovery room delirium predicts postoperative delirium after hip-fracture repair. *Anesth Analg.* 2005;101:1215–1220.

74. Duppils GS, Wikblad K. Acute confusional states in patients undergoing hip surgery. A prospective observation study. *Gerontology.* 2000; 46:36–43.

75. Inouye SK, Foreman MD, Mion LC, et al. Nurses' recognition of delirium and its symptoms: comparison of nurse and researcher ratings. *Arch Intern Med.* 2001;161:2467–2473.

76. Inouye SK, van Dyck CH, Alessi CA, et al. Clarifying confusion: the confusion assessment method. A new method for detection of delirium. *Ann Intern Med.* 1990;113:941–948.

77. Selwood A, Orrell M. Long term cognitive dysfunction in older people after non-cardiac surgery. *Br Med J.* 2004;328:120–121.

78. Dijkstra JB, Jolles J. Postoperative cognitive dysfunction versus complaints: a discrepancy in long-term findings. *Neuropsychol Rev.* 2002; 12:1–14.

79. Symes E, Maruff P, Ajani A, Currie J. Issues associated with the identification of cognitive change following coronary artery bypass grafting. *Aust N Z J Psychiatry.* 2000;34:770–784.

80. Canet J, Raeder J, Rasmussen LS, et al. Cognitive dysfunction after minor surgery in the elderly. *Acta Anaesthesiol Scand.* 2003;47:1204–1210.

81. McCusker J, Cole MG, Dendukuri N, Belzile E. Does delirium increase hospital stay? *J Am Geriatr Soc.* 2003;51:1539–1546.

82. Campbell DN, Lim M, Muir MK, et al. A prospective randomized study of local versus general anaesthesia for cataract surgery. *Anaesthesia.* 1993;48:422–428.

83. Dyer CB, Ashton CM, Teasdale TA. Postoperative delirium. A review of 80 primary data-collection studies. *Arch Intern Med.* 1995;155:461–465.

84. Parikh SS, Chung F. Postoperative delirium in the elderly. *Anesth Analg.* 1995;80:1223–1232.

85. Moller JT, Svennild I, Johannessen NW, et al. Perioperative monitoring with pulse oximetry and late postoperative cognitive dysfunction. *Br J Anaesth.* 1993;71:340–347.

86. Newton DE, Thornton C, Konieczko KM, et al. Auditory-evoked response and awareness: a study in volunteers at sub-MAC concentrations of isoflurane. *Br J Anaesth.* 1992;69:122–129.

87. Pockett S. Anesthesia and the electrophysiology of auditory consciousness. *Conscious Cogn.* 1999;8:45–61.

88. Inouye SK. Predisposing and precipitating factors for delirium in hospitalized older patients. *Dement Geriatr Cogn Disord.* 1999;10:393–400.

89. Jankowski CJ, Trenerry MR, Cook DJ, et al. Mild reductions in preoperative cognitive and functional status are associated with postoperative delirium. *Anesth Analg.* 2005;100:S–178.

90. Jankowski CJ, Trenerry MR, Cook DJ, et al. Postoperative delirium does not predict long-term postoperative cognitive dysfunction or functional decline. *Anesth Analg.* 2006;102:S–106.

91. Lundstrom M, Edlund A, Bucht G, et al. Dementia after delirium in patients with femoral neck fractures. *J Am Geriatr Soc.* 2003;51:1002–1006.

92. Muravchick S. Anesthesia for the elderly. In: Miller RD, ed. *Anesthesia.* 5th ed. Philadelphia: Churchill Livingstone; 2000:2140–2156.

93. Creasey H, Rapoport SI. The aging human brain. *Ann Neurol.* 1985; 17:2–10.

94. Severson JA. Neurotransmitter receptors and aging. *J Am Geriatr Soc.* 1984;32:24–27.

95. Wong DF, Wagner HN, Jr, Dannals RF, et al. Effects of age on dopamine and serotonin receptors measured by positron tomography in the living human brain. *Science.* 1984;226:1393–1396.

96. Trzepacz PT. Is there a final common neural pathway in delirium? Focus on acetylcholine and dopamine. *Semin Clin Neuropsychiatry.* 2000;5:132–148.

97. Gaudreau JD, Gagnon P. Psychotogenic drugs and delirium pathogenesis: the central role of the thalamus. *Med Hypotheses.* 2005;64: 471–475.

98. Uchida K, Aoki T, Ishizuka B. Postoperative delirium and plasma melatonin. *Med Hypotheses.* 1999;53:103–106.

99. Keverne EB. GABA-ergic neurons and the neurobiology of schizophrenia and other psychoses. *Brain Res Bull.* 1999;48:467–473.

100. Leavitt ML, Trzepacz PT, Ciongoli K. Rat model of delirium: atropine dose-response relationships. *J Neuropsychiatry Clin Neurosci.* 1994;6:279–284.

101. Trzepacz PT, Leavitt M, Ciongoli K. An animal model for delirium. *Psychosomatics.* 1992;33:404–415.

102. Tune LE, Egeli S. Acetylcholine and delirium. *Dement Geriatr Cogn Disord.* 1999;10:342–344.

103. Zakriya KJ, Christmas C, Wenz JF, Sr, et al. Preoperative factors associated with postoperative change in confusion assessment method score in hip fracture patients. *Anesth Analg.* 2002;94:1628–1632.

104. Kehlet H. The stress response to surgery: release mechanisms and the modifying effect of pain relief. *Acta Chir Scand Suppl.* 1989;550:22–28.

105. Kudoh A, Katagai H, Takazawa T, Matsuki A. Plasma proinflammatory cytokine response to surgical stress in elderly patients. *Cytokine.* 2001; 15:270–273.

106. Tarkowski E, Rosengren L, Blomstrand C, et al. Early intrathecal production of interleukin-6 predicts the size of brain lesion in stroke. *Stroke.* 1995;26:1393–1398.

107. Rosenberg SA, Lotze MT, Yang JC, et al. Experience with the use of high-dose interleukin-2 in the treatment of 652 cancer patients. *Ann Surg.* 1989;210:474–484; discussion 484–485.

108. Olsson T. Activity in the hypothalamic-pituitary-adrenal axis and delirium. *Dement Geriatr Cogn Disord.* 1999;10:345–349.

109. Clark RE, Brillman J, Davis DA, et al. Microemboli during coronary artery bypass grafting. Genesis and effect on outcome. *J Thorac Cardiovasc Surg.* 1995;109:249–257; discussion 257–258.

110. Pugsley W, Klinger L, Paschalis C, et al. The impact of microemboli during cardiopulmonary bypass on neuropsychological functioning. *Stroke.* 1994; 25:1393–1399.

111. Edmonds CR, Barbut D, Hager D, Sharrock NE. Intraoperative cerebral arterial embolization during total hip arthroplasty. *Anesthesiology.* 2000;93:315–318.

112. Hanning CD, Blokland A, Johnson M, Perry EK. Effects of repeated anaesthesia on central cholinergic function in the rat cerebral cortex. *Eur J Anaesthesiol.* 2003;20:93–97.

113. Jevtovic-Todorovic V, Todorovic SM, Mennerick S, et al. Nitrous oxide (laughing gas) is an NMDA antagonist, neuroprotectant, and neurotoxin. *Nat Med.* 1998;4:460–463.

114. Eckenhoff RG, Johansson JS, Wei H, et al. Inhaled anesthetic enhancement of amyloid-beta oligomerization and cytotoxicity. *Anesthesiology.* 2004;101:703–709.

115. Blokland A, Honig W, Jolles J. Long-term consequences of repeated pentobarbital anaesthesia on choice reaction time performance in ageing rats. *Br J Anaesth.* 2001;87:781–783.

116. Culley DJ, Baxter M, Yukhananov R, Crosby G. The memory effects of general anesthesia persist for weeks in young and aged rats. *Anesth Analg.* 2003;96:1004–1009.

117. Culley DJ, Baxter MG, Yukhananov R, Crosby G. Long-term impairment of acquisition of a spatial memory task following isoflurane-nitrous oxide anesthesia in rats. *Anesthesiology.* 2004;100:309–314.

118. Sapolsky RM. Glucocorticoids and hippocampal atrophy in neuropsychiatric disorders. *Arch Gen Psychiatry.* 2000;57:925–935.

119. Cosgrove DO, Jenkins JS. The effects of epidural anaesthesia on the pituitary-adrenal response to surgery. *Clin Sci Mol Med.* 1974;46: 403–407.

120. Gordon NH, Scott DB, Percy Robb IW. Modification of plasma corticosteroid concentrations during and after surgery by epidural blockade. *Br Med J.* 1973;1:581–583.

121. Hole A, Unsgaard G, Breivik H. Monocyte functions are depressed during and after surgery under general anaesthesia but not under epidural anaesthesia. *Acta Anaesthesiol Scand.* 1982;26:301–307.

122. Moller IW, Hjortso E, Krantz T, et al. The modifying effect of spinal anaesthesia on intra- and postoperative adrenocortical and hyperglycemic response to surgery. *Acta Anaesthesiol Scand.* 1984;28:266–269.

123. Schor JD, Levkoff SE, Lipsitz LA, et al. Risk factors for delirium in hospitalized elderly. *JAMA.* 1992;267:827–831.

124. Francis J, Martin D, Kapoor WN. A prospective study of delirium in hospitalized elderly. *JAMA.* 1990;263:1097–1101.

125. Huang Y. Apolipoprotein E and Alzheimer disease. *Neurology.* 2006; 66:S79–S85.

126. Rentowl P, Hanning CD. Odor identification as a marker for postoperative cognitive dysfunction: a pilot study. *Anaesthesia.* 2004;59:337–343.

127. Abildstrom H, Christiansen M, Siersma VD, Rasmussen LS. Apolipoprotein E genotype and cognitive dysfunction after noncardiac surgery. *Anesthesiology.* 2004;101:855–861.

128. Iohom G, Szarvas S, Larney V, et al. Perioperative plasma concentrations of stable nitric oxide products are predictive of cognitive dysfunction after laparoscopic cholecystectomy. *Anesth Analg.* 2004;99: 1245–1252.

129. Rasmussen LS, Christiansen M, Hansen PB, Moller JT. Do blood levels of neuron-specific enolase and S-100 protein reflect cognitive dysfunction after coronary artery bypass? *Acta Anaesthesiol Scand.* 1999;43:495–500.

130. Richards M, Deary IJ. A life course approach to cognitive reserve: a model for cognitive aging and development? *Ann Neurol.* 2005;58:617–622.

131. Satz P. Brain reserve capacity on symptom onset after brain injury: a formulation and review of evidence for threshold theory. *Neuropsychology.* 1993;7:273–295.

132. Inouye SK. Delirium in hospitalized older patients: recognition and risk factors. *J Geriatr Psychiatry Neurol.* 1998;11:118–125; discussion 157–158.

133. Inouye SK, Charpentier PA. Precipitating factors for delirium in hospitalized elderly persons. Predictive model and interrelationship with baseline vulnerability. *JAMA.* 1996;275:852–857.

134. Inouye SK, Viscoli CM, Horwitz RI, et al. A predictive model for delirium in hospitalized elderly medical patients based on admission characteristics. *Ann Intern Med.* 1993;119:474–481.

135. Inouye SK, Bogardus ST, Jr, Charpentier PA, et al. A multicomponent intervention to prevent delirium in hospitalized older patients. *N Engl J Med.* 1999;340:669–676.

136. Ritchie K, Polge C, de Roquefeuil G, et al. Impact of anesthesia on the cognitive functioning of the elderly. *Int Psychogeriatr.* 1997;9:309–326.

137. Dodds C, Allison J. Postoperative cognitive deficit in the elderly surgical patient. *Br J Anaesth.* 1998;81:449–462.

138. Morrison RS, Magaziner J, Gilbert M, et al. Relationship between pain and opioid analgesics on the development of delirium following hip fracture. *J Gerontol A Biol Sci Med Sci.* 2003;58:76–81.

139. Martin NJ, Stones MJ, Young JE, Bedard M. Development of delirium: a prospective cohort study in a community hospital. *Int Psychogeriatr.* 2000;12:117–127.

140. Dubois MJ, Bergeron N, Dumont M, et al. Delirium in an intensive care unit: a study of risk factors. *Intensive Care Med.* 2001;27: 1297–1304.

141. Gaudreau JD, Gagnon P, Roy MA, et al. Association between psychoactive medications and delirium in hospitalized patients: a critical review. *Psychosomatics.* 2005;46:302–316.

142. Brauer C, Morrison RS, Silberzweig SB, Siu AL. The cause of delirium in patients with hip fracture. *Arch Intern Med.* 2000;160:1856–1860.

143. Koenig HG, George LK, Stangl D, Tweed DL. Hospital stressors experienced by elderly medical inpatients: developing a Hospital Stress Index. *Int J Psychiatry Med.* 1995;25:103–122.

144. Lynch EP, Lazor MA, Gellis JE, et al. The impact of postoperative pain on the development of postoperative delirium. *Anesth Analg.* 1998;86:781–785.

145. Kaneko T, Takahashi S, Naka T, et al. Postoperative delirium following gastrointestinal surgery in elderly patients. *Surg Today.* 1997;27:107–111.

146. Leung JM, Sands LP, Mullen EA, et al. Are preoperative depressive symptoms associated with postoperative delirium in geriatric surgical patients? *J Gerontol A Biol Sci Med Sci.* 2005;60:1563–1568.

147. Seitz W, Luebbe N, Bechstein W, et al. A comparison of two types of anaesthesia on the endocrine and metabolic responses to anaesthesia and surgery. *Eur J Anaesthesiol.* 1986;3:283–294.

148. Punnonen R, Viinamaki O. Vasopressin release following operation upon the vagina performed under general anaesthesia or epidural analgesis. *Surg Gynecol Obstet.* 1983;156:781–784.

149. Pflug AE, Halter JB. Effect of spinal anesthesia on adrenergic tone and the neuroendocrine responses to surgical stress in humans. *Anesthesiology.* 1981;55:120–126.

150. Bonnet F, Harari A, Thibonnier M, Viars P. Suppression of antidiuretic hormone hypersecretion during surgery by extradural anaesthesia. *Br J Anaesth.* 1982;54:29–36.

151. Berggren D, Gustafson Y, Eriksson B, et al. Postoperative confusion after anesthesia in elderly patients with femoral neck fractures. *Anesth Analg.* 1987;66:497–504.

152. Gustafson Y, Brannstrom B, Berggren D, et al. A geriatric-anesthesiologic program to reduce acute confusional states in elderly patients treated for femoral neck fractures. *J Am Geriatr Soc.* 1991;39:655–662.

153. Price CC, Garvan CW, Monk TG. Neurocognitive performance in older adults with postoperative cognitive dysfunction. *Anesthesiology.* 2003;99: A50.

154. Newman MF, Kirchner JL, Phillips-Bute B, et al. Longitudinal assessment of neurocognitive function after coronary-artery bypass surgery. *N Engl J Med.* 2001;344:395–402.

155. McKhann GM, Grega MA, Borowicz LM, Jr, et al. Is there cognitive decline 1 year after CABG? Comparison with surgical and nonsurgical controls. *Neurology.* 2005;65:991–999.

156. Rasmussen LS, Steentoft A, Rasmussen H, et al. Benzodiazepines and postoperative cognitive dysfunction in the elderly. ISPOCD Group. International Study of Postoperative Cognitive Dysfunction. *Br J Anaesth.* 1999;83:585–589.

157. Levkoff SE, Evans DA, Liptzin B, et al. Delirium. The occurrence and persistence of symptoms among elderly hospitalized patients. *Arch Intern Med.* 1992;152:334–340.

158. Magaziner J, Simonsick EM, Kashner TM, et al. Predictors of functional recovery one year following hospital discharge for hip fracture: a prospective study. *J Gerontol.* 1990;45:M101–M107.

159. Murray AM, Levkoff SE, Wetle TT, et al. Acute delirium and functional decline in the hospitalized elderly patient. *J Gerontol.* 1993;48:M181–M186.

160. Francis J, Kapoor WN. Prognosis after hospital discharge of older medical patients with delirium. *J Am Geriatr Soc.* 1992;40:601–606.

161. Dolan MM, Hawkes WG, Zimmerman SI, et al. Delirium on hospital admission in aged hip fracture patients: prediction of mortality and 2-year functional outcomes. *J Gerontol A Biol Sci Med Sci.* 2000;55:M527–M534.

162. Gruber-Baldini AL, Zimmerman S, Morrison RS, et al. Cognitive impairment in hip fracture patients: timing of detection and longitudinal follow-up. *J Am Geriatr Soc.* 2003;51:1227–1236.

163. Rudolph JL, Babikian VL, Birjiniuk V, et al. Atherosclerosis is associated with delirium after coronary artery bypass graft surgery. *J Am Geriatr Soc.* 2005;53:462–466.

164. Kalisvaart KJ, de Jonghe JF, Bogaards MJ, et al. Haloperidol prophylaxis for elderly hip-surgery patients at risk for delirium: a randomized placebo-controlled study. *J Am Geriatr Soc.* 2005;53:1658–1666.

165. Silverstein JH, Bloom HG, Cassel CK. New challenges in anesthesia: new practice opportunities. *Anesthiol Clin North America.* 1999;17:453–465.

166. Lamy PP, Wiser TH. Geriatric anesthesia. In: Katlic MR, ed. *Pharmacotherapeutic Considerations in the Elderly Surgical Patient.* Baltimore: Urban & Amp Schwartzenberg, Inc.; 1990:209–239.

167. Greenblatt DJ, Sellers EM, Shader RI. Drug therapy: drug disposition in old age. *N Engl J Med.* 1982;306:1081–1088.

168. Shafer SL. The pharmacology of anesthetic drugs in elderly patients. *Anesthesiol Clin North America.* 2000;18:1–29, v.

169. Matteo RS, Ornstein E. Pharmacokinetics and pharmacodynamics of injected drugs in the elderly. *Adv Anesthesia.* 1988;5:25–52.

170. Dundee JW, Robinson FP, McCollum JS, Patterson CC. Sensitivity to propofol in the elderly. *Anaesthesia.* 1986;41:482–485.

171. Jacobs JR, Reves JG, Marty J, et al. Aging increases pharmacodynamic sensitivity to the hypnotic effects of midazolam. *Anesth Analg.* 1995; 80:143–148.

172. Homer TD, Stanski DR. The effect of increasing age on thiopental disposition and anesthetic requirement. *Anesthesiology.* 1985;62: 714–724.

173. Marcantonio ER, Flacker JM, Wright RJ, Resnick NM. Reducing delirium after hip fracture: a randomized trial. *J Am Geriatr Soc.* 2001;49: 516–522.

174. Bogardus ST, Jr, Desai MM, Williams CS, et al. The effects of a targeted multicomponent delirium intervention on postdischarge outcomes for hospitalized older adults. *Am J Med.* 2003;114:383–390.

175. Jankowski CJ, Trenerry MR, Cook DJ, et al. Continuous peripheral nerve block analgesia and central neuraxial anesthesia are associated with reduced incidence of postoperative delirium in the elderly. *Anesthesiology.* 2005;103:A1467.

176. Okumura K. Risperidone therapy for postoperative delirium in elderly patients. *Psychogeriatrics.* 2005;5:108–111.

Postanesthesia Care Unit

Frederick E. Sieber

INTRODUCTION

The elderly are subject to similar postoperative recovery room problems as other age groups. However, few studies are currently available which specifically compare the incidence of postanesthesia care unit (PACU) complications in the elderly versus younger populations. Thus, until these comparisons are available we must use information on overall PACU complication rates and attempt to extrapolate this information to the elderly.

In a series of 17,638 ambulatory surgery patients, Chung et al. found that age greater than 65 years was associated with a 3.1% incidence of adverse events in the PACU.[1] In fact, the overall incidence of any PACU event, including excessive pain, nausea and vomiting, central nervous system (CNS) problems, cardiovascular, respiratory, and excessive bleeding, was fourfold higher in patients younger than 65 years as compared to their older counterparts.[1] And, on further analysis, adverse PACU events in ambulatory surgery did not appear to be related to age.[2] Instead, other variables such as surgical procedure, type of anesthesia, length of procedure, and preexisting medical conditions were more important determinants of adverse PACU events. However, the study of Chung et al.[1] must be interpreted with caution because the type of anesthesia in the two patient groups was not comparable. In the group of age ≥65 years, 86% of patients underwent monitored anesthetic care whereas in the group of age <65 years, 76% of patients underwent general anesthesia. Although these numbers probably paint an accurate picture of the type of anesthesia administered to these two groups of outpatients, the two groups may not be directly comparable when examining PACU complications.

In a series of 18,473 consecutive patients entering a PACU at a university teaching hospital, Hines et al. found the overall PACU complication rate was 23.7%.[3] The variables which were important determinants of adverse PACU events were similar to those observed in ambulatory surgery and included surgical procedure, type of anesthesia, length of procedure, emergency surgery, and American Society of Anesthesiologists (ASA) physical status. A specific relationship between age and adverse PACU events was not mentioned. Hines et al. found that the greatest incidence of recovery room complications occurred during orthopedic and general surgery procedures.[3] Interestingly, orthopedic and general surgery procedures are also the most common type of inpatient surgery performed on the elderly.[4]

Using the above-mentioned studies as a guideline, in Table 23-1 we list the common PACU complications across all age groups and their incidence. From this table, the reader can glean that the anesthesiologist caring for the elderly PACU patient should focus on issues surrounding nausea and vomiting, need for airway support and maintenance of adequate ventilation/respiration, cardiovascular changes, and alterations in mental status.

NAUSEA AND VOMITING IN THE ELDERLY

It is controversial whether the elderly are more susceptible to nausea and vomiting in the postoperative period. In ambulatory surgery, patients older than 65 years have a 0.69% incidence of nausea and vomiting, whereas those less than 65 years of age have a 2.73% incidence.[1] However, outpatient surgery in the elderly involves a greater percentage of procedures done under local anesthesia than their younger counterparts, which significantly influences these results. Simplified risk scores for predicting postoperative nausea and vomiting do not include age as an important risk factor.[5] However, while examining all risk factors for development of postoperative nausea and vomiting, the effect of age is not clear. This is because results have varied from center to center concerning the effects of age.[6] Early reports suggest that age is not a predictor of nausea, but does influence the incidence of postoperative vomiting.[7] In contrast, other centers report that age is inversely correlated to postoperative nausea and vomiting with a 17% decrease in the probability of postoperative nausea and vomiting for a 10-year increase in age.[8] Because the question concerning the relationship of age to postoperative nausea and vomiting is unresolved, it is probably best to utilize the same intervention strategies for postoperative nausea and vomiting in both elderly and younger patients.[9]

RESPIRATORY AND PULMONARY EVENTS

▶ Events related to inadequate ventilation/respiration in the elderly

In ambulatory surgery, the elderly have a similar incidence of PACU respiratory events as their younger counterparts despite undergoing a much greater percentage of procedures under local anesthesia (0.33% vs. 0.38% incidence in patients ≥65 years of age and patients <65 years of age, respectively).[1]

With respect to nonambulatory surgery procedures, the Anesthetic Incident Monitoring Study (AIMS) has highlighted the recovery room as an important area for the occurrence of serious adverse events. Within the AIMS registry, respiratory and airway incidents accounted for 23% and 21% of total PACU complications.[10] In

Table 23-1

Major PACU Complications in 18,473 Patients

Complications	n	Incidence (%)
Nausea and vomiting	1810	9.8
Requirement for upper airway support, including nasal, pharyngeal, or endotracheal airway	1275	6.9
Hypotension	499	2.7
Dysrhythmia	259	1.4
Hypertension (diastolic >110 mm Hg)	203	1.1
Altered mental status	111	0.6
Rule out myocardial infarction	54	0.3
Major cardiac event	52	0.3

Source: Data adapted from Ref. 3.

addition, 38% of all episodes of pulmonary edema in the PACU were secondary to airway obstruction.[10] Table 23-2 gives a thumbnail sketch of the primary causes of respiratory failure and airway incidents in the PACU using the AIMS data. Inadequate reversal of neuromuscular blockade was the most common cause of respiratory failure. Residual neuromuscular blockade, as defined by a train-of-four response less than 0.7 (T4/T1 twitch ratio), is a frequent occurrence. Residual neuromuscular blockade has been reported to occur in 26% of patients receiving pancuronium and 5.3% of patients receiving atracurium or vecuronium.[11] Others have reported much higher rates of residual paralysis (42%) in the recovery room in patients receiving vecuronium.[12] These reports are especially alarming given the evidence that partial neuromuscular blockade (train-of-four = 0.70, a level thought to represent safe recovery) does depress the hypoxic ventilatory response, even in healthy awake volunteers who have been given no other sedative drugs.[13] Furthermore, train-of-four ratios less than 0.90 are associated with pharyngeal dysfunction and possible impaired airway protection.[14] Considering the alterations in pharmacology which occur with aging (see Chap. 8), one should have a high index of suspicion for the possibility of residual neuromuscular block in the elderly PACU patient. Among the nondepolarizing neuromuscular blocking agents, cisatracurium besylate and atracurium besylate have the most reproducible recovery profile and the least affected pharmacokinetics in the elderly.[15]

Table 23-2

Respiratory and Airway PACU Events

Respiratory Failure	n (%)	Airway Incidents	n (%)
Total incidents	74	Total incidents	87
Inadequate reversal of neuromuscular block	29 (39)	Airway obstruction	59 (68)
Patient debilitated	10 (14)	Laryngospasm	18 (21)
Lung collapse; consolidation	9 (12)		
Opioid overdose	6 (8)		
Obesity	5 (7)		

Source: Data adapted from Ref. 10.

Aspiration

Aspiration in the PACU is a rare event. Within the AIMS database, 133 cases of aspiration were recorded. Only seven (5%) of these episodes occurred in the recovery room. In fact, the AIMS data support the view that the greatest risk of aspiration occurs on induction of anesthesia, not in the recovery room.[16]

The most important first line of defense in the prevention of aspiration pneumonia is preservation of swallowing function and an intact cough reflex. Studies have shown that older people swallow more slowly than younger people. Although aging is associated with slowing of the swallowing process, the integrity of the swallowing process, as defined by frequency of aspiration on radiographic studies, is not increased when comparing older to younger patients.[17] In addition, aging does not appear to affect the cough reflex. Given the above, aged persons are probably at no higher risk of aspiration in the recovery room than their younger counterparts. Rather, the attention should be focused on the patient population with comorbid conditions which may impair swallowing or the cough reflex. Both cerebrovascular disease and neurodegenerative processes cause these changes. For instance, with acute stroke the incidence of dysphagia has been reported in the range of 40–70%. Similarly, both Alzheimer disease and Parkinson disease are associated with swallowing disorders early in their course.[17] In these patients, basic aspiration precautions should be taken during their PACU stay. These include upright positioning and avoiding hyperextension of the neck.[18]

Postoperative pulmonary complications

The elderly are prone to postoperative pulmonary complications for a variety of reasons. For one, as discussed in the previous chapter on pulmonary changes with aging, marked decreases in pulmonary reserve occur in the elderly. Second, the hypoxic and hypercapnic ventilatory drive is attenuated with increasing age.[19] Third, the pharmacokinetics and pharmacodynamics of drugs are greatly altered with age. In the PACU, evidence of prolonged and residual effects from narcotics and inhalational agents is often observed.

The incidence of postoperative pneumonia, hypoxemia, hypoventilation, or atelectasis in patients greater than 69 years of age ranges from 2.1% to 10.2%.[20] While in patients 80 years of age or greater and undergoing noncardiac surgery, Liu and Leung found an overall 7% incidence of postoperative pulmonary complications consisting of pneumonia, ARDS, pulmonary embolism, or reintubation.[21] In the study by Liu and Leung, strong predictors of adverse postoperative pulmonary events included a history of congestive heart failure, arrhythmias, dementia, cerebrovascular accident, seizure, or urgent/emergent surgery. The anesthesiologist must maintain a high level of surveillance for postoperative pulmonary problems. In addition, it is important to assess the elderly patient for comorbid conditions which increase the likelihood of postoperative pulmonary events.

Several investigators have attempted to provide risk indexes to help in predicting which patients are at highest risk for postoperative pulmonary complications. These indices may also be meaningful in identifying patients at risk for pulmonary problems in the recovery room. A more in-depth discussion of the National Veterans Affairs Surgical Quality Improvement Program's risk index for predicting postoperative pneumonia[22] and the Brooks-Braun predictors of postoperative pulmonary complications[23] is covered in Chap. 5.

The risk of smoking

At present, there are few studies which address PACU morbidity in the elderly. Thus the relationship between smoking history and

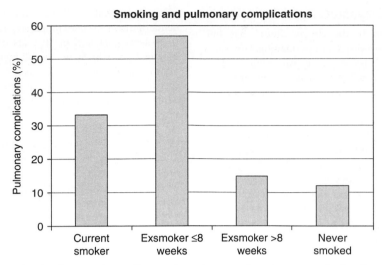

Smoking and pulmonary complications

FIGURE 23-1 The relationship between duration of preoperative smoking cessation and postoperative pulmonary complications in coronary artery bypass patients. *(Adapted from Ref. 25.)*

PACU pulmonary morbidity is unclear. A current history of smoking is associated with increased pulmonary morbidity. However, an equally important piece of information relates to how long smoking cessation must occur before an effect on pulmonary morbidity is observed. Older studies have documented that it takes at least 6 months following smoking cessation until improvement in pulmonary function tests occurs. Specifically, changes in closing volume (as a percentage of vital capacity) and closing capacity (as a percentage of total lung capacity) are not observed until 6 months following smoking cessation.[24] Warner et al., in a study of elective coronary artery bypass patients, demonstrated that pulmonary complications in those who had stopped smoking at least 6 months preoperatively were similar to those who had never smoked.[25] Warner et al.[25] also found that a minimum of 2 months of preoperative smoking cessation were necessary to see any significant decrease in pulmonary complications when compared to ongoing smokers (Fig. 23-1).

CARDIOVASCULAR COMPLICATIONS IN THE ELDERLY

To appreciate the overall picture of PACU cardiovascular complications in the elderly, it is helpful to look at both the incidence and the predictors of these complications both in PACU and postoperatively.

In ambulatory surgery patients, adverse cardiovascular events in the PACU are more common in older patients (1.06% vs. 0.41% incidence in patients ≥65 years and patients <65 years of age, respectively).[1] In the outpatient setting, hypertension accounts for over half (0.58% incidence) of the PACU cardiovascular events in the elderly, followed by bradycardia (0.17% incidence), and ischemia (0.13% incidence).

Leung and Dzankic[26] examined 601 inpatient surgical procedures in 544 consecutive patients with a mean age of 78 ± 6 years. In this study, postoperative cardiovascular complications were the leading cause of morbidity with an overall incidence of 10.3%. The complications examined included ischemic complications (new occurrence of chest pain, electrocardiogram [ECG] changes, or cardiac enzyme changes, [5.3%]), myocardial infarction (1.8%), heart failure (3.3%),

and dysrhythmias (5.9%). Leung and Dzankic then looked at predictors of these postoperative cardiac events and found that severity of preoperative comorbidity (ASA class ≥3) and clinical signs of heart failure (pre- or intraoperative) were important variables in forecasting these events. Thus, the study of Leung and Dzankic[26] shows that in the elderly inpatient surgical population of age 70 years or greater, cardiac events are common and strongly associated with presence of heart failure and severity of comorbid disease. The most common type of cardiac event is dysrhythmia and the least common is myocardial infarction. The above study was taken a step further by Liu and Leung[21] when they examined postoperative complications in patients greater than 80 years of age undergoing noncardiac, nonambulatory surgical procedures. Three hundred sixty-seven patients undergoing 410 surgical procedures were examined. The cardiovascular complications investigated were postoperative heart failure, myocardial infarction, and arrhythmias. The overall incidence of adverse postoperative cardiovascular events in patients 80 years or older was 12%. The incidence of adverse postoperative cardiovascular events was comparable between patients greater than 70 years of age and patients greater than 80 years of age (Table 23-3). In the 80-year-old population, a preoperative history of congestive heart failure (defined as a history of pulmonary edema secondary to heart failure) or arrhythmia (clinically diagnosed and documented) were strong predictors of postoperative cardiac events. Treatment and diagnosis of heart failure are important to prevent cardiovascular complications in the elderly population[27]. Further discussion of management of heart failure is covered in Chaps. 4 and 16.

Table 23-3

Incidence of Adverse Postoperative Cardiac Events in Two Age groups (%)

Event	Age ≥ 70 Years	Age ≥ 80 Years
Myocardial infarction	1.8	1.9
Heart failure	3.3	6
Dysrhythmia	5.9	7.0

Source: Data from Refs. 21 and 26.

▶ PACU management of hypotension

The treatment of hypotension in the elderly should take into account some unique aspects of this patient population. For one, it is important to be familiar with underlying comorbidities and the drugs being used to treat these conditions. Many chronic and common neurodegenerative diseases employ the use of drugs, such as levodopa, bromocriptine, and tricyclic antidepressants, which are associated with orthostatic hypotension and can have dramatic effects on blood pressure.[28] Second, drug effects should always be scrutinized. There are important changes in anesthetic drug pharmacodynamics and pharmacokinetics, which tend to prolong their residual effects. In addition, polypharmacy is a huge issue in the elderly, and one must always remain vigilant for potential drug interactions. Third, heart rate and rhythm changes have a greater impact on blood pressure in the elderly. Therefore, depending on the clinical scenario, treatment of heart rate and/or rhythm may assume precedence to initial fluid therapy. Bradycardia, in particular, can cause profound hypotension. Fourth, there is little data concerning the treatment of hypotension in the setting of diastolic dysfunction (see Chap. 16). In most surgical circumstances, a first line of treatment for hypotension is fluid administration. However, with the elderly, fluid should be cautiously administered. The use of alpha-adrenergic agents to increase the blood pressure via peripheral vasoconstriction or mixed alpha/beta agonists to both provide peripheral vasoconstriction as well as an increase in heart rate should be considered in the hypotensive elderly patient.[29] Trendelenburg position, if tolerated, is another worthwhile temporizing maneuver.

NEUROLOGIC COMPLICATIONS IN THE ELDERLY

Among all patients coming to the PACU, regardless of age, the most common neurologic complication is altered mental status which has an incidence of 0.6% (Table 23-1).[3] In ambulatory surgery, where the majority of procedures in the elderly are performed under local anesthesia, the incidence of drowsiness/sleepiness and excessive agitation are 0.13% and 0.04%, respectively (Table 23-4). This compares to their younger counterparts (<65 years of age), undergoing primarily general anesthesia, who display a 0.56% and 0.40% incidence of drowsiness/sleepiness and excessive agitation, respectively.[1] In patients greater than 70 years of age undergoing noncardiac, inpatient procedures, the overall incidence of postoperative neurologic complications is 7.7%.[4] As patients age, to 80 years or greater, the incidence of neurologic complications increases to 15%.[21] As demonstrated by Table 23-4, the incidence of postoperative change in mental status, particularly delirium and stroke, increases with age. The important preoperative predictors of these events have been consistently reported to be a preoperative history of neurologic disease, such as dementia, seizure, or stroke,[21] and poor preoperative functional status.[26]

The studies which delineate postoperative neurologic complications in the elderly do not define these events as occurring in the recovery room. The incidence of recovery room neurologic events in the elderly may be different from postoperative complications, but little data have been reported on this subject. In all likelihood stroke is probably a rare recovery room event. This inference is taken from the study of Hines et al. which does not even mention stroke as a recovery room event[3]; rather altered mental status was defined by confusion and somnolence.

▶ PACU somnolence

When evaluating PACU somnolence, the most important tenet is that delayed emergence or continued somnolence is the result of drug effects, until proven otherwise. Benzodiazepines are a prime culprit. A study by Fredman et al.[30] assessed the effect of different doses of midazolam on postoperative mental and psychomotor recovery in elderly patients undergoing brief urologic procedures. In this study, 90 geriatric patients were randomized to obtain differing amounts of preoperative midazolam. The interesting finding was that midazolam administration, regardless of the dose, significantly prolonged PACU discharge time as a result of depressed mental function. In other words, even small doses of midazolam premedication (in this study, the doses used were 0.5 and 2 mg preoperatively) have dramatic effects in determining recovery times in the elderly. Anticholinergics are another drug category classically associated with both somnolence and delirium. Many anesthetic agents affect the brain cholinergic neurotransmitter system. It has been theorized that postoperative agitation and/or somnolence may be attributed to decreased brain cholinergic activity caused by anesthetics. Historically, the anesthesia literature has attributed a major portion of abnormal emergence behavior after general anesthesia to the *central anticholinergic syndrome*[31] which has been reported to occur in 1.9–40% of patients.[32] It is certainly true that centrally acting anticholinergic agents, such as atropine or scopolamine, can profoundly affect emergence from anesthesia.[33] However, it is unclear what role other drugs used in current anesthetic practice might have in causing the central anticholinergic syndrome. The time-honored treatment for suspected central anticholinergic syndrome is the administration of a centrally acting cholinesterase inhibitor such as physostigmine. This drug can be given intravenously or intramuscularly. The initial recommended dose is the slow intravenous administration of 0.04 mg/kg.[34] Physostigmine may produce a wide variety of parasympathetic peripheral side effects. In particular, the drug should probably be avoided in asthmatics as bronchospasm can occur. The drug should always be administered under continuous ECG surveillance to monitor for the onset of bradycardia. In current anesthetic practice, it is best to reserve physostigmine for use in those cases where perioperative administration of a centrally acting anticholinergic drug has occurred in a patient displaying abnormal emergence behavior.

Table 23-4

Postoperative Neurologic Complications in the Elderly

Age Group	Type of Surgery	Incidence of Neurologic Complications	Specific Neurologic Complications	Incidence of Specific Neurologic Complications
All ages	Inpatient		Altered mental state	0.6%
≥65	Ambulatory	0.17%	Drowsiness/ sleepiness	0.13%
			Excessive agitation	0.04%
≥70	Inpatient Noncardiac	7.7%	Delirium	6.8%
			CVA/TIA	0.9%
≥80	Inpatient Noncardiac	15%	Delirium	13.6%
			CVA	1.4%

Recovery room delirium

Recovery room confusion or delirium is a phenomenon which may occur in all age groups. PACU delirium is different from somnolence. Somnolence is defined by excessive sleepiness and is the result of drugs, until proven otherwise. Delirium is a state of confusion or disorientation which may occur in the recovery room. Furthermore, recovery room delirium should not be confused with emergence delirium. Emergence delirium refers to the immediate recovery phase after anesthesia when agitation may occur. In the pediatric population, emergence delirium has been equated with agitation on awakening.[35] Older studies in adults also used agitation as a marker for emergence delirium.[36] Emergence delirium is short lived and resolves during the recovery room time period. Recovery room delirium, on the other hand, refers to a state of confusion which is not self-limited and remains unresolved throughout the recovery room stay. Recovery room delirium has been poorly studied in the past and data on its incidence are lacking. A study by Sharma et al.[37] reports the incidence of recovery room delirium to be 44% in elderly patients following hip fracture repair.

Presently, it is unclear whether the elderly as a group are more predisposed to confusion while in the recovery room. This is because many authors have defined postoperative delirium as a hyperactive state involving agitation. However, investigators have demonstrated that both hypoactive and hyperactive forms of postoperative confusion exist. Most important, recent studies of postoperative delirium in the geriatric population report that hypoactive forms of delirium are more prevalent than hyperactive forms.[38] This suggests that previous studies may have underreported recovery room delirium.

The importance of recognizing recovery room delirium comes from studies which demonstrate that recovery room delirium is a strong predictor of postoperative delirium occurring several days later during the hospital stay.[38] Thus, it becomes important to try and assess mental status changes in elderly recovery room patients. Current literature suggests that the two most consistent preoperative predictors of postoperative delirium are patient age and the presence of dementia.[39] Therefore, the clinician taking care of patients in the PACU should pay particular attention to the mental status of the older patient with underlying dementia.

The differential diagnosis of recovery room delirium incorporates a laundry list of possibilities. The workup and treatment is similar to postoperative delirium (see Chap. 22). For the purpose of this discussion, we focus on topics which are remediable within the recovery room environment. Table 23-5 displays treatable causes of delirium within the PACU. First, it is important to rule out the possibility of hypotension or hypoxia, both of which can lead to mental dysfunction. Second, hypothermia should be aggressively treated as it has been associated with delirium in hospitalized medical patients.[40]

Table 23-5

Treatable Causes of Delirium in the PACU

Hypoxia

Hypotension—especially shock

Hypothermia

Electrolyte imbalance or hypoglycemia—especially hyponatremia

Inadequate pain relief

Drugs—especially narcotics (meperidine), benzodiazepines, barbiturates, and NSAIDs

Third, the possibility of electrolyte imbalance or hypoglycemia should be sought. Hyponatremia, in particular, is closely associated with postoperative delirium.[41] Fourth, inadequate pain management is an important triggering mechanism for delirium. Authors have suggested that emergence delirium may be associated with untreated pain.[37,42] In addition, higher levels of pain at rest during the first three postoperative days have been associated with delirium.[43] In hip fracture patients, undertreated perioperative pain significantly increases the risk of developing delirium in frail elderly adults.[44] In contrast, prospective randomized controlled studies of elderly patients undergoing major abdominal surgery have failed to show differences in incidence of postoperative delirium despite documented differences in postoperative pain levels.[45] However, until more definitive data become available, it is still prudent to ensure that adequate pain relief is provided to the elderly patient. Lastly, drugs are oftentimes the culprit. As outlined in several nice review articles,[46] many types of medications are associated with delirium. Among drugs commonly used in anesthetic practice, sevoflurane,[36] meperidine,[45] benzodiazepines,[47] and anticholinergics[48] have been implicated in the development of delirium. In addition, polypharmacy may play a role as multiple drug interactions can compound CNS effects. One should always be tuned to the possibility of street drug and/or alcohol intoxication or withdrawal. The incidence of alcoholism is surprisingly high in the elderly population.[49]

When faced with the possibility of medication-induced delirium, the offending drugs must be discontinued and appropriate measures of supportive care instituted. Treatment strategies for postoperative delirium are reviewed in Chap. 22.

Propofol

In a review by Walder et al.,[50] a meta-analysis was performed to determine any untoward neurologic effects of propofol. Propofol was associated with a small but notable incidence of seizure-like phenomena, which may occur regardless of the presence of epilepsy. These seizure-like phenomena are probably related to rapid and abrupt decreases in the brain concentration of propofol. In any event, when seizures occur in the PACU it is important to determine whether or not these findings may be the result of propofol administration.

PAIN MANAGEMENT

Inadequate postoperative analgesia has been associated with numerous adverse events in the PACU, including hypertensive episodes, poor coughing and deep breathing, and delirium. In most circumstances, narcotics are the drugs of choice for providing analgesia in the PACU, and the use of morphine has been extensively studied in the elderly. As discussed in Chap. 25, there are many available options for management of acute postoperative pain in the elderly.

KEY POINTS

► Because the relationship of age to postoperative nausea and vomiting is unresolved, it is probably best to utilize the same intervention strategies for postoperative nausea and vomiting in both elderly and younger patients.

► Elderly patients are at high risk of sustaining postoperative pulmonary complications and respiratory failure. Inadequate reversal of neuromuscular blockade is the most common cause of respiratory failure. The most important initial maneuver in treating any patient with respiratory compromise in the PACU is to first assess airway patency as this is the most common cause of inadequate ventilation and oxygenation.

▶ Type of surgery and age appear to be the most important predictors of postoperative pulmonary complications. Once those patients have been identified, it is important for the clinician to aggressively treat these individuals using such modalities as oxygen therapy, positioning the patient to optimize ventilation, and encouraging coughing and deep breathing. If necessary, the residual effects of anesthetic drugs may be reversed.

▶ Cardiovascular complications are the leading cause of morbidity in the elderly.

▶ Treatment and diagnosis of heart failure in the elderly is important because of the strong relationship between failure and postoperative events. Diastolic heart failure assumes increasing importance in the elderly population.

▶ Treatment of PACU hypotension in the elderly should take into account underlying comorbidity and the drugs used to treat these diseases.

▶ The most common neurologic complication is altered mental status and may include somnolence or delirium. When evaluating PACU somnolence, the most important tenet is that delayed emergence or continued somnolence is the result of drug effects, until proven otherwise. Presently, it is unclear whether the elderly as a group are more predisposed to confusion while in the recovery room.

KEY ARTICLES

▶ Kluger MT, Bullock MF. Recovery room incidents: a review of 419 reports from the anaesthetic incident monitoring study (AIMS). *Anaesthesia*. 2002;57:1060–1066.

▶ Rooke G. Autonomic and cardiovascular function in the geriatric patient. *Anesthesiol Clin North America*. 2000;18:31–46.

▶ Bitsch M, Foss N, Kristensen B, Kehlet H. Pathogenesis of and management strategies for postoperative delirium after hip fracture: a review. *Acta Orthop Scand*. 2004;75:378–389.

▶ Alagiakrishnan K, Wiens CA. An approach to drug induced delirium in the elderly. *Postgrad Med J*. 2004;80:388–393.

REFERENCES

1. Chung F, Mezei G, Tong D. Adverse events in ambulatory surgery. A comparison between elderly and younger patients. *Can J Anaesth*. 1999;46:309–321.
2. Chung F, Mezei G, Tong D. Preexisting medical conditions as predictors of adverse events in day-case surgery. *Br J Anaesth*. 1999;83:262–270.
3. Hines R, Barash PG, Watrous G, O'Connor T. Complications occurring in the postanesthesia care unit: a survey. *Anesth Analg*. 1992;74:503–509.
4. Dzankic S, Pastor D, Gonzalez C, Leung JM. The prevalence and predictive value of abnormal preoperative laboratory tests in elderly surgical patients. *Anesth Analg*. 2001;93(2):301–308.
5. Apfel CC, Kranke P, Eberhart LH, et al. Comparison of predictive models for postoperative nausea and vomiting. *Br J Anaesth*. 2002;88:234–240.
6. Apfel CC, Laara E, Koivuranta M, et al. A simplified risk score for predicting postoperative nausea and vomiting: conclusions from cross-validations between two centers. *Anesthesiology*. 1999;91:693–700.
7. Koivuranta M, Laara E, Snare L, Alahuhta S. A survey of postoperative nausea and vomiting. *Anaesthesia*. 1997;52:443–449.
8. Pierre S, Benais H, Pouymayou J. Apfel's simplified score may favorably predict the risk of postoperative nausea and vomiting. *Can J Anaesth*. 2002;49:237–242.
9. Apfel CC, Korttila K, Abdalla M, et al. A factorial trial of six interventions for the prevention of postoperative nausea and vomiting. *N Engl J Med*. 2004;350:2441–2451.
10. Kluger MT, Bullock MF. Recovery room incidents: a review of 419 reports from the anaesthetic incident monitoring study (AIMS). *Anaesthesia*. 2002;57:1060–1066.
11. Berg H, Roed J, Viby-Mogensen J, et al. Residual neuromuscular block is a risk factor for postoperative pulmonary complications. A prospective, randomized, and blinded study of postoperative pulmonary complications after atracurium, vecuronium, and pancuronium. *Acta Anaesthesiol Scand*. 1997;41:1095–1103.
12. Baillard C, Gehan G, Reboul-Marty J, et al. Residual curarization in the recovery room after vecuronium. *Br J Anaesth*. 2000;84:394–395.
13. Eriksson LI. The effects of residual neuromuscular blockade and volatile anesthetics on the control of ventilation. *Anesth Analg*. 1999;89:243–251.
14. Eriksson LI, Sundman E, Olsson R, et al. Functional assessment of the pharynx at rest and during swallowing in partially paralyzed humans: simultaneous videomanometry and mechanomyography of awake human volunteers. *Anesthesiology*. 1997;87:1035–1043.
15. Cope TM, Hunter JM. Selecting neuromuscular-blocking drugs for elderly patients. *Drugs Aging*. 2003;20:125–140.
16. Kluger MT, Short TG. Aspiration during anaesthesia: a review of 133 cases from the Australian anaesthetic incident monitoring study (AIMS). *Anaesthesia*. 1999;54:19–26.
17. Marik PE, Kaplan D. Aspiration pneumonia and dysphagia in the elderly. *Chest*. 2003;124:328–336.
18. Oh E, Weintraub N, Dhanani S. Can we prevent aspiration pneumonia in the nursing home? *J Am Med Dir Assoc*. 2004;5:174–179.
19. Kronenberg RS, Drage CW. Attenuation of the ventilatory and heart rate responses to hypoxia and hypercapnia with aging in normal men. *J Clin Invest*. 1973;52:1812–1819.
20. Jin F, Chung F. Minimizing perioperative adverse events in the elderly. *Br J Anaesth*. 2001;87(4):608–624.
21. Liu LL, Leung JM. Predicting adverse postoperative outcomes in patients aged 80 years or older. *J Am Geriatr Soc*. 2000;48:405–412.
22. Arozullah AM, Khuri SF, Henderson WG, Daley J. Participants in the National Veterans Affairs Surgical Quality Improvement Program. Development and validation of a multifactorial risk index for predicting postoperative pneumonia after major noncardiac surgery. *Ann Intern Med*. 2001;135:847–857.
23. Brooks-Braun J. Predictors of postoperative pulmonary complications following abdominal surgery. *Chest*. 1997;111:564–571.
24. Buist AS, Sexton GJ, Nagy JM, Ross BB. The effect of smoking cessation and modification on lung function. *Am Rev Respir Dis*. 1976;114: 115–122.
25. Warner MA, Offord KP, Warner ME, et al. Role of preoperative cessation of smoking and other factors in postoperative pulmonary complications: a blinded prospective study of coronary artery bypass patients. *Mayo Clin Proc*. 1989;64:609–616.
26. Leung JM, Dzankic S. Relative importance of preoperative health status versus intraoperative factors in predicting postoperative adverse outcomes in geriatric surgical patients. *J Am Geriatr Soc*. 2001;49:1080–1085.
27. Hunt SA, Baker DW, Chin MH, et al. ACC/AHA guidelines for the evaluation and management of chronic heart failure in the adult: executive summary. A report of the American College of Cardiology/American Heart Association task force on practice guidelines (committee to revise the 1995 guidelines for the evaluation and management of heart failure): developed in collaboration with the International Society for Heart and Lung Transplantation; endorsed by the Heart Failure Society of America. *Circulation*. 2001;104:2996–3007.
28. Burton DA, Nicholson G, Hall GM. Anaesthesia in elderly patients with neurodegenerative disorders: special considerations. *Drugs Aging*. 2004;21:229–242.
29. Rooke G. Autonomic and cardiovascular function in the geriatric patient. *Anesthesiol Clin North America*. 2000;18:31–46.
30. Fredman B, Lahav M, Zohar E, et al. The effect of midazolam premedication on mental and psychomotor recovery in geriatric patients undergoing brief surgical procedures. *Anesth Analg*. 1999;89:1161–1166.
31. Schneck HJ, Rupreht J. Central anticholinergic syndrome (CAS) in anesthesia and intensive care. *Acta Anaesthesiol Belg*. 1989;40:219–228.
32. Cook B, Spence AA. Post-operative central anticholinergic syndrome. *Eur J Anaesthesiol*. 1997;14:1–2.
33. Martin B, Howell PR. Physostigmine: going . . . going . . . gone? Two cases of central anticholinergic syndrome following anaesthesia and its treatment with physostigmine. *Eur J Anaesthesiol*. 1997;14: 467–470.

34. Rupreht J. The central muscarinic transmission during anaesthesia and recovery—the central anticholinergic syndrome. *Anaesthesiol Reanim.* 1991;16:250–258.

35. Aono J, Ueda W, Mamiya K, et al. Greater incidence of delirium during recovery from sevoflurane anesthesia in preschool boys. *Anesthesiology.* 1997;87:1298–1300.

36. Nunn J. Isoflurane as a routine anaesthetic in general surgical practice. *Br J Anaesth.* 1985;57:461–475.

37. Sharma PT, Sieber FE, Zakriya KJ, et al. Recovery room delirium predicts postoperative delirium after hip-fracture repair. *Anesth Analg.* 2005;101: 1215–1220, table of contents.

38. Marcantonio E, Ta T, Duthie E, Resnick NM. Delirium severity and psychomotor types: their relationship with outcomes after hip fracture repair. *J Am Geriatr Soc.* 2002;50:850–857.

39. Bitsch M, Foss N, Kristensen B, Kehlet H. Pathogenesis of and management strategies for postoperative delirium after hip fracture: a review. *Acta Orthop Scand.* 2004;75:378–389.

40. Francis J, Martin D, Kapoor WN. A prospective study of delirium in hospitalized elderly. *JAMA.* 1990;263:1097–1101.

41. Burns A, Gallagley A, Byrne J. Delirium. *J Neurol Neurosurg Psychiatry.* 2004;75:362–367.

42. Olympio M. Postanesthetic delirium: historical perspectives. *J Clin Anesth.* 1991;3:60–63.

43. Lynch EP, Lazor MA, Gellis JE, et al. The impact of postoperative pain on the development of postoperative delirium. *Anesth Analg.* 1998;86: 781–785.

44. Morrison RS, Magaziner J, Gilbert M, et al. Relationship between pain and opioid analgesics on the development of delirium following hip fracture. *J Gerontol A Biol Sci Med Sci.* 2003;58: 76–81.

45. Mann C, Pouzeratte Y, Boccara G, et al. Comparison of intravenous or epidural patient-controlled analgesia in the elderly after major abdominal surgery. *Anesthesiology.* 2000;92:433–441.

46. Alagiakrishnan K, Wiens CA. An approach to drug-induced delirium in the elderly. *Postgrad Med J.* 2004;80:388–393.

47. Marcantonio ER, Juarez G, Goldman L, et al. The relationship of postoperative delirium with psychoactive medications. *JAMA.* 1994;272: 1518–1522.

48. Parikh SS, Chung F. Postoperative delirium in the elderly. *Anesth Analg.* 1995;80:1223–1232.

49. Johnson I. Alcohol problems in old age: a review of recent epidemiological research. *Int J Geriatr Psychiatry.* 2000;15:575–581.

50. Walder B, Tramer MR, Seeck M. Seizure-like phenomena and propofol: a systematic review. *Neurology.* 2002;58:1327–1332.

Issues of Specific Importance to the Elderly Intensive Care Unit Patient

CHAPTER 24

Ronald Pauldine

INTRODUCTION

The aging population in western countries is expected to have a tremendous impact on demand for health-care resources affecting both the need for appropriately trained personnel and the extensive financial resources required to meet the anticipated acuity and volume of those needing care. This fact is nowhere more evident than in the realm of intensive care medicine. The demographic considerations alone are staggering. These important considerations for perioperative care in general are detailed in Chap. 1 (Demographics and Economics). From the perspective of the intensivist, by 2030, one in five Americans will be over the age of 65, with those over the age of 85 representing the fastest growing component. By 2050, this number will rise to one in four with approximately 20 million people over 85 years of age.[1] Similar trends are occurring throughout western countries. Currently, the elderly comprise about one-eighth of the population, but consume nearly 25% of the trauma and critical care resources.[2] These figures will only rise based on the predicted expansion of the elderly population as outlined above. The economic implications are obvious when one considers that critical care beds make up approximately 10–20% of the beds in an average academic health center and account for 20–30% of the hospital budget.[3] This projected increase in demand will clearly be in excess of the forecasted production of intensive care providers. The expanding need for trained critical care physicians, nurse practitioners, nurses, and technicians has been recently highlighted.[4,5]

The allocation of expensive and limited critical care resources in the future represents an extremely important and difficult challenge to governments and individual health-care organizations. In order to meet this challenge, medical providers must be concerned with furthering our understanding of critical care outcomes in the elderly as well as appreciating those areas where differences exist between the young and old, and indeed within the heterogeneous subsets of the aged themselves. This chapter focuses on the current understanding of intensive care outcomes in the elderly and emerging issues central to the care of critically ill elders. The physiology of aging and the resulting effect on physiologic reserve is of prime importance in caring for elderly patients. These physiologic considerations have been addressed in detail in other sections of this text. Where these changes impact on specific issues under consideration here, they are briefly reviewed. For in-depth discussions of age-related changes in organ function, the reader is referred to the appropriate chapter.

TRIAGE OF ELDERLY PATIENTS: ACCESS TO CRITICAL CARE

The economic implication for increased utilization of critical care resources has been outlined above. In addition, the projected shortage of critical care professionals mandates the understanding of factors that must be considered in allocation of critical care resources to the rapidly expanding elderly population. These factors are complex, in some cases not well-defined, and passionately debated. The evaluation of the patient's medical condition must be combined with the patient's desires for aggressive medical intervention. Considerations include the patient's underlying medical condition, premorbid level of function, nature of the admitting diagnosis to the intensive care unit (ICU) with regard to expected ability to reverse the process by intensive care interventions, realistic expectations to eventually return to a premorbid level of function or independent living, and the wishes of the patient to undergo the recommended treatment.[6,7] Age alone should not be the sole determinant of ICU admission.[8–11] These decisions are clearly influenced by the biases of the treating physician with regard to expected outcome. In other cases, the desires of the patient may not be known and surrogate decision makers may be unable or unwilling to make difficult decisions regarding limitation of care. While research on clinical outcomes is yielding an increasing understanding of long-term effects of critical illness in the elderly, clear recommendations are lacking. Much of the decision making with regard to treatment in this group involves important ethical considerations and potential end-of-life care decisions. These principles are discussed in Chap. 28 (Medical Ethics).

Problems involved in the decision to treat patients in the ICU have been detailed in multiple publications based on the Study to Understand Prognosis and Preferences for Outcomes and Risks of Treatments (SUPPORT).[12] Overall, the study attempted to improve end-of-life decision making and reduce the frequency of protracted and painful treatment in a cohort of patients with serious illness and a predicted preenrollment high mortality rate. The study revealed considerable problems with care in this population and failed to improve aspects of care through implementation of a defined intervention tailored to improve communication and define treatment goals and patient desires. The study notably revealed that physicians were aware of patient wishes regarding cardiopulmonary resuscitation less than half of the time—38% of patients who died spent 10 or more days in an ICU and half of conscious patients were in moderate to severe pain at least 50% of the time. Additionally, advance directives were less useful than anticipated, with problems documented with implementation and application to specific situations encountered.

In many cases, patient preference may be directed at comfort care over extension of life. Lloyd et al. surveyed a group of seriously ill patients with regard to desires for care in several scenarios.[10] They found a wide variance in patient desires for aggressive care that was most closely related to predicted quality of life after illness as well as predicted survival. Premorbid level of function was less important to these patients in influencing their decision. While age alone may bias provider decisions to seek admission to a critical care unit and elderly patients may be expected to receive less aggressive care in some settings, several studies suggest that this is not a significant factor.[8,9,11] In fact, the oldest old may have diagnoses that actually respond well to therapy. This may be explained by considering that survival to extremes of age implies good health and lack of significant systemic disease that may be expected to cause death at a younger age. This appears to be the case for elderly patients requiring mechanical ventilation for the specific diagnosis of pulmonary edema.[13]

Recent evidence suggests that use of intensive care resources may be a frequent event when the evolution of disease is considered from a longitudinal perspective. Iwashyna evaluated patterns of access to critical care by evaluating the Medicare database for admission of patients 68 years and older related to common malignancies, stroke, congestive heart failure, and myocardial infarction.[14] The findings from this study suggest that admission to the ICU is common, the use of the ICU decreases with increasing age, and a significant number of admissions (23%) are related to repeat use of ICU resources by the 3% of patients admitted to the ICU at least one time per year for 5 years. In order to achieve the best use of critical care resources, it is clear that a better understanding of outcomes is necessary for advocacy of effective therapies and more accurate discussion of likely clinical course with patients and their families.

OUTCOMES

The study of outcomes in critically ill elderly patients is difficult. The elderly, as discussed elsewhere in this text, represent a vastly heterogeneous group that defies definition by age alone. The relationship between chronological age, age-related disease, and physiologic reserve is not consistent. In practice, it is not uncommon to see vigorous octogenarians undergoing intermediate- to high-risk surgical procedures with little difficulty. On the other hand, it is with some frequency that much younger patients with severe systemic disease present for similar procedures and often do not fare as well. Clearly, the more "elderly" patient is physiologically much "younger" than their less-aged counterpart with underlying chronic illness. This heterogeneity combined with the myriad of admitting diagnoses to the ICU along with differences in the nature of medical and surgical critical care patients make interpretation of the existing literature confusing. These factors next need to be considered in the context of the outcome measured. Historically, outcome studies have focused on mortality assessed as either survival to discharge from the ICU or survival until discharge from the hospital. Most have simply examined a cohort of elderly intensive care patients without considering specific diagnoses. This outcome measure fails to take into account quality of life issues after survival of intensive care.[15] The goal of any medical intervention in the elderly should be the return to the patient's premorbid level of function or greater. Unfortunately, it is a minority of studies on critical care outcomes in the elderly that address this issue specifically. The good news is that more work is being done to examine diagnosis-specific outcomes and the long-term results of ICU stays for the elderly. Here, we consider some of the available outcome data and some specific problems with the current state of the medical literature.

Studies have been inconclusive in determining factors related to survival in elderly patients. A number of studies have reported age as exhibiting significant influence while others have failed to demonstrate a significant effect. Methodological differences in the studies, definitions of aging, duration of data collection, and lack of separation of in-hospital (ICU) mortality versus long-term survival have been suggested as possible reasons for the inability to reach meaningful conclusions.[16] Additionally, it is possible that a tendency toward less aggressive care in the elderly could contribute to lower rates of survival. In a secondary analysis of the SUPPORT data, no such association could be demonstrated.[17] The authors found that the contribution of age to mortality was small, especially when compared to the contribution of diagnosis or severity of illness as assessed by acute physiology scoring. While few studies have examined differences between various age subgroups within those considered elderly, Djaiani and Ridley demonstrated significantly decreased survival at 1 year for those over 85 years of age compared to those 70–85 years old.[18] Diagnosis and severity illness were also independent predictors of survival at 1 year.

A recent study by Somme et al. sought to differentiate variables influencing survival to discharge from the ICU and examined the effect on long-term survival after discharge from the hospital.[19] The study further separated patients into different age subgroups and suggested that age is not to be the best predictor of short-term ICU survival. However, long-term survival may be best predicted by age and preexisting level of function. They followed 410 elderly patients over the age of 75 for 2 years admitted to a single university ICU in France. The study identified three subgroups: old (75–79 years), very old (80–84 years), and oldest old (over 85 years of age). ICU survival in these groups was 68%, 75%, and 69% respectively. Three-month survival was 54%, 56%, and 51%. Patients surviving their ICU stay had far greater rates of mortality than age-matched controls in the general population. These differences, however, decreased significantly by 1-year postdischarge. Acuity of illness as assessed by Acute Physiology and Chronic Health Evaluation II (APACHE II) was the only variable associated with dying in the ICU. Age and limitation of activity before admission were the only identified determinants of long-term survival. These results are also supported by a study of 817 patients over 65 years of age who received at least 48 hours of mechanical ventilation. In this study age, functional status, and preexisting illness were associated with increased mortality at 2 months.[20] Other studies have also suggested that severity of illness is the most important predictor of ICU survival with no effect demonstrated for age.[21]

Hennessy et al. recently published a review of outcomes related to functional status and health-related quality of life (HRQOL).[16] Their review of English language literature published between 1990 and 2003 revealed only 16 studies meeting their inclusion criteria. Their criteria included patients 65 years of age or older who required admission to the ICU and underwent assessment of functional status (assessed primarily by activities of daily living [ADLs]) or HRQOL. They excluded organ transplant and cancer patients. The analysis of the 16 studies revealed methodological and definition problems that made comparison and pooling of results impossible. Problems included an inconsistent definition of the term elderly, failure to report patient data stratified into deciles of age, and inconsistency in the choice and quality of instruments used to assess HRQOL. Failure to comment on validity, reliability, or responsiveness of the various instruments was noted in almost half of the studies. The results of the studies were mixed. Ten studies reported relatively good HRQOL, overall patient satisfaction with outcome, or no change from premorbid condition. Three studies demonstrated no significant difference in preadmission and postdischarge function. Two studies have documented reduction in functional status but a preserved perception of quality of life in ICU survivors. One study that focused only on physical functioning found a reduction in HRQOL but did not include a subjective assessment. It is apparent that more quality research is needed in this area to include prospective, longitudinal trials with clearly defined groups employing validated, reliable, and responsive measures of functional status and HRQOL.

In a more recent study of quality of life before and after intensive care, Cuthbertson et al. examined 300 consecutive patients admitted to a single ICU in Scotland.[22] Patients were followed longitudinally for 1 year. A previously validated tool was used to assess HRQOL. The mean age of study patients was 60.5, with patients over 64 years of age representing 36% of all study patients. All data were not reported specifically for the over 64 cohort. However, physical and mental component scores were reported for survivors over 64 years of age and suggest decline in function for the physical component at 3 and 6 months, with a gradual return to premorbid levels at 1 year (Fig. 24-1). The mental component score shows decline at 3 months with return to premorbid levels at 6 months (Fig. 24-2). The scores for all patients admitted to the ICU were significantly lower than data for controls from the general population, suggesting a lower level of function prior to ICU admission. Comparison for the older cohort was less accurate due to lack of sufficient data from age-matched controls in the general population. It is clear that more well-designed outcome trials are needed to define the patient populations and factors that determine likelihood of benefit in utilization of critical resources by the elderly.

As outlined above, quality of life is of central importance, but small decrements in objective performance may not necessarily translate to subjective dissatisfaction on the part of patients.[23] The studies mentioned above generally reviewed data for intensive care admissions for combined diagnoses. Some investigators have studied outcomes related to specific admitting diagnoses, comorbid conditions,

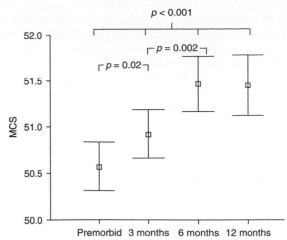

FIGURE 24-2 Differences in the mental component score (MCS) of the SF-36 between time points. The SF-36 (short form 36) is a tool for assessment of quality of life, which consists of a physical component score and a mental component score. Vitality, social function, role-emotional, and mental health make up the MCS. Data presented as error plots of means and standard errors of the means. Probability values reflect differences between time points and trends across time points. *(Reprinted with permission from Ref. 22.)*

or modalities such as use of mechanical ventilation. Highlights of some of the existing data are presented as related to affected organ systems defined below.

ORGAN SYSTEM CONSIDERATIONS FOR THE OLDER ICU PATIENT

▶ Neurologic issues—delirium in the ICU

Increasing evidence suggests that delirium in patients in the ICU is associated with increased length of stay, increased costs, increased morbidity, and increased mortality (Fig. 24-3).[24–26] Additionally, the

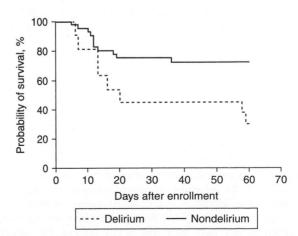

FIGURE 24-3 Survival proportion for patients with or without delirium traced with the Kaplan-Meier method (log rank test, $p = 0.003$). The dashed line represents patients with delirium; the continuous line represents patients without delirium. *(Reprinted with permission from Lin SM, Liu CY, Wang CH, et al. The impact of delirium on the survival of mechanically ventilated patients. Crit Care Med. 2004;32(11):2254–2259.)*

FIGURE 24-1 Differences in the physical component score (PCS) of the SF-36 between time points. The SF-36 (short form 36) is a tool for assessment of quality of life, which consists of a physical component score and a mental component score. Physical function, role-physical, bodily pain, and general health make up the PCS. Data presented as error plots of means and standard errors of the means. Probability values reflect differences between time points and trends across time points. *(Reprinted with permission from Ref. 22.)*

occurrence of delirium in the ICU appears to be associated with long-term cognitive decline.[25] Importantly, delirium in the ICU is frequently underdiagnosed. Recently, several methods have been validated to screen for delirium in this patient population. Appreciation of delirium is important as recognition may lead to interventions that have the potential to improve outcome. Delirium in the perioperative period has been discussed extensively in other sections of this text. Here, we consider those aspects of acute cognitive dysfunction relevant to patients in the ICU setting.

Delirium as defined by the Diagnostic and Statistical Manual IV (DSM-IV) of the American Psychiatric Association is an acute condition characterized by fluctuating changes in mental status and inattention, combined with disorganized thinking or an altered level of consciousness. Clinically, delirium can present with several different forms. It is also possible that different manifestations of delirium may have differing implications for prognosis and treatment. It is easy to identify the patient with agitation, combative behavior, or frank hallucinations. These patients with hyperactive delirium, however, represent the minority of patients with delirium in the ICU. Patients who appear quiet and peaceful are actually more likely to exhibit disordered thinking and inattention. This condition has been defined as hypoactive delirium. Further, it is the hypoactive form that is more likely to be present in elderly patients. By definition, delirium exhibits a waxing and waning course, and some patients may present with manifestations of both hyperactive and hypoactive forms. This has been defined as mixed delirium. One cohort study evaluating the prevalence of various forms of delirium in medical ICU patients found hyperactive forms present in 5% and hypoactive and mixed forms present in roughly 45% each. It is not known if these results would apply to surgical patients as well.

The pathophysiology of delirium is poorly understood and the interplay between critical illness and development of delirium is an intriguing area for further research. In general, imbalances between neurotransmitter systems involving the excitatory dopamine system and the inhibitory γ-aminobutyric acid (GABA) and acetylcholine systems are thought to be significant in the development of delirium. In acute illness, other frequently encountered mechanisms associated with altered mental status may be important, including the influence of inflammatory mediators, such as tumor necrosis factor and interleukin-1, decreased cerebral blood flow from a variety of etiologies, hypoxemia, electrolyte and metabolic disturbances, and the influence of centrally active medications, including sedatives, hypnotics, analgesics and anticholinergics.[27] In systemic inflammatory states, evidence exists that the brain may respond with local inflammatory responses.[28–30] Additionally, primary local inflammatory processes in the brain can be associated with systemic secondary inflammatory responses.[31] Therefore, the development of delirium in critical illness could result from one or a combination of various processes. It may reflect direct effects of various insults on neurotransmitter function, it may represent decreased end-organ reserve and increased susceptibility as marker of organ dysfunction during multiple organ dysfunction syndrome, It may possibly function as a source for persistent systemic inflammatory response, or it may represent an overlap of multifactorial etiologic pathways.[27]

Elderly patients in the ICU often present with many risk factors for delirium that have been previously defined for non-ICU patients. These risk factors are reviewed in Chap. 22 (Delirium and Postoperative Cognitive Dysfunction). Risk factors that have been identified specifically for ICU patients include a past medical history of hypertension and smoking, age, higher APACHE-II scores, and the use of sedative and analgesic medications.[32]

The fact that delirium in the ICU population is underrecognized has been underscored by a host of recent publications estimating the incidence of delirium in the ICU to be between 60% and 80% while being recognized only 32–66% of the time.[33,34] In this study, preexisting dementia was associated with an increased risk of developing delirium throughout all phases of hospitalization (Fig. 24-4). It is important to assess for preexisting dementia since preexisting long-term cognitive impairment is often present in elderly patients admitted to the ICU. The incidence is higher in patients admitted from nursing homes or with known impairment in activities of daily living.[34] It is, however, often difficult or impossible to assess premorbid dementia in patients admitted to the ICU compromised with an acute illness. Recently, proxy survey using the Modified Blessed Dementia Rating Scale and the Informant Questionnaire on Cognitive Decline in the Elderly has been validated to screen for the presence of dementia.[35] A survey of 912 health-care providers involved in ICU care indicated an overall appreciation of the high incidence of delirium but reflected a paucity of practitioners regularly monitoring for it.[36] Clinical practice guidelines adopted by several national organizations have recommended regular assessment for presence of delirium in ICU patients. Recently, the Confusion Assessment Method for the ICU (CAM-ICU) has been validated as an easily applied tool for serial assessment of delirium (Fig. 24-5).[37] The tool is nonverbal and has been demonstrated to be accurate in patients on mechanical ventilation with a sensitivity and specificity of greater than 95% and is highly consistent between users.[24,38] Assessment of alterations in mental status was assessed through use of the Glasgow Coma Scale or Richmond Agitation Sedation Scale (Fig. 24-6).[39]

The prognostic considerations for development of delirium in the ICU appear to be quite significant. One large prospective trial in patients on mechanical ventilation found delirium to be an independent risk factor for the need for prolonged mechanical ventilation,

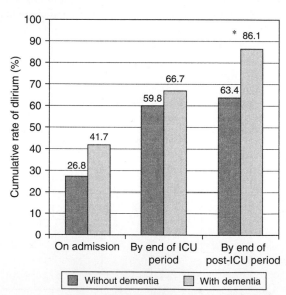

FIGURE 24-4 Cumulative rate of delirium throughout the hospital course stratified by dementia. Graph depicting the cumulative rates of delirium stratified by dementia (36 patients with dementia and 82 patients without dementia) during three separate periods of the study: on admission or baseline; by the end of the intensive care unit (ICU) period; and by the end of the post-ICU period up to 7 days. *(Reproduced with permission from Ref. 33.)*

The Confusion Assessment Method for the Intensive Care Unit (CAM-ICU)

Features and Descriptions	Absent	Present
I. Acute onset or fluctuating course*		
A. Is there evidence of an acute change in mental status from the baseline? B. Or, did the (abnormal) behavior fluctuate during the past 24 hours, that is, tend to come and go or increase and decrease in severity as evidenced by fluctuations on the Richmond Agitation Sedation Scale (RASS) or the Glasgow Coma Scale?		
II. Inattention†		
Did the patient have difficulty focusing attention as evidenced by a score of less than 8 correct answers on either the visual or auditory components of the Attention Screening Examination (ASE)?		
III. Disorganized thinking		
Is there evidence of disorganized or incoherent thinking as evidenced by incorrect answers to 3 or more of the 4 questions and inabilty to follow the commands? Questions 1. Will a stone float on water? 2. Are there fish in the sea? 3. Does 1 pound weigh more than 2 pounds? 4. Can you use a hammer to pound a nail? Commands 1. Are you having unclear thinking? 2. Hold up this many fingers. (Examiner holds 2 fingers in front of the patient.) 3. Now do the same thing with the other hand (without holding the 2 fingers in front of the patient). (If the patient is already extubated from the ventilator, determine whether the patient's thinking is disorganized or incoherent, such as rambling or irrelevant conversation, unclear or illogical flow of ideas, or unpredictable switching from subject to subject.)		
IV. Altered level of consciousness		
Is the patient's level of consciousness anything other than alert, such as being vigilant or lethargic, or in a stupor or coma? Alert: spontaneously fully aware of environment and interacts; appropriately Vigilant: hyperalert Lethargic: drowsy but easily aroused, unaware of some elements in the environment or not spontaneously interacting with the interviewer; becomes fully aware and appropriately interactive when prodded minimally Stupor: difficult to arouse, unaware of some or all elements in the environment or not spontaneously interacting with the interviewer; becomes incompletely aware when prodded strongly; can be aroused only by vigorous and repeated stimuli and as soon as the stimulus ceases, stuporous subject lapses back into unresponsive state Coma: unarousable, unaware of all elements in the environment with no spontaneous interaction or awareness of the interviewer so that the interview is impossible even with maximal prodding		
Overall CAM-ICU Assessment (Features 1 and 2 and either Feature 3 or 4): Yes___ No___		

*The scores included in the 10-point RASS range form a high of 4 (combative) to a low of –5 (deeply corratose and unresponsive). Under the RASS system, patients who were spontaneously alert, calm, and not agitated were scored at 0 (neutral zone). Anxious or agitated patients received a range of scores depending on their level of anxiety: 1 for anxious, 2 for agitated (fighting ventilator), 3 for very agitated (pulling on or removing catheters), or 4 combative (violent and a danger to staff). The scores –1 to –5 were assigned for patients with varying degrees of sedation based on their ability to maintain eye contact: –1 or more than 10 seconds, –2 for less than10 seconds, and –3 for eye opening but no eye contact. If physical stimulation was required, then the patients were scored as either –4 for eye opening or movement with physical or painful stimulation or –5 for no response to physical or painful stimulation. The RASS has excellent interrater reliability and intraclass correlation coefficients of 0.96 and 0.97, respectively, and has been validated against visual analog scale and geropsychiatric diagnoses in 2 ICU studies.[32,34]

†In completing the visual ASE, the patients were shown 5 simple pictures (previously published[35]) at 3-second intervals and asked to remember them. They were then immediately shown 10 subsequent pictures and asked to nod "yes" or "no" to indicate whether they had or had not just seen each of the pictures. Since 5 pictures had been shown to them already, for which the correct response was to nod "yes," and 5 others were new, for which the correct response was to shake their heads "no," patients scored perfectly if they achieved 10 correct responses. Scoring accounted for either errors of omission (indicating "no" for a previously shown picture) or for errors of commission (indicating "yes" for a picture not previously shown). In completing the auditory ASE, patients were asked to squeeze the rater's hand whenever they heard the letter A during the recitation of a series of 10 letters. The rater then read 10 letters from the following list in a normal tone at a rate of 1 letter per second: S, A, H, E, V, A, A, S, R, A, T. A scoring method similar to that of the visual ASE was used for the auditory ASE testing.

The table may be reproduced without permission for clinical use only (By EW et al, JAMA, 2001: 286:2707–2710)

FIGURE 24-5 CAM-ICU instrument. *(Reproduced with permission from Ref. 38.)*

abnormal cognitive function at time of discharge from the hospital, and an increased risk of death 6 months after discharge.[24] These outcomes were significant after controlling for confounding conditions such as preexisting disease, severity of illness, coma, and use of sedative and analgesic medications. As would be expected with conditions resulting in increased length of ICU stay and overall increased length of hospitalization, delirium in the ICU has been demonstrated to be associated with increased cost. A study by Mildbrandt et al. suggested a 40% increase in total cost of hospitalization for patients with one or more documented episodes of delirium.[26] The severity of delirium was associated with increasing hospital costs as well (Fig. 24-7).

Management strategies for prevention and treatment of delirium have not been well studied in the ICU. Strategies for non-ICU patients

The Richmond Agitation Sedation Scale (RASS)

Score	Term	Description	
+4	Combative	Overtly combative, violent, immediate danger to staff	
+3	Very agitated	Pulls or removes tube(s) or catheter(s): aggressive	
+2	Agitated	Frequent nonpurposeful movement, fights ventilator	
+1	Restless	Anxious but movements not aggressive or vigorous	
0	Alert and calm		
−1	Drowsy	Not fully alert, but has sustained awakening (eye opening/eye contact) to voice (> 10 seconds)	Verbal stimulaltion
−2	Light sedation	Briefly awakens with eye contact to voice (<10 seconds)	Verbal stimulaltion
−3	Moderate sedation	Movement or eye opening to voice (but no eye contact)	Verbal stimulaltion
−4	Deep sedation	No response to voice, but movement or eye opening to physical stimulation	Physical stimulaltion
−5	Unarousable	No response to voice or physical stimulation	Physical stimulaltion

Procedure for RASS assessment
1. Observe patient
   • Patient is alert, restless, or agitated
2. If not alert, state patient's name and say to open eyes and look at speaker   Score 0 to +4
   • Patient awakens with sustained eye opening and eye contact   Score −1
   • Patient awakens with eye opening and eye contact, but not sustained   Score −2
   • Patient has any movement in response to voice but no eye contact   Score −3
3. When no response to verbal stimulation, physically stimulate patient by shaking shoulder and/or rubbing sternum
   • Patient has any movement to physical stimulation   Score −4
   • Patient has no response to any stimulation   Score −5

FIGURE 24-6 The Richmond Agitation Sedation Scale. (*Reproduced with permission from Ref. 39.*)

have been examined and include nonpharmacologic interventions such as use of multidisciplinary care teams, frequent reorientation of the patient, regularly scheduled use of cognitively stimulating activities, use of sleep protocols, early mobilization and physical therapy, avoidance of urinary catheters and physical restraints, maintenance of adequate hydration, and avoidance of sensory deprivation.[40–42] While no consensus recommendations exist for the prevention and treatment of delirium in the ICU, it seems prudent to attempt to

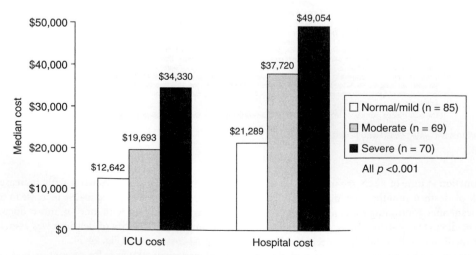

FIGURE 24-7 Medium intensive care unit (ICU) and hospital cost per patient. The histogram shows cost according to cumulative delirium severity indexes. Increasing delirium severity was significantly associated with incrementally greater ICU and hospital cost. (*Reproduced with permission from Ref. 26.*)

employ similar measures to the extent possible, given the constraints of the ICU environment. Use of weaning protocols may speed liberation from mechanical ventilation and impact the incidence of delirium. It should be noted that currently no data exist on the efficacy of these strategies in the ICU population. Prevention strategies may also include attempts to avoid use of medications known to exacerbate delirium. As mentioned previously, use of lorazepam has been associated with an increased risk of delirium, and medications with significant anticholinergic properties have been frequently implicated in contributing to delirium in hospitalized patients. Specific pharmacologic treatment of delirium is largely limited to the use of haloperidol for patients with agitation. Additionally, there is evidence that haloperidol may be associated with lower in-hospital mortality in ventilated patients.[43] Neuroleptic and atypical antipsychotic medications have the potential to prolong QT intervals, and the effect may become significant at higher doses or when combined with other medications in the ICU. Considerations should be given to monitoring the electrocardiogram (ECG) at regular intervals. Benzodiazepines are best avoided as they are more likely to worsen delirium and have several undesired effects including respiratory depression and potential for oversedation. A number of new "atypical" antipsychotic medications have found use in management of delirium in non-ICU patients including those who are institutionalized. While effective in controlling acute confusional states, the use of these medications has been associated with a small increase in mortality in this population. Use in the ICU population cannot be advocated at this time.

Respiratory considerations

The physiologic changes in the respiratory system related to aging include alterations in lung and chest wall compliance with resultant increased work of breathing, changes in closing capacity in relation to functional residual capacity (FRC) that cause an age-related increase in A-a difference, decreased diffusing capacity, alterations in ventilatory responses to hypercarbia and hypoxemia, and impaired mucociliary clearance.[44] These changes are described in detail in Chap. 5 (Pulmonary System). These alterations have the overall effect of decreasing physiologic reserve and placing the older patient at a higher risk of respiratory failure related to any insult. In addition,

ongoing disease states including primary respiratory diseases such as chronic obstructive pulmonary disease (COPD), interstitial lung disease, and pneumonia as well as nonpulmonary processes, such as congestive heart failure or neuromuscular diseases, may be superimposed. These processes may be chronic, acute or occur acutely in the setting of chronic disease and lead to respiratory compromise. Between the ages of 55 and 85, there is a tenfold increase in the incidence of acute respiratory failure requiring mechanical ventilation.[45] It is likely that age as well as the etiology of respiratory failure and other underlying comorbidities have a significant impact on outcome.[46] Figure 24-8 describes factors contributing to the development of and recovery from acute respiratory failure in the elderly. Therefore, it may not be reasonable to use age alone to determine appropriateness of initiation of mechanical ventilation in elderly patients. This decision should incorporate consideration of other age-related medical diseases, the likelihood that the clinician's judgment regarding reversibility of the current clinical situation, and the wishes of the patient or surrogate decision maker. Considering the significant cost associated with providing ventilatory support in the form of mechanical ventilation, the ability to quantify long-term benefit is of obvious significance.[15] Importantly, evidence exists that old age does not necessarily imply inability to wean successfully from mechanical ventilation. In patients over 70 years of age with admitting diagnoses of acute lung injury and adult respiratory distress syndrome, Ely demonstrated a similar proportion of survivors achieving physiologic recovery landmarks in patients over and under 70 years of age (Fig. 24-9).[47] However, age over 70 was a strong predictor of in-hospital death. Mortality rates at 28 and 180 days for patients over 70 years of age were 50% and 40%, respectively. This was twice the rate for younger patients. Older patients also spent a significantly longer time on mechanical ventilation and had a greater duration of ICU stay. In addition, older patients successfully passing a spontaneous breathing trial took longer to achieve unassisted breathing and had higher rates of reintubation. In an examination of long-term outcomes of prolonged mechanical ventilation, Chelluri et al. found an important relationship between premorbid level of function and long-term outcome.[48] Prolonged mechanical ventilation was defined as ventilatory assistance for greater than 48 hours. Premorbid function and long-term function at 1 year was determined

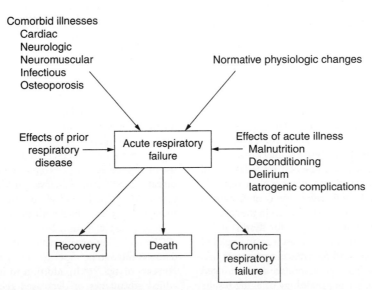

FIGURE 24-8 Causes and sequelae of acute respiratory failure. *(Reproduced with permission from Ref. 46.)*

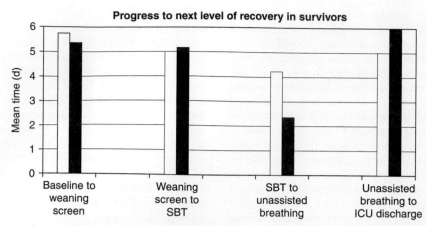

FIGURE 24-9 Histogram of the rate of progress through recovery landmarks achieved among survivors in two groups of ICU patients. White bars are patients ≥75 years of age and dark bars are patients <75 years of age. The mean time from enrollment to passing a spontaneous breathing trial (SBT) was similar between groups. The older patients took more time to progress from passing the SBT to achieving unassisted breathing and from unassisted breathing to ICU discharge. *(Adapted from Ref. 47.)*

by survey of ADLs and instrumental activities of daily living (IADLs). In this study, short-term mortality was related to severity of illness and prehospitalization functional status. Long-term mortality was associated with older age and poor prehospitalization functional status. The need for assistance with IADLs at 1 year was also associated with age and poor prehospitalization function. More than one-half of survivors required assistance with IADLs. The study included follow-up on nearly 300 survivors at 1 year after mechanical ventilation, included a mixed medical, surgical, trauma, and neurological ICU population, and adjusted for the effect of comorbid conditions on mortality over the study period.

Noninvasive positive pressure ventilation (NIPPV) may be of benefit to older patients with COPD or acute pulmonary edema.[49] Advantages of NIPPV are related to avoiding complications of invasive mechanical ventilation including tracheal injury, ventilator-associated pneumonia, and the use of heavier sedation in the elderly patient.[50] Patients who have hemodynamic instability, respiratory arrest, heavy airway secretions, agitation, upper airway obstruction, upper gastrointestinal bleeding, poor fit of the face mask, or are unable to cooperate will not be suitable candidates for NIPPV.[49] These factors will limit potential application of this mode of therapy to approximately 20% of all hospitalized patients.

▶ Cardiovascular considerations

Physiologic changes

The changes in cardiovascular physiology associated with aging are discussed in detail in Chap. 4 (Cardiovascular System). A number of these are of special interest to the intensivist. There are alterations in arterial stiffness resulting in increased pulse wave velocity throughout the vascular system, leading to increased vascular impedance and secondary changes in the myocardium including myocardial hypertrophy.[51] There is impaired diastolic relaxation contributing to the development of diastolic heart failure.[52] Alterations in the conduction system place the elderly patient at higher risk for dysrhythmia.[2] Changes in autonomic nervous system function result in an impaired ability to defend against maneuvers and pharmacologic agents that decrease sympathetic tone. Beta-adrenergic responses are attenuated in the aging myocardium as well.[52] The physiology of aging results in a net decrease in physiologic reserve, making the older patient

more susceptible to a variety of problems when facing the stress of acute illness, surgery, or trauma (Fig. 24-10). However, the increase in the incidence of disease states associated with aging is overwhelmingly the most important factor when dealing with the older patient in the ICU. Diseases such as hypertension, ischemic heart disease, valvular heart disease, and diseases of the conduction system are more prevalent in older patients and contribute significant morbidity to this population (Fig. 24-11).

The considerations discussed above for outcome studies in the elderly intensive care patient are underscored by the lack of sufficient literature addressing treatment of cardiovascular disease in older patients. Indeed, prior to 1990, age was frequently used as exclusion criterion in cardiovascular trials. More recently, patients over the age of 75 represent approximately 3.5% of the patients in coronary artery revascularization trials and approach 9% of the patients enrolled in therapeutic trials for acute coronary syndromes. Patients over the age of 75 contribute to 36% of all myocardial infarctions, 60% of myocardial infarctions-related deaths, and also have the highest incidence of heart failure.[53]

Acute coronary syndromes

Age has been demonstrated to be an independent risk factor for both ST-elevation MI and unstable angina/non-ST elevation MI.[54–56] Therapeutic benefit from standard medical therapy, including aspirin, beta-blockers, angiotensin-converting enzyme inhibitors, and nitrates, is present in the elderly and these standard pharmacologic strategies should be employed. The elderly do, however, have a greater incidence of untoward events with pharmacologic therapy including a higher incidence of gastrointestinal bleeding with aspirin therapy and an increased incidence of renal failure related to use of angiotensin-converting enzyme inhibitors.[53] In the setting of unstable angina/non-ST-elevation MI, unfractionated or low molecular weight heparin and glycoprotein IIb/IIIa inhibitors are also of therapeutic benefit albeit with an increased incidence of bleeding.[57,58]

In acute ST-elevation MI, percutaneous coronary interventions (PCI), including angioplasty and intracoronary stents, have been demonstrated to be superior to fibrinolytic therapy in patients over 70 years of age.[59,60] In addition to improved survival, PCI has the added advantages of decreased reinfarction, recurrent ischemia, and stroke when compared to fibrinolytic drug therapy alone.

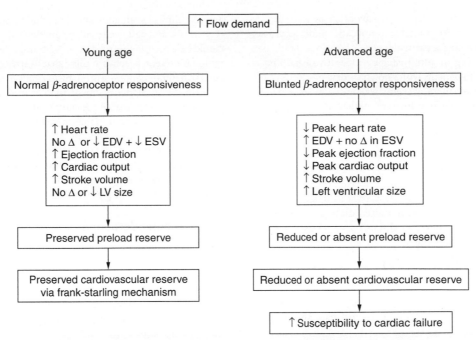

FIGURE 24-10 Cardiac response to increased flow demand in the young and the elderly. The young meet the increased flow demand primarily by β-adrenoceptor-mediated augmentation of heart rate and contractility, thus preserving preload reserve via the Frank-Starling mechanism. In contrast, the elderly employ primarily the preload reserve to augment cardiac performance, thereby losing additional cardiovascular reserve and becoming susceptible to cardiac insufficiency. EDV = end-diastolic volume; LV = Left ventricular; Δ = change. *(Reprinted with permission from Ref. 52.)*

Coronary artery bypass grafting continues to have a role in patients with left main coronary artery disease and three-vessel disease with decreased left ventricular function. However, the risk mortality of coronary artery bypass graft (CABG) surgery in patients over 75 years of age increases dramatically. In spite of demonstrated efficacy of the therapy for acute coronary syndromes in the elderly, a recent study suggested that the oldest patients are more likely to not receive guideline-recommended therapies.[61] The likelihood of therapy not being initiated was present after adjusting for patient, physician, and hospital characteristics. Interestingly, there was a variation in use of recommended therapies such that reperfusion strategies were the least likely to be employed, while differences in use of aspirin between younger and older cohorts was the smallest. This implies an influence of age on the treatment decision that is specific to each modality of therapy as opposed to a decision of whether or not to treat.

CV problems	Possible acute therapies
Unstable angina/NSEMI	ASA, β-blocker, heparin, LMWH, nitroglycerin, glycoprotein IIb/IIIa platelet inhibitor, cardiology consultation
STEMI	Percutaneous coronary intervention, fibrinolytic therapy, ASA, β-blocker, heparin, LMWH, nitroglycerin, cardiology consultation
Systolic dysfunction with heart failure	Diuretics, nitroprusside, nesiritide, nitroglycerin, inotropic agents
Diastolic dysfunction with heart failure	Diuretics, nesiritide, nitroglycerin
Atrial fibrillation—rate control	β-Blockers: metoprolol, esmolol Calcium antagonists: verapamil, diltiazem Others: digoxin, amiodarone
Atrial fibrillation—rhythm control	Amiodarone, ibutilide, electrical cardioversion
Atrial fibrillation—embolic prophylaxis	Heparin, LMWH, warfarin, ASA
Ventricular fibrillation	Advanced life support protocol
Ventricular tachycardia	Advanced life support protocol, electrical cardioversion, amiodarone, lidocaine
Aortic stenosis	Diuretics, arrhythmia management, inotropic agents, endocarditis prophylaxis, cardiology consultation
Mitral regurgitation	Diuretics, nitroprusside, nitroglycerin, arrhythmia management, inotropic agents, intra-aortic balloon pump, endocarditis prophylaxis, cardiology consultation

FIGURE 24-11 Common cardiovascular problems in the elderly ICU patients and possible acute therapies. NSEMI = non-ST-segment myocardial infarction; STEMI = ST-segment elevation myocardial infarction; LMWH = low-molecular weight heparin. *(Reprinted with permission from Ref. 53.)*

Perioperative beta blockade has been advocated as a strategy to decrease the incidence of cardiovascular complications and death associated with surgery. Whether a particular age or age alone should be a major factor in deciding to administer perioperative beta-blocker therapy is not known. In patients with known cardiac disease or major risk factors, beta-blocker therapy seems warranted as some studies have suggested potential harm in low-risk patients.[62]

Congestive heart failure

Heart failure is a frequent diagnosis in the elderly. It may be the primary reason for admission to a critical care unit or may complicate other illnesses or become an important process in the perioperative period. Heart failure may occur based on either impaired left ventricular systolic function or due to impaired diastolic relaxation of the left ventricular myocardium. As discussed previously, diastolic relaxation is impaired in the aging heart. Recalling that cardiac relaxation is an energy-requiring process, diastolic dysfunction has been observed in conditions including hypertension with left ventricular hypertrophy, ischemic heart disease, hypertrophic cardiomyopathies, and valvular heart disease. The pathophysiology and diagnostic criteria for diastolic dysfunction are discussed in Chap. 16 (Diastolic Dysfunction).

Dysrhythmia

Dysrhythmia may be the primary reason for admission to the ICU or may complicate acute illness. In some cases, the dysrhythmia may indicate significant underlying heart disease or be a marker of another comorbid process in a patient with decreased reserve. Clinical evaluation should include a search for underlying contributing factors such as acute ischemia, electrolyte abnormalities, heart failure, pulmonary embolus, acid-base disturbances, and hypoxemia. The incidence of various cardiac dysrhythmias was studied in 144,512 patients 65 years of age or older with a diagnosed cardiac dysrhythmia.[63] Atrial fibrillation was the most frequent. It was observed in 44.8% of patients compared with atrial flutter in 5.2% and supraventricular tachycardia in 3.8%. Sinoatrial node dysfunction occurred in 13.2% while complete atrioventricular block was observed in 5.8%. Cardiac arrest, ventricular tachycardia, and ventricular fibrillation occurred in 1.3%, 6.9%, and 1.3%, respectively. In symptomatic rapid atrial fibrillation with hemodynamic instability, electrical cardioversion is indicated. When the clinical situation is less tenuous, pharmacologic management should be considered. The issue of therapeutic goals in atrial fibrillation has been addressed by the Atrial Fibrillation Follow-Up Investigation of Rhythm Management (AFFIRM) trial.[64] Rate control is a reasonable therapeutic target since rhythm control strategies do not improve survival. In general, ventricular dysrhythmias can be addressed as recommended by the Advanced Cardiac Life Support guidelines. Implantable cardioverter-defibrillators may be considered for elderly patients who survive ventricular fibrillation or pulseless ventricular tachycardia (VF/VT) arrest. Bradydysrhythmia is not an infrequent event in the elderly.[65] The vast majority of pacemaker therapy is utilized in patients over the age of 65.

Valvular heart disease

The prevalence of valvular heart disease, particularly aortic stenosis and mitral regurgitation, increases with age.[53] Aortic stenosis may lead to the familiar symptoms of syncope, angina, and congestive heart failure. The only effective therapy is aortic valve replacement. Elderly patients can and do benefit from aortic valve replacement and often do well long-term. In patients with uncorrected aortic stenosis, clinical evaluation should include assessment of the degree of stenosis and left ventricular function. Pharmacologic therapy should be aimed at control of heart rate and relief of pulmonary congestion if present, keeping in mind that overly aggressive diuresis may worsen hemodynamics. Mitral regurgitation represents a complex problem. Surgical management with mitral valve replacement is associated with increased mortality rates in patients over the age of 75. Goals of medical management include relief of pulmonary congestion with diuretics and pharmacologic means to decrease the regurgitant fraction of left ventricular ejection with afterload reduction. Inotropic agents, particularly inodilators, may be beneficial. Intra-aortic balloon counterpulsation may be indicated as a bridge to valve replacement in patients deemed to be surgical candidates.

▶ Renal considerations

Age-related alterations in renal physiology are reviewed in Chap. 7 (Urinary and Hepatic Systems). Loss of nephrons results in a decrease in glomerular filtration and renal blood flow. Tubular function declines with concomitant decreases in urine-concentrating ability, hydrogen ion excretion, and sodium absorption.[51] Thirst perception is blunted as well.[66] Creatinine clearance can be estimated by the familiar equation:

$$\text{Creatinine clearance (mL/min)} = \frac{(140 - \text{age}) \times \text{body weight (kg)}}{72 \times \text{serum creatinine (mg/dL)}}$$

Creatinine clearance for women $= 0.85 \times$ above value

However, loss of muscle mass in the elderly may limit the value of serum creatinine as an accurate predictor of renal function. These changes account for an impaired ability of the geriatric patient to protect against significant dehydration and tend to decrease the clearance of drugs with renal routes of elimination.

The baseline age-related decline in renal function would seem to place the elderly patient at an increased risk for acute renal failure, especially when faced with the challenge of acute illness. Several studies have suggested that elderly ICU patients are prone to develop acute renal failure more frequently than younger patients.[67–69] However, there is some controversy regarding this finding.[70–72] When patients develop acute renal failure in the setting of sepsis, age along with use of vasoactive medications, mechanical ventilation, and renal replacement therapy are independent predictors of mortality.

As would be expected based on the physiologic changes described, hyperosmolar states are not uncommon in the elderly and are associated with high mortality.[73] They are especially frequent in institutionalized patients with a high level of functional dependency and cognitive impairment and in those with acute infections.[74]

▶ Infectious disease considerations

The elderly have number of factors predisposing them to infectious disease. Aging is associated with decline in immune competence termed *immune senescence*.[75] Declining immune function includes alterations in marrow response to infection, increases in memory T-cells, decreases in reactive T-cells, and altered patterns of interleukin-2 production. There is an increase in autoantibodies and monoclonal immunoglobulins.[2] The contribution of comorbid diseases, such as diabetes, peripheral vascular disease, and COPD, further places the elderly at risk of infection. How immune senescence interacts with age-related disease and physiologic stress is likely more important in contributing to the increased risk of infection in the older adult than is the alteration in immunity alone. Unfortunately, the mechanisms involved in age-related change of the immune system are not well-defined. These factors are further influenced by functional limitations, often associated with aging and other specific problems of the elderly, including frequent use of prosthetic devices including total joint arthroplasty, indwelling urinary catheters, and residence in chronic care facilities.[76] The presentation of various infectious diseases may also be atypical in the elderly population requiring a high index of suspicion. Often, a change in cognitive function may be the only presenting symptom of a urinary tract infection. Even in patients with life-threatening infection, fever may be the only finding at the time of initial evaluation.[77] Alternatively, fever may be absent as often as 25% of the time in elderly patients with severe life-threatening infection.[78]

Pneumonia is a particularly problematic issue in the elderly. The incidence of pneumonia is 10 times that of their younger counterparts. It represents the leading cause of death in patients over 80 years of age. In patients admitted to the ICU with pneumonia, mortality rates have been reported ranging from 13% to as high as 40%. Patterns of infection and therefore the spectrum of causative agents include community-acquired sources or those associated with chronic care facilities and those acquired in the hospital. A number of factors place the elderly patient at risk for pneumonia. Impaired swallowing in the elderly places them at increased risk for aspiration pneumonia.[79] Underlying disease, poor nutrition, residence in a chronic care facility, and cognitive impairment have all been associated with an increased risk of pneumonia.

Sepsis is a significant problem in the elderly. It is estimated that approximately 750,000 patients are affected by sepsis each year in the United States.[80] Of these, roughly two-thirds will be over the age of 65. Mortality is age dependent with mortality rates over 38% for patients over 85 years of age. Recently, recombinant human-activated protein C (drotrecogin alfa [activated] [DAA]) has been approved for use in the treatment of severe sepsis. Ely et al. studied the use of DAA in patients 75 years of age or older presenting with severe sepsis.[81] In this study, an absolute risk reduction in in-hospital mortality and mortality at 28 days was found to be 15.6% and 15.5%, respectively (Fig. 24-12). The major complication of DAA therapy is bleeding. The risk of bleeding in the study population did not differ from the risk observed for younger patients treated with DAA.

Antimicrobial therapy will be best guided based on the expected pathogen(s) and culture results, with attention to local and institutional resistance patterns and antibiotic sensitivities.[82] Appropriate

dosing of antibiotics will need to consider the likelihood of changing end-organ function in the aging patient and any specific end-organ disease especially with regard to renal function.[83] Antimicrobials can be a significant source of untoward drug effects, and the incidence and severity of drug-related adverse events increases with age.[78]

Gastrointestinal and nutritional considerations

Nutrition is of particular concern in the critically ill elderly patient. As with nearly every other organ system, functional reserve is compromised with regard to nutritional status as well. This is largely the result of changes in body composition associated with aging as well as the presence of a number of factors that place the aged at risk for malnutrition even prior to critical illness. Some of the other factors include decreased appetite, problems with dentition leading to difficulty chewing, cognitive impairment, substandard living conditions, malabsorption, and age-related disease. Malnutrition is common in the elderly occurring in up to 15% of those living in the community with higher rates found in those who are hospitalized or institutionalized.[84] Poor nutritional status has been associated with poor wound healing, pneumonia, and mortality.[2] The influence of poor nutritional status on mortality has been underscored by several recent studies. Dardaine et al. studied 116 patients of age 70 and over who received at least 24 hours of support with mechanical ventilation in an ICU.[85] Impaired nutritional status at time of admission was predictive of mortality at 6 months. In elderly patients in the general community, a body mass index less than 22 has been shown to predict mortality.[2] Low serum albumin, defined as less than 3.3 mg/dL, has been identified as an independent risk factor for all-cause mortality in the elderly and was further associated with increased length of stay and increased rate of readmission.[86] It seems prudent to include a baseline estimate of nutritional status along with assessment of functional status when addressing concerns in the elderly patient with critical illness.

Increased metabolic demands related to the stress of acute illness, surgery, or trauma may lead to a metabolic spiral with problems related to protein catabolism, decreased hepatic function, decreased immune function, impaired barrier function of skin,[87] and the gastrointestinal tract and deconditioning. Muscle mass has been shown to decrease with normal aging. This loss termed *sarcopenia* is important in decreasing protein reserve. Loss of muscle mass in critical illness is well-described and may have important implications for respiratory muscle strength during hospitalization and for rehabilitation following acute illness.[88] Given the high incidence of baseline malnutrition, early nutrition may be especially important in the elderly. Enteral nutrition is preferred; however, parenteral nutrition is indicated for patients who cannot tolerate enteral feeding. In patients requiring parenteral nutrition, glutamine supplementation may affect long-term survival.[89]

Alterations in glucose homeostasis occur with aging. Older patients have a greater likelihood of insulin resistance but also are prone to hypoglycemia. Hypoglycemia has been associated with increased mortality in the hospitalized elderly.[90,91] Insulin resistance is a feature of the postoperative stress response and response to acute illness and injury.[92] This response is magnified in older patients. Tight glucose control has been advocated for patients in the ICU and has been demonstrated to significantly decrease mortality.[93]

Biliary disease is common in the elderly and represents the most frequent indication for intra-abdominal surgery in the older population. By the age of 70, cholelithiasis and choledocholithiasis are present in approximately 33% of the U.S. population.[94] A high index of suspicion should be maintained since the presentation of significant cholecystitis

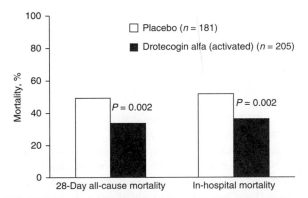

FIGURE 24-12 Histogram showing 28-day and in-hospital mortality rates according to treatment group of patients ≥75 years of age. Patients aged ≥75 years treated with drotrecogin alfa (activated), compared with placebo recipients, had absolute risk reductions in 28-day and in-hospital mortality rates. *(Reprinted with permission from Ref. 81.)*

may be atypical in the elderly, especially in those with coexisting diabetes. It follows that older patients may present to the ICU with complications of these diseases, including ascending biliary tract infection, obstructive pancreatitis, and post-ERCP pancreatitis, or following elective or emergent surgery.

▶ Complications

Elderly patients have been demonstrated to be at a higher risk for iatrogenic complications. A study of 120 patients over the age of 65 admitted to an acute service with diagnoses of congestive heart failure, acute myocardial infarction, and pneumonia noted a high incidence of iatrogenic complications (58%). Over 60% of these complications were judged to be potentially preventable.[95] Functional status at the time of admission was correlated with the likelihood of suffering an iatrogenic complication. Giraud et al. studied 400 consecutive admissions analyzing factors associated with iatrogenic complications.[96] They reported a 31% incidence of complications with 13% felt to be major. The majority of major complications included severe hypotension, respiratory distress, pneumothorax, and cardiac arrest. Patients over the age of 65 years were twice as likely to experience a major complication as younger patients.

Polypharmacy is of special concern in the elderly (see Chap. 13). Drug interactions and medication errors are a significant source of complication.

Orthopedic surgery is frequent in the elderly and orthopedic procedures, particularly total joint arthroplasty, are known to be associated with a high risk for deep venous thrombosis and pulmonary embolism. In addition, age has been considered to be an independent risk factor for thromboembolism. However, other factors including the type of surgery, comorbid disease, and functional status are important considerations in assessing the risk of deep venous thrombosis and thromboembolic complications.[97] The combination of these risks demands vigilance in deep vein thrombosis prophylaxis.

Endotracheal intubation has been associated with swallowing dysfunction postextubation. In patients intubated for longer than 48 hours, alterations in the function of mechanoreceptors and chemoreceptors in the mucosa of the pharynx and larynx, leading to pharyngeal muscle dysfunction and impaired proprioception, have been posited as possible mechanisms. Swallowing dysfunction may lead to an increased risk of aspiration of oral contents. Several studies conflict as to whether the risk of swallowing dysfunction postextubation increases with age. However, studies suggest a longer time to resolution of swallowing deficits for those with lower preadmission functional status.[98]

Following large volume resuscitation, elderly patients with sepsis have been demonstrated to mobilize fluid at a slower rate than younger patients (Fig. 24-13).[99] This has clear implications for the timing and appropriate monitoring and management of volume status in the elderly and has potential to influence the timing of transfer of patients from the ICU to lower acuity care.

CONCLUSION

The management decisions facing those caring for critically ill elderly patients are difficult and frequently not clear. The well-described alterations in physiology attributed to aging are merely a starting point. The available data suggest that while age impacts outcome, coexisting age-related disease, premorbid level of function, potential for reversibility of the acute process, and the wishes of the patient or their appointed health-care decision maker must all be carefully considered in developing treatment strategies for critically

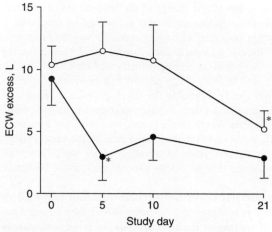

* Indicate significant change from preceding measurement.

FIGURE 24-13 Sequential measurements of excess extracellular water (ECW) in 8 elderly (open circles) and 6 young (solid circles) patients with sepsis. *(Reprinted with permission from Ref. 99.)*

ill elders. The available data suggest and emphasize the role of premorbid functional status in predicting outcome for elderly patients with critical illness. Assessment of ADLs and IADLs along with accurate estimates of nutritional status at the time of admission to the ICU is an important part of the initial evaluation of the patient. The timely, accurate, and responsible triage and treatment of our older patients in the ICU depends on defining the issues in the elderly population where interventions have the potential to improve outcome. In turn, the allocation of limited intensive care resources can be applied in the most efficient and effective manner while providing our patients and their families with realistic expectations for results of critical care interventions along with their short- and long-term outcomes.

KEY POINTS

▶ The goal of any medical intervention in the elderly should be the return to the patient's premorbid level of function or greater.

▶ Admission to the ICU should not be based on age alone. Considerations include the patient's underlying medical condition, premorbid level of function, nature of the admitting diagnosis to the ICU, realistic expectations to eventually return to a premorbid level of function or independent living, and the wishes of the patient to undergo the recommended intervention.

▶ Outcome studies involving critical care in the elderly should ideally evaluate functional outcome.

▶ It appears that survival to discharge from the ICU is most closely related to severity of illness at the time of admission, while age, prehospital functional status, and preexisting illness have the greatest effect on long-term survival.

▶ Delirium in the ICU is underrecognized and has been associated with prolonged mechanical ventilation, abnormal cognitive function at discharge, and increased risk of death.

▶ Recovery for elderly survivors of critical care is often a long process with many requiring assistance with IADLs at 1-year postdischarge.

▶ Percutaneous coronary interventions have demonstrated superiority to fibrinolytic therapy in patients over 70 years of age.

- Diastolic dysfunction is an important cause of heart failure in the elderly.

- Subgroup analysis has suggested efficacy for recombinant human-activated protein C in elderly patients with sepsis.

- Early nutritional support is an important consideration in care of the elderly as preexisting malnutrition frequently present.

KEY REFERENCES

- Rosenthal RA, Kavic SM. Assessment and management of the geriatric patient. *Crit Care Med*. 2004;32:S92–S105.

- Iwashyna TJ. Critical care use during the course of serious illness. *Am J Respir Crit Care Med*. 2004;170:981–986.

- Hennessy D, Juzwishin K, Yergens D, et al. Outcomes of elderly survivors of intensive care: a review of the literature. *Chest*. 2005;127:1764–1774.

- Cuthbertson BH, Scott J, Strachan M, et al. Quality of life before and after intensive care. *Anaesthesia*. 2005;60:332–339.

- Ely EW, Shintani A, Truman B, et al. Delirium as a predictor of mortality in mechanically ventilated patients in the intensive care unit. *JAMA*. 2004;291:1753–1762.

REFERENCES

1. Nagappan R, Parkin G. Geriatric critical care. *Crit Care Clin*. 2003;19:253–270.
2. Rosenthal RA, Kavic SM. Assessment and management of the geriatric patient. *Crit Care Med*. 2004;32:S92–S105.
3. Bekes CE, Dellinger RP, Brooks D, et al. Critical care medicine as a distinct product line with substantial financial profitability: the role of business planning. *Crit Care Med*. 2004;32:1207–1214.
4. Ewart GW, Marcus L, Gaba MM, et al. The critical care medicine crisis: a call for federal action: a white paper from the critical care professional societies. *Chest*. 2004;125:1518–1521.
5. Kelley MA, Angus D, Chalfin DB, et al. The critical care crisis in the United States: a report from the profession. *Chest*. 2004;125:1514–1517.
6. Ely EW. Optimizing outcomes for older patients treated in the intensive care unit. *Intensive Care Med*. 2003;29:2112–2115.
7. Rocker G. Controversial issues in critical care for the elderly: a perspective from Canada. *Crit Care Clin*. 2003;19:811–825.
8. Chelluri L, Grenvik A, Silverman M. Intensive care for critically ill elderly: mortality, costs, and quality of life. Review of the literature. *Arch Intern Med*. 1995;155:1013–1022.
9. Demoule A, Cracco C, Lefort Y, et al. Patients aged 90 years or older in the intensive care unit. *J Gerontol A Biol Sci Med Sci*. 2005;60:129–132.
10. Lloyd CB, Nietert PJ, Silvestri GA. Intensive care decision making in the seriously ill and elderly. *Crit Care Med*. 2004;32:649–654.
11. Kleinpell RM, Ferrans CE. Factors influencing intensive care unit survival for critically ill elderly patients. *Heart Lung*. 1998;27:337–343.
12. Phillips RS, Hamel MB, Covinsky KE, Lynn J. Findings from SUPPORT and HELP: an introduction. Study to understand prognoses and preferences for outcomes and risks of treatment. Hospitalized elderly longitudinal project. *J Am Geriatr Soc*. 2000;48:S1–S5.
13. Adnet F, Le Toumelin P, Leberre A, et al. In-hospital and long-term prognosis of elderly patients requiring endotracheal intubation for life-threatening presentation of cardiogenic pulmonary edema. *Crit Care Med*. 2001;29:891–895.
14. Iwashyna TJ. Critical care use during the course of serious illness. *Am J Respir Crit Care Med*. 2004;170:981–986.
15. Szalados JE. Age and functional status as determinants of intensive care unit outcome: sound basis for health policy or tip of the outcomes iceberg. *Crit Care Med*. 2004;32:291–293.
16. Hennessy D, Juzwishin K, Yergens D, et al. Outcomes of elderly survivors of intensive care: a review of the literature. *Chest*. 2005;127:1764–1774.
17. Hamel MB, Davis RB, Teno JM, et al. Older age, aggressiveness of care, and survival for seriously ill, hospitalized adults. SUPPORT investigators.

Study to understand prognoses and preferences for outcomes and risks of treatments. *Ann Intern Med*. 1999;131:721–728.
18. Djaiani G, Ridley S. Outcome of intensive care in the elderly. *Anaesthesia*. 1997;52:1130–1136.
19. Somme D, Maillet JM, Gisselbrecht M, et al. Critically ill old and the oldest-old patients in intensive care: short- and long-term outcomes. *Intensive Care Med*. 2003;29:2137–2143.
20. Quality of life after mechanized ventilation in the elderly study investigators. 2-month mortality and functional status of critically ill adult patients receiving prolonged mechanical ventilation. *Chest*. 2002;121:549–558.
21. Lipsett PA, Swoboda SM, Dickerson J, et al. Survival and functional outcome after prolonged intensive care unit stay. *Ann Surg*. 2000;231:262–268.
22. Cuthbertson BH, Scott J, Strachan M, et al. Quality of life before and after intensive care. *Anaesthesia*. 2005;60:332–339.
23. Montuclard L, Garrouste-Orgeas M, Timsit JF, et al. Outcome, functional autonomy, and quality of life of elderly patients with a long-term intensive care unit stay. *Crit Care Med*. 2000;28:3389–3395.
24. Ely EW, Gautam S, Margolin R, et al. The impact of delirium in the intensive care unit on hospital length of stay. *Intensive Care Med*. 2001;27:1892–1900.
25. Ely EW, Shintani A, Truman B, et al. Delirium as a predictor of mortality in mechanically ventilated patients in the intensive care unit. *JAMA*. 2004;291:1753–1762.
26. Milbrandt EB, Deppen S, Harrison PL, et al. Costs associated with delirium in mechanically ventilated patients. *Crit Care Med*. 2004;32:955–962.
27. Pandharipande P, Jackson J, Ely EW. Delirium: acute cognitive dysfunction in the critically ill. *Curr Opin Crit Care*. 2005;11:360–368.
28. Munford RS, Tracey KJ. Is severe sepsis a neuroendocrine disease? *Mol Med*. 2002;8:437–442.
29. Woiciechowsky C, Schoning B, Daberkow N, et al. Brain-IL-1beta induces local inflammation but systemic anti-inflammatory response through stimulation of both hypothalamic-pituitary-adrenal axis and sympathetic nervous system. *Brain Res*. 1999;816:563–571.
30. Rothwell NJ, Luheshi G, Toulmond S. Cytokines and their receptors in the central nervous system: physiology, pharmacology, and pathology. *Pharmacol Ther*. 1996;69:85–95.
31. Woiciechowsky C, Asadullah K, Nestler D, et al. Sympathetic activation triggers systemic interleukin-10 release in immunodepression induced by brain injury. *Nat Med*. 1998;4:808–813.
32. Dubois MJ, Bergeron N, Dumont M, et al. Delirium in an intensive care unit: a study of risk factors. *Intensive Care Med*. 2001;27:1297–1304.
33. McNicoll L, Pisani MA, Zhang Y, et al. Delirium in the intensive care unit: occurrence and clinical course in older patients. *J Am Geriatr Soc*. 2003;51:591–598.
34. Pisani MA, Redlich C, McNicoll L, et al. Underrecognition of preexisting cognitive impairment by physicians in older ICU patients. *Chest*. 2003;124:2267–2274.
35. Pisani MA, Inouye SK, McNicoll L, Redlich CA. Screening for preexisting cognitive impairment in older intensive care unit patients: use of proxy assessment. *J Am Geriatr Soc*. 2003;51:689–693.
36. Ely EW, Stephens RK, Jackson JC, et al. Current opinions regarding the importance, diagnosis, and management of delirium in the intensive care unit: a survey of 912 healthcare professionals. *Crit Care Med*. 2004;32:106–112.
37. Ely EW, Margolin R, Francis J, et al. Evaluation of delirium in critically ill patients: validation of the confusion assessment method for the intensive care unit (CAM-ICU). *Crit Care Med*. 2001;29:1370–1379.
38. Ely EW, Inouye SK, Bernard GR, et al. Delirium in mechanically ventilated patients: validity and reliability of the confusion assessment method for the intensive care unit (CAM-ICU). *JAMA*. 2001;286:2703–2710.
39. Ely EW, Truman B, Shintani A, et al. Monitoring sedation status over time in ICU patients: reliability and validity of the Richmond Agitation Sedation Scale (RASS). *JAMA*. 2003;289:2983–2991.
40. Inouye SK, Bogardus ST, Jr, Charpentier PA, et al. A multicomponent intervention to prevent delirium in hospitalized older patients. *N Engl J Med*. 1999;340:669–676.
41. Inouye SK, Bogardus ST, Jr, Williams CS, et al. The role of adherence on the effectiveness of nonpharmacologic interventions: evidence from the delirium prevention trial. *Arch Intern Med*. 2003;163:958–964.
42. Marcantonio ER, Flacker JM, Wright RJ, Resnick NM. Reducing delirium after hip fracture: a randomized trial. *J Am Geriatr Soc*. 2001;49:516–522.

43. Milbrandt EB, Kersten A, Kong L, et al. Haloperidol use is associated with lower hospital mortality in mechanically ventilated patients. *Crit Care Med.* 2005;33:226–229; discussion 263–265.

44. Zaugg M, Lucchinetti E. Respiratory function in the elderly. *Anesthesiol Clin North America.* 2000;18:47–58, vi.

45. Vincent JL, Akca S, De Mendonca A, et al. The epidemiology of acute respiratory failure in critically ill patients(*). *Chest.* 2002;121:1602–1609.

46. Sevransky JE, Haponik EF. Respiratory failure in elderly patients. *Clin Geriatr Med.* 2003;19:205–224.

47. Ely EW, Wheeler AP, Thompson BT, et al. Recovery rate and prognosis in older persons who develop acute lung injury and the acute respiratory distress syndrome. *Ann Intern Med.* 2002;136:25–36.

48. Chelluri L, Im KA, Belle SH, et al. Long-term mortality and quality of life after prolonged mechanical ventilation. *Crit Care Med.* 2004;32:61–69.

49. Heffner JE, Highland KB. Chronic obstructive pulmonary disease in geriatric critical care. *Crit Care Clin.* 2003;19:713–727.

50. Levy M, Tanios MA, Nelson D, et al. Outcomes of patients with do-not-intubate orders treated with noninvasive ventilation. *Crit Care Med.* 2004;32:2002–2007.

51. Oskvig RM. Special problems in the elderly. *Chest.* 1999;115:158S–164S.

52. Priebe HJ. The aged cardiovascular risk patient. *Br J Anaesth.* 2000;85:763–778.

53. Crispell KA. Common cardiovascular issues encountered in geriatric critical care. *Crit Care Clin.* 2003;19:677–691.

54. In-hospital mortality and clinical course of 20,891 patients with suspected acute myocardial infarction randomized between alteplase and streptokinase with or without heparin. The International Study Group. *Lancet.* 1990;336:71–75.

55. An international randomized trial comparing four thrombolytic strategies for acute myocardial infarction. The GUSTO investigators. *N Engl J Med.* 1993;329:673–682.

56. Early effects of tissue-type plasminogen activator added to conventional therapy on the culprit coronary lesion in patients presenting with ischemic cardiac pain at rest. Results of the thrombolysis in myocardial ischemia (TIMI IIIA) trial. *Circulation.* 1993;87:38–52.

57. Inhibition of platelet glycoprotein IIb/IIIa with eptifibatide in patients with acute coronary syndromes. The PURSUIT trial investigators. Platelet glycoprotein IIb/IIIa in unstable angina: receptor suppression using integrilin therapy. *N Engl J Med.* 1998;339:436–443.

58. Inhibition of the platelet glycoprotein IIb/IIIa receptor with tirofiban in unstable angina and non-Q-wave myocardial infarction. Platelet receptor inhibition in ischemic syndrome management in patients limited by unstable signs and symptoms (PRISM-PLUS) study investigators. *N Engl J Med.* 1998;338:1488–1497.

59. Berger AK, Schulman KA, Gersh BJ, et al. Primary coronary angioplasty vs. thrombolysis for the management of acute myocardial infarction in elderly patients. *JAMA.* 1999;282:341–348.

60. Weaver WD, Simes RJ, Betriu A, et al. Comparison of primary coronary angioplasty and intravenous thrombolytic therapy for acute myocardial infarction: a quantitative review. *JAMA.* 1997;278:2093–2098.

61. Rathore SS, Mehta RH, Wang Y, et al. Effects of age on the quality of care provided to older patients with acute myocardial infarction. *Am J Med.* 2003;114:307–315.

62. Lindenauer PK, Pekow P, Wang K, et al. Perioperative beta-blocker therapy and mortality after major noncardiac surgery. *N Engl J Med.* 2005;353:349–361.

63. Baine WB, Yu W, Weis KA. Trends and outcomes in the hospitalization of older Americans for cardiac conduction disorders or arrhythmias, 1991–1998. *J Am Geriatr Soc.* 2001;49:763–770.

64. Wyse DG, Waldo AL, DiMarco JP, et al. A comparison of rate control and rhythm control in patients with atrial fibrillation. *N Engl J Med.* 2002;347:1825–1833.

65. Trappe HJ, Brandts B, Weismueller P. Arrhythmias in the intensive care patient. *Curr Opin Crit Care.* 2003;9:345–355.

66. Phillips PA, Rolls BJ, Ledingham JG, et al. Reduced thirst after water deprivation in healthy elderly men. *N Engl J Med.* 1984;311:753–759.

67. Mangano CM, Diamondstone LS, Ramsay JG, et al. Renal dysfunction after myocardial revascularization: risk factors, adverse outcomes, and hospital resource utilization. The Multicenter Study of Perioperative Ischemia Research Group. *Ann Intern Med.* 1998;128:194–203.

68. de Mendonca A, Vincent JL, Suter PM, et al. Acute renal failure in the ICU: risk factors and outcome evaluated by the SOFA score. *Intensive Care Med.* 2000;26:915–921.

69. Groeneveld AB, Tran DD, van der Meulen J, et al. Acute renal failure in the medical intensive care unit: predisposing, complicating factors and outcome. *Nephron.* 1991;59:602–610.

70. Pascual J, Liano F. Causes and prognosis of acute renal failure in the very old. Madrid Acute Renal Failure Study Group. *J Am Geriatr Soc.* 1998;46:721–725.

71. Clermont G, Acker CG, Angus DC, et al. Renal failure in the ICU: comparison of the impact of acute renal failure and end-stage renal disease on ICU outcomes. *Kidney Int.* 2002;62:986–996.

72. Feest TG, Round A, Hamad S. Incidence of severe acute renal failure in adults: results of a community based study. *Br Med J.* 1993;306:481–483.

73. Bourdel-Marchasson I, Proux S, Dehail P, et al. One-year incidence of hyperosmolar states and prognosis in a geriatric acute care unit. *Gerontology.* 2004;50:171–176.

74. Weinberg AD, Pals JK, Levesque PG, et al. Dehydration and death during febrile episodes in the nursing home. *J Am Geriatr Soc.* 1994;42:968–971.

75. High KP. Infection in an ageing world. *Lancet Infect Dis.* 2002;2:655.

76. High KP, Bradley S, Loeb M, et al. A new paradigm for clinical investigation of infectious syndromes in older adults: assessment of functional status as a risk factor and outcome measure. *Clin Infect Dis.* 2005;40:114–122.

77. Marco CA, Schoenfeld CN, Hansen KN, et al. Fever in geriatric emergency patients: clinical features associated with serious illness. *Ann Emerg Med.* 1995;26:18–24.

78. Yoshikawa TT. Epidemiology and unique aspects of aging and infectious diseases. *Clin Infect Dis.* 2000;30:931–933.

79. Marik PE, Kaplan D. Aspiration pneumonia and dysphagia in the elderly. *Chest.* 2003;124:328–336.

80. Angus DC, Linde-Zwirble WT, Lidicker J, et al. Epidemiology of severe sepsis in the united states: analysis of incidence, outcome, and associated costs of care. *Crit Care Med.* 2001;29:1303–1310.

81. Ely EW, Angus DC, Williams MD, et al. Drotrecogin alfa (activated) treatment of older patients with severe sepsis. *Clin Infect Dis.* 2003;37:187–195.

82. Ferrara AM, Fietta AM. New developments in antibacterial choice for lower respiratory tract infections in elderly patients. *Drugs Aging.* 2004;21:167–186.

83. Livornese LL, Jr, Slavin D, Gilbert B, et al. Use of antibacterial agents in renal failure. *Infect Dis Clin North Am.* 2004;18:551–579, viii–ix.

84. Reuben DB, Greendale GA, Harrison GG. Nutrition screening in older persons. *J Am Geriatr Soc.* 1995;43:415–425.

85. Dardaine V, Dequin PF, Ripault H, et al. Outcome of older patients requiring ventilatory support in intensive care: impact of nutritional status. *J Am Geriatr Soc.* 2001;49:564–570.

86. Corti MC, Guralnik JM, Salive ME, Sorkin JD. Serum albumin level and physical disability as predictors of mortality in older persons. *JAMA.* 1994;272:1036–1042.

87. Bourdel-Marchasson I, Barateau M, Rondeau V, et al. A multicenter trial of the effects of oral nutritional supplementation in critically ill older inpatients. GAGE group. Groupe Aquitain Geriatrique d'Evaluation. *Nutrition.* 2000;16:1–5.

88. Griffiths RD. Muscle mass, survival, and the elderly ICU patient. *Nutrition.* 1996;12:456–458.

89. Griffiths RD, Jones C, Palmer TE. Six-month outcome of critically ill patients given glutamine-supplemented parenteral nutrition. *Nutrition.* 1997;13:295–302.

90. Kagansky N, Levy S, Rimon E, et al. Hypoglycemia as a predictor of mortality in hospitalized elderly patients. *Arch Intern Med.* 2003;163:1825–1829.

91. Shilo S, Berezovsky S, Friedlander Y, Sonnenblick M. Hypoglycemia in hospitalized nondiabetic older patients. *J Am Geriatr Soc.* 1998;46:978–982.

92. Mizock BA. Alterations in fuel metabolism in critical illness: hyperglycemia. *Best Pract Res Clin Endocrinol Metab.* 2001;15:533–551.

93. van den Berghe G, Wouters P, Weekers F, et al. Intensive insulin therapy in the critically ill patients. *N Engl J Med.* 2001;345:1359–1367.

94. Siegel JH, Kasmin FE. Biliary tract diseases in the elderly: management and outcomes. *Gut.* 1997;41:433–435.

95. Lefevre F, Feinglass J, Potts S, et al. Iatrogenic complications in high-risk, elderly patients. *Arch Intern Med.* 1992;152:2074–2080.

96. Giraud T, Dhainaut JF, Vaxelaire JF, et al. Iatrogenic complications in adult intensive care units: a prospective two-center study. *Crit Care Med.* 1993;21:40–51.

97. Keenan CR, White RH. Age as a risk factor for venous thromboembolism after major surgery. *Curr Opin Pulm Med.* 2005;11:398–402.

98. El Solh A, Okada M, Bhat A, Pietrantoni C. Swallowing disorders post orotracheal intubation in the elderly. *Intensive Care Med.* 2003;29:1451–1455.

99. Cheng AT, Plank LD, Hill GL. Prolonged overexpansion of extracellular water in elderly patients with sepsis. *Arch Surg.* 1998;133:745–751.

Assessment and Management of Acute Pain in the Elderly

Ali Chandani

INTRODUCTION

The issue of accurately assessing pain in the elderly is exceedingly important. It has been repeatedly shown that pain is undertreated in the elderly, potentially leading to sensitization of the pain pathways and development of chronic pain syndromes. Undertreated pain can lead to delirium, be both emotionally and physically disabling, and severely threaten an elderly person's functional ability.[1] Some of the limitations include impaired enjoyment of activities, impaired ambulation, impaired posture, sleep disturbance, anxiety, and depression. In addressing pain one is also addressing basic activity of daily living issues.

Techniques to manage acute postoperative pain have been poorly studied in the geriatric population. The geriatric population differs from their younger counterparts with regard to comorbidity, cognitive decline, and altered pharmacodynamic and pharmacokinetic responses to medications. This chapter attempts to review the acute pain management of geriatric patients, usually in the perioperative setting, but these principles can be generalized to other acutely painful conditions.

EVALUATION OF PAIN

The ability to adequately treat pain presupposes the ability to accurately detect the presence of pain. The underlying issue of how to best assess pain levels in the geriatric population has been sparsely studied, and there is no consensus as to the optimal tool(s) to achieve this goal. There are limitations that must be recognized when assessing pain in the elderly which include the expectation that pain is associated with aging, a fear of the meaning of pain, the belief that pain cannot be relieved, and a fear of being labeled a "complainer." In the postoperative setting there are additional factors, such as recovery from anesthesia, acute opioid administration, acute illness, and the destabilizing effects of the hospital environment, which will affect the ability to comprehend the tool being used to assess pain.

Historically, pain has been assessed using pain scales. In general, there are two main categories of pain scales. Nonverbal pain scales, such as the Visual Analog Scale (VAS), ask the patient to choose a numerical value on a defined scale that corresponds to their level of pain intensity. Because it is efficient, easily administered, and minimally intrusive, the VAS is widely used in clinical and research settings. Verbal pain scales, such as the McGill Pain Questionnaire (MPQ) or Present Pain Intensity (PPI), ask the patient to endorse certain words or adjectives that describe the qualities of their pain. The rank

values of the chosen words and adjectives are then summed or correlated to obtain a numerical pain score.

All of the pain scales in current usage were developed for a younger population, and their validity for assessing pain in the elderly population has not been verified.[2] For example, problems have been reported with the VAS and elderly patients, which include differences in pain intensity when compared with other scales and difficulty understanding and completing the scale.[3] In addition, many of these scales were developed for the assessment of chronic pain, and their ability to be valid and reliable measures of acute pain remains to be elucidated. Despite their widespread use, these scales have not been adequately studied in the acute pain setting for the elderly population.

The recent study of Gagliese et al.[4] addressed these issues, albeit with the limitations they acknowledge. They analyzed age-related patterns on three pain scales (VAS, MPQ, and PPI) in men undergoing radical prostatectomy and concluded that age-related differences in postoperative pain were better captured by verbal descriptions rather than nonverbal measures of pain intensity. This finding, along with the previously mentioned difficulties with elderly patients and the VAS, suggests that the role of the VAS in the elderly postoperative patient be limited in favor of more verbally descriptive measures of pain.

A confounding issue in assessing acute pain in the elderly population is the presence of coexisting cognitive decline or dysfunction. Dementia is an important barrier to pain assessment, and several studies have demonstrated that cognitively impaired patients receive fewer analgesics than do cognitively intact patients with similar pathology.[5,6] Many of the studies addressing the performance of the various pain scales in cognitively impaired elderly individuals have taken place in nursing home populations and have assessed chronic pain and its limitations on functionality. Whether their findings can be generalized to the acute pain setting remains to be seen.

One of the key findings from the earlier studies in this area is that cognitive impairment does not mask pain complaints.[7] While data have indicated that cognitively impaired patients tend to underreport pain, the self reports of these patients are no less valid than those of cognitively intact patients. Stated differently, cognitively impaired patients are less likely to report the presence of pain but when they do, it is a valid report and should be treated as such. Pateux et al. studied the assessment of pain in an elderly demented hospitalized patient population.[8] They compared four pain scales (horizontal VAS, vertical VAS, a French version of the MPQ, and Faces Pain Scale) with the Doloplus scale, an observational pain assessment scale developed to assess pain in older noncommunicative patients. Patients were classified using the clinical dementia rating as none, questionable, mild, moderate, and severe. Over 90% of elderly hospitalized patients with mild or moderate dementia and 40% with severe dementia were able to appropriately complete at least one of the four scales. From these data, the authors were not able to specify a clear cognitive threshold below which self-assessment scales should not be attempted.

With regard to the most appropriate scale for rating pain in the cognitively impaired elderly the studies are conflicting. The above study did not find any significant difference between the various scales. Other studies have found higher completion rates with combined visual verbal scales (e.g., MPQ).[9,10] This is consistent with the Gagliese study presented earlier in this chapter, which supports a role for more verbally based descriptions of pain as opposed to the more abstract VAS.

The observational pain scale used in the Pateux study correlated only modestly with self-assessment by patients using one of the other scales, with low scores not excluding the presence of pain. Similar findings have been seen when using other observational pain scales.[7] The role of observational pain scales should be reserved for those few patients who have demonstrated that they cannot complete a self-assessment.

The important finding raised by the above studies is that the majority of elderly cognitively impaired patients are able to validly assess their pain using a self-assessment scale. The optimal scale to use in this setting is as yet undecided; however, the data suggest that more verbally descriptive indicators of pain appear to be best understood by this population.

A salient point of the Pateux study was the finding that all four of the pain scales studied demonstrated reliability. There was a high test-retest and high interrater reliability in this cognitively impaired population. This is especially important because unreliable measurements do not effectively detect pain, and perhaps more importantly cannot measure change in pain after intervention.

▶ Clinical recommendations

When assessing an elderly patient's pain in the postoperative setting, several considerations should be taken into account. Preferably, the patient should be assessed preoperatively and the type of pain scale explained to assess their level of understanding. The presence of a family member can often be invaluable in assessing a patient's level of understanding and also provide some insight into the personality involved. A number of pain scales should be available in order that the optimal tool to assess and reassess pain is chosen. Most of the studies suggest that nonverbal scales more accurately assess pain in the elderly, and in the author's experience, the PPI scale is a simple and easy to administer tool. The PPI, a part of the MPQ, is a 5-point verbal descriptor scale with words corresponding to varying levels of pain (none = 0, mild = 1, discomforting = 2, distressing = 3, horrible = 4, and excruciating = 5). No assumptions should be made regarding a patient's ability to use a particular scale keeping in mind that apparently cognitively intact patients might not be able to understand the VAS while an obviously demented patient might be comfortable doing so. The Pateux study clearly demonstrated that up to 40% of severely demented patients were able to complete a pain self-assessment scale, so it is mandatory that every patient be given the chance to complete a self-assessment scale. The patient should be reassessed for their ability to use the chosen scale in the postanesthesia care unit (PACU) since the destabilizing effects of anesthesia, opioid administration, and unfamiliar surroundings might temporarily affect the patient's cognitive ability. The use of observational pain scales should be reserved for only three categories

of patients: intubated patients in an intensive care unit (ICU) setting; patients who are nonverbal secondary to cognitive dysfunction; and patients who are obviously unable to meaningfully interact with the provider. Later in this chapter, the issue of untreated pain and its causative relationship with delirium is addressed but it is worth keeping this in mind when assessing the patient in the PACU. Once the pain is well-controlled and the patients have demonstrated that they are able to comprehend the pain assessment tool that is going to be used, this information should be communicated to the ward. It is extremely important that the onus of pain assessment be placed on the physician and nursing staff since elderly patients will not necessarily volunteer information unless specifically asked about it. Providers should be conversant with a variety of pain scales available in order to be able to tailor their assessment to the continuum of cognitive state that is seen in the elderly population. Basic scales that every provider should be familiar with are the VAS, the PPI, and an Objective Pain Scale. The major disadvantage of this approach to pain management is that it is time and effort consuming. The initial preoperative assessment will likely require an outlay of time which is difficult in a busy practice that stresses quick turnaround times. Assessing a patient using a verbal scale takes longer than the simple "Give me a number between 1 and 10 that best describes your pain." Both physicians and nurses need to be trained to use these scales and interpret the information. The advantage, on the other hand, is improved patient outcome. As is seen later in this chapter, effective treatment of pain has both short- and long-term benefits for patients.

MANAGEMENT OF ACUTE PAIN

There are two concepts which should be understood when approaching the management of acute pain, regardless of the age of the patient. The first of these is the concept of multimodal or balanced analgesia and the second is preemptive analgesia. There are several locations along the pain pathway that can become sensitized by exposure to painful stimuli: peripheral nociceptors, dorsal horn of the spinal cord, ascending and descending tracts of the spinal cord, and thalamic and cortical regions of the brain. The use of multiple interventions, each with a different mechanism of action that targets these multiple sites, is known as multimodal therapy.[11] The concept of multimodal analgesia has been incorporated into algorithms for chronic pain. Because of the wide range of acute pain that can follow the variety of surgical procedures, there is no single recommendation that has been advocated for this setting; rather individual strategies have been shown to improve pain control following specific procedures (see ketorolac and gabapentin below). Preemptive analgesia is a theory that postulates that it is possible to limit sensitization of pain pathways by initiating appropriate pain therapy before the onset of a noxious stimulus.[12] The operative setting, in which the timing of the noxious stimulus is known in advance, represents the ideal setting in which to practice a preemptive multimodal approach to pain management.

▶ Nonpharmacologic methods

While there have been numerous case reports regarding the benefits of a wide variety of adjuvant nonmedical therapies in the management of acute postoperative pain, randomized controlled trials in this field are few and far between. Many of the nonpharmacologic pain management strategies have been shown to be effective when used in combination with drug strategies. Education programs for patients have been shown to significantly improve pain management and quality of life in the chronic pain setting.[13] The benefits of physical methods, including heat, cold, and massage, should not be overlooked as they have been shown to be effective for many patients.[14] Piotrowski et al. studied the effect of massage as an adjuvant therapy in the management of acute postoperative pain.[15] Although the use of opioid analgesics was not altered significantly by the interventions, massage appeared to improve the affective component (i.e., unpleasantness) of pain.

Some psychological maneuvers may be effective in controlling pain. Biofeedback, relaxation, and hypnosis may help some patients, although these methods require high levels of cognitive function and may not be suitable for the cognitively impaired patients. Psychologists may assess cognitive status, evaluate for the presence of mood disorders, and assist with the development of pain management strategies that may reduce pain.

Appropriate referrals to physical and occupational therapists for exercise training may significantly improve pain and improve patient function.

While it would be tempting to dismiss the nonpharmacologic methods of treating acute pain because of the lack of randomized controlled trials, it should be kept in mind that many of the pharmacologic methods also lack these same randomized controlled trials in the elderly population.

▶ Pharmacologic methods

There are a variety of pharmacologic medications that can be used in the treatment of acute pain. Because the mainstay of pain management, especially in the perioperative setting, is opioid therapy these are considered separately from the rest. Table 25-1 lists suggested dosages of nonopioid medications used in the acute pain setting.

Nonopioid therapy

Acetaminophen is the analgesic of choice in elderly patients to relieve most types of mild to moderate acute and chronic pain.[16] Scheduled dosing improves the efficacy of treatment for painful conditions. In adults, the optimal unit dose is 1000 mg with a maximal daily dosage of 3000–4000 mg, but caution is suggested in those patients with hepatic insufficiency. Even though clearance of the drug is

Table 25-1

Nonopioid Medications in the Acute Pain Setting

Drug	Class	Initial Dose/Route	Max. Dose	Uses	Comments
Acetaminophen		650–1000 mg PO Q 6 h	4000 mg/24 h	Mild to moderate pain and adjunct to NSAIDs and opioids	Monitor liver function, precaution with liver disease
Ibuprofen	COX-1 NSAID	200 mg PO Q 8 h	3200 mg/24 h	Preemptive analgesia Mild to moderate pain and adjunct to opioids	Monitor liver and renal function, monitor GI side effects
Naproxen	COX-1 NSAID	200 mg PO Q 12 h	1500 mg/24 h	Preemptive analgesia Mild to moderate pain and adjunct to opioids	Monitor liver and renal function, monitor GI side effects
Celecoxib	COX-2 NSAID	100 mg PO Q 24 h	400 mg/24 h	Preemptive analgesia Mild to moderate pain and adjunct to opioids	Higher doses associated with lower limb edema, monitor liver and renal function, monitor GI side effects, avoid with hepatic insufficiency
Ketorolac	COX-1 NSAID	15 mg IV Q 6 h	90 mg/24 h	Preemptive analgesia Moderate pain and adjunct to opioids	Limit use to 5 days, monitor liver and renal function, monitor GI side effects
Gabapentin	Anticonvulsant	100 mg PO Q 12 h	3600 mg/24 h	Preemptive analgesia	Total daily dosing based on creatinine clearance, seizure risk with abrupt withdrawal
Ketamine	NMDA antagonist	0.25–0.5 mg/kg IV then 0.25–0.5 mg/kg/h infusion during procedure 0.15 mg/kg/h IV infusion combined with opioid PCA for postoperative pain	0.5 mg/kg/h	Preemptive analgesia Adjunct to opioids	Useful in opioid-tolerant patients, psychomimetic side effects with doses higher than 0.5 mg/kg (negligible if <10 mg/h)
Bupivacaine	Local anesthetic	Up to 2.5 mg/kg SQ	0.5 mg/kg/h	Preemptive analgesia	Cardiovascular collapse and seizures with intravascular injection

reduced in the elderly, it is usually not necessary to reduce the dosage.[17] Having said this, it is common in clinical practice to use lower doses of acetaminophen in the elderly. When added to a traditional nonsteroidal anti-inflammatory agent (NSAID), acetaminophen enhances the analgesic effect and allows the use of lower doses of the NSAID for the same analgesic effect.

NSAIDs administered prior to surgical incision have been shown to improve postoperative analgesia.[18] They are an important component of a multimodal approach to pain management by limiting peripheral nociceptor input and by modulating central sensitization at the level of the spinal cord.[19] NSAIDs should be used cautiously in elderly patients, particularly those with a history of renal insufficiency, peptic ulcer disease, concurrent usage of anticoagulant or antiplatelet medication, or bleeding diathesis. Low doses of these drugs should be considered for short-term use in the acute postoperative setting. Proton pump inhibitors reduce the risk of developing peptic ulcers and should be considered if patients are to be placed on NSAIDs. Maintenance of adequate hydration appears to lower the increased risk of renal failure, and this is particularly important in the elderly population.

There are two main categories of NSAIDs referred to as cyclooxygenase (COX)-1 and COX-2 inhibitors. The COX-2 inhibitors by virtue of their decreased gastrointestinal (GI) toxicity were carving out a niche in perioperative management, especially in the orthopedic setting, before the concerns regarding increased cardiac morbidity and mortality forced their withdrawal from the market. For this reason, discussions regarding valdecoxib and rofecoxib are not addressed in this chapter.

The only remaining COX-2 type NSAID on the market is celecoxib. Recart et al. assessed the preoperative use of celecoxib, a COX-2 type of NSAID, on postoperative pain in outpatients undergoing minor ear-nose-throat surgery.[20] They found that celecoxib was more effective than placebo in reducing postoperative pain and rescue analgesic medication. However, there was no difference with respect to recovery times, patient satisfaction, and quality of recovery. Given that celecoxib is manufactured by the same company as valdecoxib, the COX-2 most widely studied in the perioperative setting, it is likely that further studies on celecoxib will be forthcoming.

Ketorolac is an intravenously formulated NSAID indicated for short-term (less than 5 days) management of moderate to severe acute pain requiring analgesia at the opioid level.[21] It has been shown to exert an opioid-sparing effect such that decreased narcotic doses provide comparable analgesia. It has the potential for decreasing glomerular filtration with subsequent acute renal failure and it increases the risk of hemorrhage due to platelet aggregation. While it has been shown to be useful, particularly in urologic surgery,[22] the above-mentioned side effects limit its utility in the elderly. As recommended for the oral NSAIDs above if used in the elderly, the dose should be decreased, length of therapy shortened, and consideration given to the concomitant use of a proton pump inhibitor.

Gabapentin. With increasing interest in central neuronal sensitization as a mechanism of chronic pain, it would seem natural that this phenomenon be investigated in the postoperative pain setting. A single preoperative dose of 1200 mg oral gabapentin has been shown to result in a substantial reduction in postoperative morphine consumption without significant side effects after radical mastectomy.[23] A dose ranging study with patients undergoing lumbar discectomy suggested the optimal preemptive dose of gabapentin to be 600 mg.[24] As the mechanism of hyperalgesia and its role in pain syndromes is better understood, there will no doubt be further research in this field and its applications to the postoperative setting.

Ketamine administered prior to surgical incision has been shown to decrease wound hyperalgesia several days after surgery and decrease postoperative pain and analgesic requirements.[25] A recent review of the perioperative use of ketamine as an adjunct to general and regional anesthesia and postoperative pain therapy[26] suggests that subanesthetic doses of ketamine in combination with general anesthesia also improves postoperative pain control. Based on an extensive review of the literature, the authors recommend a regimen as follows: 0.5 mg/kg initial slow intravenous (IV) bolus prior to skin incision followed by boluses of 0.25 mg/kg every 30 minutes or followed by an infusion of 0.5 mg/kg/h. The initial bolus can be reduced to 0.25 mg/kg for shorter, less-painful procedures. The addition of low-dose ketamine infusions combined with opioid patient-controlled analgesia (PCA) for postoperative pain control improves pain control while reducing opioid side effects. The recommended dose is 0.15 mg/kg/h as a continuous infusion, although a 1:1 ratio of ketamine to morphine as an IV PCA has also shown promise. The concern with using ketamine in the elderly, even in low doses, is the development of psychotomimetic side effects. Despite the long history of ketamine use in clinical practice, little is known about the pharmacodynamic and pharmacokinetic changes with aging; however, it has been suggested that there is a decrease in clearance and the duration of action is extended.[27] In the studies performed thus far, the incidence of side effects was dose-dependent, less likely with smaller doses (<0.15 mg/kg), and when used at an infusion at less than 10 mg/h, the incidence of cognitive impairment was negligible.

Preemptive local anesthetics, when applied to the surgical site before the onset of noxious stimuli, can have effects that outlast the presence of local anesthetic at the surgical site. Infiltration of the surgical site with the long-acting local anesthetic bupivacaine has been shown to decrease wound hyperalgesia several days following surgery.[28] A salient point with regard to the beneficial effects of local anesthetics is the timing of their administration. Local anesthetic infiltration of incision sites prior to incision reduces postoperative incisional pain following laparoscopic surgery; however, infiltration with local anesthetic at the conclusion of surgery was found to be no more effective than saline.[29]

Opioid therapy

There are difficulties with regard to making recommendations for opioid use in the elderly population, which have been concisely and well-summarized by Wilder-Smith[30] in his recent review.

The first problem, which appears to be a recurring theme in this chapter, is the relative lack of well-designed published trials on this topic. The opioid most extensively studied in elderly subjects in the postoperative setting is morphine[31,32] via the IV route, although there are pharmacokinetic studies involving fentanyl,[33,34] alfentanil,[35] sufentanil,[36] and remifentanil.[37] Few well-designed trials and even fewer comparative trials have been published, and the paucity of data precludes an evidence-based recommendation as to the best choice of therapy in the acute pain setting. Because morphine is the best-studied drug in this class, it is the focus of this chapter.

The second major problem is that elderly patients are generally more susceptible to drug side effects.[16] This is compounded by the fact that they are often concomitantly taking medications for other chronic diseases and have a higher incidence of psychiatric comorbidity (depression and dementia), predisposing them to adverse drug reactions.

Based on their previous studies,[38] Aubrun et al. devised a regimen for IV morphine titration in the PACU (Table 25-2).[39] The major advantage of the protocol is the improved safety afforded by adapting morphine titration to individual pain, allowing optimal titration in

Table 25-2

Regimen for Morphine Titration in the Elderly in PACU

Dose of intravenous morphine bolus	3 mg if >60 kg 2 mg if <60 kg
Interval between boluses	5 min
Limitations on total dose	None
VAS threshold required to administer morphine	>30 mm
Pain assessment time interval	5 min until pain relief defined as VAS ≤30 mm. If asleep consider to have adequate pain relief.
Monitoring	Respiratory rate, oxygen saturation and supplemental oxygen, sedation by Ramsey score, blood pressure, heart rate
Stop points	Respiratory rate <12 breaths/min Oxygen saturation <95% Adverse drug reaction

adult patients regardless of age. Because the titration is performed over a short period of time, the age-related changes in pharmacodynamics and pharmacokinetics are less important.

Using the protocol described above, Aubrun et al. studied 175 patients older than 70 years.[39] In comparison to 875 younger patients (mean age 45 ± 15 years), initial VAS scores were similar (74 ± 21 vs. 76 ± 20), analgesia was produced by approximately the same dose of morphine per kilogram of body weight (0.15 ± 0.10 mg/kg vs. 0.14 ± 0.09 mg/kg), and there was no significant difference in morphine-related adverse effects (13% vs. 14%, not significant [NS]), or the number of sedated patients (60% vs. 60%, NS).

This study, among others, suggests that elderly patients experience the same level of pain as their younger counterparts and initially require similar levels of intervention to achieve pain relief.

To address the issue of postoperative pain control outside of the controlled PACU setting, the Aubrun group studied 105 elderly patients (mean age 76 ± 5 years) and 224 younger patients (mean age 55 ± 11 years) undergoing total hip replacement.[31] Initial analgesia in the PACU was achieved using the above titration scale with approximately the same dose of morphine (0.15 ± 0.11 vs. 0.14 ± 0.10 mg/kg), and analgesia on the ward was achieved with subcutaneous morphine every 4 hours according to a protocol based on pain as assessed by VAS score and body weight. The elderly cohort required a significantly lower dose of morphine (mean dose 0.11 ± 0.11 mg/kg vs. 0.18 ± 0.18 mg/kg), suggesting that although initial morphine dose requirements were similar this changed during the more prolonged postoperative course of analgesia.

The above findings appear to be in agreement with the earlier work of Sear et al. who compared middle-aged and elderly patients undergoing surgery.[40] Elderly patients complained of similar initial pain intensities when compared to their younger counterparts. Although there is a reduction in the volume of distribution for morphine with age, which results in initially higher plasma drug levels, initial morphine loading doses were similar between the two groups. There was a trend toward subsequent maintenance doses being lower in the older population which is consistent with the notion that alterations in pharmacokinetics with aging decrease the clearance of morphine, thus decreasing the daily total morphine requirements.

The findings of Macintyre and Jarvis[32] perhaps offer the most relevant insight into postoperative morphine usage. They reported on the use of PCA, the current standard of postoperative opioid analgesia, and they were able to compare younger versus older patients. The key finding was that age (and not weight) was the most significant predictor of postoperative PCA morphine requirement, and that postoperative opioid requirements decrease as patient age increases. Their analysis suggested that older patients were able to use the PCA system appropriately.

A gender effect has been suggested by the observation that males use more morphine than females which correlates with the finding that sensitivity to mechanical pain has been found to increase with age, particularly in males.[41] Other studies have shown the opposite effect. In particular, the recent study of Aubrun on this topic suggests that females experience more significant postoperative pain than males and require 11% more morphine in the immediate postoperative period.[42] This sex-related difference disappeared in elderly patients. Further studies in this area are needed before any conclusions can be drawn.

The concerns raised earlier in this chapter regarding the evaluation of pain in the elderly are still valid and serve to further complicate this issue. Aubrun et al. used the VAS as an indicator of pain to tailor the titration of morphine and excluded patients with dementia or impaired mental state. Unfortunately, these comorbidities are increasingly being seen in the acute postoperative setting and this is a confounding factor.

▶ Clinical recommendations

When deciding on a pain control regimen for an elderly postoperative patient, one needs to consider the patient in the context of the surgical procedure. Certain procedures are more painful (e.g., joint replacement and thoracic or upper abdominal surgery), in particular with patient movement, physical therapy, or even respiration. These patients are candidates for more invasive methods of postoperative pain control such as epidural or continuous peripheral nerve block techniques. These are discussed in the following sections. For those patients for whom opioids are to be the primary method of pain control, morphine is the drug that has been most extensively studied. It is possible to use other opioid medications; however, meperidine in particular should be avoided. Meperidine has been shown to increase the incidence of delirium which is addressed later in this chapter. It is important to use a multimodal approach to pain control, and this would start with choosing an adjuvant NSAID which can be given orally with a sip of water prior to induction of anesthesia. There is a reluctance to use NSAIDs, particularly in the elderly population; however, lower doses of these drugs are safer and the benefits are numerous. Ibuprofen 600 mg divided three times daily is a safe starting point. The argument can be made for Celebrex 100 mg daily if ibuprofen is contraindicated. At the least, elderly patients should be given acetaminophen, starting with 2600 mg divided in four doses. Often, acetaminophen can be given in combination with ibuprofen with excellent results. Another useful adjuvant is ketamine. A single dose of 0.5 mg/kg given prior to incision followed by 0.25 mg/kg every 30 minutes till 1 hour before the end of surgery is adequate. This author has not seen an increased incidence of psychomimetic side effects; to the contrary these patients are comfortable and relaxed in the PACU. If NSAIDs have not been given, consider giving ketorolac 15 mg IV toward the end of surgery, usually after discussion with the surgeon. This is particularly useful for outpatients for whom NSAIDs are going to be an important part of the pain control regimen. The protocol outlined in Table 25-2 is a good starting point for initial titration of morphine in the PACU. The key to this protocol is individualized titration of opioid, keeping in mind that the elderly patient will likely require similar initial doses as younger patients. Once initial pain control has been achieved and it is determined that the patient is a candidate for PCA, this is the modality of choice for pain management on the ward. Continuous infusions of opioids are problematic in the elderly population, particularly in regard to oversedation. Therefore, one should probably not routinely program a basal rate for elderly patients. A rescue analgesia protocol similar to the initial titration protocol should be available on the ward for situations such as the patient falling asleep and not receiving medication for a prolonged period of time and then waking up in excruciating pain. In following a strict protocol based on continuous patient assessment, the risk of oversedation is minimized and duration of time to optimal pain control optimized. If the patient is unable to use a PCA, one should consider a protocol similar to the initial titration protocol. The major difference is that the patient is assessed every 4 hours, with morphine 2–3 mg intravenously titrated every 5 minutes till adequate pain relief is obtained. A final point with regard to postoperative pain management is the transition to oral opioids which should be accomplished as soon as feasible. Once the patient is allowed to resume a regular diet, the analgesic regimen should be converted to an oral route.

▶ Neuraxial analgesia

A confounding issue in studying the use of epidural techniques for postoperative analgesia is that in the majority of instances, the epidural is placed preoperatively, used for postoperative analgesia, and variably used intraoperatively. The question of how much the intraoperative anesthetic course affects the quality of postoperative analgesia is difficult to quantitate, especially given the contribution of preemptive analgesia which is thought to be superior with neuraxial techniques. In addition, major surgery induces a "stress response" that is substantially altered by neuraxial blockade but not by general anesthesia.[43] Again, this is going to independently affect the postoperative course.

Rodgers et al. reviewed 141 randomized trials over the previous 30 years comparing general anesthesia with spinal or epidural block.[44] Although this review covered a large number of studies on varied surgical procedures and patients with a variety of comorbidities, they showed a consistent and statistically significant reduction in postoperative morbidity and mortality with neuraxial anesthesia. In particular, they found significant reductions in risks of venous thromboembolism, myocardial infarction, bleeding complications, pneumonia, respiratory depression, and renal failure (Table 25-3). These effects were thought to be benefits of neuraxial block in general and not of a particular technique (epidural or spinal). The data showing a reduced incidence of deep venous thrombosis following hip replacement under epidural versus general anesthesia have been reported previously.[45]

Table 25-3

Advantages of Epidural Postoperative Analgesia

Advantages

Superior postoperative analgesia

Lower risk of venous thromboembolism

Lower risk of myocardial infarction

Lower risk of bleeding complications

Lower risk of pneumonia

Lower risk of respiratory depression

Lower risk of renal failure

The impact of perioperative epidural analgesia in high-risk patients undergoing high-risk surgical procedures has been studied in two large prospective randomized trials. The Veterans Affairs Cooperative Study[46] studied 1021 American Society of Anesthesiologists (ASA) III and IV patients undergoing major intra-abdominal procedures and randomized them to general anesthesia and IV opioid analgesia versus epidural plus light general anesthesia with postoperative epidural morphine. Postoperative analgesia was found to be superior with epidural morphine. In addition, patients receiving epidural morphine were noted to have a shorter intubation time and a shorter intensive care stay.

The Multicenter Australian Study of Epidural Anaesthesia (MASTER) trial[47] studied 915 patients undergoing major abdominal procedures to compare morbidity and mortality outcomes by choice of anesthetic technique. Patients were randomized either to general anesthesia and postoperative IV opioid analgesia or epidural plus light general anesthesia, with postoperative epidural analgesia using local anesthetics supplemented with opioids. There was no difference in mortality or in the incidence of major complications between the two groups with the exception of respiratory failure which occurred less frequently in the epidural subgroup (23% vs. 30%). Analysis of secondary outcomes revealed that postoperative epidural analgesia produced lower pain scores assessed by VAS during the first 3 postoperative days, in particular after coughing.

Both of the above prospective randomized trials with high-risk patients undergoing major intra-abdominal surgery concluded that morbid outcomes were not affected by the choice of anesthetic technique. However, both of the trials did show better postoperative analgesia in the epidural subgroups and concluded that many high-risk patients would receive substantial benefit from epidural analgesia. This is particularly important in the elderly who are at increased risk of inadequate analgesia, and for whom the benefits of shorter intubation times, shorter intensive care stays, and less respiratory failure are invaluable.

Block et al. performed a meta-analysis of epidural versus general anesthesia with the outcome of postoperative analgesia.[48] Their analysis included 124 randomized comparisons of epidural therapy versus parenteral opioids in adult patients. A variety of techniques were included in the analysis: thoracic epidural, lumbar epidural, and infusions containing local anesthetic, opioid, or both. The results were unequivocal. With the notable exception of thoracic epidural analgesia with opioids alone for thoracic surgery, analgesia as assessed by VAS was lower at all intervals up to the fourth postoperative day with a 30–33% reduction in pain ratings. In particular, the combination of local anesthetics and opioids provided superior analgesia.

Although these studies were not performed exclusively on elderly patients, they were not excluded from the various studies and are represented in the above meta-analysis. Because the elderly are more prone to inadequate analgesia and suffer more consequences as a result of inadequate analgesia, it would seem prudent to recommend epidural analgesia when possible in the management of these individuals.

▶ Clinical recommendations

Patient selection, type of surgery, and type of postoperative venous thromboembolism prophylaxis are the most important factors to take into account when choosing an epidural technique. Patient refusal is an obvious contraindication; however, careful explanation of the benefits of epidural analgesia is helpful in convincing a wary patient into acceptance. The majority of elderly patients are aware of their increased risk for morbidity and mortality and should be informed of the benefits of epidural analgesia. Patients with chronic pain are particularly good candidates for neuraxial techniques, and they are cognizant of the limitations of opioid analgesia. Types of surgery in which epidural techniques should be considered are thoracic surgery, any upper abdominal surgery, major lower abdominal and pelvic surgery, and hip and knee arthroplasty. The congruency of catheter insertion location to site of surgical incision is extremely important. It can be frustrating to try and make a lumbar epidural "work" for upper abdominal surgery. The dermatome in the center of the incision should be matched to the vertebral level at which the catheter is placed. Keep in mind that patients often have the head of the bed elevated postoperatively, and this gravitational effect will affect the spread of the infusing solution. For example, with a Whipple procedure, the catheter would be placed at the level of the sixth thoracic vertebra. The epidural catheter is tested preoperatively and intermittently bolused prior to incision and during the procedure (0.5% bupivacaine) in an attempt to derive the benefits of preemptive analgesia. Approximately 45 minutes before the end of the procedure, an infusion of dilute local anesthetic with opioid (e.g., 0.1% bupivacaine with 2 mcg/mL fentanyl) is started. This allows one to assess the adequacy of the infusion rate during emergence and the PACU stay and make any adjustments and treat any side effects. Doses of bupivacaine should not exceed 0.5 mg/kg/h. If the catheter is adequately placed and congruent to the surgical site, infusion rates of 6–12 mL/h should provide adequate pain relief. Patients receiving epidural infusions should be monitored postoperatively for respiratory depression and neurological dysfunction. The most common side effects associated with epidural narcotics are itching (easily treated with nalbuphine 5–10 mg IV which has less side effects than Benadryl in the elderly population) and urinary retention (requiring Foley catheter). Epidural infusions may be continued for 2–5 days. The major limiting factors are the availability of beds in a monitored setting and the need to mobilize the patient. Daily visits to patients receiving epidural infusions should assess the level of sensory and motor blockade, infection at the site of catheter placement, and presence of side effects. The widespread use of thromboembolism prophylaxis in the hospital setting has generated guidelines from the American Society of Regional Anesthesia regarding the timing of epidural catheter placement and removal. Given the increasing number of new medications being introduced and further experience with relatively new medications, it is recommended that one closely follows these guidelines which are periodically revised as new information becomes available.

The major advantage of epidural techniques is the undoubtedly superior postoperative pain relief. Further advantages of neuraxial techniques include reduction in the risk of venous thromboembolism, myocardial infarction, bleeding complications, pneumonia, respiratory depression, and renal failure. The major disadvantages are the aforementioned side effects, rare but serious neurological complications (abscess and hematoma), and the need for a dedicated service to follow the patients receiving epidurals during their hospital course. The latter issue is particularly important since it also involves training of the ward nurses who might not be familiar with epidural techniques. This involves an outlay of expense to have experienced providers, or mid-level providers at the least, to follow patients.

PERIPHERAL NERVE BLOCKADE

Peripheral nerve blocks are frequently used in elderly patients in an effort to reduce the stress response and avoid the need for general anesthesia and its deleterious effects. In addition, peripheral nerve blocks have been demonstrated to have ameliorative effects on wound hyperalgesia for days following surgery.[49]

Because the use of peripheral nerve blocks is only reemerging into the mainstream of anesthesia practice, studies of blocks in the elderly are limited to case reports and small series. Reviewing all the nerve blocks and their associated benefits is beyond the scope of this chapter; however, consideration will be given to the most commonly used techniques and those most applicable to the elderly population: interscalene nerve block, axillary nerve block, lumbar plexus block, and femoral nerve block. An excellent complete review of the studies supporting the use of the various nerve block techniques has been performed by Evans et al.[50] from which the relevant information is summarized below.

In addition to the historically used single injection techniques (lasting 6–18 hours depending on the local anesthetic used), more studies are investigating the use of continuous catheter techniques to provide prolonged postoperative analgesia. This is again an emerging field and as more studies are performed and the benefits of ultrasound facilitate easier placement of catheters, there will be more interest in the continuous catheter techniques.

▶ Interscalene nerve block

The interscalene nerve block[51] is an ideal block for surgery involving the shoulder and proximal arm, and many authors consider it the gold standard in shoulder analgesia. A number of studies have documented superior pain relief (greater than 50% reduction in VAS score) when compared with opioid analgesia for arthroscopic and open shoulder surgery,[52–53] delayed time until first analgesic use,[53] reduced total opioid requirements,[52–54] and 65–81% lower rates of postoperative nausea and vomiting.[52,53] This decreased incidence of pain and postoperative opioid use has led to further benefits including improved postoperative mood,[54] more sleep on the night after surgery,[54] faster discharge of ambulatory patients,[52] reduced patient length of stay,[55] and lower rates of unplanned hospital admission.[52,55]

All of these benefits would be of use if they are applicable to the elderly population, which they might well be, although further study in this matter is warranted. In addition, the opioid sparing effects of local anesthetics would be of particular benefit in a population that is more susceptible to medication side effects.

▶ Axillary nerve block

The axillary nerve block[56] targets the terminal branches of the brachial plexus as they surround the axillary artery, and is the most commonly performed nerve block in the United States.[57] It is indicated for surgery of the hand, wrist, and forearm. There are two prospective studies which have compared axillary block with general anesthesia in patients undergoing hand surgery.[58,59] Benefits attributed to axillary blockade include greater than 50% reduction in pain VAS score for up to 120 minutes after surgery,[60] lower in-hospital opioid requirements,[59,60] longer time until first analgesic,[60] 75% reduction in the incidence of immediate postoperative nausea and vomiting,[59,60] and quicker discharge from both the PACU and hospital.[60] There were, however, no long-term differences in pain, opioid consumption, adverse effects, or patient satisfaction between 1 and 14 days postoperatively.[60] When comparing axillary nerve block with IV regional anesthesia (IVRA) for hand surgery,[59] IVRA was associated with similar postoperative analgesia with a 30% reduction in cost, a shorter duration of recovery, and fewer PACU nursing interventions.

Lumbar plexus block

Block of the lumbar plexus within the substance of the psoas muscle provides reliable analgesia of the three main terminal nerves of the plexus: the femoral, lateral femoral cutaneous, and obturator nerves,[60] Although variably anesthetizing the more proximal nerves (the ilioinguinal, iliohypogastric, and genitofemoral nerves), this block is suited for invasive and painful procedures involving the hip and the knee.

In patients undergoing arthroscopic anterior cruciate ligament repair, an 89% decrease in opioid requirement was observed with continuous lumbar plexus block as compared with IV PCA postoperative analgesia.[61]

When comparing continuous lumbar plexus versus continuous femoral versus PCA in patients undergoing total knee arthroplasty, Kaloul et al. found that continuous nerve block techniques reduced 48-hour morphine consumption by 50%.[62] There was no difference in opioid consumption between continuous lumbar plexus and continuous femoral techniques, with the former being associated with more frequent obturator nerve block.

A number of studies have described the use of single injection lumbar plexus block for hip fractures and total hip arthroplasty with excellent results.[63,64] In comparison with subarachnoid block, patients undergoing total hip arthroplasty with lumbar plexus block experienced lower pain VAS scores and less use of opioids in the postoperative period.[65] Impressively, no patients required morphine in the first 12 hours postoperatively, only 15% of patients used morphine after 12–24 hours, and only 10% reported their pain as intense on the first postoperative day. Other studies have looked at a continuous lumbar plexus catheter technique following hip arthroplasty and uniformly documented low pain VAS scores for over 48 hours.[66,67]

The study of Turker et al.[68] demonstrated that the continuous lumbar plexus technique was as successful as a lumbar epidural in providing analgesia, minimizing opioid use, and enhancing patient satisfaction. Furthermore, they experienced an 80% reduction in the incidence of orthostatic hypotension, urinary retention, postoperative nausea and vomiting, and earlier ambulation when compared with those who received epidural analgesia. This latter finding is especially relevant since the advent of the new thromboprophylaxis agents and the association between these agents, neuraxial techniques, and epidural hematoma formation. Continuous peripheral nerve block techniques may offer an alternative to postoperative epidural analgesia for lower extremity surgery.

Femoral nerve block

The femoral nerve block is a safe and easily performed block, making itself one of the most commonly performed lower extremity peripheral nerve blocks.[68] In many cases, it is used as a less-invasive alternative to the lumbar plexus block and in comparison it preserves hip flexion but does not consistently anesthetize the obturator or lateral femoral cutaneous nerves. It is most frequently used for knee surgery. Numerous studies have shown benefits with femoral nerve block following anterior cruciate ligament (ACL) reconstruction.[69–70] When compared with placebo, femoral nerve block improved immediate postoperative analgesia,[70,72] prolonged time to first requested analgesic,[72] and reduced 24-hour morphine consumption by 45%.[72] Postoperative analgesia can be prolonged following ACL repair with a continuous femoral nerve block technique.[71]

Other studies, however, have failed to show significant postoperative analgesic benefit from a femoral nerve block after ACL reconstruction.[72,73] These conflicting findings have been somewhat resolved by the hypothesis that postoperative ACL pain is also innervated by geniculate contributions in the sciatic nerve distribution.[74] This hypothesis was validated by Williams et al. who compared combined femoral-sciatic nerve blocks versus femoral nerve block alone for ACL repair.[75] In addition to the reduced pain and analgesic requirements, this technique facilitated performing this surgery as an outpatient procedure with significant annual cost savings.

Femoral nerve blocks, both single injection and continuous catheter, have also been studied for total knee arthroplasty.[76 –77] Documented benefits include dense analgesia with up to 50% reduction in pain VAS scores for 48 hours,[79,80] up to 64% lower postoperative opioid requirements,[79,81–83] a reduced incidence of side effects,[82] and a 20% shorter hospital stay with femoral nerve catheters.[79] Additional benefits include improved short-term postoperative rehabilitation and joint mobilization.[80,82] A continuous femoral nerve infusion has been shown to provide similar analgesia with fewer side effects than a single dose of intrathecal morphine[83] or a continuous infusion of epidural local anesthetic.[79,81]

While peripheral nerve blocks have not been studied in the elderly population per se, many of the procedures in which they are widely utilized (hip and knee arthroplasty) are most commonly performed in this particular population providing indirect evidence of their benefit.

Single injection versus continuous infusion techniques

The choice of whether to perform a single injection versus a continuous catheter technique should focus on the amount of expected postoperative pain. There are centers that perform continuous techniques for patients undergoing ambulatory surgery, sending them home with infusion pumps containing local anesthetic.[78] Naturally, a follow-up mechanism should be in place regardless of whether the patient will be staying in the hospital or going home.

Clinical considerations with peripheral nerve blocks

Any surgery involving the extremities, in particular orthopedic procedures, skin grafting, amputations, and vascular procedures, should be considered for a nerve block technique. Patients are often wary of nerve block techniques for two main reasons. Firstly, they often do not like needles and are apprehensive about the discomfort associated with the nerve block itself. This can be overcome by a reassuring explanation of what to expect, explanation that limb movement with nerve stimulation is expected and not painful, infiltration of the overlying skin with local anesthetic, and judicious use of sedation when performing the block. The second main concern is awareness during the procedure. The noises of the operating room, the hard table surface, and the unfamiliarity with the surroundings can make quite a stressful experience for the patient. Reassuring the patients that they will be sedated and not be aware of the operating room is important in convincing patients to accept nerve block techniques. Nerve blocks can be performed as the sole anesthetic with supplemental sedation or in combination with a general anesthetic (via endotracheal tube or laryngeal mask airway). The decision to perform the anesthetic with supplemental sedation or in combination with a general anesthetic depends on the anxiety level of the patient, the patient's position during surgery, anticipated airway obstruction with sedation, and the extent to which the nerve block covers the proposed surgery. For example, a femoral nerve block alone is not adequate for knee arthroscopy, especially if the medial meniscus is involved (obturator nerve distribution). Options include additional obturator nerve block, local and intra-articular local anesthetic infiltration by the surgeon, or supplemental general anesthesia.

The choice of local anesthetic to use depends on the setup time required for the nerve block. Alkalinized mepivacaine 1.5% is an excellent choice for faster onset, otherwise ropivacaine 0.5% is the local anesthetic of choice. Suggested volumes of local anesthetics for single injection techniques and infusion rates for continuous catheter techniques are provided in Table 25-4. Ideally, the nerve block should be placed in the holding area prior to surgery in which case the slower onset but longer-lasting ropivacaine can be used. Typical onset times of 15–30 minutes for surgical level of anesthesia can be expected with ropivacaine with a 10-minute reduction seen when using alkalinized mepivacaine. Epinephrine diluted to 1:300,000 is used as an adjuvant in the lumbar plexus block as a marker of intravascular injection.

Following placement of the peripheral nerve catheter, alkalinized mepivacaine 1.5% can be used to initially obtain analgesia, which typically provides a surgical level of anesthesia for 4–8 hours, and at the conclusion of the procedure an infusion of ropivacaine 0.2% is begun at the rates described in Table 25-4. Managing a peripheral nerve catheter is similar to managing an epidural catheter and should be assessed daily for infection and neurological exam documented. Inadequate analgesia can be either due to catheter tip migration or inadequate spread of local anesthetic. It is important that patients with continuous peripheral nerve catheters have access to a backup modality of analgesia, should the catheter technique fail (PCA or oral opioid analgesics).

Single injection interscalene nerve block may be performed for any procedure involving the shoulder and clavicle, provided that the patient does not have any contraindications (in particular, contralateral pneumonectomy). Continuous interscalene analgesia should be considered in the following instances: shoulder arthroplasty and frozen shoulder syndromes requiring continuous motion rehabilitation techniques.

From the above studies it appears that there is no great advantage to using axillary nerve blockade over IVRA for hand surgery. For procedures expected to outlast the duration of IVRA, there are benefits of axillary nerve block compared with general anesthesia. Axillary nerve block is particularly helpful for patients having fixation of radial and ulnar fractures. An important consideration when using axillary nerve block as the sole anesthetic technique (in combination with sedation) is to ensure blockade of the musculocutaneous nerve and to supplement the second thoracic spinal nerve (T2) dermatome for tourniquet pain. It does not appear that continuous axillary nerve block techniques provide advantages over other techniques. Hip replacement is a common procedure in the elderly population, and the use of single injection lumbar plexus and sciatic nerve block in combination with general anesthesia (for

airway control in the lateral position) is a reasonable anesthetic technique. The skin overlying the incision is classically described to involve part of the twelfth thoracic spinal nerve (T12) dermatome which is not anesthetized with the lumbar plexus/sciatic nerve block combination. This incisional pain is miniscule in comparison to the benefit of absence of pain from the replaced joint, and often disappears by the first postoperative evening while the nerve block can last from 12 to 24 hours.

Knee replacement is another common procedure in the elderly. Possible anesthetic techniques involving nerve blocks include general anesthesia plus femoral nerve block for postoperative pain control, spinal anesthesia plus femoral nerve block, sedation plus lumbar plexus/sciatic nerve block combination, and sedation plus femoral/obturator/sciatic nerve block combination. Studies thus far have not demonstrated differences in pain control with continuous lumbar plexus versus continuous femoral nerve block techniques, both of which were superior to general anesthesia.

A future consideration is the development of long-acting local anesthetic agents with durations of action lasting 2–7 days.[79,80]

EFFECTS OF PAIN CONTROL ON OUTCOME

There are three main outcomes related to perioperative pain control that are discussed in this chapter: delirium, persistent pain syndromes, and cardiac morbidity. The issue of postoperative cognitive dysfunction will be addressed in a separate chapter.

There has been much interest in studying the relationship between the control of postoperative pain and the incidence of postoperative delirium. Lynch et al. demonstrated that a higher VAS pain score at rest was correlated with a higher risk of delirium over the first 3 postoperative days.[81] It is interesting to note that the method of postoperative analgesia, the type of opioid used, and the total dose of opioid were not related to the development of delirium. These findings are consistent with the study of Morrison et al. involving 541 elderly hip fracture patients, which clearly demonstrated the relationship between undertreated pain and delirium.[82] Patients who received less than 10 mg of parenteral morphine equivalents per day were more likely to develop delirium than patients who received more analgesia (relative risk [RR] 5.4, 95% confidence interval [CI] 2.4–12.3). In particular, cognitively intact patients with undertreated pain were nine times more likely to develop delirium than patients whose pain was adequately treated. The nature of opioid used did have an impact in this study with meperidine being significantly more associated with delirium than morphine (RR 2.4, 95% CI 1.3–4.5). Other risk factors for delirium were cognitive impairment, abnormal blood pressure, and heart failure. Marcantonio et al. studied the relationship of postoperative delirium with psychoactive medications.[83] They found that postoperative exposure to meperidine, in particular via the epidural route, and to benzodiazepines, particularly long-acting benzodiazepines, was associated with the development of delirium.

It has long been observed that some patients, even those without preexisting conditions, develop persistent pain following surgery.[84] Patients with chronic painful conditions, more common in the elderly population, are at risk for a more intense painful experience following surgery. In their review of acute pain therapy, Gottschalk and Wu speculate that aggressive perioperative management of pain, including preemptive multimodal therapy, can lead to long-term benefits in the form of decreased pain and speedier recovery.[85] Chronic pain after surgery can manifest as hyperalgesia and

Table 25-4

Volumes of Local Anesthetics and Infusion Rates for Peripheral Nerve Blockade

Nerve Block	Single Injection Bolus (mL)	Starting Infusion Rate (mL/h)
Interscalene	30–40	6
Femoral	20–30	8
Lumbar plexus	25–35	10

allodynia. Long-term pain is known to persist following amputation of an extremity,[86] thoracotomy,[87] mastectomy,[88] laparotomy,[89] herniorrhaphy,[90] and orthopedic procedures.[91] Even low levels of persistent pain following surgery have been associated with decreased physical and social function as well as decreased perception of overall health.[92] As mentioned earlier in this chapter, systemic opioids and N-methyl-D-aspartate (NMDA) antagonists administered prior to incision can lead to decreased wound hyperalgesia several days after surgery. Local anesthetics, when applied to the surgical site prior to incision, can have effects that outlast their presence at the surgical site. Perhaps the most widely utilized example of this phenomenon involves the use of local anesthetic cream prior to circumcision in neonatal males,[93] which resulted in a decrease in pain-related behavior at the time of vaccination. Preemptive administration of epidural opioid has led to benefits after mastectomy, thoracotomy, extremity, and abdominal surgery.[94] Use of an epidural catheter pre-, intra-, and postoperatively following amputation of an extremity led to a reduction in the development of phantom limb pain by approximately 50% in comparison to systemic opioids.[95]

Hip fracture is a common scenario in elderly patients and there is often a painful and stressful period prior to surgical intervention. In this elderly population at risk for coronary artery disease, Matot et al. prospectively studied 68 patients randomized to either receive preoperative standard analgesia (intramuscular meperidine) or continuous epidural infusion (bupivacaine and methadone).[96] The average time to surgical intervention was 27 hours. There were no differences in pain scores at rest between the two groups before surgery, but there was a marked difference in major cardiac events (myocardial infarction and heart failure). No patients in the epidural arm had major cardiac events while 7 patients (20%) in the standard group had major cardiac events including four fatalities. It should be noted that the average age of these patients was high (82.4 ± 8.1 years in epidural group vs. 81 ± 8.1 years in standard group) which would account for this extremely high rate of major cardiac events, but the finding that none of the patients in the epidural group had a major cardiac event strongly suggests a first line role for epidural analgesia in frail, elderly patients.

It is apparent that simply controlling postoperative pain has beneficial effects with regard to delirium and development of chronic pain syndromes. It goes without saying that there are beneficial effects with regard to mood, sleep patterns, and general satisfaction. As seen in the previous sections of this chapter, the modalities of pain control can have other benefits as well (e.g., epidural techniques and risk of thromboembolism) in addition to pain control. The studies showing the association between control of preoperative pain with epidural techniques and lower rates of cardiac morbidity and mortality is one example of how the choice of technique of pain control can affect patient outcome.

CONCLUSION

The main focus of this chapter is to address the issue of acute pain in the setting of the elderly patient. When assessing pain in this population, it is important to have a variety of tools to assess the pain. Some patients are able to understand and use the VAS; however, more verbally descriptive pain scales may be more reliable and better understood. The majority of cognitively impaired patients is able to comprehend and use a pain scale and should be allowed to do so. They are able to accurately report the presence of pain, and their reports should not be dismissed because of the presence of dementia. The use of observational pain scales should be reserved for those few nonverbal patients who are unable to give a description of their pain. Undertreated pain is a risk factor for the development of delirium which can be reversed by adequately treating the pain.

In the elderly population, neuraxial analgesia provides better pain control than IV opioid analgesia. While there is no difference in outcome when either method is used, the benefits of superior analgesia with decreased side effects along with the prevention of nervous system sensitization associated with neuraxial analgesia make it a better choice.

The reemergence of peripheral nerve block into the mainstream of anesthesia practice, along with the proven benefits of local anesthetics with regard to nervous system sensitization and opioid sparing, make it a useful choice for analgesia in the elderly. As more studies are performed in the elderly, it is likely that the benefits will be applicable to this population. In particular, the ability to provide analgesia comparable to epidural analgesia with regard to lower extremity surgery makes it a particularly appealing choice.

Although the choice of anesthetic technique does not make a difference with regard to mortality, there are demonstrated benefits of techniques that involve the use of local anesthetics. The institution of preemptive analgesia appears to affect the development of chronic pain syndromes, and the importance of studies showing a decreased incidence of cardiac morbidity and mortality in patients treated preoperatively with epidural analgesia cannot be overstated.

KEY POINTS

▶ Verbal pain scales appear to better assess pain in elderly populations than nonverbal scales.

▶ Cognitive decline or dementia does not preclude the majority of sufferers from using a self-assessment scale to rate their pain.

▶ There are very few settings in which observational pain scales should be utilized.

▶ Consider nonpharmacologic methods as adjuvants to pharmacologic methods in the treatment of acute pain.

▶ A multimodal approach to pain management allows lower doses of drugs to be used for reducing the incidence of side effects.

▶ Preemptive analgesia with NSAIDs, local anesthetics, anticonvulsants, and ketamine improves postoperative pain control.

▶ A strict protocol for morphine titration based on individualized pain perception in the PACU results in similar initial doses of morphine to provide initial analgesia regardless of age.

▶ Total postoperative morphine requirements on a daily basis are decreased in the elderly because of decreased clearance of the drug.

▶ Epidural techniques provide superior postoperative pain relief compared with IV opioids.

▶ Epidural techniques are associated with reductions in risk of venous thromboembolism, myocardial infarction, bleeding complications, pneumonia, respiratory depression, and renal failure.

▶ The use of nerve blocks has been shown to improve the following outcomes: immediate postoperative analgesia, time until first analgesic request, total amount of postoperative opioid use, PACU and hospital discharge times, postoperative nausea and vomiting, postoperative mood, sleep, and unplanned hospital admission.

▶ Continuous catheter techniques provide alternatives to neuraxial techniques for lower extremity surgery.

KEY ARTICLES

- ▶ Gagliese L, Katz J. Age differences in postoperative pain are scale dependent: a comparison of measures of pain intensity and quality in younger and older surgical patients. *Pain.* 2003;103:11–20.

- ▶ Pateux S, Herrmann F, Le Lous P, et al. Feasibility and reliability of four pain self assessment scales and correlation with an observational rating scale in hospitalized elderly demented patients. *J Gerontol.* 2005;60A(4):524–529.

- ▶ Kehlet H, Dahl JB. The value of "multimodal" or "balanced analgesia" in postoperative pain treatment. *Anesth Analg.* 1993;77:1048–1056.

- ▶ Woolf CJ, Chong MS. Preemptive analgesia—treating postoperative pain by preventing the establishment of central sensitization. *Anesth Analg.* 1993;77:362–379.

- ▶ Wilder-Smith OHG. Opioid use in the elderly. *Eur J Pain.* 2005;9: 137–140.

- ▶ Aubrun F, Monsel S, Langeron O, et al. Postoperative titration of intravenous morphine in the elderly patient. *Anesthesiology.* 2002; 96:17–23.

- ▶ Aubrun F, Bunge D, Langeron O, et al. Postoperative morphine consumption in the elderly patient. *Anesthesiology.* 2003;99:160–165.

- ▶ Macintyre PE, Jarvis DA. Age is the best predictor of postoperative morphine requirements. *Pain.* 1996;64:357–364.

- ▶ Rodgers A, Walker N, Schug S, et al. Reduction of postoperative mortality and morbidity with epidural or spinal anaesthesia: results from overview of randomized trials. *Br Med J.* 2000;321:1–12.

- ▶ Block BM, Liu SS, Rowlingson AJ, et al. Efficacy of postoperative epidural analgesia: a meta analysis. *JAMA.* 2003;290(18):2455–2463.

- ▶ Evans H, Steele SM, Nielsen KC, et al. Peripheral nerve block and continuous catheter techniques. *Anesthesiol Clin North America.* 2005;23:141–162.

- ▶ Liu SS, Salinas FV. Continuous plexus and peripheral nerve blocks for postoperative analgesia. *Anesth Analg.* 2003;96:263–272.

REFERENCES

1. Witte M. Pain control. *J Gerontol Nurs.* 1989;15:32ñ37.
2. Gagliese L. Assessment of pain in the elderly. In: Turk DC, Melzack R, eds. *Handbook of Pain Assessment.* New York, NY: Guilford Press; 2001:119–133.
3. Herr KA, Mobily PR. Comparison of selected pain assessment tools for use with the elderly. *Appl Nurs Res.* 1993;6:39–46.
4. Gangliese L, Katz J. Age differences in postoperative pain are scale dependent: a comparison of measures of pain intensity and quality in younger and older surgical patients. *Pain.* 2003;103:11–20.
5. Feldt S, Ryden M, Miles S. Treatment of pain in cognitively impaired compared with cognitively intact older patients with hip fracture. *J Am Geriatr Soc.* 1998;46:1079–1085.
6. Morrison RS, Siu AL. A comparison and pain and its treatment inn advanced dementia and cognitively intact patients with hip fracture. *J Pain Symptom Manage.* 2000;19:240–248.
7. Parmelee PA, Smith B, Katz IR. Pain complaints and cognitive status among elderly institution residents. *J Geriatr Soc.* 1993;41:517–522.
8. Pateux S, Herrmann F, Le Lous P, et al. Feasibility and reliability of four pain self assessment scales and correlation with an observational rating scale in hospitalized elderly demented patients. *J Gerontol.* 2005; 60A(4):524–529.
9. Ferrell BA. Pain evaluation and management in the nursing home. *Ann Intern Med.* 1995;123:681–687.
10. Krulewitch H, London MR, Shakel VJ, et al. Assessment of pain in cognitively impaired older adults: a comparison of pain assessment tools and their use by nonprofessional observers. *J Am Geriatr Soc.* 2000; 48:1607–1611.
11. Kehlet H, Dahl JB. The value of ìmultimodalî or ìbalanced analgesiaî in postoperative pain treatment. *Anesth Analg.* 1993;77:1048–1056.
12. Woolf CJ, Chong MS. Preemptive analgesia—treating postoperative pain by preventing the establishment of central sensitization. *Anesth Analg.* 1993;77:362–379.
13. Ferrell BR, Rhiner M, Ferrell BA. Development and implementation of a pain education program. *Cancer.* 1993;72(Suppl. 11);3426–3432.
14. Rhiner M, Ferrell BR, Ferrell BA, et al. A structured nondrug intervention program for cancer pain. *Cancer Pract.* 1993;1:137–143.
15. Piotrowski MM, Patterson C, Mitchinson A, et al. *J Am Coll Surg.* 2003;197(6);1037–1046.
16. Gloth FM. Pain management in older adults: prevention and treatment. *J Am Geriatr Soc.* 2001;49:188–199.
17. Bannwarth P, Pehourcq F. Pharmacologic basis for using paracetamol: pharmacokinetic and pharmacodynamic issues. *Drugs.* 2003;63(2):5–15.
18. Ochroch EA, Mardini IA, Gottschalk A. What is the role of NSAIDs in pre-emptive analgesia? *Drugs.* 2003;63:2709–2723.
19. Treede RD, Magerl W. Multiple mechanisms of secondary hyperalgesia. *Prog Brain Res.* 2000;129:331–341.
20. Recart A, Issioui T, White PF, et al. The efficacy of celecoxib premedication on postoperative pain and recovery times after ambulatory surgery: a dose ranging study. *Anesth Analg.* 2003;96(6):1631–1635.
21. Gillis JC, Brogden RN. Ketorolac: a reappraisal of its pharmacodynamic and pharmacokinetic properties and therapeutic use in pain management. *Drugs.* 1997;53:139.
22. DiBlaso CJ, Snyder ME, Kattan MW, et al. Ketorolac: safe and effective analgesia for the management of renal cortical tumors with partial nephrectomy. *Urology.* 2004;171:1062–1065.
23. Dirks J, Fredensborg BB, Christensen D. A randomized study of the effects of single-dose gabapentin versus placebo on postoperative pain and morphine consumption after mastectomy. *Anesthesiology.* 2002;97:560–564.
24. Pandey CK, Navkar DV, Giri PJ, et al. Evaluation of the optimal preemptive dose of gabapentin for postoperative pain relief after lumbar diskectomy: a randomized, double-blind, placebo-controlled study. *J Neurosurg Anesthesiol.* 2005;17(2):65–68.
25. Tverskoy M, Oz Y, Isakson A, et al. Preemptive effect of fentanyl and ketamine on postoperative pain and wound hyperalgesia. *Anesth Analg.* 1994;78:205–209.
26. Himmelseher S, Durieux ME. Ketamine for perioperative pain management. *Anesthesiology.* 2005;102:211–220.
27. Idvall J, Ahlgren I, Aronsen KR, et al. Ketamine infusions: pharmacokinetics and clinical effects. *Br J Anaesth.* 1979;51:1167–1173.
28. Hannibal K, Galatius H, Hansen A, et al. Preoperative wound infiltration with bupivacaine reduces early and late opioid requirement after hysterectomy. *Anesth Analg.* 1996;83:376–381.
29. Ke RW, Portera G, Bagous W, et al. A randomized, double-blinded trial of preemptive analgesia in laparoscopy. *Obstet Gynecol.* 1998;92:972–975.
30. Wilder-Smith OHG. Opioid use in the elderly. *Eur J Pain.* 2005;9: 137–140.
31. Aubrun F, Bunge D, Langeron O, et al. Postoperative morphine consumption in the elderly patient. *Anesthesiology.* 2003;99:160–165.
32. Macintyre PE, Jarvis DA. Age is the best predictor of postoperative morphine requirements. *Pain.* 1996;64:357–364.
33. Singleton MA, Rosen JI, Fisher DM. Pharmacokinetics of fentanyl in the elderly. *Br J Anaesth.* 1988;60:619–622.
34. Holdsworth MT, Forman WB, Killilea TA, et al. Transdermal fentanyl disposition in elderly subjects. *Gerontology.* 1994;40:32–37.
35. Lemmens HJ, Brum AG, Hennis PJ, et al. Influence of age on the pharmacokinetics of alfentanil. Gender dependence. *Clin Pharmacokinet.* 1990;19:416–422.
36. Matteo RS, Schwartz AE, Ornstein E, et al. Pharmacokinetics of sufentanil in the elderly surgical patient. *Can J Anaesth.* 1990;37:852–856.
37. Minto CF, Schnider TW, Egan TD, et al. Influence of age and gender on the pharmacokinetics and pharmacodynamics of remifentanil: I. Model development. *Anesthesiology.* 1997;86:10–23.
38. Aubrun F, Langeron O, Quesnel C, et al. Relationships between measurement of pain using visual analog score and morphine requirements during postoperative intravenous morphine titration. *Anesthesiology.* 2003;98:1415–1421.
39. Aubrun F, Monsel S, Langeron O, et al. Postoperative titration of intravenous morphine in the elderly patient. *Anesthesiology.* 2002;96:17–23.

40. Sear JW, Hand CS, Moore RA. Studies on morphine disposition: plasma concentrations of morphine and its metabolites in anesthetized middle-aged and elderly surgical patients. *J Clin Anesth.* 1989;1:164–169.

41. Pickering G, Joudan G, Eschalier A, Dubray C. Impact of age, gender, and cognitive functioning on pain perception. *Gerontology.* 2002;48:112–118.

42. Aubrun F, Salvi N, Coriat P, et al. Sex- and age-related difference in morphine requirements for postoperative pain relief. *Anesthesiology.* 2005;103(1):156–160.

43. Kehlet H. Modification of responses to surgery by neural blockade: clinical implications. In: Cousins M, Bridenbaugh P, eds. *Neural Blockade in Clinical Anesthesia and Management of Pain.* 2nd ed. Philadelphia: JB Lippincott; 1988:145–188.

44. Rodgers A, Walker N, Schug S, et al. Reduction of postoperative mortality and morbidity with epidural or spinal anaesthesia: results from overview of randomized trials. *Br Med J.* 2000;321:1–12.

45. Modig J, Borg T, Karlstrom G, et al. Thromboembolism after total hip replacement: role of epidural and general anesthesia. *Anesth Analg.* 1983;62:174–180.

46. Park WY, Thompson JS, Lee KK. Effect of epidural anesthesia and analgesia on perioperative outcome: a randomized controlled Veterans Affairs Cooperative Study. *Ann Surg.* 2001;234:560–569.

47. Rigg JRA, Jamrozik K, Myles PS, et al. Epidural anaesthesia and analgesia and outcome of major surgery: a randomized trial. *Lancet.* 2002; 359:1276–1282.

48. Block BM, Liu SS, Rowlingson AJ, et al. Efficacy of postoperative epidural analgesia: a meta-analysis. *JAMA.* 2003;290(18):2455–2463.

49. Bugedo GJ, Carcamo CR, Mertens RA, et al. Preoperative percutaneous ilioinguinal and iliohypogastric nerve block with 0.5% bupivacaine for post-herniorrhaphy pain management in adults. *Reg Anesth.* 1990;15:130–133.

50. Evans H, Steele SM, Nielsen KC, et al. Peripheral nerve block and continuous catheter techniques. *Anesthesiol Clin North America.* 2005; 23:141–162.

51. Hadzic A, Vloka JD. *Peripheral Nerve Blocks Principles and Practice.* New York, NY: McGraw-Hill; 2004:108–129.

52. Brown AR, Weiss R, Greenberg C, et al. Interscalene block for shoulder arthroscopy: comparison with general anesthesia. *Arthroscopy.* 1993;9:295–300.

53. Al-Kaisy A, McGuire G, Chan VW, et al. Analgesic effect of interscalene block using low-dose bupivacaine for outpatient arthroscopic shoulder surgery. *Reg Anesth Pain Med.* 1998;23:469–473.

54. Kinnard P, Truchon R, St-Pierre A, et al. Interscalene block for pain relief after shoulder surgery: a prospective randomized study. *Clin Orthop.* 1994;304:22–24.

55. Arciero RA, Taylor DC, Harrison SA, et al. Interscalene anesthesia for shoulder arthroscopy in a community-sized military hospital. *Arthroscopy.* 1996;12:715–719.

56. Chelly JE, Greger J, Samsam T, et al. Reduction of operating and recovery room times and overnight hospital stays with interscalene block as sole anesthetic technique for rotator cuff surgery. *Minerva Anestesiol.* 2001;67:613–619.

57. Hadzic A, Vloka JD. *Peripheral Nerve Blocks Principles and Practice.* New York, NY: McGraw-Hill; 2004:148–161.

58. Hadzic A, Vloka JD, Kuroda MM, et al. The practice of peripheral nerve blocks in the United States: a national survey. *Reg Anesth Pain Med.* 1998;23:241–246.

59. Chan VW, Peng PW, Kaszas Z, et al. A comparative study of general anesthesia, intravenous regional anesthesia and axillary block for outpatient hand surgery: clinical outcome and cost analysis. *Anesth Analg.* 2001;93:1181–1184.

60. McCartney CJ, Brull R, Chan VW, et al. Early but no long term benefit of regional compared with general anesthesia for ambulatory hand surgery. *Anesthesiology.* 2004;101:461–467.

61. Hadzic A, Vloka JD. *Peripheral Nerve Blocks Principles and Practice.* New York, NY: McGraw-Hill; 2004:218–233.

62. Matheny JM, Hanks GA, Rung GW, et al. A comparison of patient controlled analgesia and continuous lumbar plexus block after anterior cruciate ligament reconstruction. *Arthroscopy.* 1993;9:87–90.

63. Kaloul I, Guay J, Cote C, et al. The posterior lumbar plexus (psoas compartment) block and the three-in-one femoral nerve block provide

64. de Visme V, Picart F, Le Jouan R, et al. Combined lumbar and sacral plexus block compared with plain bupivacaine spinal anesthesia for hip fractures in the elderly. *Reg Anesth Pain Med.* 2000;25:158–162.

65. Biboulet P, Morau D, Aubas P, et al. Postoperative analgesia after total hip arthroplasty: comparison of intravenous patient controlled analgesia with morphine and single injection of femoral nerve or psoas compartment block: a prospective, randomized, double-blind study. *Reg Anesth Pain Med.* 2004;29:102–109.

66. Hevia-Sanchez V, Bermejo-Alvarez MA, Helvia-Mendez A, et al. Posterior block of lumbar plexus for postoperative analgesia after hip arthroplasty. *Rev Esp Anestesiol.* 2002;49:507–511.

67. Capdevila X, Macaire P, Dadure C, et al. Continuous psoas compartment block for postoperative analgesia after total hip arthroplasty: new landmarks, technical guidelines, and clinical evaluation. *Anesth Analg.* 2002;94:1606–1013.

68. Turker G, Uckunkaya N, Yavascaoglu B, et al. Comparison of the catheter technique psoas compartment block and the epidural block for analgesia in partial hip replacement surgery. *Acta Anesthesiol Scand.* 2003;47:30–36.

69. Hadzic A, Vloka JD. *Peripheral Nerve Blocks Principles and Practice.* New York, NY: McGraw-Hill; 2004:266–281.

70. Mulroy MF, Larkin KL, Batra MS, et al. Femoral nerve block with 0.25% or 0.5% bupivacaine improves postoperative analgesia following outpatient arthroscopic anterior cruciate ligament repair. *Reg Anesth Pain Med.* 2001;26:24–29.

71. Edkin BS, McCarty, Spindler KP, et al. Analgesia with femoral nerve block for anterior cruciate ligament reconstruction. *Clin Orthop.* 1999; 369:289–295.

72. Peng P, Claxton A, Chung F, et al. Femoral nerve block and ketorolac in patients undergoing anterior cruciate ligament reconstruction. *Can J Anaesth.* 1999;46:919–924.

73. Lynch J, Trojan S, Arhelger S, et al. Intermittent femoral nerve blockade for anterior cruciate ligament repair: use of a catheter technique in 208 patients. *Acta Anaesthiol Belg.* 1991;42:207–212.

74. Schwartz SK, Franciosi LG, Ries CR, et al. Addition of femoral 3-in-1 blockade to intraarticular ropivacaine 0.2% does not reduce analgesic requirements following arthroscopic knee surgery. *Can J Anaesth.* 1999; 46:741–747.

75. Frost S, Grossfeld S, Kirkley A, et al. The efficacy of femoral nerve block in pain reduction for outpatient hamstring anterior cruciate ligament reconstruction: a double blind, prospective, randomized trial. *Arthroscopy.* 2000;16:243–248.

76. Mansour NY, Bennetts FE. An observational study of combined continuous lumbar plexus and single shot sciatic nerve blocks for post-knee surgery analgesia. *Reg Anesth.* 1996;21:287–291.

77. Williams BA, Kentor ML, Vogt MT, et al. Femoral-sciatic nerve blocks for complex outpatient knee surgery are associated with less postoperative pain before same day discharge: a review of 1200 consecutive cases from the period 1996–1999. *Anesthesiology.* 2003;98:1206–1213.

78. Ng HP, Cheong KF, Lim A, et al. Intraoperative single shot ì3-in-1î femoral nerve block with ropivacaine 0.25%, ropivacaine 0.5% or bupivacaine 0.25% provides comparable 48 hr analgesia after unilateral total knee replacement. *Can J Anaesth.* 2001;48:1102–1108.

79. Edwards ND, Wright EM. Continuous low dose 3-in-1 nerve blockade for postoperative pain relief after total knee replacement. *Anesth Analg.* 1992;75:265–267.

80 Singelyn FJ, Deyaert M, Joris D, et al. Effects of intravenous patient-controlled analgesia with morphine, continuous epidural analgesia, and continuous three-in-one block on postoperative pain and knee rehabilitation after unilateral total knee arthroplasty. *Anesth Analg.* 1998; 87:88–92.

81. Dahl JB, Christiansen CL, Dauggaard JJ, et al. Continuous blockade of the lumbar plexus after knee surgery-postoperative analgesia and bupivacaine plasma concentrations: a controlled clinical trial. *Anaesthesia.* 1988;43:1015–1018.

82. Capdevila X, Barthelet Y, Biboulet P, et al. Effects of perioperative analgesic technique on the surgical outcome and duration of rehabilitation after major knee surgery. *Anesthesiology.* 1999;91:8–15.

similar postoperative analgesia after total knee replacement. *Can J Anaesth.* 2004;51:45–51.

83. Serpell MG, Millar FA, Thomson MF, et al. Comparison of lumbar plexus block versus conventional opioid analgesia after total knee replacement. *Anaesthesia.* 1991;46:275–277.

84. Tarkkila P, Tuominen M, Huhtala J, et al. Comparison of intrathecal morphine and continuous femoral 3-in-1 block for pain after major knee surgery under spinal anaesthesia. *Eur J Anaesthesiol.* 1998;15:6–9.

85. Grant SA, Nielsen KC, Greengrass RA, et al. Continuous peripheral nerve block for ambulatory surgery. *Reg Anesth Pain Med.* 2001;26:209–214.

86. Kuzma PJ, Kline MD, Calkins MD. Progress in the development of ultra-long acting local anesthetics. *Reg Anesth.* 1997;22:543–550.

87. Kopacz DJ, Allen HW, Hopf K. Extended local analgesia of bupivacaine-loaded microspheres: role of dexamethasone. *Anesth Analg.* 2001;91:S260.

88. Lynch EP, Lazor MA, Gellis JE, et al. The impact of postoperative pain on the development of postoperative delirium. *Anesth Analg.* 1998;86:781–785.

89. Morrison RS, Magaziner J, Gilbert M, et al. Relationship between pain and opioid analgesics on the development of delirium following hip fracture. *J Gerontol A Biol Sci Med Sci.* 2003;58:76–81.

90. Marcantonio ER, Juarez G, Goldman L, et al. The relationship of postoperative delirium with psychoactive medications. *JAMA.* 1994;272(19):1518–1522.

91. Perkins FM, Kehlet H. Chronic pain as an outcome of surgery. A review of predictive factors. *Anesthesiology.* 2000;93:1123–1133.

92. Gottschalk A, Wu CL. New concepts in acute pain therapy. *Ann Long Term Care.* 2004;12:18–24.

93. Sherman RA, Devor M, Jones DEC, et al. *Phantom Pain.* New York, NY: Plenum Press;1997.

94. Dajczman E, Gordon A, Kreisman H, et al. Long-term postthoracotomy pain. *Chest.* 1991;99:270–274.

95. de Vries JE, Timmer PR, Erftemeier FJ, et al. Breast pain after breast conserving therapy. *Breast.* 1994;3:151–154.

96. Gottschalk A, Smith DS, Jobes DR, et al. Preemptive epidural analgesia and recovery from radical prostatectomy: a randomized controlled trial. *JAMA.* 1998;279:1076–1082.

97. Callesen T, Kehlet H. Postherniorrhaphy pain. *Anesthesiology.* 1997;87:1219–1230.

98. Reuben SS. Preventing the development of complex regional pain syndrome following surgery. *Anesthesiology.* 2004;101:1215–1224.

99. Haythornthwaite JA, Raja SN, Fisher B, et al. Pain and quality of life following radical retropubic prostatectomy. *J Urol.* 1998;150:1761–1764.

100. Taddio A, Katz J, Ilersich AL, et al. Effect of neonatal circumcision on pain response during subsequent routine vaccination. *Lancet.* 1997;349:1123–1126.

101. Aida S, Baba H, Yamakura T, et al. The effectiveness of preemptive analgesia varies according to the type of surgery: a randomized, double-blind study. *Anesth Analg.* 1999;89:711–716.

102. Bach S, Noreng MF, Tjellden NU. Phantom limb pain in amputees during the first 12 months following limb amputation, after preoperative lumbar epidural blockade. *Pain.* 1988;33:297–301.

103. Matot I, Oppenheim-Eden A, Ratrot R, et al. Preoperative cardiac events in elderly patients with hip fracture randomized to epidural or conventional analgesia. *Anesthesiology.* 2003;98:156–163.

SECTION
7

SPECIAL TOPICS

Assessment and Management of Chronic Pain in the Elderly

Amit Sharma

Srinivasa N. Raja

INTRODUCTION

Life expectancy of humans is increasing in developed and developing countries.[1,2] The proportion of people aged 65 and above is expected to almost double by 2050 in the United States.[3] This increase in life expectancy has been achieved through improvements in the management of chronic diseases associated with middle age. Despite these impressive achievements of modern science, the incidence of degenerative conditions found in the elderly remains stable and results in significant morbidity in this subpopulation. Persistent or chronic pain is one of the most common symptoms associated with the increased burden of pathology observed with aging process.[4] For instance, 25–50% of community-dwelling seniors suffer from pain that interferes with their ability to function normally.[5,6] The prevalence of pain among patients in nursing home facilities varies from 45% to 80% in different studies.[7–9]

Despite being a common problem of elderly patients, chronic pain management in these vulnerable patients is inadequate.[10] Despite the high proportion of patients suffering from pain in the nursing home facilities, analgesics are used in only 40–50% of residents.[7–9] Multiple factors are responsible for the undertreatment of pain in the elderly. Many elderly patients relate chronic pain to negative images and stereotypes associated with long-standing psychiatric problems, futility in treatment, malingering, or drug-seeking behavior. The term persistent pain may foster a more positive attitude for patients and professionals for the many effective treatments that are available to help alleviate suffering.[4] The undertreatment by physicians may be secondary to lack of understanding of geriatric pain, difficulty in evaluating pain in elderly, and due to concerns of overtreatment and untoward side effects.[11] Since many older patients have at least one chronic condition and take multiple medications, prescribing for the senior patient in pain can be overwhelming.[12] Thus, significant improvement is needed in screening, clinical evaluation, follow-up, and attention to potential toxicities of therapy.[10]

ALTERATIONS IN PAIN SIGNALING WITH AGING

▶ Changes related to nociceptive pathways

Pain, along with other sensations such as vision, hearing, taste, smell, and touch, has significant biological implications. It helps prevent injuries and maintain homeostatic integrity, and leads to behavioral as well as emotional responses to external stimuli. Its presence is essential to the overall well-being of an individual throughout life—from the neonate to the elderly. Since the aging process is involved with the deterioration of many biological functions, it is easy to assume that these changes could affect pain perception in the elderly. Animal studies have provided some insight on this perplexing issue over the past few decades and is summarized in Table 26-1. These changes along the pain signaling pathways—nociceptive primary afferent fibers, central nervous system (CNS), and endogenous pain inhibitory system—may lead to a decrease in the sensitivity to pain in the elderly population. These physiological alterations are discussed in detail in the following sections.

▶ Changes related to prevalence

Although many authors have reported that overall prevalence of pain increases in elderly, it is often stated that self-reported pain prevalence declines in age groups beyond 60 years.[22] Possible reasons quoted for this disparity range from physiological alterations in nociception, poor reporting[23] and to an increase in stoicism.[24,25] Although some self-reported regional pain syndromes decline in prevalence in the older age groups,[24,26,27] the overall prevalence of self-reported pain remains constant with age in older people.[28] Also, while some studies have shown greater disruption of lives of elderly people suffering from chronic or persistent pain,[29,30] others have shown that despite a greater level of medical morbidity and longer duration of pain, older patients with chronic pain are not more likely to suffer from concurrent depression, are less disabled, and less somatically preoccupied than younger patients.[31]

There is a high prevalence of pain-related pathological states in elderly population. They include osteoarthritis, osteoporosis, gout, fractures of the spine, stroke, peripheral vascular diseases, peripheral neuropathy, postherpetic neuralgia (PHN), polymyalgia rheumatica, temporal arteritis, and even cancer. The coexistence of these disorders is also frequent, and many elderly patients are on multiple medications to complicate the pharmacological picture. Despite the increased prevalence of these painful disorders, there is a relative decline in pain reporting in older people. Numerous reasons have been predicted to explain this discrepancy:

1. Iatrogenic factors (sample bias): Healthier elderly population lives in the community rather than in managed care institutions, thereby reducing the incidence of pain in the general elderly population.

2. Comorbid conditions: Comorbidities such as stroke, dementia, or depression may interfere with the ability of the elderly to report pain.

3. Personal factors: It has been suggested that pain reporting in elderly might be suppressed by their concerns regarding loss of

Table 26-1

Age-Related Differences in Nociceptive Pathways

Changes in nociceptive primary afferent fibers	
Decreased density of myelinated and unmyelinated fibers	Verdu et al.[13]
Decrease in peripheral nerve conduction velocity	Verdu et al.[13]
Marked reduction in substance P and CGRP contents at various levels, causing a reduction in the density or functional integrity of nociceptive nerves	Gibson and Farrell[14]
Changes in central nervous system	
Marked loss of myelin with evidence of axonal involution, particularly in the medial lemniscal pathways	Ko et al.[15]
Decreased levels of CGRP, substance P, and somatostatin in the cervical, thoracic, and lumbar dorsal horn	Bergman et al.[16] Hukkanen et al.[17]
Progressive age-related loss of serotonergic and noradrenergic neurons in the dorsal horn, causing a change in nociceptive processing and in the function of descending modulatory pathways	Ko et al.[15] Iwata et al.[18]
Neuronal death, loss of dendritic arborization, and neurofibrillary abnormalities in cerebral cortex, midbrain, and brainstem	Pakkenberg and Gundersen[19]
Decline in the concentration and turnover of catecholamines, GABA, opioid, and serotonin receptors in the limbic system and cerebral cortex	Barili et al.[20]
Changes in endogenous pain inhibitory system	
A general age-related decline in the neural opioid- and nonopioid-dependent pain inhibitory systems	Washington et al.[21]

Source: From Ref. 14.

independence, fear to undergo unwanted investigations, treatments, or the finding of serious pathology. Also, many elderly misattribute pain syndromes to the aging process itself.

4. Physiological reasons: Reports in literature describe the possibility of age-related changes in function of nociceptive pathways that lead to reduced pain sensitivity during senescence. Laboratory studies on psychophysical indices of pain sensitivity in elderly show inconclusive results for sensory threshold for thermal or electrical stimulus.[32] At present, there exists no convincing reason to believe that the elderly population has a higher threshold or tolerance to pain.

▶ Changes related to perception and tolerance

The International Association for the Study of Pain (IASP) defines pain as an unpleasant sensory and emotional experience associated with actual or potential tissue damage, or described in terms of such damage. Pain is always subjective. Each individual learns the application of the word through experiences related to injury in early life.

Changes in pain perception threshold

Pain perception threshold is crudely defined as the intensity of a given stimulus at which it becomes painful. Once threshold is reached, adaptive or escape behaviors are activated to prevent tissue injury. Any decrease in this threshold would make an individual explicitly sensitive, whereas any increase might make an individual more prone to receive frequent injuries and also cause delay in the healing process. Although few studies described a decrease in pain threshold in the elderly,[33] a number of studies have shown that pain perception threshold is increased in the elderly. The effect of age on pain threshold intensity is variable and dependent on numerous factors like stimulus modality, site and duration of stimulation, and the area involved (Table 26-2).

Suprathreshold pain responses

As previously described, suprathreshold stimuli cause pain and lead to adaptive or avoidance behavior to limit further injury. Effect of age on suprathreshold responses has been extensively studied for thermal stimuli. With advancing age, suprathreshold pain responses are decreased, and thus the functional reserve between identification of pain and the onset of frankly injurious stimulation is reduced. This decrease in pain sensitivity at suprathreshold levels of stimulation leads to increased risk of injury in elderly. Although not much data are available for suprathreshold pain response toward nonthermal stimuli, there is some evidence that similar reactions may occur. Harkins and Chapman[48,49] in their studies involving electrical stimulation of tooth pulp showed that despite unchanged pain threshold, a significant deficit in ability to discriminate between suprathreshold shocks was observed in elderly. At present, limited data are available to generalize this observation.

Harkins and Chapman[48,49] in the above-mentioned studies also reported a significant change in willingness of the aged to report the electrical shocks as painful. *Pain*, by definition, is an unpleasant sensory and emotional experience. The unpleasantness is the hedonic dimension of pain which is considered to be closely related to stimulus intensity. In a given subject, visceral sensations are commonly described as more unpleasant than somatic sensations.[50,51] This difference is probably due to the differences in cortical processing of visceral and somatic stimulation.[52] For a given suprathreshold stimulus, ratings of pain unpleasantness are usually considered to run parallel to intensity ratings irrespective of the age of subjects.[39,47] Earlier findings of Harkins studies can be explained to some extent by the fact that threshold for electrical stimulation is probably higher in elderly, and thus same intensity stimulus may not provoke similar unpleasantness ratings.

Pain tolerance

Pain tolerance, the greatest level of pain which a subject is prepared to tolerate, has been examined in several studies. With few exceptions, majority of these studies show a decrease in the stimulus intensity requirement for development of tolerance with advancing age.[53–55] This difference in pain tolerance is probably due to age-related decrease in endogenous pain inhibitory systems.[21] Similar observations were made by Edwards et al. in their laboratory assessment of diffuse noxious inhibitory controls (DNIC) in younger and older subjects.[56] In contrary to expected response, suprathreshold pain responses are diminished in elderly population. This may be due to the fact that cognitive and secondary affective responses also play a role in modulating pain tolerance apart from endogenous pain pathway system.[57–59]

Table 26-2

Factors Affecting Pain Threshold in Elderly

Factors	Effects of Aging	References
Stimulus Modality		
Thermal stimuli	Higher threshold in elderly, especially for noncontact heat (laser, radiant) than from contact thermode application of noxious heat	Hall and Stride[34] Procacci et al.[35] Sherman and Robillard[36]
Mechanical stimuli	Equivocal results ▸ Increase in threshold ▸ No change in threshold	Jensen et al.[37] Lasch et al.[38] Pickering et al.[33] Edwards and Fillingim[39] Zheng et al.[40]
Electrical stimuli	Equivocal results ▸ No change in threshold ▸ Increase in threshold	Neri and Agazzani[41] Tucker et al.[42] Mumford[43] Lucantoni et al.[44]
Ischemic stimuli	Lower threshold in elderly	Edwards and Fillingim[39]
Stimulus Site	▸ Proximal areas (upper limb) are affected less than more distal areas (lower limb) ▸ No significant changes over back, probably due to relatively sparse distribution of nociceptors ▸ Visceral stimulation more vulnerable to age-related changes in afferent fiber density ▸ Greater sensitivity of the periosteum, hence bony prominences, for pain responses	Lautenbacher and Strian[45] Mertz[46] Lasch et al.[38] Gibson and Farrell[14]
Stimulus Area	▸ Small area stimulus affected more with age than larger area stimulation, probably due to some compensation by spatial integration at the level of the dorsal horn and cortex	Lautenbacher and Strian[45] Harkins et al.[47] Chakour et al.[48]
Stimulus Duration	▸ Decreasing duration of thermal and electrical stimuli is associated with increasingly greater pain thresholds in elderly due to some compensation by temporal summation for age-related decreases in pain acuity	Harkins et al.[47]

The function of pain as an early warning system is largely preserved in healthy older people. However, decrements of function can be identified in older people that have implications for the integrity of the pain experience as an enteroceptive sensation. Age appears to have a small but significant effect on the threshold for pain. The variability of reports of pain threshold would suggest that this effect is masked by a variety of factors that have yet to be adequately characterized. Trends within the existing literature would suggest that effects of aging on pain threshold are most likely to be apparent when stimuli are of short duration, minimal spatial extent, and delivered to the distal extent of the limbs or to the viscera. Current data for thermal stimuli are consistent with converging stimulus-response functions across the age spectrum due to more rapidly accelerating responses among older people. More studies are needed to gain further insight into the changes in pain signaling in the elderly.

▸ Changes related to postinjury protective system

Following tissue injury, there is local release of multiple chemical mediators (bradykinin, free H[+], serotonin, histamine, eicosanoids, adenosine phosphate derivatives, cytokines, excitatory amino acids, and nerve growth factors) by injured tissue, platelets, mast cells, and macrophages. In addition, there is release of calcitonin gene-related peptide (CGRP) and substance P by antidromic reflexes in nociceptive C fibers, leading to enhancement of this inflammatory response (neurogenic inflammation). Together, these mediators play an important role in mechanisms of peripheral sensitization and the initial stage of tissue repair and wound healing. The intensity of neurogenic inflammation is reduced with aging. Thus, following tissue-damaging stimuli, tissue repair and wound healing processes are slower in the elderly compared to their younger counterparts. Peripheral sensitization (increase in the excitability of nociceptors) causes development of primary hyperalgesia in proximity to tissue damage and contributes to increased pain responses. This primary hyperalgesia acts as a protective response to prevent injured area to be exposed to further tissue trauma.

As healing ensues, there is reversal of hyperalgesia. Delayed healing or repetitive afferent pain signals trigger increased excitability of neurons in the CNS instigating nociceptive firing, even with smaller intensity of stimulus. This modulation in the capacity for transmission in the nociceptive system at spinal cord level is defined as *central sensitization*. One example of this sensitization process is rapid changes in spinal cord in the context of repeated C-fiber stimuli provoking spontaneous and progressively higher intensity firing by dorsal horn neurons (windup phenomenon). Central sensitization can lead to *secondary hyperalgesia*, which is an index of dorsal horn sensitization. Even with comparable levels of spontaneous pain and flare, older people demonstrate much longer period of secondary hyperalgesia,[40] predisposing them for persistent painful symptoms.

ASSESSMENT OF PERSISTENT PAIN IN ELDERLY

For adequate pain management, assessment of etiology and severity of pain are imperative. Evaluation of pain in elderly could be delayed due to personal and social biases of patients and physicians and presence of comorbid conditions like dementia, depression, or other psychiatric or personality disorders. Numerous misconceptions avert elderly people from reporting their pain to the providers. First, many elderly people feel that pain is a sign of personal weakness or an attention-seeking device. Some feel that it is a result of punishment for their past actions. It is also believed that it might indicate the presence of severe underlying disease, diagnosis of which might make them dependent. They are also concerned that they would become addicted to pain medications. To make the circumstances worse, many health-care providers have inadequate knowledge of pain management, especially in this subgroup of population. They often rely heavily on subjective unidimensional pain scoring methods with inadequate documentation of baseline and ongoing assessments. There are also apprehensions about the elderly being excessively prone to the side effects of analgesics, and even insufficient reimbursement for the amount of time the health-care providers might have to spend with these demanding patients.[60] In these given state of affairs, it is not astounding that treatment of pain in elderly is considered to be grossly inadequate.

The assessment of pain in demented patients is even more taxing. Almost 5% of people above 65 years and 20% of those aged 80 years are suffering from dementia.[61] Its prevalence amongst nursing home patients is even higher. Often, their frequent moans and groans are considered as part of the usual aging or dementia process by their family members or hospital staff. Usual psychometric pain assessment tools are difficult to implement and not reliable. Patients with very advanced dementia cannot convey the experience of pain verbally. Under these situations, caregivers have to rely heavily on indirect pain behaviors like facial expressions (frowning, frightened face, grimacing, grinding of teeth, rapid blinking, or distorted expression), verbalization (sighing, moaning, groaning, grunting), body movements (tense body posture, fidgeting, increased pacing, rocking, restriction in movement, or gait or mobility changes), changes in interpersonal interaction (being aggressive, combative, resisting care, or withdrawn), changes in their activity pattern or routines (changes in appetite, sleep, rest pattern), and mental status changes (crying or tearful, increased confusion and irritability). Although these signs might suggest presence of pain in cognitively impaired elderly people, the measurement of intensity still remains a challenge.

Indeed, most mild to moderately demented patients can verbalize their discomfort and also participate in psychometric pain testing. The reliability of various psychometric pain testing tools was recently studied in cognitively impaired elderly population by Taylor et al.[62] In this study, reliability and validity of four selected pain intensity scales—Faces Pain Scale (FPS), the Verbal Descriptor Scale (VDS), the Numeric Rating Scale (NRS), and the Iowa Pain Thermometer (IPT)—was tested on 66 elderly people. Interestingly, FPS demonstrated a weak correlation with other scales when used with the cognitively impaired group. Test-retest reliability at a 2-week interval was found acceptable in the cognitively intact group but unacceptable for most scales in the cognitively impaired group. Both the cognitively impaired and the intact groups preferred the IPT and the VDS.[62] Similar study by Herr at al. demonstrated that VDS is the scale of choice for assessing pain intensity among older adults, including those with mild to moderate cognitive impairment.[63] Other pain intensity rating scales were also found to be psychometrically sound. Further insight into literature reaffirms the fact that cognitive impairment does not inhibit participants' ability to use a variety of pain intensity scales, but the stability issue must be considered.

In 2002, the American Geriatric Society presented its clinical guidelines for management of chronic pain in elderly.[4] These recommendations are likely to help the practitioner to improve management of pain in this population. These recommendations are summarized as follows:

1. On initial presentation or admission of any older person to any health-care service, a health-care professional should assess the patient for evidence of persistent pain.

2. Any persistent pain that has an impact on physical functions, psychosocial function, or other aspects of quality of life should be recognized as a significant problem.

3. The identified patients should undergo a comprehensive pain assessment, with the goal of detecting all potentially remediable factors. Assessment should focus on the sequence of events that led to the present pain complaint, and on establishing the diagnosis, a plan of care and likely prognosis.

4. The history at the time of initial evaluation should include details of pain problem and a description of pain in relation to impairments in physical and social functions. A thorough analgesic history, patients' attitudes and beliefs regarding pain and its management, as well as knowledge of pain management strategies should be assessed. Effectiveness of past pain-relieving treatments and side effects from various medications should be assessed. Patients' satisfaction with current pain treatment should be determined.

5. Careful physical examination of the site of reported pain, common sites for pain referral, and sites of pain in older adults should be done. Physical examination should focus on musculoskeletal system, neurological system, and physical functions.

6. Initial assessment should also include evaluation of psychological functions, social support, caregivers, family relationships, work history, cultural environment, their spirituality, and health care accessibility. Cognitive function should be evaluated for new or worsening confusion.

7. Comprehensive laboratory and other diagnostic testing should be performed to identify possible etiology.

8. For cognitively intact or mild to moderately demented patients, direct screening should be done by using a variety of terms synonymous with pain. The quantitative assessment of pain should be recorded by using a standard pain scale that is sensitive to cognitive, language, and sensory impairment. If needed, multinational pain instruments can be used. Repeated instructions might be needed due to the limited attention span or impaired cognition in these patients. Help from family members and caregivers should be utilized, when needed. Indirect indicators of ongoing persistent pain like changes in activities and functional status or various verbal and nonverbal pain-related behaviors should be noted. For older adults with moderate to severe dementia or those who are nonverbal, assessment of pain should be done via direct observation or history from caregivers.

9. The risks and benefits of various assessment and treatment options should be discussed with patients and family, with consideration for patient and family preferences in the design of any assessment or treatment strategy. Patients with persistent pain should be reassessed regularly for improvement, deterioration, or complications. The use of pain log or diary and pillboxes is encouraged to keep a track of treatment effectiveness and adequacy. A reassessment should include evaluation of analgesic and nonpharmacologic interventions, side effects, and compliance issues. It should also consider patients' preference in assessment and treatment of revisions.[4]

TREATMENT OF PERSISTENT PAIN IN ELDERLY

The medications often used to treat chronic pain can be broadly classified as typical analgesics like acetaminophen, nonsteroidal anti-inflammatory drugs (NSAIDs), and opioids; and atypical analgesics or adjuvants that encompass antidepressants (tricyclics, selective-serotonin reuptake inhibitors or SSRIs, selective norepinephrine-reuptake inhibitors or SNRIs), anticonvulsants, skeletal muscle relaxants, and others. The use of these medications require proper understanding of their mechanisms of action and their biochemical and physiologic effects (pharmacodynamics) as well as their metabolism and clearance from the body (pharmacokinetics). Effective pain management in geriatric patients requires an understanding of the physiology of aging and its effects on clinically relevant aspects of analgesic interventions.

Physiological changes in geriatrics

All systems undergo some degree of physical and physiological changes with aging. The overall effect is gradual but is characterized by uneven disintegration of the structure and functions of numerous organ systems and impairment of many regulatory processes. These age-related changes in the heart, kidneys, liver, and other organs will influence the effects of medications. These age-related changes on various organ systems are highly variable among individuals and are strongly influenced by genetic background, diet, activity level, and social habits. In general, cardiac output decreases in most elderly persons, lungs undergo emphysema-like changes, and the effectiveness of the immune system is decreased. A detailed discussion of these changes is beyond the scope of this chapter and is described well in other parts of this textbook. From the algological standpoint, changes in nervous system (as discussed earlier), hepatic and renal systems are of importance. These changes require a decrease in the dose of some medications to optimize their benefits and avoid toxicity and adverse reactions. Physiologic changes that normally occur with aging may affect the way drugs work within the body.

Pharmacodynamics

Optimum drug therapy in any age group requires a clear understanding of the physiological effects of drugs (pharmacodynamics) as well as the drug-handling capacity of the body (pharmacokinetics). The elderly population is often considered to be frail and sensitive to pain medications. Many of these effects are, in fact, a reflection of pharmacokinetic changes related to aging and not an exacerbated response at drug-receptor-response level. For example, elderly persons are physically smaller than younger adults due to loss of their muscle mass. In addition, there is an increase in the percentage of body fat with a corresponding reduction in total body water in geriatric population. This leads to lower volume of distribution and higher blood or serum concentration of drugs that are distributed in body fluids, and prolonged action of those that are distributed in fat. Thus, drugs given at adult dosing might cause untoward side effects, resulting in a false impression of higher sensitivity of this subgroup.

Pharmacokinetics

The pharmacokinetic changes that occur with aging have variable clinical significance and are difficult to predict (Tables 26-3 and 26-4).[26]

Absorption

Absorption of drugs via gastrointestinal (GI) tract, in general, is a passive process. Factors affecting this passive movement of drugs along their concentration gradient include available surface area and time of contact. Although there is a reduction in the absorptive surface area with advancing age, the motility of the GI tract is also reduced. Moreover, there is a decrease in splanchnic blood flow and an increase in gastric pH with aging. However, these changes have no significant clinical effect on drug absorption capacity, which changes little with advancing age.

The higher prevalence of few GI comorbid conditions in elderly like malabsorptive states and concomitant administration of other pharmacological agents might influence drug absorption. The prime examples of such agents are the use of antacids that causes a reduction in absorption of gabapentin and the use of laxatives that result in the reduction of the rate and extent of absorption of multiple medications.[26]

Distribution

Drug distribution is altered with increasing age. Total body water and lean body mass is decreased with proportionate increase in body fat. Thus, fat-soluble drugs are distributed more widely with prolonged elimination half-life than water-soluble drugs. The higher distribution of lipid-soluble drugs like morphine, hydromorphone, or diazepam is responsible for their longer elimination time (or prolonged half-life) in elderly. Similarly, water-soluble drugs like meperidine, gabapentin, or digoxin attain higher plasma levels in elderly due to their reduction in volume of distribution.

Serum protein binding of drugs is altered in elderly causing meaningful pharmacokinetic changes. For drugs that bound to serum proteins, an equilibrium state exists between bound (pharmacologically inactive) and free (but pharmacologically active) drug. There is a decrease in serum albumin concentration with advancing age, especially during the time of illnesses. This altered protein binding causes higher plasma free fractions of certain highly protein-bound acidic drugs like conventional NSAIDs and cyclooxygenase-2-specific inhibitors. This increases potential side effects of these medications in old age. In contrast to albumin, alpha-1 acid glycoprotein concentrations increase with advancing age. Alpha-1 acid glycoprotein is an acute phase-reactant protein that binds to certain basic drugs like lidocaine. Although this leads to some increase in plasma concentration of these drugs, their actual clinical relevance remains speculative.[26]

Metabolism

Hepatic metabolism is clinically an important rate limiting step for the elimination of most metabolized drugs. Hepatic metabolism of medications has two phases: Phase I metabolism involves oxidation and reduction by cytochrome P-450 (CYP) system, while phase II metabolism includes conjugation of drugs by glucuronidation, sulfation, acetylation, and glycine conjugation. A reduction in first-pass metabolism and rate of biotransformation of certain drugs is often seen in the elderly due to reduction in hepatic mass, hepatic blood flow, and phase I metabolism. This prolongation in hepatic metabolism causes longer duration of action of numerous pain medications like acetaminophen, salicylates, and tricyclic antidepressants (amitriptyline, nortriptyline).[26]

Elimination

Although elimination of drugs and their metabolites is lower in the elderly due to reduction in the renal plasma flow, glomerular filtration rate, and tubular secretion function; there is marked interindividual variation. Pharmacodynamic unpredictability is seen due to alteration in receptor number or their affinity and changes in second-messenger function as well as in cellular and nuclear responses.[26,64]

Commonly used medications to treat chronic pain

As mentioned, pharmacological management in geriatric population is challenging. Elderly are more susceptible to drug-related side

Table 26-3

Pharmacokinetics of Commonly Used Nonnarcotic Medications

Medication	Absorption	Distribution	Metabolism	Elimination	Concerns in Elderly
Acetaminophen 0.5–2 g	Well-absorbed via GIT T_{max} = 20–90 min	Poor PPB at therapeutic doses	Hepatic—glucuronide and sulphate derivatives. One toxic alkylating metabolite is also formed in minute amounts and is deactivated by conjugation with reduced glutathione.	Renal—85–95% excreted within 24 h $T\frac{1}{2}$ = 1.9–2.5 h	Hepatotoxicity at higher doses Avoid excessive use Encourage use of pillbox to maintain count
Aspirin*	Diffusion via GIT (unionized) High presystemic hydrolysis to salicylate T_{max} = 25 min (S) T_{max} = 4–6 h (T)	High PPB Alb = 80–90% (salicylate)	Hydrolysis to salicylate (active) by nonspecific esterases in body tissues, gut, plasma, hepatic CYP450	Excreted as salicylic acid or as glucuronidate/glycine conjugates $T\frac{1}{2}$ = 0.25 h (aspirin) $T\frac{1}{2}$ (salicylate) = 15–30 h (high dose)	▶ Higher P_c (plasma concentration) of free drug due to age-related reduction in serum albumin. Access renal functions before and during therapy
Diclofcnac† 50 mg	40% GIT‡ T_{max} = 10–40 min (S) T_{max} = 1.5–2 h (T)	High PPB Alb = 99%	Hepatic—CYP450: 2C9, 3A4 substrate	Renal—65%, bile—35% 90% excreted within 3–4 h $T\frac{1}{2}$ = 1–1.5 h	▶ GI toxicity ↑ with age. Elderly also have poor tolerance to GI ulceration or bleeding ▶ Should take with food or antacids
Ibuprofen¶ 400 mg	>80% GIT T_{max} = 1.39 h (S) T_{max} ~3 h (T)	High PPB Alb = 99%	Hepatic—CYP450: 2C9 substrate Two enantiomers: S–(+)–ibuprofen clinically active R–(+)–ibuprofen → unidirectional inversion to S-form (slower absorption → higher inversion)	Urine—mostly as hydroxyl and carboxyl conjugates. <1% is excreted unchanged 70–90% excreted within 24 h $T\frac{1}{2}$ = 2–2.5 h	▶ Caution in patients with hepatic dysfunction ▶ May cause fluid retention and peripheral edema ▶ Avoid smoking or alcohol intake ▶ Consider starting at lower doses
Indomethacin§ 25–50 mg	Well-absorbed via GIT T_{max} = 2–4 h	High PPB Alb = 90%	Hepatic—CYP450: 2C9 substrate	Renal—60%, bile/feces—33% $T\frac{1}{2}$ = 4.5 h	
Celecoxib 100–200 mg	Well-absorbed via GIT T_{max} = 2–4 h	High PPB Alb = 97%	Hepatic—CYP450: 2C9 substrate to hydroxyl, carboxyl, and glucuronidase derivatives Major metabolite = SC-62807, inactive Minor metabolite = SC-60613, inactive	<2% unchanged in urine $T\frac{1}{2}$ = 11.2–15.6 h	40% higher peak P_c in elderly Start at lower doses for patients <50 kg
Gabapentin	Oral BioAv = 60% Higher doses have lower BioAv T_{max} = 2–3 h	PPB <3%	None No hepatic enzyme induction	Renal $T\frac{1}{2}$ = 6–7 h	Higher plasma conc. in elderly with age-related ↓ in renal functions Start at lower doses
Pregabalin	Oral BioAv ≥90% T_{max} = 3 h (with food) T_{max} = 1.5 h (fasting)	PPB ~ 0	None No hepatic enzyme induction	Renal 90% unchanged 0.9% N-methyl derivative $T\frac{1}{2}$ = 6.3 h	Clearance ↓ with increasing age Related to age-related ↓ in CL_{Cr} Reduce dose in patients with compromised renal function

Table 26-3

Pharmacokinetics of Commonly Used Nonnarcotic Medications *(Continued)*

Medication	Absorption	Distribution	Metabolism	Elimination	Concerns in Elderly
Nortriptyline	Variable GI absorption BioAv = 32–79% T_{max} = 7–8.5 h	PPB = 93–95%	Hepatic—P450: 2D6 (~ 7–10 and Caucasians "poor metabolizers") Caution with concomitant use of CYP: 2D6 inhibitors: quinidine; cimetidine; other antidepressants, phenothiazines, type 1C antiarrhythmics propafenone, and flecainide; and the selective serotonin reuptake inhibitors (SSRIs)	Renal—mainly Fecal—small amount $T\frac{1}{2}$ = 18–93 h	Higher P_c of the 10-OH-NT Cardiovascular dysrhythmias Fluctuations in blood pressure Higher incidence of confusional states Lowered seizure threshold Higher incidence of photosensitivity Start smallest effective daily dose Avoid alcohol and other CNS depressants

Abbreviations: GIT = gastrointestinal tract; T_{max} = peak plasma concentration time; BioAv = bioavailability; PPB = plasma protein bound, $T\frac{1}{2}$ = plasma half-life; S = soluble/solution; T = tablet; Alb = albumin; CL_{Cr} = creatinine clearance.
*Irreversible inhibitor, †Time-dependent inhibitor, ‡Drug that escapes presytemic elimination, ¶Competitive-reversible inhibitor, §Mixed-kinetic inhibitor.

effects due to various reasons.[65,66] Differences in pharmacodynamics or pharmacokinetics, existence of polypharmacy, and presence of frequent noncompliance in this age group make pharmacotherapy even more challenging. A common theme of "start low and go slow" has been accepted and widely recommended. Commonly used therapeutic agents are discussed in the next section.

Typical agents

The commonly used pharmacological management options in the elderly include acetaminophen, NSAIDs, and opioids.

Acetaminophen Acetaminophen lacks peripheral anti-inflammatory properties but is often considered similar to NSAIDs by most. Together they are often the first-line management for nociceptive pain in all age groups. Acetaminophen is para-aminophenol derivative with analgesic and antipyretic properties. Its mechanism of action probably involves inhibition of central prostaglandin synthesis (COX-3 inhibition), thus inhibiting pyrogen-induced modulation of hypothalamic regulatory center and peripheral vasodilatation. Its pharmacokinetic properties are discussed in Table 26-3. Acetaminophen is an effective analgesic agent for the treatment of mild-moderate noninflammatory pain with its potency almost equivalent to aspirin. It lacks gastric irritability, platelet function inhibition, or uricosuric activity. Possible side effects associated with acetaminophen use include hepatic dysfunction, interstitial nephritis or renal papillary necrosis, or pancytopenia. Daily doses should be limited to 4 g to avoid any potential hepatic damage, and dose adjustments should be made in patients with history of chronic alcoholism and underlying hepatic or renal dysfunction. Two clinically important drug interactions noticed with the use of this drug include enhanced action of warfarin and sulphonylureas.

Nonsteroidal Anti-Inflammatory Drugs This is a broad category of medications that work by inhibiting the enzyme cyclooxygenase (COX). Two distinctive isoforms of this enzyme exist: Type 1

cyclooxygenase (COX-1) is present in most cells including platelets, renal tubules, and endothelium, while type 2 cyclooxygenase (COX-2) is selectively found in kidneys, CNS, and other cells following injuries and is known to be involved in production of hyperalgesia. The existence of third isoform, type 3 cyclooxygenase (COX-3), is currently debated. Clearly, most analgesic activity of this class of drugs is by inhibition of COX-2 enzyme, while inhibition of COX-1 enzyme produces unwanted side effects like damage to gastric mucosa, platelet dysfunction, and renal toxicity. This class of drugs is crudely divided into salicylates, nonselective nonsteroidal anti-inflammatory agents, and selective nonsteroidal anti-inflammatory agents. Prime example of salicylates is aspirin. Nonselective NSAIDs have variable inhibition of both COX-1 and COX-2 enzymes and include more than a dozen drugs including, but not limited to, ibuprofen, naproxen, indomethacin, ketorolac, and piroxicam. Selective NSAIDs, on the other hand, mainly block COX-2 enzyme. Currently, the only U.S. Food and Drug Administration (FDA)-approved selective NSAID medication being used is celecoxib. The other two drugs, rofecoxib and valdecoxib, have recently been removed from the market following their association with myocardial infarction. A comparative difference in pharmacokinetic properties of these medications is depicted in Table 26-3.

Efficacy of NSAIDs has been extensively studied in arthritic conditions and is discussed in Table 26-5. Although extensive head-to-head comparisons between various NSAIDs are lacking, present evidence suggests that all nonselective NSAID drugs have probably equivalent potency. The major concerning side effects of aspirin and the nonselective NSAIDs include inhibition of platelet aggregation; GI complications like dyspepsia, ulceration, bleeding, or perforation; renal insufficiency; liver damage; hypersensitivity; and CNS dysfunction like decreased attention span, loss of short-term memory, and difficulty with calculations. In order to minimize GI complications, NSAIDs should be used at smallest effective dose and for the shortest time required. Moreover, these drugs should be taken with food, and concurrent alcohol intake is strongly discouraged. The

Table 26-4

Pharmacokinetics of Commonly Used Opioid Medications

Medication	Absorption	Distribution	Metabolism	Elimination	Concerns in Elderly
Morphine	40% GI tract* T_{max} = 30 min	25–30% reversibly PPB	Liver: <5% demethylation >95% glucuronidation to M3G 50% (inactive) and M6G 15% (active but does not cross BBB)	Renal—mainly as M3G/M6G and 10% unchanged Feces—7–10% $T\frac{1}{2}$ = varies	▶ Elderly are more prone to side effects, e.g., sedation, constipation
Hydromorphone	24% GI tract* T_{max} = 30–60 min	8–19% PPB	Liver: glucuronidation >95% to H3G <5% to 6-hydroxy reduced metabolites	Renal—mostly as inactive metabolites $T\frac{1}{2}$ = 2.6 h	▶ Polypharmacy might make them more like to get unexpected responses to medications ▶ Tolerance ▶ Dependence
Oxycodone	60–87% GI tract* T_{max} = 1.6–3.2 h†	45% PPB	Liver: noroxycodone (weak analgesic) Oxymorphone (analgesic) via CYP450 2D6	Renal: 50% conjugated oxycodone 19% free oxycodone 14% conjugated oxymorphone $T\frac{1}{2}$ = 3.2–4.5 h†	▶ Abuse potential ▶ Oxycodone SR when crushed is rapidly absorbed and acts like immediate release dose
Fentanyl transmucosal	25% buccal mucosa (rapid) 25% GI tract* T_{max} = 20–40 min	Highly lipophilic PPB = 80–85% α-1 AG>Alb>Lipo	Liver and intestinal mucosa by CYP450 3A4 isoform to norfentanyl (inactive)	Renal (>90% inactive metabolites, 7% unchanged) Feces (1% unchanged) $T\frac{1}{2}$ = 40–50 min	▶ Methadone accumulates with repeated dosing, requiring a reduction in dose size or frequency on day 2–5
Fentanyl transdermal	92% skin 13–21% unbound fraction in plasma are finally achieved T_{max} = 12–24 h	Highly lipophilic PPB = 80–85% α-1 AG>Alb>Lipo	Liver CYP450 3A4 isoform to norfentanyl (inactive) by oxidative N-dealkylation	Renal (75% inactive metabolites, <10% unchanged) Feces (9% metabolites) $T\frac{1}{2}$ = 17 h (13–22)	▶ Prolonged elimination half-life of methadone warrants less frequent changes separated by at least 3–4 weeks ▶ Increased risk of seizure with tramadol at doses more than 400 mg/day
Methadone	Excellent GI absorption T_{max} = 2–3 h	PPB = major site: α-1 AG	Liver CYP 3A4	Renal and feces pH dependent urinary excretion $T\frac{1}{2}$ = 8–59 h	▶ Tramadol with TCAs—increases risk of CNS depression, seizures, psychomotor impairment, and serotonin syndrome
Tramadol	Racemic form = parent drug + M1 metabolite 75% GI tract* T_{max} = 2–3 h	PPB = only 20%	Liver via CYP 2D6 isoform (primary), 2C9 and 2D6 Chronic dosing may induce own metabolism	Mostly renal $T\frac{1}{2}$ (parent drug) = 6.3 ± 1.4 h $T\frac{1}{2}$ (M1 metabolite) = 7.4 ± 1.4 h	

Abbreviations: T_{max} = peak plasma concentration time; PPB = plasma protein bound; $T\frac{1}{2}$ = plasma half-life; M3G = morphine-3-glucuronide; M6G = morphine-6-glucuronide; BBB = blood brain barrier; H3G = hydromorphone-3-glucuronide; α-1 AG = α-1 acid glycoprotein; Alb = albumin; Lipo = lipoprotein; FF = free fraction.
*Drug that escapes hepatic and first-pass elimination.
†Depending on type of preparation like immediate-release or sustained or controlled-release.

addition of proton pump inhibitors (PPIs) or prostaglandin analog misoprostol provides some protection against GI complications. There is also evidence that selective COX-2 inhibitors have lower incidence of GI complications, and should be considered in presence of predisposing risk factors. In contrast to GI effects, both nonselective and selective NSAIDs can induce renal insufficiency by decreased renal prostaglandin synthesis, impaired renin secretion, enhanced water and sodium absorption, and interstitial nephritis.

In short, efficacy of nonselective NSAIDs and COX-2 inhibitors in the treatment of arthritic pain is almost compatible. Nonselective

NSAIDs have slightly higher predisposition toward GI complications, although both classes of medications have equivalent renal toxicities. Elderly patients are is somewhat more likely to develop these side effects due to certain physiological differences. In this subgroup, acetaminophen or aspirin should be initially tried for safety issues. Whenever possible, use of NSAIDs should be limited to smaller doses and for shorter periods.

Opioid Analgesics Opiates are the drugs derived from opium, while the term opioid is broader and includes all naturally and synthetically

Table 26-5

Evidence-Based Management of Osteoarthritis

Therapy in OA	Systematic Review Results	Reference(s)
Acetaminophen	Acetaminophen and OA: 10 RCTs including 1712 patients Effective and safe agent for pain relief due to OA. Although safer, it is less effective than NSAIDs. For safety reasons it should be the first-line treatment for OA	Zhang et al.[68]
Nonselective NSAIDs	NSAIDs in OA of the hip: 43 RCTs, 17 included for MA No clear recommendations for the choice of specific NSAID therapy in hip OA	Towheed et al.[69]
	NSAIDs in OA of the knee: 23 trials (10,845 patients) NSAIDs can reduce short-term pain in OA of the knee slightly better than placebo Long-term use of NSAIDs for OA is not recommended due to concerns of serious adverse effects	Bjordal et al.[70]
	NSAIDs (including COX-2 inhibitors) versus acetaminophen: 7 studies NSAIDs are statistically superior in reducing pain compared with acetaminophen for symptomatic OA Safety is not statistically different between NSAIDs and acetaminophen-treated groups	Lee et al.[71]
	Best NSAID/worst NSAID: 43 RCTs included No recommendations for the choice of specific NSAID therapy due to poor data	Towheed and Hochberg[72]
	Comparison of NSAIDs: 18 studies Tenoxicam is better tolerated than piroxicam, diclofenac, and indomethacin No other difference noted	Riedemann et al.[73]
Selective NSAIDS	GI safety with celecoxib: UGI tolerability of therapeutic dosages of celecoxib was significantly better than diclofenac	McKenna et al.[74]
	GI safety with rofecoxib: 20 RCTs (removed from market) Lower incidence of PUBs with rofecoxib treatment, in patients with or without risk factors	Watson et al.[75]
	GI safety with valdecoxib: 8 studies (removed from market) At less than 8-mg doses, valdecoxib has lower rate of upper gastrointestinal ulcer complications than therapeutic doses of nonselective NSAIDs	Goldstein et al.[76]
	Cost-effectiveness of COX-2 inhibitors: naproxen 500 mg twice daily versus once daily coxib COX-2 Inhibitors provide an acceptable incremental cost-effectiveness ratio only in the subgroup of patients with a history of bleeding ulcers	Spiegel et al.[77]
Antidepressants	Antidepressants could be effective for pain associated with osteoarthritis	Fishbain[78]
Topical agents	Topical NSAIDS: 25 studies, almost 1500 patients Effective and safe in treating chronic musculoskeletal conditions for 2 weeks	Mason et al.[79]
	Topical NSAIDS: 13 trials, representing 1983 patients No evidence of efficacy compared to placebo after 2 weeks, long-term use not supported	Lin et al.[80]
Dietary supplements	Glucosamine therapy: 20 studies with 2570 patients No long-term benefit for pain (when taking for 2–3 months) Questionable improvement in functional status	Towheed et al.[81]
	S-adenosylmethionine: 11 Studies As effective as NSAIDs in reducing pain and improving functional limitation in OA without the adverse effects often associated with NSAID therapies	Soeken et al.[82]
	Glucosamine and chondroitin in knee OA: 15 RCTs included Structural and symptomatic improvement, further studies suggested	Richy et al.[83]
	Herbal therapy in OA: 5 studies (four different herbal interventions) Avocado/soybean unsaponifiables showed beneficial effects on functional index, pain, intake of NSAIDs and global evaluation	Little et al.[84]
	Fish oil in arthritis: promising anti-inflammatory effects in RA, efficacy in OA unclear Meta-Analysis—395 individual patients Dietary fish oil supplementation for 3 months significantly reduced tender joint count and morning stiffness The relative improvements in the other outcome variables did not reach statistical significance	Fortin et al.[85]

Table 26-5

Evidence-Based Management of Osteoarthritis *(Continued)*

Therapy in OA	Systematic Review Results	Reference(s)
Physical modalities	Low level laser therapy in OA: 5 trials included, 112 patients randomized to laser, 85 to placebo laser No clear benefit, limited by poor data	Brosseau et al.[86]
	Ultrasound for OA of the knee: 3 trials including 294 participants Ultrasound therapy has no benefit over placebo or short-wave diathermy for hip or knee OA	Welch et al.[87]
	TENS in OA: 7 trials eligible; 6 used TENS, 1 used acupuncture like TENS (AL-TENS), 148 patients TENS groups versus 146 placebo TENS and AL-TENS are shown to be effective in pain control over placebo	Osiri et al.[88]
Patient education	PET versus NSAIDS: 19 PET with 32 treatment arms and 28 NSAID trials with 46 treatment arms Patient education interventions provide additional benefits that are 20–30% as great as the effects of NSAID treatment for pain relief in OA	Superio-Cabuslay et al.[89]
Behavioral therapy	Cognitive behavior therapy in chronic pain: 25 trials Significantly greater changes for the domains of pain experience, cognitive coping and appraisal (positive coping measures), and reduced behavioral expression of pain No significant differences in mood/affect, cognitive coping and appraisal (negative, e.g., catastrophization), and social role functioning.	Morley et al.[90]
Interventional therapies	Corticosteroid/hyaluronic acid injections for OA of the knee: 26 trials, 1721 participants Short-term benefit in treatment of knee OA is well-established, and few side effects have been reported Longer-term benefits could not be confirmed	Bellamy et al.[91]
	Viscosupplementation for OA of the knee: 37 trials hyaluronic/hylan vs. placebo, 9 trials with corticosteroids, and 5 trials with NSAIDs Effective treatment with beneficial effects on pain, function, and patient global assessment; especially at the 5–13-week postinjection period. Unclear data but no major safety issues. The response to hyaluronic acid products appears more durable than corticosteroids	Bellamy et al.[92]
	Corticosteroid injections for OA of the knee: 10 trials Short-term (up to 2 weeks) improvement in symptoms Significantly longer (16–24 weeks) improvement was also shown in two methodologically sound studies A dose equivalent to 50 mg of prednisone may be needed to show benefit at 16–24 weeks	Arroll and Goodyear-Smith[93]
	Corticosteroid injections for OA of the knee: 5 trials, 312 patients Improvement in pain up to 3–4 weeks	Godwin and Dawes[94]
	Hyaluronic acid injections for OA of the knee: 20 RCTs IA injection of hyaluronic acid has therapeutic efficacy and safety for the treatment of OA of the knee	Wang et al.[95]
	Hyaluronic acid injections for OA of the knee: 22 RCTs Small effect when compared with an intra-articular placebo Significant publication bias suggested in current literature on the subject Highest-MW hyaluronic acid may be more efficacious in treating knee OA than lower MW analogues	Lo et al.[96]

Abbreviations: RCT = randomized controlled trial; MA = meta-analysis; OA = osteoarthritis; SAMe = S-adenosylmethionine; PET = patient education trials; PUBs = upper GI perforations, symptomatic gastroduodenal ulcers, and upper GI bleeding; IA = intra-articular.

produced peptides that bind to opioid receptors. These receptors predominantly include mu, delta, and kappa receptors. These receptors are distributed at various supraspinal, spinal, and peripheral sites. Commonly used oral opioid analgesics include morphine-like agonists or mu-receptor agonist (codeine, morphine, oxycodone, meperidine, hydrocodone, and fentanyl), weak mu-receptor agonist-monamine reuptake inhibitor (tramadol), and mixed agonist-antagonist (kappa agonists like pentazocine, nalbuphine, butorphanol). Opioids are considered to be the most potent analgesic medications with possible abuse potential. They are extensively being used in the treatment of acute postoperative pain control as well as for the management of chronic pain of malignancies. Their long-term use in the treatment of chronic nonmalignant pain has been challenged, but recent clinical trials demonstrate their effectiveness in musculoskeletal and neuropathic pain states.[97–99] Pharmacokinetics of these medications and concerns associated with their usage in elderly population are discussed in Table 26-4.

Common adverse reactions are

▶ CNS—euphoria, dysphoria, syncope, blurred vision, dependence, addiction

▶ GI—nausea, vomiting, constipation, biliary tract spasm, anorexia, delayed gastric emptying

▶ Cardiovascular—hypo- or hypertension, bradycardia, chest wall rigidity, dysrhythmias

▶ Pulmonary—bronchospasm, laryngospasm, respiratory arrest

▶ Genitourinary—urinary retention, ureteral spasm

▶ Allergic—pruritus, urticaria

Atypical agents, adjuvants, or coanalgesics

Antidepressants Although classically used to treat depression, many antidepressant medications have shown efficacy in the treatment of neuropathic pain syndromes. Two distinct classes are often discussed in relation to pain management:

Tricyclic antidepressants (TCAs) TCAs (e.g., amitriptyline, nortriptyline, desipramine, or imipramine) have a characteristic three-ring nucleus and resemble phenothiazines chemically. They are mixed norepinephrine and serotonin uptake inhibitors along with several other properties, including autonomic actions and downregulation of beta-receptor sensitivity. Most tricyclics are incompletely absorbed and undergo significant first-pass metabolism. Their volume of distribution is large due to their high protein binding and relatively high lipid solubility. They are metabolized by transformation of the tricyclic nucleus and alteration of the aliphatic side chain. An important fact to understand is that monodemethylation of tertiary amines leads to active metabolite formation. For example, monodemethylation of amitriptyline forms nortriptyline. Since nortriptyline has a safer side-effect profile than amitriptyline, it might be beneficial to consider nortriptyline as the "tricyclic of choice" for pain management. Pharmacokinetic properties of nortriptyline are discussed in Table 26-3, including concerns in the elderly population.

Although effective antidepressant actions of tricyclics take days to weeks, receptor blockade and hence pain response is relatively quick. Indeed, the analgesic effects may occur partly through their antidepressant effects but they also work by mechanisms that are independent of mood effects. These mechanisms include increased activity of serotonin and norepinephrine in descending nociceptive inhibitory pathways or spinal N-methyl-D-aspartate (NMDA) receptor antagonism. They also bind to opioid receptors and enhance potency of coadministered opioid medications. It is strongly felt that TCAs are useful in treating burning, aching, or dysesthetic component of neuropathic pain than lancinating or shooting variety.

Common side effects are

▶ Antimuscarinic (blurred vision, constipation, urinary hesitancy, confusion)

▶ Cardiovascular (orthostatic hypotension, conduction defects, arrhythmias)

▶ Metabolic-endocrine (weight gain, sexual disturbances)

▶ Neurologic (sedation, seizures)

▶ Psychiatric (aggravation of psychosis, withdrawal syndrome)

▶ Sympathomimetic (tremor, insomnia)

TCAs do not have addiction potential, but sudden discontinuation of drug might precipitate withdrawal symptoms. Also, with prolonged use, tolerance to anticholinergic and sedative effects is seen without any decrease in their analgesic properties. Desipramine has the best pharmacokinetic and side-effect profile of all TCAs. Due to arrhythmia potentials, a baseline electrocardiography (ECG) is recommended in elderly with history of conduction abnormalities.

TCA overdose is potentially dangerous. Caution is advised in patients with underlying depression. When clinical depression is suspected, prescriptions should be limited to amounts less than 1.25 g, or 50 dose units of 25 mg, on a no refill basis, and timely psychiatric involvement is encouraged. The drugs must be kept away from children.[100]

Serotonin norepinephrine reuptake inhibitor (SNRI) This class of antidepressants (e.g., venlafaxine, milnacipran, and duloxetine) blocks the reuptake of both serotonin (5-HT) and norepinephrine with differing selectivity. Whereas milnacipran blocks 5-HT and norepinephrine reuptake with equal affinity, duloxetine has a tenfold selectivity for 5-HT and venlafaxine a 30-fold selectivity for 5-HT. Clinically, venlafaxine seems to be the least well-tolerated (serotonergic adverse effects and hypertension) than duloxetine and milnacipran.[101] Venlafaxine is the most investigated of these new drugs and has shown to be effective in the treatment of different kinds of pain, with side-effect profile significantly better than TCAs. Other drugs in this category have been less extensively studied but have shown promising results in preliminary studies.[102-104]

Others Two other classes of antidepressants have been projected to be helpful for pain management. These include noradrenergic and specific serotoninergic antidepressants or NSSA (e.g., mirtazapine) and noradrenaline reuptake inhibitors or NRI (e.g., reboxetine).[100] At present, inadequate literature exists to recommend these medications for frequent usage. If routine medications have failed, a trial of these newer agents may be considered.

Membrane Stabilizers

Antiepileptic drugs (AEDs) AEDs reduce neuronal hyperexcitability in damaged areas of the CNS or peripheral nervous system (PNS) and include gabapentin, carbamazepine, oxcarbazepine, lamotrigine, topiramate, and tiagabine. They are used either alone or with opioids and other analgesics in the management of neuropathic pain. In contrast to TCAs, most AEDs are considered to be more efficacious for lancinating or shooting variety of neuropathic pain. Although their exact mechanisms of action in the management of neuropathic pain is uncertain, they seem to cause ion channel (i.e., calcium, sodium) modulation, γ-aminobutyric acid (GABA) inhibition, neuronal cell membrane stabilization, and/or NMDA receptors activation. They can be categorized further based on these properties into sodium or calcium channel blockers.

Sodium channel blockers. AEDs with sodium channel blocking properties that have been used in pain management include carbamazepine, oxcarbazepine, and lamotrigine. Carbamazepine is an iminostilbene derivative structurally related to TCAs used in the treatment of trigeminal neuralgia, thalamic poststroke pain, diabetic neuropathy, and PHN. It is usually started in doses of 100 mg twice a day and increased on a weekly basis by additional 200 mg up to a maximum of 1600 mg/day. Therapeutic range of analgesic effects is around 3–14 mcg/mL. Carbamazepine is primarily metabolized by liver. Its onset of action is around 3–4 days with half-life of 25–65 hours. Its common side effects include sedation, dizziness, gait abnormalities, exfoliative dermatitis or Stevens-Johnson syndrome, and hematologic changes. Blood counts should be initially at the beginning of therapy, bimonthly for the next 6 months and then six monthly thereafter. Oxcarbazepine is a keto-analogue of carbamazepine with safer side-effect profile and does not require serial blood testing. Due to these significant benefits, it is increasingly being used to treat trigeminal neuralgia. It is usually prescribed at the initial doses of 300 mg twice a day and increased by additional 600 mg weekly up to 2400 mg total. Therapeutic serum concentration is in the range of 15–30 mcg/mL. Its pharmacologic properties resemble carbamazepine. The only concerning side effect beyond somnolence or dizziness is hyponatremia which is likely to occur in the first 3 months of therapy. Lamotrigine acts as sodium channel blocker and also prevents release of glutamate. Started at 25–50 mg at bedtime, it is then escalated slowly to 300–500 mg/day, as tolerated. This drug is being used to treat trigeminal neuralgia, cold-induced pain as in the setting of peripheral vascular disease or trauma, diabetic neuropathy, and human immunodeficiency virus (HIV) polyneuropathy. It is metabolized in the liver and more than 90% is excreted in urine. Common side effects seen with lamotrigine use include somnolence, dizziness, and a rash.

Calcium channel blockers. Gabapentin, a structural analog of the neurotransmitter GABA, is the best-studied AED for neuropathic pain management. There is some suggestion that it possibly works by binding to L-type Ca channel alpha 2/delta-subunit. Its pharmacokinetic properties are discussed in Table 26-3. Gabapentin is efficacious for lancinating or shooting as well as burning, aching, and dysesthetic variety of neuropathic pain. Mellegers et al. recently published a meta-analysis of 35 studies involving 727 patients and concluded that gabapentin seems to be effective in multiple painful neuropathic conditions.[103] The authors also pointed out that effectiveness of AEDs may be reduced if adequate doses are not tried. Similarly, rapid dose escalation of these medications may be associated with increased CNS side effects. Thus, slow upward titrations are recommended until analgesia is achieved or side effects are observed. It is usually started in doses of 300 mg at bedtime and increased by additional 300 mg weekly up to a maximum of 2400 mg/day in three divided doses. Other uses of gabapentin include treatment of painful muscle spasms in patients with spinal cord injury and multiple sclerosis. An analogue of gabapentin, pregabalin, has been recently introduced that can be titrated more rapidly than gabapentin, and its beneficial effects on neuropathic pain can be observed within a day to a week of initiation of treatment.[104,105] The suggested dose is 75 mg twice a day or 50 mg three times a day. The dose can be increased to 300 mg/day in divided doses within a week based on efficacy and tolerability.

Common adverse reactions are

- CNS—somnolence, dizziness, ataxia, fatigue, depression, nystagmus, hyperkinesias, dyskinesia, dysarthria, paresthesia
- Pulmonary—rhinitis, pharyngitis, coughing, bronchospasm
- Cardiovascular—hypotension, angina pectoris, arrhythmia, palpitation
- GI—dry mouth, dyspepsia, constipation, increased appetite, gingivitis
- Genitourinary—impotence
- Skin—abrasion, pruritus

Local anesthetics Although both lidocaine and mexiletine act as sodium channel blockers, it is easier to consider them under separate subcategory than AEDs due to significant pharmacologic differences. Topical lidocaine can also act as local anesthetic to reduce pain, hyperalgesia, or allodynia. It is often used in the management of PHN, intercostal neuralgia, postthoracotomy pain, and meralgia paresthetica. Intravenous lidocaine infusion has been used as a therapeutic tool in the treatment of a variety of neuropathic pain syndromes like spinal cord injury pain,[108] central pain,[109] radiculopathies,[110] and PHN.[111]

Usual dose of lidocaine is 1–5 mg/kg. Potential side effects include bradycardia and hypotension.

Mexiletine is an oral analogue of lidocaine. Some studies had shown that a positive response to intravenous lidocaine could be valuable in selecting patients for oral therapy with mexiletine.[112] Mexiletine was often given in doses of 150–450 mg orally every day in the treatment of diabetic neuropathy, thalamic stroke pain, myotonia, and spasticity. In clinical trials, efficacy of this drug has been substandard.

Miscellaneous Agents Many other classes of drugs are also used in the management of pain. They include skeletal muscle relaxants, glucocorticoids, antispasmodic agents, antihistamines, benzodiazepines, topical agents like capsaicin or lidocaine, and bisphosphonates.

▶ Nonpharmacologic treatment

Numerous nonpharmacological therapies like physical activity, interventional techniques, cognitive-behavioral therapy, transcutaneous electrical nerve stimulation (TENS), heat or cold therapy, massage, and acupuncture have been tried with some success in pain management. Due to minimal associated risks, they should be utilized as adjunctive modalities with ongoing pharmacological interventions. The physical therapy program would help improve their gait, motor strength, flexibility, and endurance. This eventually improves their activity of daily living and self-dependence. Many interventional techniques like epidural steroid injections, trigger point injections, intra-articular hyaluronidase injections, facet rhizotomies have recently gained acceptance in the treatment of acute and chronic pain. Their short-term benefits are commonly seen but their long-term results have not been studied extensively. Certain procedures like neurolytic celiac plexus block, epidural neurolysis, vertebroplasty, or kyphoplasty are increasingly being used in the management of cancer pain and have shown promising results in palliative care. If usual therapeutic maneuvers have not been successful, a timely consultation to an international expert should be considered in this regard.

COMMON PAIN SYNDROMES IN ELDERLY

Pain can be classified in various ways. A common method is based on its potential mechanism—nociceptive, neuropathic, and psychogenic or mixed pain. *Nociception* is the physiological process of activation of neural pathways by stimuli that are potentially or actually damaging to tissue. The conscious experience produced by such stimulus-induced activation of afferent neural pathways is classified as nociceptive pain. Examples of nociceptive pain include musculoskeletal pain (osteoarthritis, rheumatoid arthritis), ischemic or vascular pain (Raynaud disease), myofascial pain, and visceral pain (urolithiasis, chronic pancreatitis). Neuropathic pain, on the contrary, is initiated or caused by a primary lesion or dysfunction in the PNS or CNS. Examples of neuropathic pain include diabetic neuropathy, cervical or lumbar radiculitis, PHN, thalamic syndrome, poststroke central pain, and postspinal cord injury pain. Psychogenic pain has no clear organic etiology and occurs in the presence of psychiatric or personality disorders like depression, hypochondriasis, or hysteria. Finally, certain conditions present with a mixed picture of these three categories of pain (mixed pain) like cancer pain, in which a growing tumor can involve somatic tissues as well as nerves, and patients' pain experience can be further modulated by presence of depression. We discuss some of these pain conditions pertinent to elderly population in the following section.

▶ Somatic pain

Arthritic- or bone-related pain

As per the 2004 U.S. Census report, the 2-year average data from 2001–2002 showed that almost 30% males and 40% females above age 65 suffer from arthritic symptoms. These numbers are almost comparable to heart disease (37% in males, 27% in females) and hypertension (47% in males, 52% in females). Apart from pain, arthritis is also responsible for significant disability in elderly people. In 1999, almost 6.8 million of older Americans were suffering from chronic disabilities, and arthritis is a leading cause of this loss of freedom. Considering the cost of diagnosis; nonpharmacologic, pharmacologic, and surgical interventions; and lost productivity, arthritis is one of the most expensive and debilitating diseases in the United States.[113] Osteoarthritis is the commonest arthritic condition affecting the elderly population and is discussed later.

Osteoarthritis Osteoarthritis is primarily a disease of the cartilage characterized by progressive deterioration and loss of articular cartilage, accompanied by a proliferation of new bone and soft tissue in and around an involved joint. These changes become more prominent with age, typically affecting weight-bearing joints asymmetrically. It commonly involves knees, hips, feet, the distal interphalangeal joints, the first carpometacarpal joints, and the cervical and lumbar spine. Clinical symptoms of osteoarthritis commonly include early-morning joint stiffness lasting for about 30 minutes, gel phenomenon (stiffness while sitting which disappears with movement), constant pain, loss of joint movement or functional limitation, joint instability or deformity, and joint crepitations. Physical examination will often show monoarthritis or asymmetric oligo/polyarthritis, presence of bony swellings of the joint margins (Heberden nodes, Bouchard nodes), mild synovitis, joint effusion, joint deformity, and even objective neurological abnormalities with spine involvement.

Assessment beyond a good history and thorough physical examination includes radiographs and microscopic evaluation of joint fluid aspirate. Routine laboratory work is usually normal as are erythrocyte sedimentation rate (ESR), serum rheumatoid factor, and antinuclear antibodies test (ANA). ESR might be elevated in patients with moderate to severe synovitis. Radiographs of the involved joints show a variable picture of being normal in the initial stages but showing narrowing of the joint space, subchondral bone sclerosis, subchondral cysts, and osteophytes as the disease progresses. Joint fluid aspirate is straw-colored with good viscosity and is typically noninflammatory or minimally inflammatory; generally the white blood cell count is less than 2000/mcL, with most cells being mononuclear.

Since osteoarthritis is one of the commonest pain syndromes affecting the elderly population, a detailed discussion of the benefits of different treatment modalities is presented in Table 26-5. The following recommendations have been made by the American Pain Society:

- ▶ Analgesic and anti-inflammatory medications are important but should be used concurrently with nutritional, physical, educational, and cognitive-behavioral interventions.
- ▶ Clinicians should consider efficacy, adverse side effects, dosing frequency, patient preference, and cost in selecting medications for pain management.
- ▶ Acetaminophen is the medication of first choice for mild pain, although it does not provide any benefit when peripheral inflammation is a causative factor for the pain.

- ▶ COX-2 selective NSAID is the first choice for patients with moderate to severe pain and/or inflammation, but should be avoided in hypertension or renal disorders. A regular low-dose aspirin should be prescribed to patients at risk for cardiovascular events.
- ▶ Nonselective NSAIDs should be considered if the above-mentioned treatment modalities fail, only after a risk analysis of the GI complications. Proton pump inhibitor or misoprostol should also be prescribed if these factors exist.
- ▶ Intra-articular hyaluronic acid injection into the knee should be considered at anytime during the course of illness in patients who are unresponsive to the above therapies.
- ▶ Intra-articular steroids should be considered in presence of significant inflammatory flare anytime during the course of illness.
- ▶ When NSAIDs or acetaminophen are ineffective alone, consider addition of low-dose tramadol.
- ▶ Opioids should be considered only when other management steps have failed.
- ▶ Nonpharmacologic interventions like cognitive-behavioral strategies, attaining ideal body weight, exercise, physical/occupational therapy, and assisted devices should be utilized throughout the management.
- ▶ Surgical interventions are reserved as a terminal consideration.[114]

Osteoporosis Osteoporosis or brittle bone disease is the most common and debilitating metabolic bone disease characterized by marked reduction in bone mass per unit volume with normal bone chemical composition. The pathophysiology of the disease involves an imbalance between bone formation and resumption (remodeling). In elderly osteoporotic patients, the rate of bone resorption exceeds the rate of bone formation due to underlying modeling or metabolic derangements. This progressive loss of bone density predisposes the patients toward fractures, progressive spinal deformity, as well as decreased skeletal function. Vertebrae, wrist bones, humerus, and tibia are particularly prone to fractures. Fractures involving the hip are associated with increased morbidity and mortality, while compression fractures of the vertebra are associated with kyphotic deformity called *dowagers hump* with or without significant pain, neurological symptoms, and debilitation. Thus, pain in osteoporosis could originate from fractures, spinal deformities, and even compressive radiculopathy (neuropathic/mixed picture).

Two distinct varieties of the disease are identified in elderly population. In type 1 osteoporosis, there is a disproportionate loss of trabecular bone in association with fractures of the vertebrae and distal forearm. This subtype of disease is often seen in middle-aged, postmenopausal women, and is associated with low serum estrogen, normal serum calcium, and low or normal serum parathyroid hormone levels. Predisposing factors for type 1 osteoporosis include white race, small stature, sedentary lifestyle, low calcium intake, low weight-bearing regimen, cigarette smoking, and excessive alcohol consumption. On the other hand, type 2 osteoporosis or senile osteoporosis is seen in men and women above age 75, and is associated with fractures of the femoral neck, proximate humerus, proximal tibia, and pelvis. This subtype is often characterized by high serum parathyroid hormone levels.

Evaluation of osteoporosis includes a thorough history and physical examination and a complete laboratory panel testing to detect underlying etiologies like thyrotoxicosis, hyperparathyroidism, or hypogonadism. Radiographic imaging techniques are not helpful in the initial stages of the disease as any significant changes can only be observed after almost one-third bone density loss has occurred;

however, they are helpful in detecting fractures. The diagnostic value of dual-energy x-ray absorptiometry is beyond the scope of discussion in this chapter. Treatment often involves prevention of ongoing loss of bone mass, measures to increase bone density, and treatment of any underlying secondary contributors. Most cases are managed by the primary care physician, and referral to an interventional pain clinic or spine surgeon is made in the setting of vertebral compression fractures or progressive neurological deterioration. Treatment options for osteoporosis are mainly preventative and include:

1. *Oral calcium:* At least 1–1.5 g of oral elemental calcium is given every day. Calcium supplementation alone has a small positive effect on bone density. The present evidence suggests a trend toward reduction in vertebral fractures, but it is unclear if calcium reduces the incidence of nonvertebral fractures.[115]

2. *Vitamin D supplementation:* Vitamin D analogs alfacalcidol and calcitriol are superior to native vitamin D in preventing bone loss and spinal fractures in primary osteoporosis, including post-menopausal women.[116]

3. *Exercise:* Aerobics, weight bearing, and resistance exercises are all effective in increasing the bone density of the spine in post-menopausal women. Walking is also effective on the hip.[117] Efficacy of resistance exercise for increasing or maintaining lumbar spine and femoral neck bone mass density in premenopausal women has recently been questioned.[118]

4. *Removal of secondary risk factors:* Appropriate management of endocrine disorders when present is important in the management of osteoporosis.

5. *Hormone replacement therapy:* Low-dose oral or transdermal estrogen in postmenopausal women with or without progesterone and androgen therapy in hypogonadal men has been recommended.

6. *Bisphosphonates:* The overall risk reduction for hip fractures in post-menopausal women with alendronate therapy is around 55%.[119] Despite some differences in bone density response, different bisphosphonates have comparable reduction in the risk of vertebral fractures over 3 years.

7. *Calcitonin:* In doses greater than 250 IU every week, calcitonin reduces the risk of vertebral fracture, although its effect on nonvertebral fracture remains uncertain.[120] It is more cost effective than etidronate, but its cost-effectiveness versus alendronate remains inconclusive.[121]

8. *Fluoride:* Although fluoride has an ability to increase bone mineral density at the lumbar spine, it does not result in a reduction in vertebral fractures. Increasing the dose of fluoride increases the risk of nonvertebral fractures and GI side effects without any effect on the vertebral fracture rate.[122] Overall, the efficacy of fluoride in the management of osteoporosis is unclear.

9. *Thiazide diuretics:* In patients with high turnover osteoporosis with hypercalciuria and secondary hyperparathyroidism, thiazide diuretics are recommended.

10. *Percutaneous techniques:* Vertebroplasty and kyphoplasty are percutaneous interventional techniques used to restore vertebral body strength or stability (vertebroplasty) or height (kyphoplasty) by injection of bone cement. They are increasingly being used in the treatment of vertebral body fractures.

11. *Surgery:* Surgery is usually reserved as a last option for severe cases with marked functional limitation.

Muscular or myofascial pain

Myofascial pain is crudely defined as a soft tissue pain of unclear etiology. It is most frequently found in the head, neck, shoulders, extremities, and low back, and is more prevalent in women than men. A painful condition that is defined by the presence of active trigger points is called *myofascial pain syndrome*. Myofascial trigger points are frequently identified in patients with chronic head and neck pain, for example, temporo-mandibular joint disorders, neck pain after a whiplash injury, cervicogenic headaches, and tension-type headache.

▶ Visceral pain

Pain arising from visceral structures is often poorly localized and described as dull, aching, or boring in nature, and tightness, pressure-like, discomfort, or squeezing in character. It is often accompanied by associated symptoms or signs of autonomic response like excessive sweating, changes in heart rate or blood pressure, or vasomotor responses. Angina, myocardial infarction, vascular pain, chronic pelvic pain, and genitourinary pain are all examples of visceral pain. Although detailed discussion of each of these diseases is beyond the scope of this chapter, the mechanism of this distinct variety of pain is probably worth mentioning. Stimuli inducing visceral pain often differ from those eliciting somatic pain. Although cutting or crushing of internal organs is usually nonpainful, stretching, ischemia, or chemical irritations can illicit visceral pain mechanisms. There also exists a differential response to these stimuli to various internal systems with serosal membranes being more sensitive to irritable incitements than actual viscera. Another remarkable phenomenon associated with visceral pain is referred pain or transferred pain. Although during the initial stages, visceral pain is vague and poorly localized, it can become well-demarcated to a specific somatic site with time, despite no true involvement of this somatic structure with the injury process. Examples of such pain include referred shoulder pain associated with angina symptoms. Possible explanations for this referred pain include convergence-facilitation and reflex arc. The convergence-facilitation theory involves stimulation of an irritable focus in the spinal cord by visceral inputs causing facilitation of somatic inputs. The convergence-facilitation mechanisms are often associated with presence of hyperalgesia in the involved somatic region. The reflex arc theory involves actual development of algogenic conditions in the peripheral area causing subsequent excitement of peripheral nociceptors. By either mechanism, referred pain helps physicians to identify the possible visceral structures involved and direct investigations and therapy accordingly.

▶ Neuropathic pain

Classic examples of neuropathic pain are postherpetic neuralgia (PHN) and diabetic neuropathy. Other diseases with predominant neuropathic pain include postamputation pain syndrome, complex regional pain syndrome, nerve root disorders (including spinal stenosis), spinal cord injury-related pain, and poststroke pain. For the purpose of discussion, PHN is discussed here. PHN is the most common chronic debilitating sequela of shingles or herpes zoster (HZ). Following an episode of chickenpox (Varicella) earlier in life, the varicella-zoster virus becomes dormant in sensory ganglia throughout the CNS. Later in life, the virus can get reactivated and precipitate a local recrudescence (shingles or HZ) characterized by unilateral vesicular eruptions in a dermatomal distribution accompanied by severe local pain. The precipitating factors for shingles include age and immunosuppression. In the United States, as many as 500,000 new cases of shingles are being diagnosed yearly.

Pain may precede the development of lesions in HZ by 48–72 hours. This initial pain might last for approximately 30 days after the onset of the rash, and is called acute herpetic neuralgia. If this pain persists beyond 4–6 months, it is considered as PHN. It is to be noted that PHN can sometimes develop in HZ patients even in the absence of a history of acute herpetic neuralgia. PHN has been estimated to affect 1 million Americans and accounts for substantial suffering and reduction in quality of life. It is been estimated that as many as 50% of elderly patients who have had shingles may develop PHN.[123] The disease is often diagnosed clinically based on burning, throbbing, or occasionally sharp or shooting pain in a dermatome distribution with or without allodynia. The two most commonly affected sites include thoracic area and trigeminal division of the upper face. Objective evidence of herpes lesions in the past like scaling, scarring, and hypo- or hyperpigmentation in the same dermatome might add to the diagnostic value, although they may be absent (*zoster sine herpete*).

Significant attention has been focused on efforts to reduce the incidence of this disease in the recent past. The most important measure is administration of antiviral medications as early as possible to treat acute HZ. A meta-analysis of five randomized clinical trials on the use of acyclovir to prevent PHN in immunocompetent adults showed that treatment of HZ with 800 mg/day of oral acyclovir within 72 hours of rash onset may reduce the incidence of residual pain at 6 months by 46%.[124] Since severe acute pain associated with shingles is an independent risk factor for later development of PHN, reducing the severity or duration of this pain may help reduce PHN incidence. The use of anticonvulsant drugs (gabapentin or pregabalin) or opioid medications is an additional promising analgesic approach for reducing the risk of PHN in HZ beyond that achieved by antiviral agents.[125]

Evidence-based treatment of PHN at present includes the oral use of opioids,[98] tricyclic antidepressants,[126,127] and gabapentinoids.[128–131] Topical therapy with lidocaine patches[132,133] and capsaicin is similarly supported. Intrathecal administration of methylprednisolone appears to be associated with high efficacy, but its safety requires further evaluation.[134] Interventional local anesthetic blocks play a minor role in control of acute exacerbations during the disease course, but their long-term benefits are unproven.

▶ Cancer pain

Pain related to malignancies is often a therapeutic challenge. Many cancers are more prevalent in the elderly. Cancer-related pain could be nociceptive—originating from tumor involving soft tissue or bone, visceral—produced by a tumor causing obstructive symptoms, neuropathic—tumor involvement of CNS or PNS, or mixed. World Health Organization (WHO) guidelines are often used for treating cancer pain. In general, physicians are more aggressive in pharmacotherapy, and early institution of opioid medications is not uncommon. Many interventional techniques like neurolytic blocks or intrathecal pump implantation are being used more often to provide optimal care.

SUMMARY

Management of pain in the elderly is often demanding. Despite the higher prevalence, pain is undertreated in this population. A fair understanding of pharmacological and physiological differences is required to provide safe care in this subgroup. Elderly people are more sensitive to most pain medications than their younger counterparts, and the lowest dose of the safest medication for the shortest possible time should be prescribed whenever possible. Because of the potential for adverse effects, the elderly should be followed

closely and more frequently. Nonpharmacological management options should also be explored as complementary therapies. The goals of therapy should include pain control as well as achievement of satisfactory functional level. Despite the inherent problems, pain management in the elderly is a rewarding experience.

KEY POINTS

▶ Treatment of pain in the elderly remains inadequate due to its poor understanding amongst physicians.

▶ There are numerous changes in pain signaling and perception with advancing age. A clear understanding of these variations is required to optimize treatment of pain in the elderly.

▶ Assessment of pain in the elderly imposes many challenges due to associated comorbid conditions (like dementia) and their strong personal views regarding pain.

▶ Various physiological changes in the elderly alter pharmacokinetics of analgesic medications, predisposing them for untoward side effects, if used improperly.

▶ Pain conditions in the elderly can be divided into four broad categories: somatic, visceral, neuropathic, and cancer-related pain. In any given patient, a combination of these might exist making the treatment plan more challenging.

▶ Osteoarthritis is the commonest somatic pain, and postherpetic neuralgia is a common neuropathic pain state in the elderly.

KEY REFERENCES

▶ AGS Panel on Persistent Pain in Older Persons. The management of persistent pain in older persons. American Geriatrics Society. *J Am Geriatr Soc.* 2002;50(6):1–20.

▶ Barkin RL, Barkin SJ, Barkin DS. Perception, assessment, treatment, and management of pain in the elderly. *Clin Geriatr Med.* 2005;21(3):465–490, v.

▶ Gagliese L, Melzack R. Chronic pain in elderly people. *Pain.* 1997;70:3–14.

▶ Gloth FM, III. Pain management in older adults: prevention and treatment. *J Am Geriatr Soc.* 2001;49(2):188–199.

▶ Jakobsson U, Klevsgard R, Westergren A, Hallberg IR. Old people in pain: a comparative study. *J Pain Symptom Manage.* 2003;26(1):625–636.

REFERENCES

1. Centers for Disease Control and Prevention, National Center for Health Statistics, National Vital Statistics System; Grove RD, Hetzel AM. Vital statistics rates in the United States, 1940–1960. Washington: U.S. Government Printing Office; 1968; life expectancy trend data available at http://www.cdc.gov/nchs/about/major/dvs/mortdata.htm.
2. Arias E, Anderson RN, Kung HC, et al. Deaths: final data for 2001. National vital statistics reports. Vol. 52, no. 3. Hyattsville, Maryland: National Center for Health Statistics; 2003.
3. U.S. Census Bureau. "Older Americans 2004: Key Indicators of Well-Being." 2004http://www.agingstats.gov/chartbook2004/healthstatus.html.
4. AGS Panel on Persistent Pain in Older Persons. The management of persistent pain in older persons. American Geriatrics Society. *J Am Geriatr Soc.* 2002;50(6):1–20.
5. Crook J, Rideout E, Browne G. The prevalence of pain complaints among a general population. *Pain.* 1984;18:299–314.
6. Magni G, Marchetti M, Moreschi C, et al. Chronic musculoskeletal pain and depressive symptoms in the National Health and Nutrition Examination. I. Epidemiologic follow-up study. *Pain.* 1993;53:163–168.

7. Roy R, Michael T. A survey of chronic pain in an elderly population. *Can Fam Physician*. 1986;32:513–516.

8. Sengstaken EA, King SA. The problems of pain and its detection among geriatric nursing home residents. *J Am Geriatr Soc*. 1993;41:541–544.

9. Ferrell BA, Ferrell BR, Osterweil D. Pain in the nursing home. *J Am Geriatr Soc*. 1990;38:409–414.

10. Chodosh J, Solomon DH, Roth CP, et al. The quality of medical care provided to vulnerable older patients with chronic pain. *J Am Geriatr Soc*. 2004;52(5):756–761.

11. Von Roenn JH, Cleeland CS, Gonin R, et al. Physician attitudes and practice in cancer pain management: a survey from the Eastern Cooperative Oncology Group. *Ann Intern Med*. 1993;119:121–126.

12. Van Nostrand JF, Furner SE, Suzman R, eds. Health data on older Americans: United States, 1992. *Vital and Health Statistics. Series 3: Analytic and Epidemiological Studies*. No. 27. Hyattsville, MD: National Center for Health Statistics; 1993.

13. Verdu E, Ceballos D, Vilches JJ, Navarro X. Influence of aging on peripheral nerve function and regeneration. *J Peripher Nerv Syst*. 2000;5(4):191–208.

14. Gibson SJ, Farrell M. A review of age differences in the neurophysiology of nociception and the perceptual experience of pain. *Clin J Pain*. 2004; 20(4):227–239.

15. Ko ML, King MA, Gordon TL, Crisp T. The effects of aging on spinal neurochemistry in the rat. *Brain Res Bull*. 1997;42(2):95–98.

16. Bergman E, Johnson H, Zhang X, et al. Neuropeptides and neurotrophin receptor mRNAs in primary sensory neurons of aged rats. *J Comp Neurol*. 1996;375(2):303–319.

17. Hukkanen M, Platts LA, Corbett SA, et al. Reciprocal age-related changes in GAP-43/B-50, substance P and calcitonin gene-related peptide (CGRP) expression in rat primary sensory neurones and their terminals in the dorsal horn of the spinal cord and subintima of the knee synovium. *Neurosci Res*. 2002;42(4):251–260.

18. Iwata K, Fukuoka T, Kondo E, et al. Plastic changes in nociceptive transmission of the rat spinal cord with advancing age. *J Neurophysiol*. 2002; 87(2):1086–1093.

19. Pakkenberg B, Gundersen HJ. Neocortical neuron number in humans: effect of sex and age. *J Comp Neurol*. 1997;384(2):312–320.

20. Barili P, De Carolis G, Zaccheo D, Amenta F. Sensitivity to ageing of the limbic dopaminergic system: a review. *Mech Ageing Dev*. 1998;106(1-2): 57–92.

21. Washington LL, Gibson SJ, Helme RD. Age-related differences in the endogenous analgesic response to repeated cold water immersion in human volunteers. *Pain*. 2000;89(1):89–96.

22. Helme RD, Gibson SJ. The epidemiology of pain in elderly people. *Clin Geriatr Med*. 2001;17(3):417–431.

23. Klinger L, Spaulding S. Chronic pain in the elderly: is silence really golden? *Phys Occup Ther Geriatr*. 1998;15:1–17.

24. Gibson SJ, Helme RD. Age-related differences in pain perception and report. *Clin Geriatr Med*. 2001;17(3):433–456.

25. Gagliese L, Melzack R. Chronic pain in elderly people. *Pain*. 1997; 70:3–14.

26. Beyth RJ, Shorr RI. Medication use. In: Duthie EH, ed. *Practice of Geriatrics*. 3rd ed. Philadelphia: WB Saunders; 1998.

27. Jakobsson U, Klevsgard R, Westergren A, Hallberg IR. Old people in pain: a comparative study. *J Pain Symptom Manage*. 2003;26(1):625–636.

28. Urwin M, Symmons D, Allison T, et al. Estimating the burden of musculoskeletal disorders in the community: the comparative prevalence of symptoms at different anatomical sites, and the relation to social deprivation. *Ann Rheum Dis*. 1998;57(11):649–655.

29. Sternberg RA. Survey of pain in the United States: the Nuprin pain report. *Clin J Pain*. 1986;2:49–53.

30. Reyes-Gibby CC, Aday L, Cleeland C. Impact of pain on self-rated health in the community-dwelling older adults. *Pain*. 2002;95(1-2): 75–82.

31. Thomas E, Peat G, Harris L, et al. The prevalence of pain and pain interference in a general population of older adults: cross-sectional findings from the North Staffordshire Osteoarthritis Project (NorStOP). *Pain*. 2004;110(1-2):361–368.

32. Harkins SW, Price DD. Assessment of pain in elderly. In: Turk D, Melzack R, eds. *Handbook of Pain Measurement and Assessment*. New York: Guilford Press; 1992:315–351.

33. Pickering G, Jourdan D, Eschalier A, Dubray C. Impact of age, gender, and cognitive functioning on pain perception. *Gerontology*. 2002;48(2):112–118.

34. Hall KR, Stride E. The varying response to pain in psychiatric disorders: a study in abnormal psychology. *Br J Med Psychol*. 1954;27(1-2):48–60.

35. Procacci P, Bozza G, Buzzelli G, Della Corte M. The cutaneous pricking pain threshold in old age. *Gerontol Clin (Basel)*. 1970;12(4):213–218.

36. Sherman ED, Robillard E. Sensitivity to pain in relationship to age. *J Am Geriatr Soc*. 1964;12:1037–1044.

37. Jensen R, Rasmussen BK, Pedersen B, et al. Cephalic muscle tenderness and pressure pain threshold in a general population. *Pain*. 1992;48(2):197–203.

38. Lasch H, Castell DO, Castell JA. Evidence for diminished visceral pain with aging: studies using graded intraesophageal balloon distension. *Am J Physiol*. 1997;272(1 Pt. 1):G1–G3.

39. Edwards RR, Fillingim RB. Age-associated differences in responses to noxious stimuli. *J Gerontol A Biol Sci Med Sci*. 2001;56(3):M180–M185.

40. Zheng Z, Gibson SJ, Khalil Z, et al. Age-related differences in the time course of capsaicin-induced hyperalgesia. *Pain*. 2000;85(1-2):51–8.

41. Neri M, Agazzani E. Aging and right-left asymmetry in experimental pain measurement. *Pain*. 1984;19(1):43–48.

42. Tucker MA, Andrew MF, Ogle SJ, Davison JG. Age-associated change in pain threshold measured by transcutaneous neuronal electrical stimulation. *Age Ageing*. 1989;18(4):241–246.

43. Mumford JM. Pain perception in man on electrically stimulating the teeth. In: Soulairac A, Cahn J, Charpentier J, eds. *Pain*. London: Academic Press; 1968:224–229.

44. Lucantoni C, Marinelli S, Refe A, et al. Course of pain sensitivity in aging: pathogenetical aspects of silent cardiopathy. *Arch Gerontol Geriatr*. 1997; 24(3):281–286.

45. Lautenbacher S, Strian F. Similarities in age differences in heat pain perception and thermal sensitivity. *Funct Neurol*. 1991;6(2):129–135.

46. Mertz H, Fullerton S, Naliboff B, Mayer EA. Symptoms and visceral perception in severe functional and organic dyspepsia. Gut. 1998 Jun;42(6):814-22.

47. Harkins SW, Price DD, Martelli M. Effects of age on pain perception: thermonociception. *J Gerontol*. 1986;41(1):58–63.

48. Chakour MC, Gibson SJ, Bradbeer M, Helme RD. The effect of age on A delta- and C-fibre thermal pain perception. *Pain*. 1996;64(1):143–152.

49. Harkins SW, Chapman CR. Detection and decision factors in pain perception in young and elderly men. *Pain*. 1976;2(3):253–264.

50. Harkins SW, Chapman CR. The perception of induced dental pain in young and elderly women. *J Gerontol*. 1977;32(4):428–435.

51. Strigo IA, Bushnell MC, Boivin M, Duncan GH. Psychophysical analysis of visceral and cutaneous pain in human subjects. *Pain*. 2002;97(3):235–246.

52. Verne GN, Robinson ME, Price DD. Hypersensitivity to visceral and cutaneous pain in the irritable bowel syndrome. *Pain*. 2001;93(1):7–14.

53. Petzke F, Harris RE, Williams DA, et al. Differences in unpleasantness induced by experimental pressure pain between patients with fibromyalgia and healthy controls. *Eur J Pain*. 2005;9(3):325–335.

54. Woodrow KM, Friedman GD, Siegelaub AB, et al. Pain tolerance: differences according to age, sex and race. *Psychosom Med*. 1972 Nov–Dec; 34(6):548–556.

55. Walsh NE, Schoenfeld L, Ramamurthy S, et al. Normative model for cold pressor test. *Am J Phys Med Rehabil*. 1989 Feb; 68(1):6–11.

56. Edwards RR, Doleys DM, Fillingim RB, et al. Ethnic differences in pain tolerance: clinical implications in a chronic pain population. *Psychosom Med*. 2001 Mar–Apr; 63(2):316–323.

57. Edwards RR, Fillingim RB, Ness TJ. Age-related differences in endogenous pain modulation: a comparison of diffuse noxious inhibitory controls in healthy older and younger adults. *Pain*. 2003;101(1-2):155–165.

58. Neumann W, Kugler J, Seelbach H, Kruskemper GM. Effects of nondirective suggestions on pain tolerance, pain threshold, and pain intensity perception. *Percept Mot Skills*. 1997;84(3 Pt. 1):963–966.

59. Neumann W, Kugler J, Pfand-Neumann P, et al. Effects of pain-incompatible imagery on perception of pain, heart rate, and skin resistance. *Percept Mot Skills*. 1997;84(3 Pt. 1):939–943.

60. van den Hout JH, Vlaeyen JW, Peters ML, et al. Does failure hurt? The effects of failure feedback on pain report, pain tolerance and pain avoidance. *Eur J Pain*. 2000;4(4):335–346.

61. Barkin RL, Barkin SJ, Barkin DS. Perception, assessment, treatment, and management of pain in the elderly. *Clin Geriatr Med*. 2005;21(3): 465–490, v.

62. Blair KA. Aging: physiological aspects and clinical implications. *Nurse Pract*. 1990;15(2):14–16, 18, 26–28.

63. Taylor LJ, Harris J, Epps CD, Herr K. Psychometric evaluation of selected pain intensity scales for use with cognitively impaired and cognitively intact older adults. *Rehabil Nurs*. 2005;30(2):55–61.

64. Herr KA, Spratt K, Mobily PR, et al. Pain intensity assessment in older adults: use of experimental pain to compare psychometric properties and usability of selected pain scales with younger adults. *Clin J Pain*. 2004;20(4):207–219.

65. Wijeratne C, Shome S, Hickie I, Koschera A. An age-based comparison of chronic pain clinic patients. *Int J Geriatr Psychiatry*. 2001;16(5):477–483.

66. Rochon PA, Gurwitz JH. Drug therapy. *Lancet*. 1995;346(8966):32–36.

67. Gloth FM, III. Pain management in older adults: prevention and treatment. *J Am Geriatr Soc*. 2001;49(2):188–199.

68. Zhang W, Jones A, Doherty M. Does paracetamol (acetaminophen) reduce the pain of osteoarthritis? A meta-analysis of randomized controlled trials. *Ann Rheum Dis*. 2004;63(8):901–907. Epub 2004 Mar 5.

69. Towheed T, Shea B, Wells G, et al. Analgesia and non-aspirin, non-steroidal anti-inflammatory drugs for osteoarthritis of the hip. *Cochrane Database Syst Rev*. 2000;(2):CD000517.

70. Bjordal JM, Ljunggren AE, Klovning A, et al. Non-steroidal anti-inflammatory drugs, including cyclo-oxygenase-2 inhibitors, in osteoarthritic knee pain: meta-analysis of randomized placebo controlled trials. *Br Med J*. 2004;329(7478):1317. Epub 2004 Nov 23.

71. Lee C, Straus WL, Balshaw R, et al. A comparison of the efficacy and safety of nonsteroidal anti-inflammatory agents versus acetaminophen in the treatment of osteoarthritis: a meta-analysis. *Arthritis Rheum*. 2004;51(5):746–754.

72. Towheed TE, Hochberg MC. A systematic review of randomized controlled trials of pharmacological therapy in osteoarthritis of the hip. *J Rheumatol*. 1997;24(2):349–357.

73. Riedemann PJ, Bersinic S, Cuddy LJ, et al. A study to determine the efficacy and safety of tenoxicam versus piroxicam, diclofenac, and indomethacin in patients with osteoarthritis: a meta-analysis. *J Rheumatol*. 1993;20(12):2095–2103.

74. McKenna F, Arguelles L, Burke T, et al. Upper gastrointestinal tolerability of celecoxib compared with diclofenac in the treatment of osteoarthritis and rheumatoid arthritis. *Clin Exp Rheumatol*. 2002;20(1):35–43.

75. Watson DJ, Yu Q, Bolognese JA, et al. The upper gastrointestinal safety of rofecoxib vs. NSAIDs: an updated combined analysis. *Curr Med Res Opin*. 2004;20(10):1539–1548.

76. Goldstein JL, Eisen GM, Agrawal N, et al. Reduced incidence of upper gastrointestinal ulcer complications with the COX-2 selective inhibitor, valdecoxib. *Aliment Pharmacol Ther*. 2004;20(5):527–538.

77. Spiegel BM, Targownik L, Dulai GS, Gralnek IM. The cost-effectiveness of cyclooxygenase-2 selective inhibitors in the management of chronic arthritis. *Ann Intern Med*. 2003;138(10):795–806.

78. Fishbain D. Evidence-based data on pain relief with antidepressants. *Ann Med*. 2000;32(5):305–316.

79. Mason L, Moore RA, Edwards JE, et al. Topical NSAIDs for chronic musculoskeletal pain: systematic review and meta-analysis. *BMC Musculoskelet Disord*. 2004;5:28.

80. Lin J, Zhang W, Jones A, Doherty M. Efficacy of topical non-steroidal anti-inflammatory drugs in the treatment of osteoarthritis: meta-analysis of randomized controlled trials. *Br Med J*. 2004;329(7461):324. Epub 2004 Jul 30.

81. Towheed TE, Maxwell L, Anastassiades TP, et al. Glucosamine therapy for treating osteoarthritis. The Cochrane Database of Systematic Reviews. 2005;(2):CD002946.pub2. DOI: 10.1002/14651858.CD002946.pub2.

82. Soeken KL, Lee WL, Bausell RB, et al. Safety and efficacy of S-adenosylmethionine (SAMe) for osteoarthritis. *J Fam Pract*. 2002; 51(5):425–430.

83. Richy F, Bruyere O, Ethgen O, et al. Structural and symptomatic efficacy of glucosamine and chondroitin in knee osteoarthritis: a comprehensive meta-analysis. *Arch Intern Med*. 2003;163(13):1514–1522.

84. Little CV, Parsons T, Logan S. Herbal therapy for treating osteoarthritis. The Cochrane Database of Systematic Reviews. 2000;(4):CD002947. DOI: 10.1002/14651858.CD002947.

85. Fortin PR, Lew RA, Liang MH, et al. Validation of a meta-analysis: the effects of fish oil in rheumatoid arthritis. *J Clin Epidemiol*. 1995;48(11):1379–1390.

86. Brosseau L, Welch V, Wells G, et al. Low level laser therapy (classes I, II, and III) for treating osteoarthritis. *Cochrane Database Syst Rev*. 2003; (2):CD002046.

87. Welch V, Brosseau L, Peterson J, et al. Therapeutic ultrasound for osteoarthritis of the knee. Cochrane Database Syst Rev. 2001;(3): CD003132.

88. Osiri M, Brosseau L, McGowan J, et al. Transcutaneous electrical nerve stimulation for knee osteoarthritis. The Cochrane Database of Systematic Reviews. 2000;(4):CD002823. DOI: 10.1002/14651858.CD002823.

89. Superio-Cabuslay E, Ward MM, Lorig KR. Patient education interventions in osteoarthritis and rheumatoid arthritis: a meta-analytic comparison with nonsteroidal antiinflammatory drug treatment. *Arthritis Care Res*. 1996;9(4):292–301.

90. Morley S, Eccleston C, Williams A. Systematic review and meta-analysis of randomized controlled trials of cognitive behavior therapy and behavior therapy for chronic pain in adults, excluding headache. *Pain*. 1999;80(1-2):1–13.

91. Bellamy N, Campbell J, Robinson V, et al. Intraarticular corticosteroid for treatment of osteoarthritis of the knee. *Cochrane Database Syst Rev*. 2005;(2):CD005328.

92. Bellamy N, Campbell J, Robinson V, et al. Viscosupplementation for the treatment of osteoarthritis of the knee. *Cochrane Database Syst Rev*. 2005;(2):CD005321.

93. Arroll B, Goodyear-Smith F. Corticosteroid injections for osteoarthritis of the knee: meta-analysis. *Br Med J*. 2004;328(7444):869. Epub 2004 Mar 23.

94. Godwin M, Dawes M. Intra-articular steroid injections for painful knees. Systematic review with meta-analysis. *Can Fam Physician*. 2004;50:241–248.

95. Wang CT, Lin J, Chang CJ, et al. Therapeutic effects of hyaluronic acid on osteoarthritis of the knee. A meta-analysis of randomized controlled trials. *J Bone Joint Surg Am*. 2004;86-A(3):538–545.

96. Lo GH, LaValley M, McAlindon T, Felson DT. Intra-articular hyaluronic acid in treatment of knee osteoarthritis: a meta-analysis. *JAMA*. 2003;290(23):3115–3121.

97. Watson CP, Babul N. Efficacy of oxycodone in neuropathic pain: a randomized trial in postherpetic neuralgia. *Neurology*. 1998;50:1837–1841.

98. Raja SN, Haythornthwaite JA, Pappagallo M, et al. Opioids versus antidepressants in postherpetic neuralgia: a randomized, placebo-controlled trial. *Neurology*. 2002;59(7):1015–1021.

99. Kalso E, Edwards JE, Moore RA, et al. Opioids in chronic non-cancer pain: systematic review of efficacy and safety. *Pain*. 2004;112(3): 372–380.

100. Potter WZ, Hollister LE. Antidepressant agents. In: Katzung BG, ed. *Basic and Clinical Pharmacology*. 9th ed. New York: Lange Medical Books/McGraw-Hill Medical Publishing Division; 2004.

101. Stahl SM, Grady MM, Moret C, Briley M. SNRIs: their Pharmacology, clinical efficacy, and tolerability in comparison with other classes of antidepressants. *CNS Spectr*. 2005;10(9):732–747.

102. Mattia C, Paoletti F, Coluzzi F, Boanelli A. New antidepressants in the treatment of neuropathic pain. A review. *Minerva Anestesiol*. 2002; 68(3):105–114.

103. Gutierrez MA, Stimmel GL, Aiso JY. Venlafaxine: a 2003 update. *Clin Ther*. 2003;25(8):2138–2154.

104. Barkin RL, Barkin S. The role of venlafaxine and duloxetine in the treatment of depression with decremental changes in somatic symptoms of pain, chronic pain, and the pharmacokinetics and clinical considerations of duloxetine pharmacotherapy. *Am J Ther*. 2005;12(5):431–438.

105. Mellegers MA, Furlan AD, Mailis A. Gabapentin for neuropathic pain: systematic review of controlled and uncontrolled literature. *Clin J Pain*. 2001;17(4):284–295.

106. Dworkin RH, Corbin AE, Young JP, Jr, et al. Pregabalin for the treatment of postherpetic neuralgia: a randomized, placebo-controlled trial. *Neurology*. 2003;60(8):1274–1283.

107. Rosenstock J, Tuchman M, LaMoreaux L, et al. Pregabalin for the treatment of painful diabetic peripheral neuropathy: a double-blind, placebo-controlled trial. *Pain*. 2004;110(3):628–638.

108. Finnerup NB, Biering-Sorensen F, Johannesen IL, et al. Intravenous lidocaine relieves spinal cord injury pain: a randomized controlled trial. *Anesthesiology*. 2005;102(5):1023–1030.

109. Attal N, Gaude V, Brasseur L, et al. Intravenous lidocaine in central pain: a double-blind, placebo-controlled, psychophysical study. *Neurology.* 2000;54(3):564–574.

110. Medrik-Goldberg T, Lifschitz D, Pud D, et al. Intravenous lidocaine, amantadine, and placebo in the treatment of sciatica: a double-blind, randomized, controlled study. *Reg Anesth Pain Med.* 1999;24(6): 534–540.

111. Rowbotham MC, Reisner-Keller LA, Fields HL. Both intravenous lidocaine and morphine reduce the pain of postherpetic neuralgia. *Neurology.* 1991;41(7):1024–1028.

112. Galer BS, Harle J, Rowbotham MC. Response to intravenous lidocaine infusion predicts subsequent response to oral mexiletine: a prospective study. *J Pain Symptom Manage.* 1996;12(3):161–167.

113. Gabriel SE, Matteson EL. Economic and quality-of-life impact of NSAIDs in rheumatoid arthritis: a conceptual framework and selected literature review. *Pharmacoeconomics.* 1995;8(6):479–490.

114. Simon LS, Lipman AG, Jacox AK, et al. Pain in osteoarthritis, rheumatoid arthritis, and juvenile chronic arthritis. 2nd ed. Glenview, IL: American Pain Society (APS); 2002:179. (Clinical practice guideline; no. 2).

115. Shea B, Wells G, Cranney A, et al. Osteoporosis Methodology Group; Osteoporosis Research Advisory Group. Calcium supplementation on bone loss in postmenopausal women. *Cochrane Database Syst Rev.* 2004;(1):CD004526.

116. Richy F, Schacht E, Bruyere O, et al. Vitamin D analogs versus native vitamin D in preventing bone loss and osteoporosis-related fractures: a comparative meta-analysis. *Calcif Tissue Int.* 2005;76(3):176–186. Epub 2005 Feb 7.

117. Bonaiuti D, Shea B, Iovine R, et al. Exercise for preventing and treating osteoporosis in postmenopausal women. *Cochrane Database Syst Rev.* 2002;(3):CD000333.

118. Kelley GA, Kelley KS. Efficacy of resistance exercise on lumbar spine and femoral neck bone mineral density in premenopausal women: a meta-analysis of individual patient data. *J Womens Health (Larchmt).* 2004;13(3):293–300.

119. Papapoulos SE, Quandt SA, Liberman UA, et al. Meta-analysis of the efficacy of alendronate for the prevention of hip fractures in postmenopausal women. *Osteoporos Int.* 2005;16(5):468–474. Epub 2004 Sep 21.

120. Cranney A, Tugwell P, Zytaruk N, et al. Osteoporosis Methodology Group and the Osteoporosis Research Advisory Group. Meta-analyses of therapies for postmenopausal osteoporosis. VI. Meta-analysis of calcitonin for the treatment of postmenopausal osteoporosis. *Endocr Rev.* 2002;23(4):540–551.

121. Coyle D, Cranney A, Lee KM, et al. Cost effectiveness of nasal calcitonin in postmenopausal women: use of Cochrane Collaboration methods for meta-analysis within economic evaluation. *Pharmacoeconomics.* 2001; 19(5 Pt. 2):565–575.

122. Haguenauer D, Welch V, Shea B, et al. Fluoride for the treatment of postmenopausal osteoporotic fractures: a meta-analysis. *Osteoporos Int.* 2000;11(9):727–738.

123. Bowsher D. Post-herpetic neuralgia in older patients. Incidence and optimal treatment. *Drugs Aging.* 1994;5(6):411–418.

124. Jackson JL, Gibbons R, Meyer G, Inouye L. The effect of treating herpes zoster with oral acyclovir in preventing postherpetic neuralgia. A meta-analysis. *Arch Intern Med.* 1997;157(8):909–912.

125. Dubinsky RM, Kabbani H, El-Chami Z, et al. Practice parameter: treatment of postherpetic neuralgia: an evidence-based report of the Quality Standards Subcommittee of the American Academy of Neurology. *Neurology.* 2004;63:959–965.

126. McQuay HJ, Tramer M, Nye BA, et al. A systematic review of antidepressants in neuropathic pain. *Pain.* 1996;68(2-3):217–227.

127. Volmink J, Lancaster T, Gray S, Silagy C. Treatments for postherpetic neuralgia—a systematic review of randomized controlled trials. *Fam Pract.* 1996;13(1):84–91.

128. Rowbotham M, Harden N, Stacey B, et al. Gabapentin for the treatment of postherpetic neuralgia: a randomized controlled trial. *JAMA.* 1998; 280(21):1837–1842.

129. Rice AS, Maton S. Postherpetic Neuralgia Study Group. Gabapentin in postherpetic neuralgia: a randomized, double blind, placebo controlled study. *Pain.* 2001;94(2):215–224.

130. Serpell MG. Neuropathic Pain Study Group. Gabapentin in neuropathic pain syndromes: a randomized, double-blind, placebo-controlled trial. *Pain.* 2002;99(3):557–566.

131. Parsons B, Tive L, Huang S. Gabapentin: a pooled analysis of adverse events from three clinical trials in patients with postherpetic neuralgia. *Am J Geriatr Pharmacother.* 2004;2(3):157–162.

132. Galer BS, Rowbotham MC, Perander J, et al. Topical lidocaine patch relieves postherpetic neuralgia more effectively than a vehicle topical patch: results of an enriched enrollment study. *Pain.* 1999;80(3):533–538.

133. Rowbotham MC, Davies PS, Verkempinck C, et al. Lidocaine patch: double-blind controlled study of a new treatment method for postherpetic neuralgia. *Pain.* 1996;65(1):39–44.

134. Hempenstall K, Nurmikko TJ, Johnson RW, et al. Analgesic therapy in postherpetic neuralgia: a quantitative systematic review. *PLoS Med.* 2005;2(7):e164. Epub 2005 Jul 26.

Anesthesia Management of the Patient with Dementia

Barbara Eckel
Manfred Blobner

INTRODUCTION

Dementia is a slowly progressing loss of mental abilities, which exceeds the normal age-related decline of brain efficiency, and therefore is classified as a disease. Above all, memory and the ability to solve everyday problems are impaired. In addition, sensory and thought disturbance, disorientation, as well as personality changes develop with prolonged illness.[1]

Dementia at an advanced age is the most frequent cause for escalation in the level of daily care requirements, since the elderly also decline physically as a consequence of their illness. Usually, it involves a gradual and progressive process of decline, which can be modified by medication, however, not be cured. The life expectancy of Alzheimer's disease patients averages 8 years from the onset and diagnosis; few live up to 20 years later.[2]

For senile dementia, apart from Alzheimer's disease with late onset, there are many known causes, for example, arteriosclerosis and its consequences, Parkinson's, Lewy body, and reversible dementia.

During preoperative evaluation of demented patients, problems may arise from lack of insight, understanding, and ability to cooperate. Frequently, consent and history cannot be obtained from the patient any longer, so the family members and responsible guardians are included in the physician-patient relationship. This also applies to consideration of possible medication interactions and pathophysiological changes.

EPIDEMIOLOGY

Dementia is unevenly distributed over age groups. Within the group of 60–70-year-olds, dementia is hardly of significance; only about 1–2% is afflicted. Beyond the age of 70, however, the percentage affected rises sharply. While, within the group of 70–80-year-olds, the percentage remains at approximately 5–7%; nearly one-fifth of the 80–90-year-old seniors (15–20%) is afflicted. Of the 90–95-year-olds, one-third is stricken.[3]

Twelve million people in Germany are already older than 65 years; of these currently 1.2 million suffer a progressive dementia. About 800,000–900,000 will advance to the moderately severe and grave stages of the disease, when independent living becomes no longer possible. Today, of all patients with difficulties and in need of assistance with routine care, probably about 70% suffer from dementia.[4] The average cost for care of these patients in the United States, whether in family home or in a nursing facility, is about US $47,000 per year.[5]

For Germany, the projected estimate for care of all advanced dementia patients is US $40 billion per year. In Germany, one anticipates the cost, depending on disease stage, as between €5100 and 92,000 per patient per year.[6]

For the year 2000 already a total budget of approx. €18 billion in direct services was expended.[7] Without change in health-care policies, expenditures would rise to €26.4 billion by the year 2020. Family members' indirect care contributions and time invested are not even accounted for. As a result of extended life expectancy, population case numbers are anticipated to rise over the next decades. Consequently, the World Health Organization (WHO) addresses Alzheimer's disease as "one of the most significant medical problems the world faces today."

It is important to differentiate between normal memory loss with respect to aging, and clinical dementia. Normal, age-related decrease of cognitive abilities may include slight memory deficits and small impairments of other cognitive processes, which do not significantly impair the ability to function in daily life. Typically, the learning of new information decreases in efficiency, whereas distant memory is less affected.[8]

The various forms of dementia include Alzheimer's disease, vascular-mediated or multi-infarct dementia, Parkinson's and associated dementia (including Lewy body dementia and progressive supranuclear paralysis), frontal dementia, and reversible dementia. Alzheimer's disease is the most frequent cause of dementia and accounts for 60–80% of diagnoses.[9] Vascular dementia constitutes a further 10–20%, while Parkinson's accounts for approximately 5% of total dementias. As causes for the remaining cases of chronic dementia, one may consider alcohol abuse, pharmaceutical side effects, depression, or other cerebral illnesses. With elderly patients, Parkinson's associated with Lewy body dementia is observed just as frequently as vascular dementia.[10] Due to the high incidence of cardiovascular risk factors in senior patients, mixed forms of dementia are the rule rather than the exception.

In regard to all these dementia forms, with the exception of Alzheimer's disease, there are no investigations into the effects of dementia on anesthetic management and related pharmaceutical interactions, nor vice versa, the effect of anesthesia on the disease process. The discussion of the less-frequently diagnosed forms of dementia is brief. Our attention focuses on Alzheimer's, since some investigations into this disease exist, documenting the reciprocal effect of dementia and anesthesia, and because this illness has overwhelmingly the highest incidence.

DIAGNOSIS

If dementia is suspected, it is critical for the elderly, their families, and society at large to seek early diagnosis and care. Usually, entry into the medical system is via a family doctor or primary care practitioner. Unfortunately, up to 75% of dementia cases are not recognized.[11]

The diagnosis of dementia is obtained clinically, using cognitive tests. Based on the criteria of the 4th edition of the American Psychiatric Association's Diagnostic and Statistic Manual (DSM-IV, see Fig. 27-1),[1] the most frequently used diagnostic test for dementia is the Mini-Mental Status Test (MMST) (see Chap. 12).[12]

The maximum score attainable for the MMST is 30 points. A score below 24 suggests the diagnosis of dementia. The MMST has a sensitivity of 87%, and a specificity of 82% among the White population.[13] The diagnostic ability of the MMST is limited when testing patients with moderate dementia, low literacy, impaired motor function or linguistic abilities, or uncorrected eyesight.[12,14]

Another easily accessible test, which is relatively independent of educational, cultural and, linguistic background is the Mini Cog test, which consists of a clock/signal test, and the repetition of three unrelated random words (see Chap. 12).[15] Patients who can repeat all three words are not considered demented; if they cannot repeat the words, they are diagnosed as such. If they can repeat one or two words, they are classified according to the clock/signal test. Normal rating depends on whether the patient is able to point out a given time correctly.[15] Sensitivity and specificity generally correspond to the MMST.[16] The Mini-Cog Test is so simple, quick, and easy that it can be easily administered, even in exceptional cases within the context of a preanesthetic consultation.

There are also substantially more complex psychometric and cognitive tests available which are able to recognize more subtle forms of dementia. However, these tests can be expensive and time consuming. In addition to the evaluation of cognitive function, a thorough general, physical, and neurological exam is essential, emphasizing the assessment of focal neurological deficits or parkinsonian symptoms. With some dementias, laboratory testing and imaging diagnostics are valuable. These are discussed when reviewing the specifics of different dementia forms.

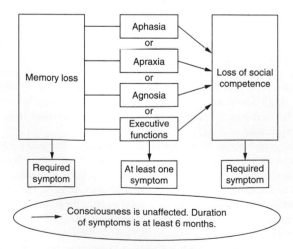

FIGURE 27-1 Diagnostic criteria for dementia according to the American Psychiatric Association Diagnostic and Statistical Manual (DSM-IV).

DEMENTIA FORMS

▶ Vascular dementia

This diagnosis, due to lack of specific diagnostic criteria, is often not definitive. A vascular dementia with cognitive deficits is likely after stroke with sudden onset and slow progression, a diagnosed preexisting stroke, or imaged ischemic brain areas.[17] Frequently, vascular dementia is associated with regional areas of cerebral ischemia, and is particularly common with lacunar infarction cases.

Of note, microvascular lesions may cause more cognitive deficits than larger areas of infarction after stroke.[18]

▶ Parkinson-associated dementia

Patients suffering from Parkinson's have nearly a six times increased risk of developing dementia compared to a healthy control group.[19] This means that approximately 30% of all Parkinson's patients will succumb to dementia.[20] Lewy body dementia is most frequently associated with Parkinson's, and is the second most significant neurodegenerative dementia following Alzheimer's disease.[21] Typical clinical symptoms associated with Parkinson's generally are a slowly progressing dementia with fluctuating changes in cognitive abilities, constant visual hallucinations, and the spontaneous motor/coordination difficulties of Parkinson's disease. Neuropathologically, this form of dementia is defined by the occurrence of Lewy bodies in the brain stem and cortex.[21]

As Parkinson's, Lewy body dementia and Alzheimer's often overlap; clinically and histopathologically, it is difficult to differentiate between these diseases. Clinical criteria for the identification of Lewy body dementia are being defined. It seems that fatigue or more than 2 hours of sleep during the day, "vacant stares," and foggy thought processes are typical for Lewy body dementia.[22]

▶ Frontal lobe dementia

Frontal lobe dementia represents a very rare cause of dementia. These patients demonstrate significant deficits regarding executive functions and uninhibited behavior. Cognitive deficits are mild early on, and are often denied by the patients.[23] A subgroup of frontal lobe dementia is represented by Pick disease, which is characterized by Pick bodies in neocortex and hippocampus. The patients exhibit language anomalies such as logorrhea, echolalia, and the repetition of clichés.[24]

▶ Reversible dementia

Apart from the classical, progressive dementia, there is also potentially reversible dementia. Possible causes are medications (e.g., anticholinergics, psychopharmacological drugs, sedatives), alcohol (intoxication, withdrawal), metabolic disturbances (thyroid malfunctions, electrolyte disturbances, liver and kidney insufficiency), depression, reversible structural changes in the brain (tumor, chronic subdural hematoma, meningitis, normal pressure hydrocephalus), and others. The most common causes are medications, depression, and metabolic alterations.[25] Before diagnosing an irreversible, progressive senile dementia, the possibility of a reversible dementia must be precluded. Although reversible, in many cases, regaining normal cognitive abilities is not always achieved. Elective operations must be postponed until the cause of dementia is elucidated and any indicated treatment instituted.

▶ Alzheimer's disease

In 1907, German neuropathologist Alois Alzheimer (1864–1915) described the typical symptoms of this syndrome later bearing his name, referring to a 51-year-old female patient as "a woman with rapidly deteriorating memory, apparently dysfunctional in her home, dragging items back and forth, hiding them, and occasionally delusional that someone wants to kill her, she acts out with loud screaming."[26] After 4 years of illness, the woman died following progressive decline, disorientation, aphasia, apraxia, and memory deficits. With the advent of the use of silver dye staining, Alzheimer described the characteristic findings of neurofibrillary tangles and neuritic plaques in an atrophied brain. Since the initial description of these histological changes, a clinical dementia before the age of 65 was usually defined as Alzheimer's disease. Dementia in older persons was attributed to vascular causes and defined as senile dementia. Alzheimer's disease is a progressive, fatal neurodegenerative illness, which manifests itself with degradation of cognitive abilities and memory, increasing inability to master the requirements of daily life, multiple diverse neuropsychiatric symptoms, and personality and behavior changes.

More than 12% of all seniors over 65 years are stricken by this illness.[27]

Risk factors

The cause of Alzheimer's disease is multifactorial. The most significant risk factor to develop this illness is, and remains, older age.[28] A municipal study documented an annual Alzheimer's incidence rate of 0.6% for all inhabitants between 65 and 69 years, 1% between 70 and 79 years, 2.0% between 75 and 79 years, 3.3% between 80 and 84 years, and 8.4% for all persons older than 85 years.[29] Another important risk-factor is a positive family history. Family members, first-degree related to an Alzheimer's sufferer, have a 10–30% increased risk of developing the disease themselves.[30] The risk for close relatives decreases when the patient is of advanced age at the onset of the disease.[31] It should be pointed out that family members' illness risk between ages 50 and 54 is the highest with a risk ratio of 19.7, compared to a relative at age 90 with a risk ratio of 1.2.

It is established that there is a genetic component to the pathogenesis of Alzheimer's disease. It is also possible to differentiate between genetic risk factors responsible for either the late or the early onset of Alzheimer's disease.

Five to ten percent of all Alzheimer's cases occur at a younger age (<65 years). These are usually familial, genetically predisposed, and autosomal dominant with nearly 100% penetrance.[32] The first gene identified for Alzheimer's disease codes for the amyloid-precursor protein (APP), located on chromosome 21.[33]

This mutation is also found in patients with Down syndrome, who typically develop a dementia syndrome early on. There are 16 known mutations on the APP gene, all located in the proximity of the interface of the γ-secretase.[34]

Further genetic changes leading to an early onset of Alzheimer's disease are presenelin1 (PSN1) on chromosome 14 and presenelin2 (PSN2) on chromosome 1. On these two genes, new mutations are continuously being discovered. The number of known mutations with PSN1 already constitutes 130.[34]

The occurrence of Alzheimer's disease in patients older than 65 years may partially be genetically predisposed. However, for the disease to manifest itself, further risk factors are necessary. The apolipoprotein E4 (Apo E4) genotype seems to predispose to later development of Multi-infarct Alzheimer's disease.[35,36] In the Rotterdam study, which included a population-based cohort of approximately 8000 participants, 162 persons had the E4/E4 genotype carrier compared with 3989 E3/E3 carriers, and the E4/E4 genotype was associated with an eight times increased relative risk to develop Alzheimer's disease.[37] Next to Apo E4 , hypercholesterolemia and arterial hypertension are

further independent, additive risk factors. Interestingly enough, the risk accompanying the treatable risk factors is higher than that of ApoE4.[38] Other risk factors include head trauma with loss of consciousness,[39] low literacy, history of depression,[40] female gender,[41] smoking,[42,43] low thyroid-stimulating hormone (TSH) with euthyroid metabolism,[44] hyperlipidemia,[43] and possibly also exposure to organic solvents. Although the study results are partially contradictory in regard to diabetes mellitus as a risk factor for Alzheimer's disease, there are increasing references that insulin resistance may be a risk factor.[45]

Another risk factor is the angiotensin-converting enzyme (ACE) genotype. In a meta-analysis of 23 studies, the risk as a function of the genotype was increased (odds ratio [OR] 1.27, confidence interval [CI] 1,1–1,47).[46] The studies analyzed in this meta-analysis were quite diverse, and the results require further confirmation.

Another controversial topic is whether previous exposure to anesthesia actually affects the onset of Alzheimer's disease and its incidence. So far, results of the few completed studies are contradictory. The few available clinical studies, which actually examined the connection between anesthesia and previous operations, are based on very small patient groups. Besides, none of these are prospective, randomized, and double-blind. Bohnen et al. showed in a retrospective case control study of 252 Alzheimer's patients that neither the cumulative anesthesia time nor the number of anesthetics were associated with an increased risk for Alzheimer's disease.[47] A further case control study of 115 patients confirmed this result.[48] In another study by Bohnen et al., the cumulative anesthesia time (general anesthesia and regional anesthesia combined) before the age of 50 correlates with the age of the confirmed diagnosis of Alzheimer's disease. This study demonstrated a negative correlation, that is, the longer the cumulative anesthesia, the earlier was the onset of Alzheimer's.[49] In summary, these three studies show no effect on the incidence, but a negative correlation in regard to the time of diagnosis, for example, an earlier onset of disease symptoms.[47–49] However, considering the above-mentioned study limitations, this may only be considered a preliminary result.

Pathogenesis

Even today, nearly 100 years after the first description of Alzheimer's disease, science is far from comprehensively understanding the pathogenesis of this illness. In the following section, some current hypotheses are presented which are based on histological investigations of Alzheimer's patients and animal experiments involving transgenic mice with a genetic predisposition to Alzheimer's disease.

Since the discovery of the presence of β amyloid $(A\beta)$[50] in the neuritic plaques, the hypothesis of the amyloid cascade was proposed as a cause for Alzheimer's disease. This means that an imbalance in the $A\beta$ metabolism leads to the aggregation and deposit of $A\beta$ which represents the main cause for neuron failure and neuron dysfunction (see Fig. 27-2) This leads to dementia. $A\beta$ is formed from enzymatic splitting of APP. The proteases involved are the α-, β-, and γ-secretases. The α-secretase splits the larger part of the APP into two longer fragments. A smaller portion of the APP is split by the β- and/or γ-secretases into short peptides, thereby producing the 42 amino acids long split product $A\beta_{1-42}$. $A\beta_{1-42}$ is considered the critical pathophysiological factor in the emergence of Alzheimer's disease. One assumes that in patients suffering from Alzheimer's disease, the equilibrium between splitting is shifted in favor of the latter by the α-secretase and by the β- and/or γ-secretase, resulting in more $A\beta_{1-42}$.

This theory is accepted by most Alzheimer's researchers, although there is one smaller group which considers the neurofibrillary tangles and its main component, tau, central in the pathogenesis of Alzheimer's disease.

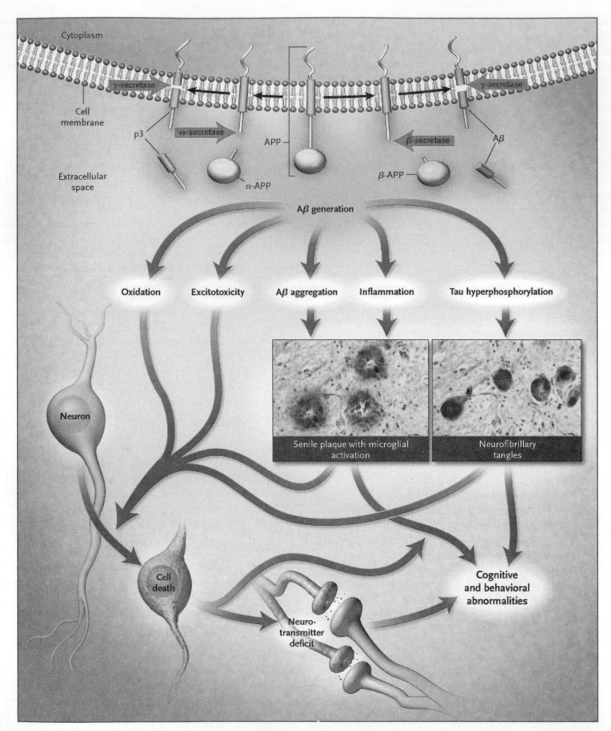

FIGURE 27-2 Pathophysiology of Alzheimer's disease.

Many experimental findings support the Aβ hypothesis. Remarkably, the Alzheimer's disease-related mutations on APP, PSN1, and PSN2 deposit Aβ either by increased production of the pathological $A\beta_{42}$ or by Aβ aggregation. In addition, neuronal degeneration takes place in the proximity of the amyloid plaques, and Aβ can produce in vivo and in vitro neurodegeneration.[51] Because neurodegeneration and inflammation processes can also develop without plaques, it is presently under discussion whether indeed plaques or rather soluble Aβ peptides

and/or Aβ-derived diffusible ligands (ADDLs) cause the pathogenesis of Alzheimer's disease, and later deposits and inflammation processes only constitute the final product of pathogenesis. This hypothesis is supported by animal experimental data with transgenic mice, observing cognitive deficits in those with increased $A\beta_{42}$ levels before amyloid deposits occured.[52] Recently, it was also documented that Aβ is instrumental in the production of neurofibrillary tangles. In summary, the Aβ seems superior to the tau hypothesis.

Secondary consequences seem to be oxidation and fat peroxidation, glutamatergic excitotoxicity, inflammation, and activation of the apoptosis cascade (Fig. 27-2). According to current scientific opinion, cognitive deficits are essentially due to end-stage neuronal failure and imbalance of neurotransmitters.

The cholinergic nervous system has been most intensively investigated. The ascending cholinergic strands degenerate toward the cerebral cortex.[53] Also, acetylcholine depletion has been described.

Pathology

The atrophied brains of Alzheimer's patients are marked by extracellular $A\beta$ deposits, intracellular neurofibrillary tangles, and neuronal losses (see Fig. 27-2), particularly in the hippocampus, the substantia innominata, the locus coeruleus, and the temporoparietal and frontal cortex.[54] An association exists between their spread and density and the character and severity of the dementia.

Amyloid plaques consist of quasicrystalline deposits of $A\beta$.[55] These neuritic plaques are clearly distinguishable from healthy tissue. The neurofibrillary tangles are formed by hyperphosphorylated tau monomers. The tau protein is a component of the neural cytoskeleton. It is an axonal protein involved in microtubule assembly. Normally, an equilibrium exists between the phosphorylated tau protein kinases and dephosphorylated protein phosphatases.

The physiological tau protein is phosphorylated only in five places and can deposit itself on the microtubule. Alzheimer's disease, and other dementia forms, create a surplus of protein kinases; the tau protein is hyperphosphorylated and can no longer bind to microtubules.[56] These hyperphosphorylated tau monomers couple and merge into the double helix (paired helical filament [PHF]). This process is chemically no longer reversible, nor is its pathophysiological correlate. These deposits store themselves in neurons first. After first producing disturbances in cell function, they proceed to cause cell failure.[57]

These deposits lead to progressive neuron loss, beginning in the entorhinal cortex, with eventual spread across the entire brain cortex. The cholinergic system in particular is affected early in this process. Deposits occur years before the initial symptoms first present.[57]

In practice, these histopathological findings are not used in the diagnosis of Alzheimer's as they are only observed postmortem, and although typical, they are not specific to Alzheimer's disease.[58]

The pathophysiological changes with associated deficits in neuronal function, as well as cell failure, lead to alterations of the neurotransmitter systems in the brain. All neurotransmitter systems are not equally stricken. The cholinergic system seems to be affected the greatest.

Mutations of neurotransmitters in the brain of patients with Alzheimer's disease

With Alzheimer's, glucose conversion in the brain is reduced. This is significant for neurotransmission, as the most important cerebral neurotransmitters such as acetylcholine, glutamate, aspartate, γ-aminobutyric acid (GABA), and glycine are synthesized from glucose. With early occurring familial forms, the reduced glucose metabolism does not correlate with reduced oxygen consumption in contrast to later developing forms. It can be deduced that there is no energy deficit with early occurring forms in contrast to later developing forms.[59]

As alluded to previously, different neurotransmitter systems are impaired to various degrees by Alzheimer's disease: cholinergic system > serotonergic system > excitatory amino acids > GABAnergic system > noradrenergic system > neuropeptide > dopaminergic system.[60] Acetylcholine (ACh) contributes substantially to learning and memory processes,[61] and regulates with noradrenaline, the regional microcirculation in the brain.[62] With Alzheimer's, severe degenerative changes are observed in the cholinergic transmitter system.

The most stricken are the long cholinergic ascending fiber systems which originate from the nucleus basalis of Meynert and target cortical regions as well as strands from the medial septum core to the hippocampus.[63] The number of nicotinic acetylcholine receptors (nAChR) is reduced in the cerebral cortex of Alzheimer's patients.[64] Also, the muscarinic AChR seems affected by the reduced number of receptors. Additional to the reduction of receptor density, less ACh is being produced. This lack of ACh correlates with the severity of the dementia.[65] It is possible that the downward regulation of the nicotinic AChR precedes neurodegeneration. One $A\beta$ binds to seven nAChR, whereby the Ca^{++} influx and the ACh release are decreased. Consecutive reduction of the nicotinic signal transduction and an increased vulnerability of neurons are among some of the factors which explain the deficits in memory function.[66,67]

Serotonergic fiber systems of the raphe nucleus are severely affected by neurodegenerative processes. Interestingly, serotonin transmission rises with the reduced number of receptors.[63]

A short pulsating release of glutamate is necessary for important processes of learning and memory,[68] whereas a prolonged release of glutamate may be excitotoxic,[69] and cause cell failure. Glutamate can affect N-methyl-D-aspartate (NMDA), α-amino-3-hydroxy-5-methyl-4-isoxazole propionic acid (AMPA), kainate, or mGluR1 receptors with neurotoxic consequences. The selective neuronal cell death with Alzheimer's disease, however, is essentially caused by NMDA receptor activation.[70] By inhibiting the NMDA receptor-dependent neurotransmission, $A\beta$ can impair the synaptic plasticity in the brain, and thus affect learning and memory processes.[71]

The glutamatergic system of the brain is substantially impaired with Alzheimer's disease. The number of NMDA receptors is severely reduced.[72] Some studies demonstrated a reduction of the glutamine synthetase and of the glutamate transportation by $A\beta$, whereby reduced reabsorption of glutamate could lead to increased glutamate levels, and thus to cytotoxicity.[71] Glutamate is decarboxylated to GABA. Messenger RNA (mRNA) expression of the glutamate decarboxylase in Alzheimer's disease patients is about 50% higher,[73] which causes increased GABA-ergic neurotransmission.[74] One theory asserts that the increased GABA levels affect presynaptic GABA type A ($GABA_A$) receptors causing chronic depolarization block and subsequent neuronal destruction. GABA-ergic deafferentation develops along with degeneration of neural systems.[75] Some authors attribute the reduced number of $GABA_A$ receptors primarily to a reduction of the total number of neurons caused by generalized neurodegeneration. Other researchers showed a reduction of the $GABA_A$ receptors[76] in several postmortem studies, particularly in cortical structures themselves. It seems that there is not a generalized reduction of the $GABA_A$ receptors, but the specific reduction of individual subunits, for example, the a5 subunit.[77,78]

Diagnosis

Although the diagnosis of Alzheimer's disease is clinically derived, the final confirmation rate is rather high. In one study, the clinical diagnosis of Alzheimer's disease was histologically confirmed after death in 92 of 106 patients (87%).[79] The basis of a dementia diagnosis is the criteria.[1]

The diagnosis of Alzheimer's disease is based on criteria by the United States of America National Institutes of Health-National

Institute of Neurology and Communicative Disorders and Stroke.[80] In accordance, the diagnosis is divided into three groups: definite (clinical diagnosis with histological confirmation), probable (typical clinical symptoms without histological confirmation), possible (e.g., typical clinical symptoms but no differential diagnosis possible, no histological confirmation).

The typical sensitivity and specificity for the diagnosis of a probable Alzheimer's disease using these criteria is about 0.65 and 0.75.[81] The classical symptoms are memory loss,[82] speech difficulties,[83] visual/spatial deficit,[84,85] as well as affective disorders and abnormal social behavior. Changes in motor abilities, senses, gait instability, and convulsions do rarely occur in the final stage of the illness.[80] At the beginning of the disease, higher activities of daily living are impaired, for example, writing out bank checks or using public transportation; with the illness progressing, additional, simple activities of daily living are affected such as food intake, hygiene, and the use of a toilet.[86] During the progression of the illness, behavior disturbances increase.[87] Personality changes and apathy are noticeable early on, and are permanent. Only in the later phases of the illness do patients exhibit psychotic symptoms, becoming agitated, sometimes even aggressive.[88]

According to the International Statistical Classification of Diseases, 10th revision (ICD-10), three severity levels are distinguished[89]:

▶ Slight: lowered learning of new material; with still independent lives, complicated daily tasks or leisure activities are no longer possible.

▶ Moderate: only well-learned and familiar material remembered, new information can be kept only briefly, memories are clouded; independent life hardly still possible, everyday life activities strongly reduced.

▶ Severe: heavy memory loss and inability to retain new information, only fragments of long-term memory remain; void of comprehensible trains of thought.

When suspecting Alzheimer's disease, a thorough history provides important clues for the diagnosis. As Alzheimer's patients frequently deny cognitive problems, significant attention is given to family members' observations. If patients themselves report cognitive losses, another cause for the symptoms is assumed; most frequently depression is the basis. Despite increasing advances in imaging procedures, the diagnostic algorithm for Alzheimer's begins with a cognitive test battery. It is important to consider the previously existing cognitive status and education, since a relative deficit in a well-educated person does not automatically lead to an absolute, measurable deficit. In contrast, a low intelligence could lead to an overinterpretation of cognitive deficits. Therefore, the evaluation of cognitive abilities is of importance in the process. Most frequently, the MMST[12] and the user-friendly Mini-Cog Test are used.

It is recommended to preclude vitamin B_{12} deficiency and hypothyroidism[90] by laboratory testing. Routinely, a blood screen is administered[90] to determine urea, electrolytes, blood sugar, and liver function parameters in the serum. There are typical changes in the cerebrospinal fluid of Alzheimer's patients. The level of the tau protein is increased[91] and the level of Aβ with the protein end of 42 (Aβ_{42}) is decreased.[92,93] In one study, the measurement of these proteins showed a positive predictive value of over 90% for Alzheimer's disease. Other studies examined the ratios of tau and Aβ_{42},[94] and demonstrated that the tau protein—contrary to Aβ_{42}—can differentiate between Alzheimer's disease and Lewy body dementia.[95] A definitive role of these levels in the cerebrospinal fluid is not yet clarified for the diagnosis of Alzheimer's disease.[96]

The role of diagnostic imaging is unclear. Presently, despite insufficient evidence, a computed tomography (CT) investigation of the brain or a magnetic resonance tomography (MRT) is recommended.[90] At the beginning of a dementia workup, it should be emphasized, as previously mentioned, that diagnostic criteria are sufficient for diagnosis of Alzheimer's disease without additional imaging. However, this does not apply to the early forms, which in the future may first be diagnosed with advanced imaging procedures, and then possibly treated at an earlier stage.[97,98] Further indications are the exclusion of structural causes for dementia, for example, chronic subdural hematoma, cerebrovascular changes, including stroke and tumors. The typical, radiologic changes with Alzheimer's disease are initially an atrophy of the entorhinal cortex, followed by extension into other limbic structures such as amygdala and hippocampus. Progressively larger structures also atrophy, for example, a majority of the cortical areas of the temporal and parietal lobes as well as the frontal lobe.[99] Because with Alzheimer's disease, brain metabolism is clearly reduced, positron emission tomography (PET) offers a sensitive procedure for imaging these changes. A study of 146 patients with cognitive deficits showed a promising sensitivity for Alzheimer's and other neurodegenerative diseases. The progression of cognitive deficits after a negative PET scan was near absent over a 3-year follow-up.[100] In a more recent study, the advantage of PET scans was demonstrated over standard cognitive tests during the early phase of Alzheimer's disease.[101] As long as there are only symptomatic and no definitive therapies for Alzheimer's disease, such investigations might add to the worry of patients, and should therefore only be administered if necessary with discretion and for prevention studies.

Therapy, pharmaceutical intervention

The therapy of Alzheimer's disease can be grouped into experimental and established procedures. However, even with established pharmaceuticals, only a stabilization of the process and/or a delay in progression of the illness is possible. Presently, a chance for cure does not exist. At this time, acetyl cholinesterase inhibitors are the standard therapy for slight to moderate cases of Alzheimer's disease.[102,103] With Alzheimer's disease, this therapeutic concept is based on the fact that by inhibition of acetyl cholinesterase the concentration of ACh in the synaptic gap increases, thereby increasing cholinergic transmission despite depletion of ACh receptors, leading to improvement of cognitive function. Because of minor toxicity and a longer duration of effectiveness, now only anticholinergics of the second generation such as donepezil, rivastigmine, and galantamine are prescribed. These pharmaceuticals can slow the degeneration of cognitive abilities and behavioral symptoms.[104]

The NMDA receptor antagonist Memantine is the second most frequently used antidementia drug. This medicine is used for moderate to severe stages. It is assumed that Memantine reduces glutamatergic excitotoxicity, and can positively affect the functioning of hippocampus neurons.[105] Since Memantine acts as a noncompetitive antagonist, the NMDA receptors remain fully available for glutamate-induced learning and memory processes, but protected from the excitatory effects of glutamate. In a randomized double-blind study, the advantage of Memantine over a placebo was well-documented with moderate to severe stages of Alzheimer's disease.[106] Also, combining Memantine with acetyl cholinesterase inhibitors has proven successful.[107] The extent of clinical improvement with Memantine is limited. Only minor improvements or stabilization of the disease were accomplished. Side effects were rarely observed.

The most frequently used nonspecific nootropic is *Ginkgo biloba* special extract. It causes a strong inhibition of the free radical-induced lipid peroxidation (radical inhibitors), membrane stabilization, normalization of the cerebral energy metabolism after hypoxic damage, antagonistic effects on platelet-activating factor (PAF), as well as a possible influence on the aggregation of Aβ.[108]

Newer therapy initiatives are less concerned with controlling the symptoms, but aim to delay the underlying neurodegenerative processes of the illness. These newer approaches have applied advances in knowledge over the emergence and pathophysiology of Alzheimer's disease. Referring to the pathophysiology discussed above, there are many therapy innovations (see Table 27-1). A very promising concept is immunization with Aβ.[114] Due to some cases of encephalitis, a clinical study was terminated.[113] However, the analysis of the remaining patients concluded that those who had formed antibodies against Aβ had slowed the progression of the disease.[112] Anti-inflammatory therapy with nonsteroidal anti-inflammatory drugs (NSAIDs) (diclofenac,[118] rofecoxib, and naproxen[117]) or prednisone[116] could not demonstrate an advantage over placebo, and is not recommended at this time. Epidemiological data suggest a possible benefit of an estrogen replacement for postmenopausal women. Randomized placebo-controlled clinical studies could not determine any benefit of such therapy.[120,121] One study even documented negative effects from estrogen administration.[123] Therefore, estrogen replacement is, at present, not recommended. Therapy with GABA$_A$ agonists is also conceivable, since GABA$_A$ activation reduces the neurotoxicity resulting from Aβ.[124] Additionally, it has been shown that the GABA$_A$ agonists carbamazepine, phenytoin, and valproic acid reduce neurotoxic effects of Aβ by stabilization of intracellular calcium levels.[125]

However, clinical trials of Alzheimer's therapy with GABA$_A$ agonists showed improvement of the psychomotor symptoms, for example, agitation or fear rather than that of cognitive abilities.[76]

This is even more surprising given that with Alzheimer's patients, postsynaptic GABA$_A$ receptors and interstitial GABA$_A$ levels increase, and thereby induce chronic depolarization and neural degeneration.[71] Indeed, Fastbom's study reports protective effects of benzodiazepines by influencing GABA$_A$ receptors with potentiation of GABA$_A$-ergic neurotransmission, causing glutamatergic inhibition and thus neuroprotection.[126]

Apart from the therapy of cognitive deficits with Alzheimer's disease, treatment is also targeted toward neuropsychiatric symptoms, as they occur in at least 80% of all Alzheimer's patients.[88] These behavioral symptoms are initially not pharmacologically treated, but when they are persistent and cause further impairment of the patient (not the responsible guardian!) one adopts drug therapy. Since there are few substantial randomized studies for the therapy of behavioral symptoms,[104] one must evaluate the recommendations of smaller, partially nonrandomized studies. The indications and reciprocal effects with anesthesia are shown for the individual substance groups in Table 27-2.

ANESTHESIA PREPARATION

First, it is important to identify the demented patient, since up to 75% of dementia cases are not recognized by the family doctor.[11] Additionally, if suspected, the anesthetist can administer the Mini-Cog Test. With clearly demented and/or already diagnosed patients, the preanesthetic consultation must be conducted with sensitivity and patience. The time span, in which demented patients can concentrate, is usually reduced. Patients become frequently annoyed with repeated posing of questions, or if they feel that they cannot answer them. Repeated questions may also create the impression that the anesthetist is incompetent, arousing more uncertainties in the patient. Even if the anesthetist addresses questions to family members or the responsible guardian, demented patients may quickly become agitated. In such cases, it is best to settle the patient by having them perform a concrete task, which might as well be part of a cognitive test. Nevertheless, it is essential to speak with family members, since the patient frequently is not competent to answer anesthesia-related questions in regard to medical and drug history. Also, it is imperative to secure a legal guardian's consent for these patients, except in emergency situations.

During the anesthesia preparation of patients with Lewy body dementia, as with patients with Parkinson's, typical cardiopulmonary and gastroenterological problems have to be considered: specifically swallowing, apnea due to autonomic dysfunction, and lack of muscle control in the upper respiratory system, thereby increasing the risk of aspiration. Moreover, thoracic rigidity, as well as orthostatic hypotension occur frequently.[127]

Anti-Parkinson medication should be administered just before the operation and as immediately as possible afterwards, because L-dopa has a very short half-life (1–3 hours). Unfortunately, the medication is only available orally. Frequently, patients with Alzheimer's received acetyl cholinesterase inhibitors. Particularly at the beginning of therapy, one needs to ask about symptoms of gastrointestinal side effects. Depending on which medications are taken, one can count on 17–48% of patients experiencing nausea and 10–27% vomiting, along with the associated aspiration risk in the context of anesthesia and/or an electrolyte imbalance. Of all acetyl cholinesterase inhibitors, donepezil has the smallest emetic potential.[128–130] Some important medications used in dementia therapy and their preoperative are shown in Table 27-2.

Table 27-1

Possible Therapeutic Approaches in Therapy of Alzheimer's Disease

Pathophysiology	Potential Intervention Options
Increased production of Aβ	α-Secretase activators β-Secretase inhibitors[109] γ-Secretase inhibitors[110] Statin therapy[111]
Increased deposit of Aβ	Amyloid immunization[112–114] Chelating agents (clioquinol)[115] Activation of proteins which dismantle amyloid plaques
Tau hyperphosphorylation	GSK (tau protein kinase-I-glycogensynthasekinase-3b)-inhibitors Lithium
Local inflammation reaction	Nonsteroidal anti-inflammatory agents[116–118]
Oxidative damage	Antioxidants (vitamin E,[119] estrogen[120,121])
Nerve cell loss	NGF (nerve growth factor), NGF-producing implants, NGF stimulators

Source: From Ref. 122.

Table 27-2

Therapy of Behavioral and Psychic Symptoms of Dementia

Target Symptoms	Substance Group	Medication (Example)	Interactions with General Anesthesia
Cognitive deficiency	Acetylcholinesterase inhibitors	Donepezil, rivastigmine, galantamine	Increased sensitivity with muscle relaxants and lengthening of the neuromuscular blockade Increased cholinergic side effects in patients taking cholinergic agents and β-receptor blockers.
Cognitive deficiency	NMDA-receptor-antagonists	Memantine	Side effects of anticholinergics and dopaminergic agonists increased, decreased effects of barbiturates and neuroleptics
Aggression, paranoid syndrome, anxiety/restlessness, (hallucinations)	Atypical narcoleptics	Risperidone, olanzapine	Inhibitor of α-adrenergic, cholinergic, and dopaminergic Receptors Vasodilatation, hypotension risk with inhalation anesthetics, spinal anesthesia, or volume loss ↑
Motor or fearful anxiety, (aggression)	Classic, low, and medium potent neuroleptics	Melperone, pipamperone	
Hallucinations, paranoid syndrome, (aggression, anxiety)	Classic, highly potent neuroleptic	Haloperidol	Sedative and hypnotic indications?
Fear, (agitation, strain/stress, panic)	Benzodiazepines	Alprazolam, lorazepam, buspirone	Increased effect of anesthetics
Depressive symptoms, fear, (decrease of motivation, loss of initiative)	Serotonin reuptake inhibitor	Sertraline, citalopram	Catecholamine reuptake reduced Effect of indirect sympathomimetics reduced, direct sympathomimetics increased; increased effect of opiates, hypnotics, sedatives Combination with serotoninergic agonists to be avoided (serotonin syndrome)
	Nontricyclic antidepressives	Trazodone	
Agitation, (aggression, various behavioral symptoms)	Anticonvulsives	Carbamazepine, zolpidem	Interactions with barbiturates, relaxants, and opioids
Sleep disturbances, disruption in sleep and wake cycles	Neuroleptics	Melperone prothipendyl	

Source: From Ref. 108.

Premedication should be considered only with appreciation of drug interactions. Slight sedation with benzodiazepine is often indicated in these patients. Due to increased risk of aspiration, an antacid may be advantageous with Parkinson-associated Lewy body dementia. For these patients, metoclopramide and droperidol are contraindicated due to their antidopaminergic action.[127]

TYPE OF ANESTHESIA

The advantages or disadvantages of either regional or general anesthesia for demented patients have yet to be investigated. However, a meta-analysis of 24 studies examining the postoperative incidence of cognitive deficits after spinal versus general anesthesia did not demonstrate any advantages of either anesthetic technique.[131] This confirms the results of the largest study to date with 438 elderly patients.[132] Ultimately, the anesthetist weighs the decision for or against a regional technique based on individual medical history and the patient's ability to cooperate. The possible influences of various general anesthesia procedures (total intravenous anesthesia vs. balanced anesthesia with volatile anesthetics) on the dementia process are not yet known.

INDUCTION AND MAINTENANCE OF GENERAL ANESTHESIA

A specific type of anesthesia induction is not required with dementia patients except to bear in mind possible alterations in pharmacokinetics as a result of patient's medical history, age, and characteristics. Patients with Parkinson-associated Lewy body dementia do require attention. Their increased risk of aspiration warrants a rapid sequence induction. With Parkinson's it is critical to avoid medications which lead to an exacerbation of the illness, for example, phenothiazine, butyrophenone (inclusive DHBP), and metoclopramide. With patients who take monoamine oxidase (MAO) inhibitors, one needs to be aware of medication interactions with anesthetics.[133] Inhalation anesthetics have complex effects on dopamine concentrations in the brain. They inhibit synaptosomal dopamine transport and increase the extracellular dopamine concentration, which in turn may depress transmission.[134]

Due to the smaller arrhythmogenicity, newer inhalation anesthetics (with exception of desflurane) should be used. Among intravenous anesthetics, propofol exhibits, in theory, the most favorable side-effect profile in regard to Parkinson's disease. However, there have also been reports of ketamine use without problems. Ketamine, in theory, may be contraindicated, based on its sympathomimetic characteristics.[135] Individual case reports describe parkinsonian effects with thiopental, a reason why this intravenous anesthetic should not be used.[58] Regarding muscle relaxants, including succinylcholine, there are no restrictions.[133] Muscle rigidity, as described in healthy patients after opioids, is most likely caused by presynaptic inhibition of dopamine release.[136] Indeed, these symptoms have been observed after opioid administration, particularly higher morphine dosages.[133]

For other dementia forms, there are presently no universal recommendations regarding general anesthesia. In patients with vascular dementia, the particulars of medical history have to be examined. During anesthesia and surgery, patients of similar risk profile (arterial hypertension, diabetes, and arteriosclerosis) are essentially treated like all other vascular patients. Specifically, the mean arterial blood pressure should not deviate any more than ± 20% from the average value of the last days, so as not to risk decreased brain perfusion, due to modified autoregulation by the arterial hyper tension in the brain.

Apart from gastrointestinal side effects of acetyl cholinesterase inhibitors, they also significantly affect the duration of muscle relaxants in Alzheimer's patients. The effective onset of succinylcholine is shortened and the effective duration is extended. In addition, other cholinergic side effects may occur, for example, bradycardia and hypotonia. This may be especially prominent in patients already taking cholinergic agents and β-receptor blockers.[108]

With patients taking Memantine, the side effects of L-dopa, dopaminergic agonists and anticholinergics may be enhanced. The effect of barbiturates and neuroleptics can be weakened. Due to the danger of a drug-induced psychosis, ketamine is ill-advised with patients taking Memantine.

Generally, elderly patients require fewer anesthetic medications due to alterations in pharmacokinetics and pharmacodynamics. Since with older patients the minimum alveolar concentration (MAC) is reduced, it can be assumed generally also .[137] The need for intravenous anesthetics is generally lower with older patients.[138]

The half-life of various medications commonly given by anesthesiologists such as diazepam, digoxin, lidocaine, vecuronium, aminoglycoside, and propanolol is altered as a result of an increased volume of distribution and reduced renal and hepatic elimination. Albumin synthesis is lower with elderly patients, whereas the alpha glycoprotein synthesis is increased. This would modify the bioavailability of a multitude of protein-bound medications.[139]

A further important question is with regard to the potential pharmacodynamics of different sedatives, hypnotics, and opioids caused by the mutated receptor composition in the brain of demented patients. Generally, the sensitivity of most receptors, including β-adrenergic, seems to be reduced. β-Adrenergic receptors are endogenously blocked, which leads to a reduced response both with agonist and antagonist medications.[137]

According to most recent investigations, volatile anesthetics directly affect various receptors in brain and spinal cord.[140] With Alzheimer's disease, these receptors are frequently changed in quantity, composition, and regional distribution. This may result in modified pharmacodynamics of volatile anesthetics. GABA is the most important inhibiting neurotransmitter in the brain. GABA$_A$ receptors are activated exactly the same by volatile anesthetics, as the similarly inhibiting glycine receptors. The GABA$_A$ receptors are reduced in Alzheimer's disease, and could thus cause increased neural activity. In order to counteract this effect, an increased concentration of volatile

anesthetic would be needed. Actually, an increased MAC-value for isoflurane was discovered when studying transgenic mice with predisposition to Alzheimer's disease.[141] However, whether these animal results can be transferred to humans requires further investigation.

In contrast, the brain-activating nAChR are inhibited by volatile anesthetics. This could reduce the existing, diminished cholinergic neurotransmission even further, and possibly worsen cognitive function. This contradicts some clinical[47,48] and one experimental[142] study.

The excitatory glutamate receptors (NMDA, AMPA, kainic acid) are inhibited by volatile anesthetics. The inhibition on the NMDA receptor could again affect cognition favorably, because the NMDA-receptor antagonist (e.g., Memantine) plays a substantial role in the therapy of moderate to severe forms of dementia. This would confirm the results of the previously mentioned studies.

The multiple interactions of different neurotransmitter systems in a healthy person are complex, and are not yet completely understood despite today's intensive research. Also, the exact actions of volatile and other anesthetics still are the subject of current investigations. It is very difficult to study the consequences of alterations in neurotransmission as occur in Alzheimer's and other diseases, for example, their effect on anesthesia, and vice versa, their effect on dementia. Initially, animal experiments and hopefully future clinical studies will provide more explanations, despite difficult challenges.

REGIONAL ANESTHESIA

There are no investigations specifically examining the effects of regional anesthesia on demented patients. Due to possible changes in peripheral neurotransmission, specific changes in the effects of local anesthetics are to be anticipated, although without appropriate studies this remains speculation.

Until such investigations are made, the administration of regional anesthesia in demented patients is exactly like any other elderly patient, according to their age and circumstances. Thus, a somewhat higher level of block results with older patients with spinal anesthesia, despite adjustment to individual body size.

POSTOPERATIVE MANAGEMENT

The principal question for elderly patients is whether an anesthetic affects postoperative intellectual capacity, and whether this effect is limited to general anesthesia or also applies to regional anesthesia. Moreover, it is important to examine how particular patients with preexisting cognitive deficits respond to anesthesia, and whether a previous anesthetic exposure can cause future dementia syndromes. There are no investigations into anesthesia effects on postoperative cognitive abilities in Parkinson's patients; however, an increased incidence of postoperative hallucinations and confusion are reported.[143] This could also be relevant to the Parkinson-associated Lewy body dementia.

Examination of postoperative cognitive deficits (POCD) suggests that exposure to general anesthesia is a possible risk factor for cognitive deficits. POCD occurs at a frequency of 25.8% 1 week after the operation, and then at 9.9% 3 months later.[144] The anesthesia is usually blamed without considering other possible POCD causes, for example, the operation, the hospital transport, infections, or the underlying disease. Unfortunately, a preexisting cognitive deficit often represents an exclusion criterion for such studies. Only one investigation into POCD also included patients with preexisting cognitive deficits, and determined an increased risk for POCD in this group, exactly as for patients with depression and over 75 years of age.[145] However, the study included only 140 patients and the result may not be representative. In addition, the cause of POCD could not be clarified.

An increased cumulative number of anesthetics and thus an extended anesthetic exposure time leads, according to a few, smaller retrospective studies, to an earlier onset of Alzheimer's disease, but not to an increased incidence.[47–49] Finally, the question whether anesthesia accelerates or facilitates the occurrence of Alzheimer's disease cannot be clarified with the patient, since Alzheimer's patients are usually operated on as emergencies and are not able to consent.

An elective study of anesthesia without operation in order to examine the pure anesthetic effect is not plausible. The only randomized double-blind study, which investigated the sole influence of an isoflurane monoanesthesia on cognition, was accordingly performed with transgenic mice (APP23 of mice), predisposed to develop Alzheimer's disease. Interestingly, this study demonstrated that a 2-hour anesthetic with 1 MAC isoflurane improved the cognitive abilities of the Alzheimer's mice. This improvement was assessed as a reduction, as with Alzheimer's patients, of their fearfulness.[142] These results from the animal laboratory cannot be directly transferred to humans, rather they permit the conclusion along with the results of clinical studies, that according to current scientific evidence, anesthetics do not appear to be harmful.

KEY POINTS

▶ The various forms of dementia include Alzheimer's disease, vascular-mediated or multi-infarct dementia, Parkinson's and associated dementia (including Lewy body dementia and progressive supranuclear paralysis), frontal dementia, and reversible dementia. Alzheimer's disease is the most frequent cause of dementia and accounts for 60–80% of diagnoses.

▶ The diagnosis of dementia is obtained clinically, using cognitive tests.

▶ The cause of Alzheimer's disease is multifactorial. The most significant risk factor to develop this illness is, and remains, older age. It is established that there is a genetic component to the pathogenesis of Alzheimer's disease. It is also possible to differentiate between genetic risk factors responsible for either the late or the early onset of Alzheimer's disease.

▶ Many experimental findings support the β-amyloid hypothesis as the cause of Alzheimer's.

▶ The atrophied brains of Alzheimer's patients are marked by extracellular β-amyloid deposits, intracellular neurofibrillary tangles, and neuronal losses particularly in the hippocampus, the substantia innominata, the locus coeruleus, and the temporoparietal and frontal cortex.

▶ Different neurotransmitter systems are impaired to various degrees by Alzheimer's disease: cholinergic system > serotonergic system > excitatory amino acids > GABAnergic system > noradrenergic system > neuropeptide > dopaminergic system.

▶ At this time, acetyl cholinesterase inhibitors are the standard therapy for slight to moderate cases of Alzheimer's disease. The NMDA receptor antagonist Memantine is the second most frequently used antidementia drug. The most frequently used nonspecific nootropic is *Ginkgo biloba* special extract. Apart from the

therapy of cognitive deficits with Alzheimer's disease, treatment is also targeted towards neuropsychiatric symptoms, as they occur in at least 80% of all Alzheimer's patients.

▶ The principle question for elderly patients is whether an anesthetic affects postoperative intellectual capacity, and whether this effect is limited to general anesthesia or also applies to regional anesthesia. Moreover, it is important to examine how particular patients with preexisting cognitive deficits respond to anesthesia, and whether a previous anesthetic exposure can cause future dementia syndromes. Both animal and clinical studies suggest that anesthetics do not appear to be harmful.

KEY ARTICLES

▶ Corey-Bloom J. The ABC of Alzheimer's disease: cognitive changes and their management in Alzheimer's disease and related dementias. *Int Psychogeriatr.* 2002;14(Suppl. 1):51–75.

▶ Cummings JL. Alzheimer's disease. *N Engl J Med.* 2004;351:56–67.

REFERENCES

1. DSM-IV-TR, APA Press, Washington DC, 2000.
2. Sloane PD, Zimmerman S, Suchindran C, et al. The public health impact of Alzheimer's disease, 2000–2050: potential implication of treatment advances. *Ann Rev Public Health.* 2002;23:213–231.
3. Bickel H. Dementia syndrome and Alzheimer disease: an assessment of morbidity and annual incidence in Germany. *Gesundheitswesen.* 2000;62:211–218.
4. Lämmler G, Herms J, Hanke B. Demenz. In: Hanke B. (Hrsg) Neurogeriatrie auf einen Blick. Berlin: Blackwell Verlag; 2003.
5. Whitehouse PJ. Pharmacoeconomics of dementia. *Alzheimer Dis Assoc Disord.* 1997;11(Suppl. 5):S22–S32; discussion S-3.
6. Hallauer J, Schons M, Smala A, Berger K. Untersuchung von Krankheitskosten bei Patienten mit Alzheimer-Erkrankung in Deutschland. Gesundhökon Qualmanag; 2000;5:73–S79.
7. Hallauer J, Berger K, Ruckdäschl S. Nationale und internationale Untersuchungsergebnisse. In: Kurz A (Hrsg). *Weißbuch Demenz.* Stuttgart: Thieme; 2002:20–S23.
8. Petersen RC, Smith G, Kokmen E, et al. Memory function in normal aging. *Neurology.* 1992;42:396–401.
9. Bachman DL, Wolf PA, Linn R, et al. Prevalence of dementia and probable senile dementia of the Alzheimer type in the Framingham Study. *Neurology.* 1992;42:115–119.
10. Rahkonen T, Eloniemi-Sulkava U, Rissanen S, et al. Dementia with Lewy bodies according to the consensus criteria in a general population aged 75 years or older. *J Neurol Neurosurg Psychiatry.* 2003;74: 720–724.
11. Gifford DR, Cummings JL. Evaluating dementia screening tests: methodologic standards to rate their performance. *Neurology.* 1999;52: 224–227.
12. Folstein MF, Folstein SE, McHugh PR. "Mini-mental state." A practical method for grading the cognitive state of patients for the clinician. *J Psychiatr Res.* 1975;12:189–198.
13. Crum RM, Anthony JC, Bassett SS, Folstein MF. Population-based norms for the Mini-Mental State Examination by age and educational level. *JAMA.* 1993;269:2386–2391.
14. Freidl W, Schmidt R, Stronegger WJ, et al. Mini mental state examination: influence of sociodemographic, environmental and behavioral factors and vascular risk factors. *J Clin Epidemiol.* 1996;49:73–78.
15. Borson S, Scanlan J, Brush M, et al. The mini-cog: a cognitive "vital signs" measure for dementia screening in multi-lingual elderly. *Int J Geriatr Psychiatry.* 2000;15:1021–1027.
16. Borson S, Scanlan JM, Chen P, Ganguli M. The Mini-Cog as a screen for dementia: validation in a population-based sample. *J Am Geriatr Soc.* 2003;51:1451–1454.
17. Hachinski VC, Iliff LD, Zilhka E, et al. Cerebral blood flow in dementia. *Arch Neurol.* 1975;32:632–637.

18. White L, Petrovitch H, Hardman J, et al. Cerebrovascular pathology and dementia in autopsied Honolulu-Asia Aging Study participants. *Ann N Y Acad Sci.* 2002;977:9–23.
19. Aarsland D, Andersen K, Larsen JP, et al. Risk of dementia in Parkinson's disease: a community-based, prospective study. *Neurology.* 2001;56:730–736.
20. Stern Y, Marder K, Tang MX, Mayeux R. Antecedent clinical features associated with dementia in Parkinson's disease. *Neurology.* 1993;43: 1690–1692.
21. McKeith IG, Galasko D, Kosaka K, et al. Consensus guidelines for the clinical and pathologic diagnosis of dementia with Lewy bodies (DLB): report of the consortium on DLB international workshop. *Neurology.* 1996;47:1113–1124.
22. Ferman TJ, Smith GE, Boeve BF, et al. DLB fluctuations: specific features that reliably differentiate DLB from AD and normal aging. *Neurology.* 2004;62:181–187.
23. Clinical and neuropathological criteria for frontotemporal dementia. The Lund and Manchester Groups. *J Neurol Neurosurg Psychiatry.* 1994; 57:416–418.
24. Neary D, Snowden JS, Northen B, Goulding P. Dementia of frontal lobe type. *J Neurol Neurosurg Psychiatry.* 1988;51:353–361.
25. Clarfield AM. The reversible dementias: do they reverse? *Ann Intern Med.* 1988;109:476–486.
26. Alzheimer A. Über eine eigenartige Erkrankung der Hirnrinde. Allgemeine Zeitschrift fur Psychiatrie und Psychisch-gerichtliche Medizin. 1997;64:146–148.
27. Hebert LE, Scherr PA, Bienias JL, et al. Alzheimer disease in the US population: prevalence estimates using the 2000 census. *Arch Neurol.* 2003; 60:1119–1122.
28. Evans DA. The epidemiology of dementia and Alzheimer's disease: an evolving field. *J Am Geriatr Soc.* 1996;44:1482–1483.
29. Hebert LE, Scherr PA, Beckett LA, et al. Age-specific incidence of Alzheimer's disease in a community population. *JAMA.* 1995;273: 1354–1359.
30. van Duijn CM, Clayton D, Chandra V, et al. Familial aggregation of Alzheimer's disease and related disorders: a collaborative re-analysis of case-control studies. EURODEM Risk Factors Research Group. *Int J Epidemiol.* 1991;20(Suppl. 2):S13–S20.
31. Green RC, Cupples LA, Go R, et al. Risk of dementia among White and African American relatives of patients with Alzheimer disease. *JAMA.* 2002;287:329–336.
32. Higgins GA, Jacobsen H. Transgenic mouse models of Alzheimer's disease: phenotype and application. *Behav Pharmacol.* 2003;14:419–438.
33. Tanzi RE, Gusella JF, Watkins PC, et al. Amyloid beta protein gene: cDNA, mRNA distribution, and genetic linkage near the Alzheimer locus. *Science.* 1987;235:880–884.
34. Bertram L, Tanzi RE. The current status of Alzheimer's disease genetics: what do we tell the patients? *Pharmacol Res.* 2004;50:385–396.
35. Corder EH, Saunders AM, Strittmatter WJ, et al. Gene dose of apolipoprotein E type 4 allele and the risk of Alzheimer's disease in late onset families. *Science.* 1993;261:921–923.
36. Henderson AS, Easteal S, Jorm AF, et al. Apolipoprotein E allele epsilon 4, dementia, and cognitive decline in a population sample. *Lancet.* 1995; 346:1387–1390.
37. Slooter AJ, Cruts M, Hofman A, et al. The impact of APOE on myocardial infarction, stroke, and dementia: the Rotterdam Study. *Neurology.* 2004;62:1196–1198.
38. Kivipelto M, Helkala EL, Laakso MP, et al. Apolipoprotein E epsilon4 allele, elevated midlife total cholesterol level, and high midlife systolic blood pressure are independent risk factors for late-life Alzheimer disease. *Ann Intern Med.* 2002;137:149–155.
39. Fleminger S, Oliver DL, Lovestone S, et al. Head injury as a risk factor for Alzheimer's disease: the evidence 10 years on; a partial replication. *J Neurol Neurosurg Psychiatry.* 2003;74:857–862.
40. Green RC, Cupples LA, Kurz A, Auerbach S, Go R, Sadovnick D, Duara R, Kukull WA, Chui H, Edeki T, Griffith PA, Friedland RP, Bachman D, Farrer L (2003) Depression as a risk factor for Alzheimer disease: the MIRAGE Study. Arch Neurol 60:753-9.
41. Fratiglioni L, Grut M, Forsell Y, et al. Prevalence of Alzheimer's disease and other dementias in an elderly urban population: relationship with age, sex, and education. *Neurology.* 1991;41: 1886–1892.

42. Juan D, Zhou DH, Li J, et al. A 2-year follow-up study of cigarette smoking and risk of dementia. *Eur J Neurol.* 2004;11:277–282.
43. Luchsinger JA, Mayeux R. Cardiovascular risk factors and Alzheimer's disease. *Curr Atheroscler Rep.* 2004;6:261–266.
44. van Osch LA, Hogervorst E, Combrinck M, Smith AD. Low thyroid-stimulating hormone as an independent risk factor for Alzheimer disease. *Neurology.* 2004;62:1967–1971.
45. Craft S, Watson GS. Insulin and neurodegenerative disease: shared and specific mechanisms. *Lancet Neurol.* 2004;3:169–178.
46. Elkins JS, Douglas VC, Johnston SC. Alzheimer disease risk and genetic variation in ACE: a meta-analysis. *Neurology.* 2004;62:363–368.
47. Bohnen NI, Warner MA, Kokmen E, et al. Alzheimer's disease and cumulative exposure to anesthesia: a case-control study [see comments]. *J Am Geriatr Soc.* 1994;42:198–201.
48. Gasparini M, Vanacore N, Schiaffini C, et al. A case-control study on Alzheimer's disease and exposure to anesthesia. *Neurol Sci.* 2002;23: 11–14.
49. Bohnen N, Warner MA, Kokmen E, Kurland LT. Early and midlife exposure to anesthesia and age of onset of Alzheimer's disease. *Int J Neurosci.* 1994;77:181–185.
50. Masters CL, Simms G, Weinman NA, et al. Amyloid plaque core protein in Alzheimer disease and Down syndrome. *Proc Natl Acad Sci U S A.* 1985;82:4245–4249.
51. Verdile G, Fuller S, Atwood CS, et al. The role of beta amyloid in Alzheimer's disease: still a cause of everything or the only one who got caught? *Pharmacol Res.* 2004;50:397–409.
52. Van Dam D, D'Hooge R, Staufenbiel M, et al. Age-dependent cognitive decline in the APP23 model precedes amyloid deposition. *Eur J Neurosci.* 2003;17:388–396.
53. Boncristiano S, Calhoun ME, Kelly PH, et al. Cholinergic changes in the APP23 transgenic mouse model of cerebral amyloidosis. *J Neurosci.* 2002;22:3234–3243.
54. Perl DP. Neuropathology of Alzheimer's disease and related disorders. *Neurol Clin.* 2000;18:847–864.
55. Hartmann T, Beyreuther K. Molekulare Pathologie, Teil 2. In: Kurz A (Hrsg). *Demenzen. Grundlagen und Klinik.* Stuttgart: Thieme; 2002; S99–S105.
56. Frölich L, Sandbrink R, Hoyer S. Molekulare Pathologie, Teil 1. In: Kurz A (Hrsg). *Demenzen. Grundlagen und Klinik.* Stuttgart: Thieme; 2002: S98–S105.
57. Braak H, Braak E. Neuroanatomie. In: Kurz A (Hrsg). *Demenzen. Grundlagen und Klinik.* Stuttgart: Thieme; 2002:S118–S129.
58. Arendt T. Neuronale Pathologie. In: Kurz A (Hrsg). *Demenzen. Grundlagen und Klinik.* Stuttgart: Thieme; 2002:S106–S111.
59. Hoyer S. Oxidative energy metabolism in Alzheimer brain. Studies in early-onset and late-onset cases. *Mol Chem Neuropathol.* 1992;16:207–224.
60. Gsell W, Strein I, Riederer P. The neurochemistry of Alzheimer type, vascular type and mixed type dementias compared. *J Neural Transm Suppl.* 1996;47:73–101.
61. Drachman DA, Noffsinger D, Sahakian BJ, et al. Aging, memory, and the cholinergic system: a study of dichotic listening. *Neurobiol Aging.* 1980;1:39–43.
62. Sato A, Sato Y. Cholinergic neural regulation of regional cerebral blood flow. *Alzheimer Dis Assoc Disord.* 1995;9:28–38.
63. Gsell W, Moll G, Sofic E, Riederer P: Cholinergic and monoaminergic neurotransmitter systems in patients with Alzheimer's disease and senile dementia of the Alzheimer type: A critical evaluation. In: Maurer K (Hrsg). *Dementias—Neurochemistry, Neuropathology, Neuroimaging, Neuropsychology, Genetics.* Braunschweig: Vieweg; 1993:S25–S43.
64. Nordberg A. Nicotinic receptor abnormalities of Alzheimer's disease: therapeutic implications. *Biol Psychiatry.* 2002;49:200–210.
65. Baskin DS, Browning JL, Pirozzolo FJ, et al. Brain choline acetyltransferase and mental function in Alzheimer disease. *Arch Neurol.* 1999;56:1121–1123.
66. Kihara T, Shimohama S. Alzheimer's disease and acetylcholine receptors. *Acta Neurobiol Exp (Wars).* 2004;64:99–105.
67. Wang HX, Fratiglioni L, Frisoni GB, et al. Smoking and the occurrence of Alzheimer's disease: cross-sectional and longitudinal data in a population-based study. *Am J Epidemiol.* 1999;149:640–644.
68. Collingridge GL, Singer W. Excitatory amino acid receptors and synaptic plasticity. *Trends Pharmacol Sci.* 1990;11:290–296.

69. Myhrer T. Adverse psychological impact, glutamatergic dysfunction, and risk factors for Alzheimer's disease. *Neurosci Biobehav Rev.* 1998; 23:131–139.

70. Greenamyre JT, Young AB. Excitatory amino acids and Alzheimer's disease. *Neurobiol Aging.* 1989;10:593–602.

71. Butterfield DA, Pocernich CB. The glutamatergic system and Alzheimer's disease: therapeutic implications. *CNS Drugs.* 2003;17:641–652.

72. Greenamyre JT. The role of glutamate in neurotransmission and in neurologic disease. *Arch Neurol.* 1986;43:1058–1063.

73. Boissiere F, Faucheux B, Duyckaerts C, et al. Striatal expression of glutamic acid decarboxylase gene in Alzheimer's disease. *J Neurochem.* 1998;71:767–774.

74. Hertz L, Drejer J, Schousboe A. Energy metabolism in glutamatergic neurons, GABAergic neurons and astrocytes in primary cultures. *Neurochem Res.* 1988;13:605–610.

75. Marczynski TJ. GABAergic deafferentation hypothesis of brain aging and Alzheimer's disease revisited. *Brain Res Bull.* 1998;45:341–379.

76. Lanctot KL, Herrmann N, Mazzotta P, et al. GABAergic function in Alzheimer's disease: evidence for dysfunction and potential as a therapeutic target for the treatment of behavioural and psychological symptoms of dementia. *Can J Psychiatry.* 2004;49:439–453.

77. Armstrong DM, Sheffield R, Mishizen-Eberz AJ, et al. Plasticity of glutamate and GABAA receptors in the hippocampus of patients with Alzheimer's disease. *Cell Mol Neurobiol.* 2003;23:491–505.

78. Rissman RA, Mishizen-Eberz AJ, Carter TL, et al. Biochemical analysis of GABA(A) receptor subunits alpha 1, alpha 5, beta 1, beta 2 in the hippocampus of patients with Alzheimer's disease neuropathology. *Neuroscience.* 2003;120:695–704.

79. Gearing M, Mirra SS, Hedreen JC, et al. The Consortium to Establish a Registry for Alzheimer's Disease (CERAD). Part X. Neuropathology confirmation of the clinical diagnosis of Alzheimer's disease. *Neurology.* 1995;45:461–466.

80. McKhann G, Drachman D, Folstein M, et al. Clinical diagnosis of Alzheimer's disease: report of the NINCDS-ADRDA Work Group under the auspices of Department of Health and Human Services Task Force on Alzheimer's Disease. *Neurology.* 1984;34:939–944.

81. Chui H, Lee AE. Clinical criteria for dementia subtypes. In: Brodaty H (Hrsg). *Evidence Based Dementia Practice.* Oxford, England: Blackwell Science; 2002:S106–S119.

82. Pillon B, Deweer B, Agid Y, Dubois B. Explicit memory in Alzheimer's, Huntington's, and Parkinson's diseases. *Arch Neurol.* 1993;50:374–379.

83. Price BH, Gurvit H, Weintraub S, et al. Neuropsychological patterns and language deficits in 20 consecutive cases of autopsy-confirmed Alzheimer's disease. *Arch Neurol.* 1993;50:931–937.

84. Esteban-Santillan C, Praditsuwan R, Ueda H, Geldmacher DS. Clock drawing test in very mild Alzheimer's disease. *J Am Geriatr Soc.* 1998;46:1266–1269.

85. Kirk A, Kertesz A. On drawing impairment in Alzheimer's disease. *Arch Neurol.* 1991;48:73–77.

86. Galasko D, Bennett D, Sano M, et al. An inventory to assess activities of daily living for clinical trials in Alzheimer's disease. The Alzheimer's Disease Cooperative Study. *Alzheimer Dis Assoc Disord.* 1997;11(Suppl. 2): S33–S39.

87. Kawas CH. Clinical practice. Early Alzheimer's disease. *N Engl J Med.* 2003;349:1056–1063.

88. Mega MS, Cummings JL, Fiorello T, Gornbein J. The spectrum of behavioral changes in Alzheimer's disease. *Neurology.* 1996;46:130–135.

89. Förstl H, Calabrese P. Alzheimer-Demenz: Diagnose, Symptome und Verlauf. In: Förstl H (Hrsg). *Lehrbuch der Gerontopsychiatrie und psychotherapie.* Berlin: Springer; 2003:3–6.

90. Knopman DS, DeKosky ST, Cummings JL, et al. Practice parameter: diagnosis of dementia (an evidence-based review). Report of the Quality Standards Subcommittee of the American Academy of Neurology. *Neurology.* 2001;56:1143–1153.

91. Andreasen N, Minthon L, Davidsson P, et al. Evaluation of CSF-tau and CSF-Abeta42 as diagnostic markers for Alzheimer disease in clinical practice. *Arch Neurol.* 2001;58:373–379.

92. Clark CM, Xie S, Chittams J, et al. Cerebrospinal fluid tau and beta-amyloid: how well do these biomarkers reflect autopsy-confirmed dementia diagnoses? *Arch Neurol.* 2003;60:1696–1702.

93. Sunderland T, Linker G, Mirza N, et al. Decreased beta-amyloid1-42 and increased tau levels in cerebrospinal fluid of patients with Alzheimer disease. *JAMA.* 2003;289:2094–2103.

94. Maddalena A, Papassotiropoulos A, Muller-Tillmanns B, et al. Biochemical diagnosis of Alzheimer disease by measuring the cerebrospinal fluid ratio of phosphorylated tau protein to beta-amyloid peptide42. *Arch Neurol.* 2003;60:1202–1206.

95. Gomez-Tortosa E, Gonzalo I, Fanjul S, et al. Cerebrospinal fluid markers in dementia with lewy bodies compared with Alzheimer disease. *Arch Neurol.* 2003;60:1218–1222.

96. Galasko D. Cerebrospinal fluid biomarkers in Alzheimer disease: a fractional improvement? *Arch Neurol.* 2003;60:1195–1196.

97. Adak S, Illouz K, Gorman W, et al. Predicting the rate of cognitive decline in aging and early Alzheimer disease. *Neurology.* 2004;63:108–114.

98. Killiany RJ, Gomez-Isla T, Moss M, et al. Use of structural magnetic resonance imaging to predict who will get Alzheimer's disease. *Ann Neurol.* 2000;47:430–439.

99. Braak H, Braak E. Neuropathological stageing of Alzheimer-related changes. *Acta Neuropathol (Berl).* 1991;82:239–259.

100. Silverman DH, Small GW, Chang CY, et al. Positron emission tomography in evaluation of dementia: regional brain metabolism and long-term outcome. *JAMA.* 2001;286:2120–2127.

101. Zamrini E, De Santi S, Tolar M. Imaging is superior to cognitive testing for early diagnosis of Alzheimer's disease. *Neurobiol Aging.* 2004;25:685–691.

102. Doody RS, Stevens JC, Beck C, et al. Practice parameter: management of dementia (an evidence-based review). Report of the Quality Standards Subcommittee of the American Academy of Neurology. *Neurology.* 2001;56:1154–1166.

103. Small GW, Rabins PV, Barry PP, et al. Diagnosis and treatment of Alzheimer disease and related disorders. Consensus statement of the American Association for Geriatric Psychiatry, the Alzheimer's Association, and the American Geriatrics Society. *JAMA.* 1997;278:1363–1371.

104. Cummings JL. Alzheimer's disease. *N Engl J Med.* 2004;351:56–67.

105. Parsons CG, Danysz W, Quack G. Memantine is a clinically well tolerated N-methyl-D-aspartate (NMDA) receptor antagonist—a review of preclinical data. *Neuropharmacology.* 1999;38:735–767.

106. Reisberg B, Doody R, Stoffler A, et al. Memantine in moderate-to-severe Alzheimer's disease. *N Engl J Med.* 2003;348:1333–1341.

107. Tariot PN, Farlow MR, Grossberg GT, et al. Memantine treatment in patients with moderate to severe Alzheimer disease already receiving donepezil: a randomized controlled trial. *JAMA.* 2004;291:317–324.

108. Hirsch RD. Pharmacotherapy of patients with dementia. *Internist (Berl).* 2003;44:1584–1596.

109. Koelsch G, Turner RT, III, Hong L, et al. Memapsin 2, a drug target for Alzheimer's disease. *Biochem Soc Symp.* 2003;70:213–220.

110. Xu M, Lai MT, Huang Q, et al. Gamma-Secretase: characterization and implication for Alzheimer disease therapy. *Neurobiol Aging.* 2002;23:1023–1030.

111. Petanceska SS, DeRosa S, Olm V, et al. Statin therapy for Alzheimer's disease: will it work? *J Mol Neurosci.* 2002;19:155–161.

112. Hock C, Konietzko U, Streffer JR, et al. Antibodies against beta-amyloid slow cognitive decline in Alzheimer's disease. *Neuron.* 2003;38:547–554.

113. Orgogozo JM, Gilman S, Dartigues JF, et al. Subacute meningoencephalitis in a subset of patients with AD after Abeta42 immunization. *Neurology* 2003;61:46–54.

114. Schenk D, Barbour R, Dunn W, et al. Immunization with amyloid-beta attenuates Alzheimer-disease-like pathology in the PDAPP mouse. *Nature.* 1999;400:173–177.

115. Ritchie CW, Bush AI, Mackinnon A, et al. Metal-protein attenuation with iodochlorhydroxyquin (clioquinol) targeting Abeta amyloid deposition and toxicity in Alzheimer disease: a pilot phase 2 clinical trial. *Arch Neurol.* 2003;60:1685–1691.

116. Aisen PS, Davis KL, Berg JD, et al. A randomized controlled trial of prednisone in Alzheimer's disease. Alzheimer's Disease Cooperative Study. *Neurology.* 2000;54:588–593.

117. Aisen PS, Schafer KA, Grundman M, et al. Effects of rofecoxib or naproxen vs. placebo on Alzheimer disease progression: a randomized controlled trial. *JAMA.* 2003;289:2819–2826.

118. Scharf S, Mander A, Ugoni A, et al. A double-blind, placebo-controlled trial of diclofenac/misoprostol in Alzheimer's disease. *Neurology.* 1999;53:197–201.

119. Sano M, Ernesto C, Thomas RG, et al. A controlled trial of selegiline, alpha-tocopherol, or both as treatment for Alzheimer's disease. The Alzheimer's Disease Cooperative Study. *N Engl J Med.* 1997;336:1216–1222.

120. Henderson VW, Paganini-Hill A, Miller BL, et al. Estrogen for Alzheimer's disease in women: randomized, double-blind, placebo-controlled trial. *Neurology.* 2000;54:295–301.

121. Mulnard RA, Cotman CW, Kawas C, et al. Estrogen replacement therapy for treatment of mild to moderate Alzheimer disease: a randomized controlled trial. Alzheimer's Disease Cooperative Study. *JAMA.* 2000;283:1007–1015.

122. Diel J, Kurz A. Innovative kausale Therapieverfahren. In: Förstl H (Hrsg). *Antidementiva.* München, Jena: Urban & Fischer; 2003:S211–S230.

123. Shumaker SA, Legault C, Rapp SR, et al. Estrogen plus progestin and the incidence of dementia and mild cognitive impairment in post-menopausal women: the Women's Health Initiative Memory Study: a randomized controlled trial. *JAMA.* 2003;289:2651–2662.

124. Louzada PR, Lima AC, Mendonca-Silva DL, et al. Taurine prevents the neurotoxicity of beta-amyloid and glutamate receptor agonists: activation of GABA receptors and possible implications for Alzheimer's disease and other neurological disorders. *Faseb J.* 2004;18:511–518.

125. Mark RJ, Ashford JW, Goodman Y, Mattson MP. Anticonvulsants attenuate amyloid beta-peptide neurotoxicity, Ca2+ deregulation, and cytoskeletal pathology. *Neurobiol Aging.* 1995;16:187–198.

126. Fastbom J, Forsell Y, Winblad B. Benzodiazepines may have protective effects against Alzheimer disease. *Alzheimer Dis Assoc Disord.* 1998;12:14–17.

127. Kalenka A, Hinkelbein J. Anaesthesia in patients with Parkinson's disease. *Anaesthesist.* 2005;54:401–409; quiz 10–11.

128. Corey-Bloom J. The ABC of Alzheimer's disease: cognitive changes and their management in Alzheimer's disease and related dementias. *Int Psychogeriatr.* 2002;14(Suppl. 1):51–75.

129. Raskind MA, Peskind ER, Wessel T, Yuan W. Galantamine in AD: A 6-month randomized, placebo-controlled trial with a 6-month extension. The Galantamine USA-1 Study Group. *Neurology.* 2000;54: 2261–2268.

130. Rogers SL, Farlow MR, Doody RS, et al. A 24-week, double-blind, placebo-controlled trial of donepezil in patients with Alzheimer's disease. Donepezil Study Group. *Neurology.* 1998;50:136–145.

131. Wu CL, Hsu W, Richman JM, Raja SN. Postoperative cognitive function as an outcome of regional anesthesia and analgesia. *Reg Anesth Pain Med.* 2004;29:257–268.

132. Rasmussen LS, Johnson T, Kuipers HM, et al. Does anaesthesia cause postoperative cognitive dysfunction? A randomized study of regional versus general anaesthesia in 438 elderly patients. *Acta Anaesthesiol Scand.* 2003;47:260–266.

133. Nicholson G, Pereira AC, Hall GM. Parkinson's disease and anaesthesia. *Br J Anaesth.* 2002;89:904–916.

134. el-Maghrabi EA, Eckenhoff RG. Inhibition of dopamine transport in rat brain synaptosomes by volatile anesthetics. *Anesthesiology.* 1993;78:7 50–756.

135. Hetherington A, Rosenblatt RM. Ketamine and paralysis agitans. *Anesthesiology.* 1980;52:527.

136. Wand P, Kuschinsky K, Sontag KH. Morphine-induced muscular rigidity in rats. *Eur J Pharmacol.* 1973;24:189–193.

137. Solca M, Salvo I, Russo R, et al. Anaesthesia with desflurane-nitrous oxide in elderly patients. Comparison with isoflurane-nitrous oxide. *Minerva Anestesiol.* 2000;66:621–626.

138. Muravchick S. Anaesthesia for the aging patient. *Can J Anaesth.* 1993;40:R63–R73.

139. Paxton JW, Briant RH. Alpha 1-acid glycoprotein concentrations and propranolol binding in elderly patients with acute illness. *Br J Clin Pharmacol.* 1984;18:806–810.

140. Campagna JA, Miller KW, Forman SA. Mechanisms of actions of inhaled anesthetics. *N Engl J Med.* 2003;348:2110–124.

141. Eckel B, Riemenschneider M, Ohl F, et al. MAC of isoflurane is increased in transgenic mice with Alzheimer's disease-like pathology. In: *Anesthesiology:* San Francisco;2003:A901.

142. Eckel B, Ohl F, Riemenschneider M, et al. Effects of isoflurane anesthesia on cognitive performance in mouse model of Alzheimer disease. *Anesthesiology.* 2005;submitted.

143. Golden WE, Lavender RC, Metzer WS. Acute postoperative confusion and hallucinations in Parkinson disease. *Ann Intern Med.* 1989;111:218–222.

144. Møller JT, Cluitmans P, Rasmussen LS, et al. Long-term postoperative cognitive dysfunction in the elderly ISPOCD1 study. ISPOCD investigators. International Study of Post-Operative Cognitive Dysfunction. *Lancet.* 1998;351:857–861.

145. Ancelin ML, de Roquefeuil G, Ledesert B, et al. Exposure to anaesthetic agents, cognitive functioning and depressive symptomatology in the elderly. *Br J Psychiatry.* 2001;178:360–366.

Legal Issues of Importance to the Elderly

Kevin Gerold

CHAPTER 28

INFORMED CONSENT

The need to obtain informed consent arises from a physician's ethical obligation to assist patients in making a choice from among the therapeutic alternatives consistent with good medical practice.[1] The notion of informed consent is an important, but relatively recent principle to the practice of medicine. In 1984, Jay Katz characterized that "disclosure and consent, except in the most rudimentary fashion, are obligations alien to medical thinking and practice.[2]" In ancient and medieval times, a formal consent process was unnecessary because the physician's ability to affect a cure relied heavily on his ability to inspire the patient's faith and confidence in a treatment, provide comfort, and offer hope; even if doing so required using deceit and manipulation. The patient's role in the therapeutic process was passive. Informed consent as we interpret it today did not emerge until in the early 1900s when doctors reluctantly began to abandon their long-held authoritarian doctor-relationship and gradually accepted a growing social expectation that they disclose to their patients matters relating to their care and treatment; even if this included informing the patient of a dire prognosis.

The legal concept on informed consent is rooted within the ethical principle of autonomy. Justice Cardozo stated in 1914, "Every human being of adult years and sound mind has the right to determine what shall be done with his own body . . ."[3] The need to obtain informed consent arises because our society holds that legally competent patients have the right of self-determination in matters relating to their health, and it prohibits physicians from substituting their judgment for that of the patient in matters relating to care and treatment.

Legal liability for failing to obtain informed consent arose originally under the tort of battery. Battery is a civil wrong arising from an intentional and wrongful physical contact with a person without his or her consent that entails some injury or offensive touching.[4] In 1905, a physician-surgeon in Minnesota was the first sued successfully for battery. In Mohr v. Williams,[5] a patient consented to surgery for a diseased condition of the right ear. While the patient was under anesthesia, the surgeon determined that the right ear was not serious enough to require surgery, and determined that the left ear was more seriously diseased and required surgical treatment. Without waking the patient and obtaining her permission to operate on the left ear, the surgeon proceeded to perform the necessary operation. The operation was performed skillfully and the outcome was successful. For failing to obtain prior consent, the patient sued the surgeon under the tort of battery and the jury awarded the patient $14,322.50 (this amount was reduced to $39.00 on retrial). When reviewed by the Supreme Court of Minnesota, the court acknowledged that the left ear was diseased, that it required operation, that the operation was performed skillfully, and that the physician-surgeon acted in good faith and without an evil intent. Nonetheless, the court concluded that performing an operation on a patient without consent was wrong, and as such, was unlawful. This legal remedy for a lack of informed consent persisted until the 1960s when courts began to view battery as too strong a legal remedy for failures of informed consent, and now reserve it for limited cases where a physician might fail to obtain any consent. Today, nearly all states view a failure to obtain informed consent as a breach of the doctors' professional duty to their patient, and apply a negligence test.

Under a negligence theory, the legal obligation to obtain informed consent arises from a duty of physicians to exercise due care in their conduct toward others from which injury may result.[6] The duty to obtain informed consent is excused only when: (1) an emergency condition exists, the patient is unconscious, or is otherwise incapable of consenting, and the failure to treat poses an imminent harm; and (2) in rare circumstances when the risk of disclosure would pose such a serious psychological threat of detriment to the patient as to be medically contraindicated.[1]

States differ in how they define the duty expected of physicians when obtaining informed consent. About one-half of states apply a "reasonable patient" standard. These states require physicians to provide the patient with information that a reasonable patient would require in order to make an informed decision. The remaining states apply a "reasonable physician" standard. These states require physicians to provide information that reasonable physicians would provide normally to their patients when obtaining informed consent.

Informed consent is not the act of having the patient sign a consent form. Rather, it is the dialogue that takes place between a physician and the patient prior to engaging in a proposed plan treatment or procedure. It includes the material aspects of their diagnosis and proposed treatment that will enable a reasonable patient to consider his or her options, including having no treatment, and enable them to make an educated conclusion in the context of their needs and values.

A physician may delegate the process of obtaining informed consent to others, but always retains responsibility for the adequacy of the consent. Once informed consent is obtained, practitioners should document the discussion in the medical record. The value of a signed informed consent document is that it creates a legal presumption that the consent was informed and makes it difficult for plaintiff-patients to allege that they were not informed of the risks and alternatives of a procedure or treatment plan. Having a patient sign a consent form never excuses the physician's obligation to inform the patient, personally or through others, about the plan of treatment or a proposed procedure.

The essential steps to fulfill informed consent requirements are outlined in Table 28-1. Information generally considered material and necessary for a patient to make an informed decision includes: (1) the diagnosis; (2) the nature and purpose of the proposed treatment or procedure, the probability and severity of its risks, and whether those risks would be temporary or permanent; and (3) viable treatment alternatives. When describing the proposed treatment, it is unnecessary to describe the details or technical or mechanical means of performing an operation or procedure, and it is unnecessary to inform patients of what they already know. The discussion should occur in the patient's preferred language, and plain language terms are preferable to medical terms. If the patient requires an interpreter, the physician should obtain one who is sufficiently fluent in the language and culture to express the subtleties necessary for patients to understand their medical condition and treatment.

An emerging aspect of informed consent is whether physicians are required to include their own experience or outcomes with a proposed treatment or procedure. As studies increasingly demonstrate, reductions in morbidity and mortality are achievable when treatments such as cardiac surgery and cancer treatments are performed in specialized centers; it is anticipated that disclosing the physicians or centers success with a proposed treatment as compared to other physicians or centers will become an additional element of the informed consent discussion. Also unclear is whether physicians are required to disclose information about their own health status when that condition may affect the treatment plan or affect the patient's risk. A Maryland court held recently that a physician had a duty to disclose to patients that he was infected with human immunodeficiency virus (HIV+), even though the risk of transmitting the infection was small.[7]

To ensure the adequacy of consent, physicians should ensure that they take the time to engage in a dialogue with the patient about their diagnosis and the proposed treatment plan. The dialogue should take place using plain language terms and, if necessary, in a language that the patient will understand. If subjected to legal scrutiny, the courts will evaluate the adequacy of the discussion in the context of a reasonable patient or physician. A *reasonable person* at law is someone who exercises the qualities of attention, knowledge, intelligence, and judgment which society requires of its members for the protection of their own interests and the interests of others. The reasonable person is a fictitious person, who is never negligent and whose conduct is always up to standard.[8] By applying a reasonable person test, the courts do not expect physicians to defend themselves against a specific patient who might assert that she would not have undergone a proposed treatment or procedure had they been made aware of a complication omitted while obtaining consent.

The legal burden for a plaintiff-patient to assert the failure of informed consent is high and, in general, it is unusual to file a lawsuit for negligent consent alone (Table 28-2). When appropriate, lawyers may add negligent consent to a lawsuit alleging medical malpractice.

The best strategy to avoid legal allegations of not obtaining informed consent is to adhere to the standards of good medical practice. Prior to initiating a plan of treatment or engaging in a procedure, physicians must take the time to inform patients of their diagnosis, prognosis, reasonable therapeutic options including no treatment, and make recommendations as to what the physician believes to be the best plan of care. If the physician chooses to forego consent because: (1) an emergency condition exists, the patient is incapable of consenting, and the failure to treat poses an imminent harm; or (2) when the risk of disclosure poses such a serious psychological threat of detriment to the patient as to be medically contraindicated, then the physician should document these special circumstances in the medical record. If the patient has diminished capacity or is unable to provide an informed consent, then the physician has an obligation to obtain informed consent from the patient's surrogate decision-maker. In cases where the patient has diminished capacity, yet retains the ability to make informed decisions, it may be proper to obtain the patients permission to engage family members or friends in the discussion to aid the patient in arriving at an informed decision. In rare circumstances where the patient is unable to make an informed decision and a legally authorized surrogate decision-maker is unavailable, physicians must seek the appointment of a court-appointed guardian to protect the patient's interests.

Table 28-1

Essential Steps to Fulfill the Informed Consent Requirements

Provide the patient with the information about a treatment plan or procedure that a reasonable person would require to make an informed decision.

It is unnecessary to provide information already known to the patient.

Take time to answer questions and address specific concerns that a particular patient may have while making an informed decision.

Recognize that a signed consent form is not informed consent. Signed documents indicate only that the patient agreed to go forward with a plan of care. A signed consent form makes it more difficult for a patient to assert a claim of negligent informed consent.

Providing care in an emergency does not require consent. When providing care in an emergency and without consent, document the need for emergency treatment in the medical record.

A physician is permitted to limit the scope of discussion relating to consent when, in the physician's opinion, the risk of disclosure poses such a serious psychological threat of detriment to the patient as to be medically contraindicated. Under this condition, this decision should be documented in the medical record.

A clinical institution's responsibility is to verify that a signed consent form appears in the chart before engaging in medical care. It is not obligated to determine adequacy of the consent.

Table 28-2

Legal Elements for Alleging Negligent Informed Consent

1. Physician failed to inform patient adequately of material risks before engaging in a treatment plan or performing a procedure.
2. A reasonable patient, if informed of the material risks, would not have consented to the proposed treatment or procedure.
3. The adverse consequences left undisclosed went on to occur and the patient was injured as a result of the treatment or procedure.
4. There was not an emergency need for treatment for the procedure.

EVALUATING CAPACITY TO MAKE AN INFORMED CHOICE

▶ Introduction

Inherent in the patient's right of self-determination and a physician's obligation to obtain informed consent prior to medical treatment is an assumption that a patient possesses the capacity to make an informed choice.[9,10] Competent patients are entitled to information that permits them to deliberate among choices concerning their treatment and express a choice. The doctrine of informed consent acknowledges that the consequences of a physician's explanation may be a patient's' refusal of medical treatment and his or her assumption of risk for the consequences of that decision.[11–13] It is, therefore, imperative that physicians protect patients' right to autonomy by assessing patients' abilities to understand and appreciate the information provided as well as the ability to arrive at a reasoned decision.

Although age per se does not reduce competence, a relationship exists between advanced age and decision-making ability. The incidence of dementia increases with age, especially among the "old-old" (those older than 85 years of age), and the increased incidence of chronic illness, an increased susceptibility to medications and their side effects, and other risk factors combine to cause an increased incidence of cognitive incapacity among the elderly.

Medicine, law, psychiatry, philosophy, and other disciplines have all developed competing theories of competence. The law requires that all adult patients are presumed competent unless a court declares them incompetent and evaluates it broadly in two ways.[14] Some persons are deemed incompetent as a matter of law (*de jure* or per se incompetence). Per se incompetents include infants and young children because they are considered to lack the decision-making capacity because of their immature cognitive abilities and judgments. Other persons are declared incompetent by court order (*de facto* incompetence) after a formal inquiry into their actual capacities and a determination that they lacked the requisite functional abilities to make decisions on their own behalf. *De facto* incompetents include patients in coma, the severely mentally-impaired, and those with severe mental illness. When a court makes a determination of incompetence, it declares that a person is unable to act in his or her best interest and appoints a guardian to intervene on his or her behalf. Declaring a patient incompetent to make health-care decisions is a serious legal matter and is potentially more intrusive and liberty-depriving than a criminal conviction.[15]

In the past, when a patient's capacity to make informed decisions was in question, courts traditionally viewed competence in broad terms; the person was either competent or not competent.[16] More recently, courts have begun viewing competency in contextual terms; mentally-ill persons may be incompetent to manage financial affairs, but competent to make their own health-care decisions.[17]

Competency to make informed decisions relating to health care is not a bright-line matter but instead is nuanced in shades of gray, making legal determinations difficult. Many authors now distinguish between the assessments of decision-making capacity, which are conducted by health-care professionals using various capacity assessment instruments (Table 28-3), and determinations of competence, which are legal determinations made by courts. In clinical practice, a determination that a patient lacks decision-making capacity has nearly the same consequences as a legal determination of incompetence. A patient's cognitive ability to understand and reason may change during the course of their hospitalization or as a consequence of their condition or treatment. As a result, their capacity to make informed decisions may change.

Table 28-3

Capacity Assessment Instruments

Mini-Mental Status Examination (MMSE)

MacArthur Competence Assessment Tool (MacCAT-T)

Edelstein's Hopemont Capacity Assessment Inventory

Neurobehavioral Cognitive Status Examination

Dementia Rating Scale

Wechsler Adult Intelligence Scale

Geriatric Depression Scale

Center for Epidemiological Studies Depression Scale

Short Psychiatric Evaluation Schedule

Global Deterioration Scale

Alzheimer Disease Assessment Scale

Brief Cognitive Rating Score

Cambridge Mental Disorders of the Elderly Examination

Dementia of the Alzheimer Type Inventory

Dementia Diagnostic Screening Questionnaire

Mental Status Questionnaire

AARP Executive Cognitive Function measure (ECF)

Source: From Ref. 11.

Distinguishing between decision-making capacity and incapacity can be difficult. When caring for the elderly or patients with an acute illness or injury, the ability to identify a patient's impaired capacity to make informed health-care decisions may not be obvious. In most cases, these determinations of capacity are nearly always made by physicians, determinations are reviewed rarely,[17] and these assessments take place often without the patient's awareness or consent.[18] There are several contexts in which a physician is likely to question a patient's capacity (see Table 28-4).[19]

▶ Determining incompetence and incapacity

Legal incompetence or incapacity is defined through the five legal maxims (see Table 28-5). "Incompetence (or incapacity) constitutes a status of the individual that is defined by functional deficits (due to mental illness, mental retardation, or other medical conditions)

Table 28-4

When to Assess Decision-Making Capacity

Patient presents with abrupt changes in mental status

When a patient refuses recommended treatment

When consenting to treatment that is especially invasive, experimental, or risky

When a patient displays one or more risk factors associated with impaired decision making, such as a neurologic or psychiatric diagnosis; comorbid clinical factors such as anxiety, depression, sleep deprivation, and sepsis; situational factors such as inpatient hospitalization or the need for urgent surgery; and advanced age.

Source: From Ref. 10.

Table 28-5

Five Maxims of Legal Competence

Legal Competence is related to, but not the same as, Impaired Mental Status

Based on the patient's functional deficits

Depends on the functional demands imposed on the patient

Legal Incompetence depends on the consequences of the decision

Legal Incompetence can change with the patient's condition, clinical situation, or circumstance

Source: From Ref. 10.

judged to be sufficiently great that the person currently cannot meet the demands of a specific decision-making situation, weighed in the light of its potential consequences."[20] The actual determination of competence cannot be accomplished by applying a simple formula or assessment tool alone.[21]

While mental illness, mental retardation, and cognitive impairments may increase the likelihood that a patient is incompetent, such conditions do not create a presumption of incompetence. Evaluating a cognitive impairment requires an understanding of the information that a patient is expected to consider, an appreciation of the patient's ability to evaluate the information presented in the context of one's circumstance, and the patient's ability to reason with the information to arrive at an expressed choice. Deficits in these abilities can only be evaluated in the context of the decision-making demands of the specific clinical situation.

It is unlikely that an anesthesiologist will be called upon to make a formal determination of competence or capacity prior to a patient making informed decisions. It is important, however, that all anesthesiologists recognize their obligation to respect patients' right to make their own decisions and identify patients who may have an impaired ability to make an informed decision. If during a patient interview, the physician develops a suspicion that the patient may lack the capacity to make an informed decision, then the physician should obtain a formal evaluation of the patient's competency prior to obtaining consent. In the absence of an emergency condition, patients who appear to lack the functional abilities to make an informed decision (Table 28-6) or under circumstances that invite the need to evaluate a patient's ability to choose (see Table 28-4) should have a formal evaluation of competency before undertaking a treatment plan. When confronted with a patient of questionable competence, practitioners

Table 28-6

Functional Abilities Related to Competence

The ability to express a choice

The ability to understand information relevant to treatment decision making

The ability to appreciate the significance of information in the context of one's own situation, especially the details of one's illness and the probable consequences of available treatment options

The ability to reason with relevant information so as to engage in a logical process of weighing treatment options

Source: From Ref. 12.

should avoid the inclination to turn immediately to the patient's surrogate decision-maker to make decisions on the patient's behalf.

ADVANCED HEALTH-CARE DIRECTIVES

▶ Introduction

Historical developments have complicated medical decision-making for seriously-ill patients. The former culture of medical paternalism has given way to patient's rights to autonomy and informed consent. Increasingly complex technologies enable us now to extend life using artificial means, but cannot necessarily restore patients to their prior level of functioning. Determining the best plan of care for patients requires that health-care practitioners consider each patient's values and preferences, how that patient views the quality and quantity of life, and to make sound medical judgments of medical appropriateness.[22] The complexity of these decisions is made more difficult when patients lose the capacity to make their own decisions and someone else must make decisions on their behalf. The medical, legal, and ethical communities have increasingly turned to advance directives to resolve the uncertainties in these circumstances.

In 1992, in an effort to encourage hospitalized patients to express advance directives, Congress enacted the Patient Self-Determination Act.[23] The act requires hospitals, nursing homes, home health agencies, and hospice programs to provide written information concerning patients' rights under State law as to medical decisions, including the right to formulate advance directives. Despite this mandated effort encouraging the execution of advance directives, only 10–25% of patients complete an advance directive, and these documents are regularly ignored by health-care practitioners. There is also a wide disparity among age groups. Approximately 5% of adults under age 40 have advance directives, while an estimated 70% of the elderly population has them.[22] Interestingly, physicians as a group are no more likely to execute advance directives than is the general population. However, when physicians are surveyed, they describe a preference for limiting medical interventions for themselves in the event of a serious or life-threatening illness.[24]

In the spring of 2005, the end-of-life decision-making for Terri Schiavo, a Florida woman in a persistent vegetative state, played out as a public spectacle and a tragedy for her and her husband. Mr. Schiavo's private feud with his wife's parents over his continued attempts to discontinue the administration of fluids and nutrition delivered artificially through a feeding tube was taken to the media, the courts, the Florida legislature, Florida Governor Jeb Bush, the U.S. Congress, and President Bush. After more than 7 years of litigation involving nearly 20 judges, Mrs. Schiavo's case caused a reexamination of issues that most physicians, lawyers, and bioethicists considered well settled since the 1976 New Jersey Supreme Court decision in the case of Karen Quinlan and later by the 1990 U.S. Supreme Court decision in the case of Nancy Cruzan.[25]

In 1976, the New Jersey Supreme Court ruled in the case of Karen Quinlan that care providers, including physicians, could not be held civilly or criminally responsible for the death of a patient that resulted from the removal of life-sustaining treatment to a patient determined and confirmed by a hospital ethics committee, to have "no reasonable possibility of returning to a cognitive, sapient state."[26] In the Quinlan case, doctors were reluctant to honor the family's request to discontinue her artificial ventilation for fear that they would be liable for her death. The Quinlan case encouraged states to enact "living will" statutes that provided legal immunity to physicians who honored patients' written advance directives specifying their medical care if they became incompetent to make their own decisions. It also encouraged hospitals to establish ethics committees to resolve end-of-life decision disputes between practitioners and families without going to court.

In 1990, the U.S. Supreme Court affirmed a Missouri Supreme Court case involving Nancy Cruzan and determined that it was permissible to discontinue artificial feeding based on the patient's right of self-determination.[27] In the Cruzan case, the Missouri Court held that only the patient herself could make such a decision, but if a patient becomes unable to express her decision, then those speaking on her behalf, including parents, could express her wishes using "clear and convincing" evidence of prior expressions of a choice. The U.S. Supreme Court upheld the Missouri Court's requirement for a clear and convincing threshold in order to "err on the side of life." The Court's ruling made no legal distinction between artificially delivered fluids and nutrition and other medical interventions such as ventilator support. The consequence of Cruzan case was a movement encouraging people to create documents such as proxy or durable powers of attorney forms designating an agent to make decisions on their behalf in the event they become unable to do so. All states recognize delegation forms and many states grant decision-making authority to family members, even if the patient has not made a prior delegation.

Although the majority of Americans believed that the Terri Schiavo case represented an intrusion of politics into medical decision-making and well-defined law, it highlights the reality that most people do not wish to remain in a persistent vegetative state kept alive by nutrition delivered through a feeding tube. The publicity generated by this case spoke to the need for families to discuss openly their medical wishes among each other and hopefully sign an advanced directive or designate a health-care agent.

Advance health-care directives are legal documents that are more commonly used in medical settings than in the courts. "This is how it should be"—medical decisions are private matters best left to patients, assisted by their physicians. Advance health-care directives enable agents, surrogates, and families to act on the patient's behalf at times of incapacity. The Shiavo case highlights a widely held belief in medicine and in law that the courts should remain the place of last resort to resolve disputes between patients and care providers. The emotional toll upon all parties can be enormous and the delays significant. The legal remedies are often "clumsy, intrusive, overbearing, and counterproductive. Doctors don't want to litigate health care. Patients don't want it. And . . . lawyers and judges probably don't want it either."[28]

Following the Terri Shiavo case, the law remains clear and incompetent patients retain an interest in self-determination. Physicians should encourage health-care agents to act on the patient's best interest, and make treatment decisions consistent with what they believe the patient would want if they were expressing a choice for themselves. If decision-makers cannot determine the patient's choice, then care providers should base treatment decisions on what a reasonable person would want under same or similar circumstances.[25]

▶ Creating advance directives

Advance health-care directives are legal documents intended to assist care providers with clarifying the uncertainties of medical decision-making and extend patient self-determination under circumstances of incapacity. They are personal contingency plans that provide guidance to family members, friends, and care providers on how to make medical choices in the event of decisional or communicating incapacity. Advance health-care directives are created by statutory expressions by a decisionally competent adult, and may be in the form of a living will or a durable power of attorney for health care. An advance health-care directive, or living will, is a legal expression made by persons intending to direct their medical treatment in advance of future incapacity. It is patients' instruction to their care providers about medical decisions that may occur in the future. Alternatively, a durable power of attorney for health care appoints another person as health-care decision-maker for the patient in the event of future incapacity. Most are made in writing, but some states permit the creation of advance directives orally by making their directives known to their treating physician. For example, Texas law states, "a competent, qualified patient who is an adult may issue a directive (i.e., a living will) by a non-written means of communication." Maryland law permits oral expressions and Florida law permits oral or written statements. When a patient expresses an advance health-care directive orally, physicians should document the directive in the medical record and should consider having the patient and a witness sign the entry.

Early forms of advance directives were usually in the form of a living will. Living wills, or declarations, are death with dignity directives recognized in law in 47 states. Living wills provide specific instructions to attending physicians and other care providers about medical treatments in the event of a patient's incapacity. Often, they instruct attending physicians as to how to provide or withhold death-delaying procedures and when to implement comfort-only care in the event of a terminal condition. The authority of a living will is not uniform among the states. Some states (Missouri and Illinois) do not permit the withdrawal of artificial hydration and nutrition under the terms of a living will if doing so would result in death. Forty-one states have passed enabling legislation permitting the withholding of sustenance. States where the law has not addressed this issue include Arkansas, California, the District of Columbia, Kansas, Massachusetts, Michigan, Montana, North Dakota, Rhode Island, and Wyoming.[28] The advantage of living wills is that they communicate directly with the care providers and do not require the presence of a third party to act on the patient's behalf. Their limitation is that they do not provide instructions for unforeseen circumstances. For this reason, lawyers increasingly encourage persons to replace living wills with a durable power of attorney for health care.

The durable power of attorney for health care is replacing the living will as the advance directive of choice because it permits persons to delegate any or all medical decisions, routine and end-of-life care, to a proxy or agent automatically upon their incapacity to make their own decisions. The durable power of attorney usually terminates if or when the patient regains the ability to express an informed choice. The designated health-care agent authorized under a durable power of attorney is permitted to confer with attending physicians, review medical records, and act on incompetent patients' behalf to make treatment decisions consistent with what the patients would have decided on their own. Although they represent a broad grant of authority, the ability to revoke a durable power of attorney is quite simple. In addition to the traditional means of physical destruction, some jurisdictions (Delaware, Iowa, and Nebraska) provide for oral revocation, irrespective of mental state. In these states, once revoked, the durable power is terminated no matter how implausible or inopportune the revocation may be.

Physicians who may disagree with a patient's advance health-care directive should avoid the temptation to disregard them and unilaterally provide care contrary to the patient's or the agent's wishes. Physicians and other practitioners who disregard an advance directive and substitute their own judgments for that of the patients or their surrogate expose themselves to assertions of battery or the intentional infliction of emotional harm. If disagreements about the best plan of care occur between care providers and families, agents, or surrogates, then every attempt should be made to reconcile them, using an appropriate mediator, if necessary. An ethics committee may be helpful in these situations. If a health-care practitioner is unable to carry out the instructions described in an advance directive or is unwilling to execute the wishes of a health-care agent, then the practitioner is obligated to find a willing successor and resign in a nonjudgmental manner. To avoid any assertion of abandonment, it is important to maintain continuity of care during the transition and document its occurrence in the medical record.

▶ Perioperative do-not-resuscitative orders

One manifestation of an advance directive that anesthesiologists will encounter, particularly when caring for the elderly, is a do-not-resuscitate (DNR) order. Its purpose is to preserve a patient's right of self-determination by limiting the use of modern-day technology during the terminal phase of illness. Although widely accepted in general medical practice since the 1970s, surgeons and anesthesiologists generally suspended a patient's DNR when in the operating room (OR) and postoperatively until the 1990s.

Advocates for suspending DNR orders when patients come to surgery have attempted to avoid the sometimes difficult issue of distinguishing resuscitation from routine anesthetic or surgical care. Arguments for revoking the DNR order include the uncertainty about what constitutes "resuscitation" in the OR. Providing anesthesia and performing surgery routinely involve actions many physicians would consider acts of resuscitation, such as tracheal intubation, mechanical ventilation, the administration of blood products and intravenous fluids, and administering medications to correct arrhythmias or to elevate blood pressure. They reason that resuscitative-type measures when performed in the OR have more favorable outcomes when the inciting event is witnessed and/or the need for resuscitation is iatrogenic. Other reasons to err on the side of resuscitation include the avoidance of feeling responsible for a patient's death or to avoid the unfounded legal concerns such as being liable for negligence.

Arguments for continuing to honor a patient's DNR request in the OR acknowledge the need to balance the burdens associated with surgery against the benefits of undergoing the procedure (Table 28-7). The burdens of anesthesia and surgery include outcomes that may result in diminished functional or cognitive capacities. At the end of life, surgery may offer palliative benefits to patients who will not survive long-term, or in whom resuscitation will not benefit. For example, a patient with obstructing esophageal cancer may benefit from a gastrostomy to permit feeding and improve the quality of life, but may not wish the surgical team to resuscitate him in the event a cardiac arrest occurred during or after the procedure.

In response to changing social values, the American Society of Anesthesiologists published statements in 1993 and 1994 advocating

the reevaluation of a surgical patient's DNR order rather than its automatic revocation.[29,30] These position statements encourage members of the surgical team to meet with patients before surgery and negotiate a resuscitation care plan in the event such care becomes necessary. When terminally-ill patients were asked about how they wanted their DNR interpreted during the perioperative period, nearly all wanted to participate in a discussion about what would occur. The options available to the surgical team include (Table 28-8): (1) suspending the DNR during the perioperative period; (2) initiating a procedure-directed order that permits or forbids specific interventions such as tracheal intubation, postoperative mechanical ventilation, chest compressions, defibrillation or cardioversion, the administration of vasoactive medications, or the insertion of invasive hemodynamic monitors; (3) initiating a goal-directed order set that prioritizes outcomes rather than procedures. Goal-directed outcomes recognize that patients consider treatments in terms of outcomes, and it may be more effective to discuss goals of treatment rather than specific procedures. By prioritizing outcomes, the surgical care team can exercise their clinical judgment to direct specific interventions to achieve the patient's goals. A goal-directed approach should explore the burden the patient is willing to accept, the benefit the patient hopes to gain from undergoing the procedure, and the likelihood of success.

Since the goal of medical therapy and surgical procedures is to provide benefits meaningful to the patient, it is important to discuss DNR orders in the context of the proposed surgery. Anesthesiologists recognize that up to 46% of patients may be unaware that a DNR order exists in their medical record, even when they are competent.[31] The approach to discussing how to modify a DNR order for the perioperative period will depend on the type of surgery, the patient's condition and personal values, and the beliefs held by the surgical care team. Discussions should include pertinent caregivers such as surgeons, intensivists, primary care practitioners, and nurses, and when finalized, all members of the care team should be able to abide by the agreement.

Anesthesiologists unable to abide by patients' request or the request of their surrogate on medical or moral grounds should withdraw in a nonjudgmental manner and provide for an alternative anesthesiologist in a timely manner. If proposed modifications of the DNR conflict with "generally accepted standards of care, ethical practice, or institutional policies, then the anesthesiologist should voice such concerns and present the situation to the appropriate institutional body."[28] Under circumstances where an alternative practitioner is unavailable within a time necessary to prevent further morbidity or to limit suffering, the conflicted practitioner should proceed with providing care with reasonable adherence to the patient's directives while

---

Table 28-7

Withholding DNR in the Operating Room

When DNR is judged to be of no benefit medically to the patient

When a competent patient or her surrogate indicates that they do not want resuscitation, even if the need arises to perform it

---

Table 28-8

Do-Not-Resuscitate Orders in the Perioperative Period

Full Resuscitation—suspend the DNR during the perioperative period

Procedure Directed, Limited Resuscitation—determine in advance a mutually agreeable list of specific resuscitative interventions that can be used, if necessary, during the perioperative period

Goal Directed, Limited Resuscitation for temporary and reversible conditions—provide resuscitative measures for temporary and reversible events that may occur during the perioperative period

Goal Directed, Limited Resuscitation consistent with the patient's expressed goals and values—provide resuscitative measures that promote the patient's goals and values being mindful of the patient's treatment goals and personal values. Doing so is in accordance with the American Medical Association's principles of medical ethics.[32]

An exception to an anesthesiologist's obligation to clarify patients' wishes regarding their care is an emergency situation requiring immediate intervention. In the absence of a clear instruction not to treat, the surgical care team should reach a consensus as to the medical benefit or futility of different treatment alternatives. In times of uncertainty, it is reasonable to err on the side of continuing to provide care until a patient's preferences are known. Legally, physicians should view stopping and not starting ineffective treatments as the same.[29] Withholding and withdrawing life-support modalities are ethically and legally equivalent actions and the consideration given to making these decisions is the same.[32]

MEDICAL FUTILITY IN THE PERIOPERATIVE PERIOD

▶ Introduction

Medical futility refers to interventions that are unlikely to provide any significant benefit to the patient. In contrast to informed consent and advanced health-care directives which emphasize a patient's right to choose from among medically acceptable treatment options, including the right to refuse further treatment, medical futility concerns itself with a physician's obligation to withhold care that is determined to be without therapeutic benefit. The ethical authority to make judgments regarding the futility of specific treatments rests with the medical profession as a whole, not with individual physicians at the bedside, and determinations of futility at the bedside should conform to generally accepted standards of care.

The concept of medical futility dates back to ancient Hippocratic writings, which suggested three major goals for medicine: cure; relief of suffering; and the refusal to treat those who are "overmastered" by their diseases.[33] Until the latter half of the twentieth century, determining when patients were "overmastered" by their disease was a reasonably easy task. With the advent of cardiopulmonary resuscitation, mechanical ventilation, and medications to support blood pressure, it became necessary for physicians and patients to examine what being "overmastered" by illness meant. Ethicists within the medical community began to question what could be done as opposed to what should be done.[34] In 2000, Helft and his colleagues posited that "futile care in hospitals is still very much an issue," but then claimed that the argument was moot because "doctors today are no more empowered to declare a treatment futile unilaterally than they were 15 years ago."[35]

Futility today may be viewed as quantitative, where the likelihood of benefit to the patient is exceedingly small, or qualitative, where the quality of benefit from the intervention is exceedingly small. In both instances, futility considers the prospect of whether a particular medical intervention or treatment will serve the patient's interest.[36] Concerns about medical futility arise, in part, from the conflict between the ability of the technological advances in medicine to permit physicians to keep critically-ill patients alive longer, and the reality that such treatment is often unable to cure or resolve the patient's underlying condition. Interventions that support blood pressure, provide respiration, provide nutrition, or treat infection may prolong life, but may not succeed in restoring patients to a condition that permits them a meaningful and dignified existence.

Determinations of medical futility do not attempt to address the issue of rationing patient care because it does not involve an analysis of cost or a consideration of allocating available resources. The analysis of futility asks the question, "What is the likelihood that a specific intervention will benefit the patient," without contemplating "How much does this treatment cost," or "Who else might benefit from this treatment." Medical futility determinations are also unable to contemplate experimental interventions because an analysis of futility requires the evaluation of evidence to arrive at a conclusion that a proposed treatment provides no significant likelihood of conferring a reasonable benefit. Experimental treatments, by their nature, are considered experimental because the effects of the intervention are unknown.

Medical futility is an issue that is well-developed in the ethics of medicine, and the medical profession instructs its physicians on how to proceed when such circumstances arise. The American Medical Association's Code of Medical Ethics provides specific guidance as to a physician's obligation in matters of futility. It instructs physicians that when "further intervention to prolong the life of a patient becomes futile, (they) have an obligation to shift the intent of care toward comfort and closure." It recognizes that the process of arriving at a determination of futility requires making value judgments, that such decision-making should consider the "patient's or proxy's assessments of worthwhile outcome," and take "into account the physician's or other provider's perception of intent in treatment, which should not be to prolong the dying process without benefit to the patient or to others with legitimate interests." Determinations of futility must "also take into account community and institutional standards, which in turn may have used physiological or functional outcome measures."[37] When disagreements arise between physician and the patient or proxy about whether care is futile, efforts to resolve the disagreement should occur using a process that affords the patient a form of due process (see Table 28-9).

In some circumstances, it may be medically appropriate to continue interventions deemed futile temporarily in order to assist patients or their families to come to terms with the gravity of their

---

Table 28-9

Seven Steps to Declaring Futility in Specific Cases

1. Make earnest attempts in advance to deliberate and negotiate prior understandings between patient or proxy and the physician on what constitutes futile care for the patient, and what falls within acceptable limits for the physician, the family, and possibly, the institution.

2. To the extent possible, decision-making should occur between the patient or proxy and the physician.

3. If disagreements arise, parties should attempt to negotiate or mediate their differences in order to reach an acceptable agreement, using the assistance of consultants if necessary.

4. If the parties cannot resolve their differences, then the parties should involve the assistance of an institutional committee such as an ethics committee.

5. If the institutional review process supports the patient's position and the physician remains unpersuaded, then the physician should arrange to transfer the patient to the care of another physician.

6. If the process supports the physician's position, and the patient or proxy remains unpersuaded, then the family may arrange transfer to another institution.

7. If the patient cannot be transferred, then the physician and the institution are not obligated to provide the intervention.

situation or to provide time to reach a point of personal closure. For example, it may be appropriate to continue mechanical ventilation or renal dialysis in a terminally-ill patient in order for family members to consult with members of the clergy or to allow family members to arrive from another state so that they may visit the patient one last time. At all times, it is important to reassure the patient or proxy that everything possible is being done to ensure the patient's comfort and dignity.

Although the ethics and the medical community have achieved a clear consensus on how to proceed in matters relating to medical futility, the issue remains unexplored in law. Experience demonstrates that nearly all disagreements between patients or proxies and physicians are resolved successfully using the due process approach described above. In rare cases, physicians' attempts at withholding medical care have been challenged in the courts.

On February 10, 1994, the United States Court of Appeals for the Fourth Circuit ruled that the federal Emergency Medical Treatment and Active Labor Act (EMTALA)[38] obligated physicians to provide treatment, in the form of ventilator support, to an encephalic infant when she presented to the emergency department.[39] The narrowly interpreted ruling upheld that EMTALA's plain language intent requirement was to provide emergency care to all patients presenting to an emergency department. In doing so, the court overruled the physician's medical judgment in order to accommodate the treatment goals and desires of the patient's family and signaled the "uphill effort to harness professional judgment, technology, and human emotion in the service of rational medical care."[40]

Recent efforts by state legislators in Virginia and Maryland have attempted to balance the patients' right to make their own health-care decisions weighed against a physician's obligation to forego futile care. In 1992, Virginia amended its Health Care Decisions Act to include the following provision, "Nothing in this article shall be construed to require a physician to prescribe or render medical treatment to a patient that the physician determines to be medically or ethically inappropriate."[41] While the statute does not define what constitutes what is medically or ethically appropriate, it serves to acknowledge the concept of physician autonomy.[42] A statute similar to Virginia's appears in Maryland's Health Care Decisions Act.[43] Enacted in 1993, the Act includes specific language that codifies physicians' right to decline treating patients when doing so would be contrary to their medical judgment. Section 5-611 provides: "Nothing in this subtitle may be construed to require a physician to prescribe or render medical treatment to a patient that the physician determines to be ethically inappropriate . . . or . . . medically ineffective. It provides further that a physician may withhold or withdraw medically ineffective treatment if the physician and a second physician certify in writing that the treatment is medically ineffective, and the patient or surrogate is informed of the decision." The Maryland law goes further than Virginia's law by providing a definition of medically ineffective treatment under the statute: "Medically ineffective treatment means that, to a reasonable degree of certainty, a medical procedure will not: (1) Prevent or reduce the deterioration of the health of an individual; or (2) Prevent the impending death of an individual." It remains uncertain as to how state courts will interpret these laws if challenged and whether federal laws such as EMTALA will preempt states' efforts to address this important issue.

Until future court challenges define more clearly the legal limits of a physician's obligation to withhold futile care, physicians and hospitals should continue to work within existing ethical and professional guidelines to balance medical obligations with a patient's right of self-determination.

KEY POINTS

▶ Information generally considered necessary for a patient to make an informed decision includes: (1) the diagnosis; (2) the nature and purpose of the proposed treatment or procedure, the probability and severity of its risks, and whether those risks would be temporary or permanent; and (3) viable treatment alternatives.

▶ If the physician chooses to forego consent because: (1) an emergency condition exists, the patient is incapable of consenting, and the failure to treat poses an imminent harm; or (2) when the risk of disclosure poses such a serious psychological threat of detriment to the patient as to be medically contraindicated, then the physician should document these special circumstances in the medical record.

▶ If the patient has diminished capacity or is unable to provide an informed consent, then the physician has an obligation to obtain informed consent from the patient's surrogate decision-maker.

▶ It is important that all anesthesiologists recognize their obligation to respect a patient's' right to make own decisions and identify patients who may have an impaired ability to make an informed decision.

▶ If during a patient interview, the physician develops a suspicion that a patient may lack the capacity to make an informed decision, then the physician should obtain a formal evaluation of the patient's competency prior to obtaining the patient's consent.

▶ Incompetent patients retain an interest in self-determination. Physicians should encourage health-care agents to act on the patients' best interest and make treatment decisions consistent with what they believe the patient would want if they were expressing a choice for themselves.

▶ Physicians who may disagree with a patient's advance health-care directive should avoid the temptation to disregard them and unilaterally provide care contrary to the patient's or the agent's wishes.

▶ In terms of do-not-resuscitate perioperative orders, the options available to the surgical team include: (1) suspending the DNR during the perioperative period; (2) initiating a procedure-directed order that permits or forbids specific interventions; (3) Initiating a goal-directed order set that prioritizes outcomes rather than procedures.

▶ Until the legal limits of a physician's obligation to withhold futile care are clearly defined, physicians and hospitals should continue to work within existing ethical and professional guidelines to balance medical obligations with a patient's right of self-determination.

KEY REFERENCES

▶ Grisso T, Applemaum PS. *Assessing competence to consent to treatment, a guide for physicians and other health professionals.* New York: Oxford University Press; 1998:18–31.

▶ Annas GJ. "Culture of Life" politics at the bedside—the case of Terri Schiavo. *N Eng J Med.* 2005;352:16.

▶ Krohm C, Summers S. *Advance health care directives: a handbook for professionals.* Chicago: American Bar Association; 2002.

▶ Committee on Ethics of the American Society of Anesthesiologists. Perioperative DNR orders to limit resuscitation. In: Syllabus on Ethics, American Society of Anesthesiologists. Available at: http://www.asahq.org/publicationsAndServices/EthicsSyllabus. pdf. Accessed January 20, 2006.

► American Society of Anesthesiologists. Ethical guidelines for the anesthesia care of patients with do-not-resuscitate orders or other directives that limit care. Available at: http://www.asahq.org/ publicationsAndServices/standards/09.html. Accessed January 20, 2006.

► Jecker NS. Futility. Ethics in Medicine. Seattle, Washington: University of Washington School of Medicine; 1998. Available at: http://depts.washington.edu/bioethx/topics/futil.html. Accessed January 23, 2006.

REFERENCES

1. Council on Ethics and Judicial Affairs. § 8.08, Informed consent. In: *Code of Medical Ethics.* Chicago: American Medical Association; 1997: 120–122.

2. Katz J. *The Silent World of Doctor and Patient.* Baltimore, Md: Johns Hopkins Press; 1984.

1. Scholendorff v. Society of New York Hospital, 211 N.Y. 125, 105 N.E. 92 (1914).

4. *Black's Law Dictionary.* 6th ed. St Paul: West Publishing; 1990. Battery; p. 152.

5. Mohr v. Williams, 95 Minn. 261, 104 N.W. 12 (1905).

6. *Black's Law Dictionary.* 6th ed. St Paul: West Publishing; 1990. Negligence; p. 1032.

7. Faya v. Almaraz, 329 Md. 435 (1993).

8. Restatement (Second) of Torts § 283: Conduct of a reasonable man: The standard. (1965).

9. Pollock SG. Life and death decisions: who makes them and by what standards? *Rutgers Law Rev.* 1989;47:507.

10. Annas GJ, Densberger JE. Competence to refuse medical treatment: autonomy versus paternalism. *Toledo Law Rev.* 1984;15:568.

11. Cantor NL. A patient's decision to decline life-saving medical treatment: bodily integrity versus the preservation of life. *Rutgers Law Rev.* 1973; 26:237.

12. Natanson v. Kline. 350 P.2d 1093, 1104 (1960).

13. Moujan M, Walkow MM. informed consent-legal competency not determinative of a person's ability to consent to medical treatment—Miller v. Rhode Island Hospital, 625 A.2d 778 (R.I. 1993). *Suffolk Univ Law Rev.* 1994;28:271.

14. Gorman WF. Testamentary capacity in Alzheimer's disease. *Elder Law J.* 1996;4:227.

15. Meyer RG, Landis ER, Hays JR. *Law for the Psychotherapist.* New York: Norton;1988:89–113.

16. Lo B. Assessing decision-making capacity. *Law Med Health Care.* 1994; 18:194.

17. Margolis WM. The doctor knows best: patient capacity for health care decision making. *Oregon Law Rev.* 1992;71:919–921.

18. Applebaum PS, Grisso TG. Assessing patients' capacities to consent to treatment. *N Engl J Med.* 1988;319:1635.

19. Weyrauch S. Decision making for incompetent patients: who decides and by what standards? *Tulsa Law J.* 2000;35:770.

20. Grisso T, Applemaum PS. *Assessing Competence to Consent to Treatment, a Guide for Physicians and Other Health Professionals.* New York: Oxford University Press; 1998:18–31.

21. Kapp MB, Mossman D. Measuring decisional capacity: cautions on the construction of a "capacitometer." *Psychol Public Policy Law.* 1996;2:80.

22. Post LF, Blustein J, Dubler NN. The doctor-proxy relationship: an untapped resource: introduction. *J Law Med Ethics.* 1999;27(1):5–12.

23. Patient Self-Determination Act, 42 USCA §1395cc(f) (1992).

24. Brunetti L, Carperos S, Westlund R. Physicians attitudes toward living wills and cardiopulmonary resuscitation. *J Gen Intern Med.* 1991;6:323.

25. Annas GJ. "Culture of Life" politics at the bedside—the case of Terri Schiavo. *N Engl J Med.* 2005;352:16.

26. In re Quinlan, 70 N.J.10, 355 A2d 647 (1976).

27. Cruzan v. Director, MDH, 497 U.S. 261 (1990).

28. Krohm C, Summers S. *Advance Health Care Directives: A Handbook for Professionals.* Chicago: American Bar Association; 2002.

29. Committee on Ethics of the American Society of Anesthesiologists. Perioperative DNR orders to limit resuscitation. In: *Syllabus on Ethics.* American Society of Anesthesiologists. Available at: http://www. asahq.org/ publicationsAndServices/EthicsSyllabus.pdf. Accessed January 20, 2006.

30. American Society of Anesthesiologists. Ethical guidelines for the anesthesia care of patients with do-not-resuscitate orders or other directives that limit care. Available at: http://www.asahq.org/publicationsAndServices/ standards/09.html. Accessed January 20, 2006.

31. Van Norman G. Do-not-resuscitate orders during anesthesia and urgent procedures. Ethics in Medicine. Seattle, Washington: University of Washington School of Medicine. 1998. Available at: http://depts.washington.edu/ bioethx/topics/dnrau.html. Accessed January 23, 2006.

32. Council on Ethics and Judicial Affairs. § 2.20, Withholding or withdrawing life-sustaining medical treatment. In: *Code of Medical Ethics.* Chicago: American Medical Association; 1997:39–41.

33. Jecker NS. Knowing when to stop: the limits of medicine. *Hastings Cent Rep.* 1991;21:5–8.

34. Schuster DP. Everything that should be done—not everything that can be done (editorial). *Am Rev Respir Dis.* 1992;145:508–509.

35. Helft PR, Siegler M, Lantos J. The rise and fall of the futility movement. *N Engl J Med.* 2000;343:293–296.

36. Jecker NS. Futility. Ethics in Medicine. Seattle, Washington: University of Washington School of Medicine. 1998. Available at:http://depts. washington.edu/bioethx/topics/futil.html. Accessed January 23, 2006.

37. Council on Ethics and Judicial Affairs. § 2.035, Informed Consent. In: *Code of Medical Ethics.* Chicago: American Medical Association; 1997:8.

38. 42 U.S.C. § 1395dd (1988 & Supp. V 1993).

39. In re Baby K, 16 F.3d at 593–94.

40. Greenhouse L. Court order to treat baby with partial brain prompts debate on costs and ethics. The New York Times. 1994 Feb 20. Available at:http://query.nytimes.com/gst/fullpage.html?sec=health&res= 9E07E4DD123BF933A15751C0A962958260. Accessed January 23, 2006.

41. VA. CODE ANN. § 54.1–2990 (Michie 1994).

42. Daar JF. Medical Futility and implications for physician autonomy. *Am J Law Med.* 1995;21:221–240.

43. MD. CODE ANN., HEALTH-GEN. §§ 5–601 to -618 (1994).

INDEX

Page numbers followed by *f* or *t* indicate figures or tables, respectively.